Woman-Centered Care in Pregnancy and Childbirth

Edited by

SARA G. SHIELDS, M.D., M.S.
Clinical Associate Professor of Family Medicine and Community Health
University of Massachusetts
Family Health Center
Worcester, MA, USA

and

LUCY M. CANDIB, M.D.
Professor of Family Medicine and Community Health
University of Massachusetts
Family Health Center
Worcester, MA, USA

Forewords by
Wendy Savage and Stephen Ratcliffe

Radcliffe Publishing
Oxford • New York

Radcliffe Publishing Ltd
18 Marcham Road
Abingdon
Oxon OX14 1AA
United Kingdom

www.radcliffe-oxford.com

Electronic catalogue and worldwide online ordering facility.

British Library Cataloguing in Publication Data

A catalogue record for this book is available from the British Library.

ISBN-13: 978 184619 161 9

Typeset by Pindar NZ, Auckland, New Zealand
Printed and bound by Cadmus Communications, USA

Contents

We dedicate this book to all those committed to making each birth a treasured and empowering experience in a woman's life.

Series Editors' Introduction

A new clinical method, which has been developed during the 1980s and 1990s, has attempted to regain the balance between curing and caring. It is called the Patient-Centered Clinical Method and has been described and illustrated in *Patient-centered Medicine: transforming the clinical method*.[1] In the 2003 book, conceptual, educational and research issues were elucidated in detail. The patient-centered conceptual framework from that book is used as the structure for each book in the Series introduced here; it consists of six interactive components to be considered in every patient–practitioner interaction.

The first component is to assess the two modes of ill health: disease and illness. In addition to assessing the disease process, the clinician explores the patient's illness experience. Specifically, the practitioner considers how the patient feels about being ill, what the patient's ideas are about the illness, what impact the illness is having on the patient's functioning, and what he or she expects from the clinician.

The second component is an integration of the concepts of disease and illness with an understanding of the whole person. This includes an awareness of the patient's position in the life cycle and the proximal and distal contexts in which they live.

The third component of the method is the mutual task of finding common ground between the patient and the practitioner. This consists of three key areas: mutually defining the problem; mutually defining the goals of management/treatment; and mutually exploring the roles to be assumed by the patient and the practitioner.

The fourth component is to use each visit as an opportunity for prevention and health promotion. The fifth component takes into consideration that each encounter with the patient should be used to develop the helping relationship; the trust and respect that evolves in the relationship will have an impact on other components of the method. The sixth component requires that, throughout the process, the practitioner is realistic in terms of time, availability of resources and the role of collaborative teamwork in patient care.

However, there is a gap between the description of the clinical method and its application in practice. The series of books, presented here, attempts to bridge that gap. Written by international leaders in their field, the series represents clinical explications of the patient-centered clinical method. Each volume deals with a common and challenging problem faced by practitioners. In each book, current thinking is organized in a similar way, reinforcing and illustrating the patient-centered clinical method. The common format begins with a description of the burden of illness, followed by chapters on the illness experience, the whole person, finding common ground, and the patient–practitioner relationship.

The book series is international, to date representing Norway, Canada, New Zealand, the USA, England and Scotland. This is a testament to the universality of the values and concepts inherent in the patient-centered clinical method. We feel that an international definition of patient-centered practice is being established and is represented in this book series.

The vigor of any clinical method is proven in the extent to which it is applicable in the clinical setting. It is anticipated that this series will inform further development of the clinical method and move thinking forward in this important aspect of medicine.

Moira Stewart, Ph.D.
Judith Belle Brown, Ph.D.
Thomas R. Freeman, M.D., C.C.F.P.
November 2009

REFERENCE

1 Stewart M, Brown JB, Weston WW, *et al.*, editors. *Patient-centered Medicine: transforming the clinical method*. 2nd ed. Oxford: Radcliffe Medical Press; 2003.

Foreword

Woman-Centered Care in Pregnancy and Childbirth is a unique book which focuses on the needs of the woman at these important and life-changing times in her life. Birth is such a miraculous process which can make or mar a woman's subsequent life and yet so often the process of antenatal care or the assembly line provision of abortion care appears mechanistic and uncaring to the user. Miscarriage and induced abortion are the commonest events and procedures carried out but in the UK are often neglected in undergraduate teaching for medical students and barely acknowledged in the midwifery curriculum. These are well dealt with here, as is infertility. The holistic approach of the whole book and the inclusion of preconceptual care, health promotion and discussion about the complex issues of unnecessary caesarean section makes this an ideal reference book for every medical and midwifery school library – indeed every public library.

This is an immense piece of work, which despite the differences in the way that healthcare is organised in the USA, has great relevance to the practice of midwives, the few GP obstetricians still practicing and all obstetricians practicing in the UK.

The use of clinical and psychosocial data about patients and their caregivers in many of the chapters to underpin the theoretical discussion of the topic is unusual but will make this book more accessible to medical and midwifery students, as well as doctors and midwives. The style is clear and informative and many women, social workers and health visitors may also find it a fascinating book to read. What comes across strongly is the wealth of experience and compassion of the two main authors and their colleagues.

Although the majority of the references are to US publications there are references to practice in other countries and this up-to-date and comprehensive reference list will be of enormous help to British practitioners. Michael Klein's chapter on how to examine the evidence when trying to practice in an evidence-based way is particularly useful.

This book brings a new perspective to the reproductive care of women in the 21st century and I hope it will receive the same recognition, use and impact as did *Effective Care in Pregnancy and Childbirth*[1] in the latter half of the 20th century.

Professor Wendy Savage, M.R.C.O.G.
Honorary Visiting Professor, Middlesex University
November 2009

Preface

We attend births in a conventional tertiary care hospital in the USA and face all the challenges of doing normal births in that setting in the 21st century. In the course of this work during the last 15 years together, we realized we were talking about births differently from other colleagues and paying attention to details in prenatal care that were not a part of teachings in the standard obstetric or maternity care textbooks. We knew that midwives passed this lore down among themselves, but had never seen a text trying to teach from this perspective. The doula movement and Penny Simkin in particular have heightened awareness within the women's health movement on empowering women in the course of labor – we wanted to teach that approach to clinicians who could make a difference by offering woman-centered care from the first visit through postpartum care. And to those family doctors like ourselves, some of whom practice the patient-centered clinical method of Stewart *et al.*, we wanted our book to encompass ongoing woman-centered care spanning the time before pregnancy, between pregnancies, and afterwards, as well as the care of children and partners. From these very ambitious hopes, this book is born.

Sara G. Shields
Lucy M. Candib
November 2009

About the Editors

Sara G. Shields, M.D., M.S., is a Clinical Associate Professor of Family Medicine and Community Health at the University of Massachusetts and the Family Health Center of Worcester. Her interest in women's health and maternity care began during her undergraduate time at Harvard thanks to a course in Biology and Women's Issues and the experience of providing labor support at her sister's home birth in rural Kentucky with a lay midwife. After completing her A.B. in English and pre-medical studies, Sara attended medical school at the University of California at San Francisco, where she found her niche working in urban under-served multicultural communities with young families. She combined all these interests in her family medicine residency at the University of Rochester, based in a community health center (CHC) setting, and then a fellowship in maternal and child health at Brown University, where she did clinical work in a CHC and received a master's degree in community health with research on continuity of care in labor. Her fellowship finished in 1994 with the birth of her daughter, Maggie, in a birthing center attended by a midwife and discharged home after six hours; her son Dan's birth in 1996 was more complicated with his brief stay in intensive care and his later infancy and childhood affected by chronic asthma. Since 1995, Sara has provided and taught maternity care at the University of Massachusetts, with her clinical practice based in an urban CHC where she can do full-spectrum family medicine. Her special interests are in teaching the basics of labor support, understanding labor dystocia, supporting breastfeeding, and teaching in the Advanced Life Support in Obstetrics program, as well as teaching about doctors' experiences of family members' illnesses. Sara hopes to stay in her current position long enough to be multigenerational in maternity care, emulating Lucy by attending the births of women whose mothers she attended in childbirth. She lives in Northborough, Massachusetts with her husband Bruce Fishbein and their two teenagers.

Lucy M. Candib, M.D., is a family doctor who has taught and practiced family medicine, including obstetrics, at the Family Health Center of Worcester, an urban neighborhood health center, in central Massachusetts, since 1976. This site offers residency-training within the Family Medicine Residency of the University of Massachusetts Medical School where she is a Professor of Family Medicine and Community Health. Within the context of long-term doctor-patient relationships, Lucy has applied feminist principles in a multicultural setting and has focused attention on the concerns of women trainees and practitioners. She has lectured widely on the topics of sexual abuse and violence against women. She introduced a feminist critique of medical theory in numerous articles and in her book, *Medicine and the Family: A Feminist Perspective* (Basic Books, 1995). In 1995 she won a Fulbright grant to teach family medicine in Ecuador and in 2004 continued as a Fulbright Senior Specialist to the University of Loja in Ecuador. Lucy is on the steering committee for the Wonca Working Party on Women and Family Medicine and manages the group's listserve, a forum connecting women family physicians around the world. (Wonca is the World Organization of Family Doctors.) She runs workshops to help family medicine educators overcome obstacles in their writing as part of her work within the Society of Teachers of Family Medicine. She is a committed champion of empowerment strategies in multiple areas of clinical family medicine: in women's health, in cross-cultural care, within the care of well families, in the care of diabetes and other chronic illnesses, as well as woman-centered maternity care. Lucy has attended births for at least a dozen women whom she had delivered and at least once had delivered both mother and father! She lives in Worcester, Massachusetts with her life partner, Richard Schmitt, with whom she birthed two children, Addie and Eli – now young adults – by cesarean section and vaginal birth after cesarean (VBAC).

Acknowledgments

We would like to express our deep thanks to the staff of the Family Health Center of Worcester and to our colleagues both there and in the wider family medicine community in Worcester who supported us while writing this book and cared for our patients when we were unavailable. Many other family medicine colleagues around the USA and elsewhere who are dedicated to providing healthy birthing experiences for all families have also inspired our work over the years. Nurses, medical assistants, and perinatal advocates too numerous to name have joined us in this work and made the day-to-day practice of woman-centered care possible in a busy culturally diverse practice. We are also indebted to Andy Dzaugis and Rosemary Leary of the Homer Gage Medical Library at the Memorial Campus of the UMass Memorial Hospital who made every resource available with lightning efficiency and great cheer. Of course, our families (Sara's – Bruce and Dan Fishbein and Maggie Shields – and Lucy's – Richard and Eli Schmitt and Addie Candib) provided endless emotional and practical support to enable us to make this dream into a real book. Lastly, the women we care for at Family Health and in the hospital maternity setting have taught us what it means to "do" woman-centered care – a gift for which we will always be grateful.

List of Permissions

Box 4.2 South Community Birth Program: Working with Community Doulas. Permission for use granted by South Community Birth Program: www.scbp.ca

Box 4.3 Possible Childbirth Fears that May Impact Labor Progress. From Simkin P. *The Labor Progress Handbook: early interventions to prevent and treat dystocia.* 2nd ed. New York: Blackwell; 2005. Permission granted.

Figure 5.1 Where are you right now? From: Runkle A. *In Good Conscience: a practical, emotional and spiritual guide to deciding whether to have an abortion.* 1st ed. San Francisco: Jossey-Bass Publishers; 1998. Permission granted directly from Anna Runkle.

Box 5.2 Starting Points. From Singer J. Options counseling: techniques for caring for women with unintended pregnancies. *J Midwifery Womens Health.* 2004; **49**: 235–42. Permission obtained from Elsevier via Science Direct.

Box 5.7 Standards for a Family-Centered Perinatal Education. From: Westmoreland MH, Zwelling E. Innovative perinatal education management service: developing a family-centered, hospital-based perinatal education program. *J Perinat Educ.* 2000; **9**(4): 28–39. Reprinted with permission, compliments of the *J Perinat Educ*, which is published by Lamaze International, www.lamaze.org.

Figure 7.1 Interconnectedness of the system of interventions in maximin obstetrics. Adapted from Brody H, Thompson JR. The maximin strategy in modern obstetrics. *J Fam Pract.* 1981; **12**: 977–86. Permission granted from Dowden Health Media.

Figure 7.2 Conceptual model of factors affecting the occurrence of cesarean section for dystocia in healthy nulliparous women. From Lowe NK. A review of factors associated with dystocia and cesarean section in nulliparous women. *J Midwifery Womens Health.* 2007; **52**: 216–28. Used with permission from Elsevier.

Quotation on pages 461–2 from Enkin MW, Keirse MJNC, Neilson J, *et al. A Guide to Effective Care in Pregnancy and Childbirth.* New York: Oxford University Press; 1995. By permission from Oxford University Press.

Introduction

Woman-Centered Care in Pregnancy and Childbirth adapts the patient-centered clinical method, developed by Stewart *et al.*,[1] to pregnancy and childbirth – fundamental human events that are central moments in women's lives. This book promotes the vision of pregnancy and childbirth as normal human experiences. The childbearing experience – including pre-conception, pregnancy diagnosis, pregnancy, labor and delivery, and the postpartum period including breastfeeding – brings about enormous changes in a woman's life. The physical, psychosocial, and developmental changes have very wide ranges of normality, especially across social and cultural dimensions, but can also extend into areas of severe pregnancy-related symptoms or frank pathological conditions. A woman-centered approach must be flexible enough to address this entire range of possibilities, including the experiences of women who choose not to carry a pregnancy or women who undergo miscarriage. A woman-centered approach must also be applicable to the variety of maternal conditions around the world – to women living in a variety of family structures, to women from many cultures, to women at risk from their position in society and their positions in their families. The patient-centered clinical method is a supple framework on which to build an approach to woman-centered care encompassing this broad range of women's reproductive experiences.

This book is unique in offering a single text suitable for primary care maternity clinicians and trainees in multiple fields – family physicians, nurse practitioners, women's health clinicians, midwives, obstetrical nurses, and obstetricians committed to offering woman-centered care. The text applies the clinically powerful and research-supported model of patient-centered care to the normal process of pregnancy and birth – an expansion of the approach to a normal developmental process in women's lives, beyond previous applications to various chronic illnesses. The text incorporates dozens of vignettes describing how a varied group of clinicians approach the specifics of woman-centered maternity care, working with many different women and their families from a variety of social, cultural, and economic situations, who face both normal and problematic challenges over the course of prenatal care, birth, and the postpartum period. The stories of these clinicians and patients are composites of our real-life experiences in teaching and delivering maternity care in a community health center in the USA. We have also invited colleagues in family medicine and midwifery from the USA and Canada to join us in writing sections of this book, enabling us to broaden the focus beyond our own experience. The collaborators have provided a public health and international perspective on woman-centered maternity care and a critical analysis of the impact of evidence-based medicine on the conduct of contemporary obstetrical care.

But why woman-centered care? Why not stick to patient-centered care? Why not family-centered care? In today's consumerist medical marketplace, is care not already focused on the woman? Are not maternity units already family-centered? Applying the concept of patient-centered care to contemporary pregnancy and birth led us to the question: who or what is at the center of maternity care in today's systems? Historically, the medical approach to pregnancy and childbirth and women's health focused on pathology and subjected women's bodies to medical scrutiny. Medicine's preoccupation with pathology has meant that obstetrics has increasingly become a specialty dedicated to looking for disease in pregnancy and preventing bad outcomes in obstetrics by increasing surgical intervention. Prenatal "care" is transformed into surveillance for incipient disease. Attention during labor is centered on fetal "monitoring" for abnormalities in the fetal heart pattern. Preoccupation with malpractice suits has understandably heightened obstetrical concerns about birth outcomes, thus increasing the likelihood of making the leap to intervention. At the same time, the forces for increasing technological surveillance are unopposed: the pressure for modernity which privileges technology over simplicity in all aspects of life; the competition for technical superiority (as opposed to quality) as a way to attract consumers and professionals; and the institutional pressures on hospitals to reduce human labor costs by using machines for surveillance. As a result, pregnancy and birth have become less patient-centered and more technology-centered and physician-controlled.

Why not family-centered care? In family medicine, it is customary to talk about family-centered maternity care, in which practitioners steadily incorporate strategies to include the father, and possibly other family members including siblings, in birth practices. Thirty years ago family-oriented birth attendants had to fight for the right to get fathers and other family members in the delivery room. Nowadays, these practices are standard in North American hospitals: fathers cut the cord; mothers, sisters, aunts, and grandmothers can play roles in labor support; husbands can stay overnight during the postpartum period; and healthy siblings are allowed to visit. During labor, the nursing staff often help integrate the father of the baby into some assigned role – coach, timer, masseur, physical supporter – or, at a minimum, hand-holding bystander. Nevertheless, in spite of this involvement of family members, the organizational system of care, with its internal structure and values, with doctors at the helm, remains in control; labor and delivery are dangerous processes that require medical "management." Women and their partners are attracted to facilities that offer the appearance of family centeredness, but they are unaware that the family is not, in fact, at the center of care.

Family-centeredness has several other problems, as pointed out by Midmer over 15 years ago.[2] First is the reliance on the standard nuclear family as normative. The idealized family is composed of an English-speaking married couple who are employed and able-bodied with no problems with drugs or alcohol, and no conflicts;

they are "nice." (And in the USA they have health insurance.) Single women, obese women, divorced women, pregnant adolescents, lesbian women, women on public assistance, women who do not speak English, women with histories of drugs or alcohol or victimization do not fit these norms; all pose "red flags." Hospital staff are uncertain how to be family-centered when they do not know how to recognize who is "family" for the woman, when the woman is different ethnically, socially, or otherwise from the hospital staff. Individual nurses work hard to overcome these barriers, but often the institutions and the other hospital staff do not make it easy to give the woman the care she deserves within the context of her choice of family.

A second problem with family-centeredness is the issue of power and control within the family itself. We know that many pregnant women have a history of physical, sexual, or emotional abuse, as high as 44%.[3] A portion of pregnant women are in *currently* abusive relationships – perhaps up to 10% – and still more are in relationships where the power is asymmetrical, where men exert emotional control over the lives of the women and children. Family-centered maternity care is hard-pressed to carry out screening for violence and victimization in the relationship while at the same time trying to integrate men into what is often an uncomfortable setting for them. When the labor nurse (or any maternity provider) senses a problem between a laboring woman and the father of the baby, she appropriately focuses her attention on trying to make sure that the woman is safe. She knows intuitively that being "family-centered" does not make sense if a woman is at risk. She might, for instance, be suspicious of the man who will not let the woman receive pain medication during labor because "his baby" is not going to "get drugs." Thus a central problem with the notion of "family-centered maternity care" is the dissonance between the image of the family as the ideal setting to receive an infant and the reality that families are often harmful to women and children.

The other competitor for center stage is the fetus. Despite our best efforts, technology, supposedly the handmaiden to clinical care, has diverted our attention away from the pregnant woman herself, toward representations of the fetus – biochemical, visual, and electrical. First, the decision to have genetic screening or amniocentesis puts chemical results from the fetus at the focal point. Later, a routine ultrasound unwraps the mystery of who is within and supplies each pregnant woman with a photograph (and if desired for purchase, a video with music) of her unborn infant. And in labor, like a television in the living room, or a computer screen on the desk, the electronic fetal monitor magnetically diverts the eye and the mind away from the laboring woman. Make no mistake: women desperately want and demand these technologies. But the overall impact is to make each pregnancy and birth less woman-centered and more focused on the fetus. In early pregnancy, ultrasound images showing fetal parts can be used to discourage a woman from terminating an unplanned pregnancy that might not be best for her or for any resulting child at that time. Later in pregnancy when the technology is ideally used to establish fetal well-being, the detection of minor abnormalities can produce a level of maternal anxiety that cannot be allayed until the delivery. Here the fetal-centricity of the technology can work against the woman's best interests. During labor, the thrust of technology has focused attention on the fetal monitor and its continuous recording of the fetal heart rate in relation to contractions. Both for nurses[4] and for doctors doing maternity care,[5] surveillance through electronic fetal monitoring has come to signify obstetrical care itself. "Central" monitoring, enabling overview of multiple patients at once, replicates the "panopticon" vision of prison imagined by Foucault – all are being watched.[5] Attention and decisions revolve around the interpretation of this visual electronic data. In response to variations in the monitoring strip, the mother rolls this way and that, puts on an oxygen mask, and submits to a variety of measuring devices all focused on fetal well-being. Thus fetus-centered care, or "fetocentric" care, obscures the pregnant woman. She is not the principal actor in birth, but rather the imperfect vehicle transporting the most valuable player.

Around the world, midwifery has been the primary countervailing force against the medicalization of pregnancy and childbirth. In the UK, New Zealand, and Australia, midwives are primary caregivers for many or most normal births,[6,7] and midwifery is a growing force in Canada.[8] Even in the USA, the number of live births attended by midwives has increased in the last 20 years.[9] For most of the past 30 years, however, obstetrical nursing within hospitals has been increasingly co-opted into the management of fetal surveillance, and the human aspect of nursing care has been constricted by the intrinsic dynamic of the technology, staffing concerns, and nursing's own concerns about malpractice. Midwifery's role in hospitals has been restricted, and many midwives choose practice in birthing centers outside of hospitals. The public is hard-pressed to understand how to make choices about childbirth, and apart from the few who make choices to avoid technology on principle, most US women must follow the pattern of their insurance coverage and have their pregnancies and births monitored in the hospital environment. While home birth is common in the Netherlands, and has recently received increasing recommendation in the UK, it is the source of ridicule in US obstetrical circles. Without exposure to home births or alternative birthing centers, trainees in medicine and nursing lack exposure to alternative views of pregnancy and birth, and women as consumers are unaware that their prenatal and delivery care will not be focused on them as persons but rather on the avoidance of risk. When women hear that the safety of their babies is at stake, they will abide by whatever interventions their doctors recommend, unaware that risk avoidance is not the same as promoting the normal processes of labor and birth.

The public as well has fallen in love with obstetrical technology. An ultrasound to see the baby and determine its sex; an epidural as soon as possible to make childbirth painless; a fetal monitor throughout labor so that no change in fetal heart rate will go undetected – all have become almost universal procedures increasingly expected by consumers, already familiar with these processes from births on television or from visiting friends and relatives having babies. Only veritable Luddites question or oppose these routines, despite lack of a good evidence base that routine ultrasound and fetal monitoring improve perinatal outcome. Consumers (and truly they are consumers at the point of insisting on their "rights") now expect and demand these procedures; practitioners worry that *not* using such technology exposes clinicians to malpractice.

Technology and specialization – two forces that emerged to dominate medicine in the 20th century – have coincided to deflect the focus of childbearing from the woman herself to the preoccupation with pathology and the means of preventing, detecting, and treating abnormalities in the process. Labor pain becomes conflated with pathological pain from injury, making pain relief, defined by pain scales, the goal of treatment. Instead of patient-controlled labor and birth approaches, the ideal of woman-centered childbirth has become increasingly redefined as childbirth without pain. Epidural anesthesia – the "Cadillac" of obstetrical anesthesia – is now used in 68% of deliveries in the USA and reaches 75% in some hospitals;[10] Canadian rates have also increased.[11] The disappearance of the woman herself from medical attention might have gone unnoticed except for criticism from feminist circles whose concerns birthed the women's health movement and led to the woman-centered text *Our Bodies Ourselves*[12] and the very recent book on pregnancy, *Our Bodies, Ourselves: pregnancy and birth*,[13] both by the Boston Women's Health Book Collective. In these books women inform, educate, and empower other women to take charge of their own healthcare and explain the available options, options they might not hear about in medical settings.

At the same time, scattered individual practitioners, families, and communities have tried to withstand the technical and depersonalizing forces, but relatively few women benefit from these efforts. Lay reactions to professional and technical control of childbirth promoted a return to home births for a small number of women. But few doctors or nurses attempt to bring such a low-tech approach into the technical sphere of modern obstetrics. Within hospitals, some advocates in midwifery and family medicine have tried to promote more humanistic care inside the technical environment. Nevertheless, woman and couple-centered labor coaching strategies, beginning with the Lamaze approach in the 1950s and extending to Penny Simkin's work *The Labor Progress Handbook*,[14] have been accessible primarily to middle and upper class women, and then only to those who pursued the idea of such strategies themselves.

So the question arises: can such technologies be used to *foster* a woman-centered approach? The only answer at the moment is a guarded "perhaps" – and maybe "sometimes." The mixed blessing is apparent as we consider how evidence-based medicine in obstetrics care may be able to benefit the individual pregnant woman. As early as the mid-1980s, Chalmers and Enkin's seminal work, *Effective Care in Pregnancy and Childbirth*, drew attention to the need for maternity care to follow more rigorous, objective, scientific principles of medical care and be less anecdotally based.[15] The resultant push for "levels of evidence" and meta-analyses of trials has led to more scientifically sound guidelines from organizations such as the American College of Obstetricians and Gynecologists (ACOG), which finally published guidelines supporting the option of intermittent fetal heart auscultation for women in labor and no routine episiotomy;[16,17] similarly, the UK has published guidelines for normal birth.[18] In addition, in hospitals that establish and follow protocols for indications for cesarean including postpartum audits, cesarean rates are lower than in hospitals that do not have such guidelines. Systems of care that standardize certain aspects of maternity care *can* lead to better perinatal outcomes but must be applied in a patient-centered way. The key to woman-centered perinatal care is to apply evidence-based care in a personalized, relational way without turning such guidelines into another excuse for application of impersonal, provider-centered technology.

As family physicians providing maternity care in this complex environment, we wrote and edited this book to offer another approach to the normal processes involved in prenatal and delivery care for women and their families. We promote the practice of maternity care in the context of the woman – where she comes from, where her partner comes from, the family they are creating and how this baby fits into that context. Using both case vignettes and personal narratives, we wanted to honor birth as the life-changing moment for the woman and her family, all who came before and all who come after. We also wanted to recognize and honor the experience of practitioners deeply involved in the process of providing maternity care. Our goal was to combine practical, woman-centered, evidence-based perspectives that trainees and full-fledged clinicians can apply in the busy context of everyday clinical practice. We believe that applying the patient-centered clinical method to maternity care will strengthen the healing relationship and ultimately ease the provider's care and lead to the woman's self-empowerment.

The book is organized to reflect the elements of the patient-centered clinical method. In Part One we address the magnitude of the problem – the lack of woman-centered reproductive care. To reflect our perspective that the essential problem is a *human* problem, not a set of abstract issues, we introduce the experiences of various providers, focusing primarily on Larisa Foster, a recently trained maternity care provider in family medicine, who confronts the lack of woman-centered care in her practice environment. She finds that the problem has many facets, particularly in the USA, where significant public health issues prevail: limited access to reproductive health services, excess prematurity and low birth weight in the setting of wide health disparities, and poorly served subgroups of women. Beyond socioeconomic and ethnic disparities, teenage women, older women and obese women encounter systemic problems in obtaining respectful maternity care. Larisa and her colleagues face an additional complexity in trying to deliver woman-centered care; while they have adopted the language and approach of evidence-based medicine (EBM), seeing this as the way to provide the best care to women, they need to understand how the location, conduct, and analysis of EBM research might actually serve the high-technology system from which it developed. EBM's promise of an unbiased truth remains unfulfilled. Thus today's practitioners of maternity care, illustrated by Larisa, face enormous challenges in embracing and enacting the goal of woman-centeredness.

The remainder of the book proposes the woman-centered approach to these issues, beginning in Part Two, in two sections, first with a strategy to understand the woman's experience of the normal process of pregnancy and childbirth, and then applying this to the "illness experience" of pregnancy when problems occur. We explore the application of the patient-centered clinical method using the four dimensions of women's feelings, ideas, function, and expectations across the phases of pregnancy, from diagnosis, through each trimester, to labor and birth, and the postpartum period. We introduce the clinical stories of a number of women of varying ages, ethnicities, social classes, and levels of education and experience to demonstrate the wide range of normal. For women with either intended or unplanned pregnancies, sensitive counseling at the moment of "diagnosis" of pregnancy addresses the above four dimensions to elucidate the range of potential reactions to pregnancy. When a woman plans to keep a pregnancy, the woman-centered clinical method explores questions like: What are this woman's feelings about this pregnancy and at this point in pregnancy? How does she understand or explain what is happening to her and her body over the course of pregnancy and birth? How does pregnancy at various points affect her function, either at home or at work? What are her expectations of her healthcare provider and the healthcare system during this process? With each woman's individual responses to these questions, clinicians can begin to alleviate fears, correct misconceptions, encourage discussion of disappointment or discouragement, and provide compassionate concern and empathic listening.

The second section of Part Two underscores exploring the subjective experience of pregnancy when medical problems occur. When women experience abnormal pregnancy such as miscarriage, the diagnosis of fetal anomalies, preterm labor and delivery, or emergency cesarean section, woman-centered clinicians still need to elicit each woman's feelings, ideas, functions, and expectations. Pregnancy losses, including the loss of the normal pregnancy experience, are sources of grief, like other losses, but may also be assaults on a woman's self-esteem. Infertility and miscarriage may lead to feelings of guilt or incompetence as a woman. The woman-centered method of care, by eliciting such feelings, leads to a more complete treatment plan for the difficult pregnancy. A woman's model of illness about why things happen in pregnancy also needs to be explored and validated or gently corrected, as such beliefs may influence her behavior regarding her medical care. The demands of such care may accelerate in a problem pregnancy, significantly affecting a woman's daily functions and her capacity to fulfill other roles besides expectant mother. Finally, the woman-centered clinician who understands these dimensions can then more fully explore the woman's expectations of the healthcare system during an abnormal pregnancy. Women may expect and indeed demand high levels of technological intervention with a "do everything you can" attitude, or women may prefer to "let nature take its course" and avoid invasive treatments. Eliciting and finding common ground about such preferences is the key to the woman-centered understanding of the experience of pregnancy problems.

Part Three, divided into three sections, explores pregnancy within the context of women's development, both in the immediate or proximal context of her world and family in Sections One and Two, and then, in Section Three, within the more expansive context of the woman's culture. We see how pregnancy fits into the lives of many different women across the spectrum of the normal developmental experience of pregnancy. Woman-centered care recognizes that the timing of the first pregnancy makes an irreversible change in a woman's individual development. Whether the pregnancy is planned or unplanned, whether she is single or has a partner of the same or different gender, pregnancy is a fundamental directional choice in her adult development, changing forever her relationship to her family of origin and her connection to her education or her work. A pregnant woman and her partner must examine whether they have shared goals about the future of the family and prepare themselves for the potential physical, emotional, and social changes, including changes in gender roles, that pregnancy, birth, and breastfeeding can imply for the couple. Women from vulnerable populations with certain life experiences face varying challenges in pregnancy: the lesbian mother, the abused mother, the addicted mother, the imprisoned mother. These women require that the woman-centered clinician have a heightened attention to their safety as well as awareness of the dynamics of power, stigma, blame, and betrayal. Violence and victimization are writ large throughout this text, not only in Part Three. We have chosen this history for several women in our vignettes (6 out of 33) because abuse is so common; this number also reminds providers that evaluation of many common prenatal and intrapartum issues should include attention to the possibility of past and/or present victimization.

In the third section of Part Three, we introduce women from many cultures to develop a woman-centered approach to pregnancy and birth in the larger context of culture and community. Clinicians in developed countries usually encounter cultural issues in pregnancy when caring for immigrant women, or women from specific ethnic groups within their country. Culture and community play an enormous role in setting the stage for understanding the meaning and practices around pregnancy and the expectations around birth and mothering. The complexity of possibilities among life-cycle events, timing of events, immigration, and culture makes generalization about cultural context problematic. Nevertheless, familiarity with a woman's culture and the heterogeneity within that culture is essential to woman-centered maternity care. Women from different cultures have different expectations of labor and birth; likewise, cultures put specific gendered expectations on men for this family event. To best address these needs, the woman-centered clinician needs a working knowledge of the various geographic and cultural communities within the larger residential area where she or he practices and extensive familiarity with the vulnerabilities of specific groups to maternal morbidity, prematurity, and infant mortality. Cultural and socioeconomic factors are among the distal forces that shape the community environments where women become pregnant and deliver.

Part Four addresses the specific process of finding common ground in the care of pregnant, laboring, and postpartum women. This process requires that the woman-centered clinician interpret and navigate the often conflicting, widely divergent worlds of professional medicine and lay experience. Expanding the previously limited concept of the birth plan beyond the intrapartum period to encompass the entire process of pregnancy, birth, and parenting offers providers a tool for educating, empowering, and encouraging the woman and her family through the birth process. The birth plan addresses common symptoms in pregnancy, incorporates planning for labor support, maintains a broad understanding and approach to pain and analgesia, keeps open the flexibility to deal with emergencies, and recognizes the necessity of culturally appropriate postpartum support. Establishing plans for consultation proactively, in the event of complications during the course of pregnancy or labor and delivery, is another type of system-wide birth plan. The process of consultation with its requirement for three-way communication between the woman, the primary provider, and the consultant requires dedicated attention and a special focus on communication. The ideal consultation occurs when both the referring primary provider and the consultant remain woman-centered.

Part Five, on prevention and health promotion, first addresses the importance of woman-centeredness in pregnancy planning, including suitable contraception counseling for the woman not desiring pregnancy and options counseling to approach an unplanned pregnancy, both tailored to a woman's needs. Pregnancy itself is an ideal time to focus on health promotion and disease prevention since many of the traditional behaviors that clinicians ask of pregnant women are good for a woman's overall long-term health, such as balanced nutrition, avoidance of tobacco and alcohol, adequate rest, and exercise. Prenatal care also usually includes an emphasis on prevention of problems through risk assessment and risk reduction or avoidance. Woman-centered risk assessment takes stock not only of a woman's potential vulnerabilities, but also of the strengths she and her family bring to the process of pregnancy. We use the method of finding common ground first to explore both the complex pregnancy-related risk issues involved in genetic screening and later to illustrate lifelong health promotion about potential chronic disease. Health promotion depends on the process of empowering the woman herself. Group prenatal visits are a relatively new strategy where women engage in prenatal care together with a clinician and health educator and take charge of learning and their own health through support and connection with other women. This and other comprehensive approaches to health promotion require the involvement of support staff, childbirth educators, office systems, information systems, and delivery settings. Providers can also work collaboratively with institutional systems to foster mother-friendly and baby-friendly hospital routines and programs that both prevent errors and promote healthy outcomes for mothers and infants.

Part Six deals with the establishment and maintenance of the relationship between the pregnant woman and her clinician and addresses the trajectory, expectations, challenges, and rewards in the longitudinal care of families through this life-cycle experience. The relationship between the woman-centered provider and the pregnant woman and her family, as she defines it, evolves over the course of the childbearing year. While providing relationship-centered care characterized by compassion, empathy, and caring, the clinician must stay constantly attuned to the issues of power – including safety and trust; healing and connectedness; and continuity, constancy, and communication. Such relationships require a broad tolerance for uncertainty, a high level of self-awareness by the provider, and a sensitivity to how the dynamics of transference and counter-transference affect the feelings, ideas, function, and expectations both of the woman and of the provider himself or herself.

Providers must also find woman-centered ways to relate to the woman's partner, whether a lesbian partner or the father of the baby, and to the woman's extended support system. Assuring the safety of the woman and the baby is a part of this process. When the woman desires the involvement of the father of the baby, the woman-centered provider can proactively foster this involvement into the routines of prenatal care, labor, birth, lactation, and infant care. The conscious and thoughtful participation of the baby's father in caring activities for the pregnant woman sets the stage for a man to take on a nurturing role as father. The provider must also reflect on the significance of his or her own gender and how that might play into the pregnant woman's strengths or vulnerabilities, as well as the provider's own. Finally, Part Six addresses the clinician's own experience of providing woman-centered maternity care: the joy and satisfaction of attending a birth and helping to make it an affirming event for the woman. The multiple personal tensions involved in shouldering the availability and responsibility for maternity care are addressed in Part Seven.

The final segment, Part Seven, focuses on the themes of time, teamwork, and wise stewardship of resources – key elements of being realistic in the practice of woman-centered care in pregnancy and birth. The dimension of time is important in the provision of prenatal care in the office, in the overall approach to labor and delivery, and in developing a satisfactory system for obstetrical coverage for deliveries. Such systems are central in enabling providers to offer woman-centered maternity care over the long term because of the potential and real conflicts between providers' own personal and family needs and their ongoing responsibilities for women's care. The development of woman-centered teams requires attention to collaboration with colleagues and staff in the office, at the hospital, on the labor floor, and in other departments. Some complex problems, such as a woman with a chronic illness delivering a premature infant, or a pregnant woman with problematic substance abuse, will require coordination and communication among multiple kinds of consultants, case workers, nurses, therapists, and educators for the best outcome. The wise stewardship of resources requires a critical viewpoint about the appropriate use of technology, and serious evaluation of the nature of risks involved in the use, misuse, or avoidance of technical interventions in pregnancy and delivery.

Part Seven introduces the idea that the worldwide acceleration in the rate of cesarean section is recognizable as a *syndemic*, a complex and widespread phenomenon in population health produced by multiple reinforcing conditions. While it seems impossible to imagine that this tide could be reversed, a variety of forces are at work to do just that: activism for woman-centered decision-making; demand for human over technical approaches; movement for the empowerment of women in their health; mobilization of consumers; promotion of national and international recognition of the extremely high costs of technical solutions at the expense of other health priorities; and finally preferential education of increasing numbers of primary care maternity clinicians (midwives and family doctors) over specialty-focused providers.

Throughout this book we have tried to portray the women and their providers as real people. However, the stories are not stories of specific women but rather composites of real events that have happened to many different women and families. The women's names are completely fictitious; we tried to use names that were typical of the age and culture of the women described. For brevity and familiarity, we have chosen to use the provider-centered shorthand of gravidity and parity numbers (e.g. G3P2, meaning a woman who has been pregnant three times and has had two births) to introduce several of the multiparous women, acknowledging that this nomenclature is not how women describe themselves. Because women's stories unfold throughout the book, but readers may not read the chapters sequentially, we have provided complete "vignettes" of each woman's history in the Appendix.

The doctors' and midwives' names are fictitious as well. At times we refer to the doctor by his or her first name and at times as Dr. Miller or Dr. Epps. We deliberately use varied levels of formality because some women in their care are more comfortable with formality and will use the title *doctor* while others prefer the informality and familiarity of the first name. Larisa and Judith and Helen and Harmony consistently prefer to use their first names in their practice; Jonathan Rosen and Greg Diamond can go either way depending on what feels right to them; Dr. Miller, Dr. Epps, Dr. Burman and Dr. Rao usually use their titles and expect that their patients will be comfortable with that choice. We assume that conversations among providers themselves would occur on a first-name basis. "Biographies" of all the named providers are also offered in the Appendix. Occasionally, a provider from the past or a provider in an anonymous setting goes unnamed deliberately; unfortunately, real women often do not know the name of the person who is treating them.

We have consolidated most of the women and practitioners into two practices in a medium-sized city: a well-established woman-centered group private practice, Woman-Centered Community Family Practice, where Larisa joins Judith, Helen (a midwife), and Dr. Rao; and the community health center where Drs. Miller, Burman, and Epps practice with an obstetrical nurse practitioner, Harmony. Greg Diamond is an obstetrician consultant at the community hospital where they attend deliveries; he also teaches at a university hospital in the nearby big city where a resident, Dr. Thibeault, is training. Applying the method of patient-centered care to the interactions between these doctors and the many women for whom they care in the course of this book, we tried to bring alive the personal experience of providing and receiving woman-centered care of pregnancy and birth.

We know that many readers are already sensitive to the needs of the women in their care and are worried about the problems in contemporary maternity care. We hope that this book can clarify for these practitioners a model for keeping the woman at the center of the birth experience. Finally, by presenting woman-centered care as a solution to the troubled maternity care environment, we hope that this book helps make woman-centered maternity care a reality for women and their families having babies in the 21st century.

Sara G. Shields
Lucy M. Candib
November 2009

REFERENCES

1 Stewart M, Brown JB, Weston WW, *et al.*, editors. *Patient-centered Medicine: transforming the clinical method.* 2nd ed. Oxford: Radcliffe Medical Press; 2003.

2 Midmer DK. Does family-centered maternity care empower women? The development of the woman-centered childbirth model. *Fam Med.* 1992; **24**: 216–21.

3 Rodriguez MA, Heilemann MV, Fielder E, *et al.* Intimate partner violence, depression, and PTSD among pregnant Latina women. *Ann Fam Med.* 2008; **6**: 44–52.

4 Sandelowski M. *Devices & Desires: gender, technology, and American nursing.* Chapel Hill, N.C.: UNC Press; 2000.

5 Arney WR. *Power and the Profession of Obstetrics.* Chicago: University of Chicago Press; 1982.

6 National Health Services. NHS maternity statistics, England: 2006–7. 2008 [cited January 16, 2009]. Available from: www.ic.nhs.uk/statistics-and-data-collections/hospital-care/maternity/nhs-maternity-statistics-england:-2006-2007

7 New Zealand Health Information Service. *Report on Maternity: maternal and newborn information 2004.* Ministry of Health; 2007.

8 British Columbia Perinatal Health Program. *Caesarean Birth Task Force Report 2008.* British Columbia Perinatal Health Program; 2008.

9 Martin J, Hamilton B, Sutton P, *et al.* Births: final data for 2006. *Natl Vital Stat Rep.* 2009; **57**: 1–102.

10 Menacker F, Martin J. Expanded Health Data from the New Birth Certificate, 2005. *Natl Vital Stat Rep.* 2008; 56: 1–24.

11 CIHI. Giving birth in Canada: regional trends from 2001–2 to 2005–6. 2007 [cited January 10, 2009]. Available from: http://secure.cihi.ca/cihiweb/dispPage.jsp?cw_page=AR_1106_E

12 Boston Women's Health Book Collective. *Our Bodies, Ourselves: a new edition for a new era.* New York: Touchstone; 2005.

13 Boston Women's Health Book Collective. *Our Bodies, Ourselves: pregnancy and birth.* New York: Simon and Schuster; 2008.

14 Simkin P. *The Labor Progress Handbook: early interventions to prevent and treat dystocia.* 2nd ed. New York: Blackwell; 2005.

15 Chalmers I, Enkin M, Keirse M, editors. *Effective Care in Pregnancy and Childbirth, Volume I: Pregnancy; Volume II: Childbirth.* New York: Oxford University Press; 1989.

16 ACOG. ACOG Practice Bulletin no.70. Clinical management guidelines for obstetrician-gynecologists. Intrapartum fetal heart rate monitoring. *Obstet Gynecol.* 2005; **106**: 1453–60.

17 ACOG. ACOG Practice Bulletin No. 71. Episiotomy. Clinical management guidelines for obstetrician-gynecologists. *Obstet Gynecol.* 2006; **107**: 957–62.

18 National Collaborating Centre for Women's and Children's Health. Intrapartum care: care of healthy women and their babies during childbirth. 2007 [cited May 13, 2008]. Available from: www.nice.org.uk/nicemedia/pdf/IntrapartumCareSeptember2007mainguideline.pdf

PART ONE

The Magnitude of the Problem

CHAPTER 1

Introduction

Sara G. Shields and Lucy M. Candib

Dr. Larisa Foster is a family doctor who has just finished her residency and is joining Woman-Centered Community Family Practice (WCCFP). She entered residency with a focus on women's health and empowerment but has since learned that many women live in areas where they have little control over options in contraception and abortion. Larisa trained in high-tech interventional obstetrics but worries that she has not learned how to pay attention to the woman herself during prenatal care, labor, delivery, and the postpartum period. She is not sure she really understands about women's issues in lactation, and has not yet had children of her own, so cannot refer to her own experience. She wonders how to be woman-centered with women from different cultures and women whose life experiences are as different as a pregnant 16-year-old who has run away from home and a married professional woman in her thirties having a baby. Larisa is looking for help in forming her own personal strategies in working with women now that she is out of training and can shape her own practice pattern. (*See* full biography of Larisa in the Appendix.)

Larisa faces the task of any health provider just beginning in clinical practice – how best to pull together the vast array of knowledge about general public health issues and individual clinical scenarios and fit these into a care plan for unique patients seeking her services. She needs not only to recognize the medical aspects of specific health and disease patterns but also to be familiar with the fields of epidemiology and public health. These dynamic disciplines – reflecting today's medical culture, practices, and norms – attempt to understand illness and disease, health and well-being, interventions and outcomes by measuring health statistics, following trends, and looking for attributable causes and explanations.

Larisa's responsibility as a clinician thus is to understand the wider epidemiologic trends that affect what she does, the conclusions she draws, and the recommendations she makes to individual patients as she conducts woman-centered care. Her training has taught her to review statistics objectively, but she must also analyze the tremendous impact of the wider sociologic and cultural trends on healthcare and look at them with attention to individual women's needs. Her woman-centered focus will provide a truly balanced review of both her knowledge and the limits of her knowledge. She hopes to be able to look critically at the interventional approach promoted in her training, and offer her patients choices based on their needs and wishes rather than feeling pressured to base her decisions primarily on avoidance of litigation. She knows that excellent communication with patients will be her best defense against malpractice suits.

Using Larisa's story as the framework, this part will explore how traditional systems of maternity care fail to address the individual needs of women and families in several critical arenas: pregnancy planning, preterm birth prevention, pregnancy in older women, the obesity epidemic, labor and delivery issues including the cesarean epidemic, and postpartum issues. We will also situate the discussion of woman-centered care within an international perspective on perinatal public health.[1] Finally, we will examine how the current push toward evidence-based medicine might potentially support but, as yet, lacks a woman-centered perspective.

Examination of important perinatal public health issues in the world's industrialized countries reveals both established conditions that have been resistant to medical interventions and emerging conditions that increasingly affect the health of our communities. Individual women whose stories will appear later in this book become the statistics when their pregnancies get complicated. The US current maternity care system, in which Larisa trained, is a technologic birthing model that uses labor induction, epidural analgesia, continuous electronic fetal monitoring (EFM), and cesarean delivery as a roadmap for improved safety in maternity care. This model increasingly dominates labor and delivery wards in industrialized countries, as well as urban centers in developing countries, yet has made little headway in improving certain perinatal health outcomes. Nevertheless, without hard evidence, both practitioners and patients around the world are under the impression that this evolving technological system is actually better and safer for women and babies. The purpose of this part of the book is not to explain the data behind each perinatal trend, but rather to look briefly at the data, and then reframe the questions to seek more woman-centered approaches to certain trends now emerging as significant issues in perinatal public health.

CHAPTER 2

Pregnancy Planning Services

Marji Gold

During her second week in practice, Larisa encountered a 17-year-old woman, Zoë, who had decided she wanted to have an abortion. The teen chose Larisa over the older partners in the practice as she thought the young doctor might be more supportive of her decision. During medical school, Larisa always thought she would be a family physician who would offer medication abortion to her patients as part of her general primary care practice. She enjoyed an opportunity to see abortions covered by national health insurance in Canada during an elective rotation in women's health in Toronto. But she became caught up learning so many other things during residency and never found a mentor to help her figure out how to integrate abortion care into her practice. In her new practice, Larisa learned quickly about the problems that women faced in her community around reproductive choice. Her practice was in a conservative county where the school board had consistently opposed sex education in the schools. The area was 50 miles from a metropolitan area where abortion was available, in a state with strict laws about teenagers and parental consent and with a state legislature considering even stricter regulations about abortion in the future. Larisa learned that teenagers were concerned about confidentiality in obtaining birth control at local pharmacies, had trouble getting to the city for birth control or abortion services, and lacked solid understanding of their contraceptive choices. Uninsured patients were unable to afford either medication or surgery for abortion and had few options. Larisa spent a long time trying to figure out how to help Zoë with the unwanted pregnancy. Although she could not yet offer the service in her practice, she was able to share what she did know about abortion with Zoë.

This chapter addresses the problems facing physicians like Larisa who want to offer reproductive health services to women in primary care yet face multiple barriers. Especially in the USA, but even in countries with less restrictive climates toward abortion, such barriers include the unavailability of contraception in various regions (particularly more rural areas), judgmental attitudes toward teen sexuality, the local and regional political landscape of reproductive healthcare, and the lack of provider training and availability for abortion services. In spite of an increasing array of contraceptive choices and options for pregnancy termination, the choices for individual women may remain dramatically limited. Larisa's woman-centered counseling about pregnancy options recognizes how these all of these issues interact to restrict Zoë's reproductive choices.

Woman-centered reproductive care clearly links unintended pregnancy with a need for better education about family planning and unrestricted access to different contraception methods. Internationally, unintended pregnancy and access to contraception are closely related to abortion rates, both legal and illegal. European countries such as Belgium and the Netherlands with universal access to effective contraception and legal abortion have the world's lowest unintended pregnancy rates and abortion rates.[2] By contrast, half of all pregnancies in the USA are unintended, and nearly half of women with an unintended pregnancy terminate the pregnancy.[3] For US women during the first decade of this century, the polarized politics around reproductive health have curtailed comprehensive sexuality education for teenagers such as Zoë, with federal funding limited to abstinence-only sexuality education.[4] A meta-analysis of the few randomized trials of abstinence-only methods suggests that this strategy results in an increase in teen pregnancy,[5] which appears to be borne out by statistics during this time period.

Across Europe, teen pregnancy rates have decreased in recent decades.[6] Generally, countries with accessible contraceptive services have lower teen pregnancy rates.[6] In the UK there is less regional variation in teen pregnancy and abortion rates than in the USA,[6] suggesting less variation in access to contraception and to abortion services. A national coordinated strategy in the UK to reduce teen pregnancy rates appears to have been successful; however, these rates still surpass other Western European countries.[7] Even in countries with national health insurance, poverty dramatically affects a woman's risk of teen pregnancy; for instance, in Scotland, poor teens have four times the rate of pregnancy as their less deprived counterparts.[8] In Canada, poor women in certain provinces that have limited abortion services have to travel at personal expense to find such services,[9-11] and immigrants within the first three months of arrival are uninsured, limiting their access.

For Larisa, even if her US community encouraged more comprehensive teen sexuality education, access to contraception could still be a stumbling block for girls and women like Zoë. Multiple barriers to such access include: lack of insurance, limited public funding resources for uninsured women, concerns about privacy, transportation, and restrictions in prescription coverage or dispensing rules. The increasing number of women without insurance along with a reduction in public funding combine to leave many US women of reproductive age without financial assistance for contraception.[4] Despite recent enhanced public programs in some states designed to provide contraceptive care to more low-income women, such plans still cover only half of women needing such services.[12] Overall, public funding for such services has not kept pace with the need. Although more insurance plans now include contraceptive method coverage than a decade ago,[4] barriers to effective use of contraception exist even for insured women. For instance, the out-of-pocket cost or co-pay for birth control pills remains high for many women, and many insurance plans allow only one pack of pills to be dispensed at a time, despite evidence that giving women a year's worth of pills saves money and prevents unintended pregnancy.[13]

If Zoë had had access to contraception, she still may have had an unintended pregnancy due to contraceptive failure. A woman-centered approach to such pregnancies avoids blaming women for neglecting to use birth control, recognizing the realities not only of access to contraception but also of contraceptive failure. Almost half of women with unintended pregnancies have used some contraceptive method during the month in which the pregnancy occurred.[3]

Zoë's age affects her risk of unintended pregnancy and access to abortion. Although the declines in abortion rates and in teenage pregnancy rates in the last decade[3] appear as public health successes, these rates – across all socioeconomic levels – are higher in the USA than in other developed countries.[4] A closer look at racial and economic disparities in these rates reveals how certain subgroups of women fall far short of "achieving their reproductive goals."[3] For instance, the rate of both abortion and unintended pregnancy among poor and minority women in the USA increased between 1994 and 2000. Although teenage pregnancy rates decreased overall in this time frame, the proportion of teen pregnancies that were unintended actually increased.[3] High teen pregnancy rates also occur disproportionately among poor or less educated women in countries like Australia.[14] Zoë also faces the other significant political aspect of reproductive healthcare for teenagers in both Canada and the USA: the burden of restrictive parental notification laws that exist in many states or provinces.[9]

Even if she lives in a place without these restrictions, Zoë may not have access to abortion services. Over one-third of US women live in a county without an abortion provider, and even one-third of US metropolitan areas lack an abortion provider, requiring some women to travel up to five hours to find abortion services.[15] Even if a woman can find a provider, she may lack financial access to the services, again related to geography: only 17 states use state funds to provide medically necessary abortions; public funding through Medicaid pays for just 13% of abortions.[16] These issues of access occur even in countries with national insurance: for instance, in Australia, public funding is limited for abortion. Most women either need to access private services or at least pay an out-of-pocket fee,[17] and up to two-thirds of women do not receive public services due to capacity limits. Additionally, access to safe abortions is an issue for women not living in metropolitan areas.[17] Even in Canada, where abortion is legal, rural women have difficulty finding abortion services; most abortions are still done in hospitals rather than clinics; only one-third of hospitals offer abortions; and, as noted above, poor women's access is constrained by limited provincial funding.[9-11]

In developing countries, limited healthcare availability and restrictive abortion laws combine in a deadly way. Unmet needs for contraception lead to more unintended pregnancies and subsequently unsafe abortions, with the concomitant risks of infection and death.[18] Although the Millennium Development Goals (*see* Chapter 9) include empowering women and improving maternal health, the framework neglects addressing the significant health issue of unsafe abortion.[19,20]

In spite of her formal training about the types of abortion procedures and their safety for the woman, Larisa faces other barriers to effective reproductive care for her patients. Two specific developments in reproductive care, emergency contraception and medical abortion, remain underutilized in the USA due to political forces affecting access and training. Although safe off-label use of standard oral contraceptive pills for emergency contraception has been known for decades, federal approval of a brand method did not happen until 1999. Politics further delayed the drive to make this method available without a prescription, despite evidence that over-the-counter availability prevents unintended pregnancy and does not lead to misuse.[21,22] Even though pharmacists are able to dispense the medication without a doctor's prescription, many are reluctant to do so and even refuse to do so,[23] do not have accurate information about the medication, or do not have the medication in stock.[24-6] Finally, despite extensive studies in both the USA and other countries, medical abortion remains limited, although slowly increasing in availability.[27]

In sum, until women around the world have access to widespread education around sexuality and contraception; convenient, free access to contraceptive services; removal of restrictive rules limiting access to contraceptive methods and abortion for teenagers; and change in the cultural climate around unplanned pregnancy, they will be burdened by unplanned and unwanted pregnancies that could have been prevented. Woman-centered reproductive care begins with these essential components.

CHAPTER 3

Preterm Birth and Health Disparities

Richard Long

Dr. Simon Miller is an experienced family doctor who has worked for nearly 20 years at the community health center across town from Woman-Centered Community Family Practice. He has had a long interest in cross-cultural medicine and has worked hard to make sure that immigrants coming to the health center get culturally competent care. He has also been concerned about the extent of violence and victimization he sees in women's lives. In recent years he has become interested particularly in addiction issues and has chosen to become involved with obstetrical care at the state prison and with an innovative substance abuse program for pregnant women that follows them inside and outside the prison system. (*See* full biography of Simon in Appendix.)

His first new patient one morning was Tonya Butler, a 28-year-old G4P3 African-American woman with a high school education coming for her first prenatal visit at 14 weeks. During her initial health history, Dr. Miller noted that Tonya was smoking almost a pack a day. Her previous obstetrical history revealed that her first baby, born at term, weighed 6 lb (2.73 kg); her second was born at 35 weeks weighing 3 lb (1.36 kg) and then died of Sudden Infant Death Syndrome (SIDS) at four months. Her third child was born at 37 weeks weighing 5 lb (2.27 kg). Dr. Miller thought that Tonya was again at risk for a preterm birth and possibly a small-for-gestational-age infant. The only modifiable risk factor that he knew of was her smoking. Dr. Miller asked Tonya if she thought she might want to use the prenatal period as a good time to give up smoking since it is harmful to the fetus. Tonya replied, "All you doctors are on my case about the smoking. I smoked for all three of my pregnancies. After all the stuff I went through, it's no wonder I smoke. They tried to say my baby died of crib death [SIDS] because I smoke. But my other two babies were fine." Dr. Miller, reflecting on how best to respond to this, did not want Tonya to think that he too blamed her for the SIDS death. (*See* full vignette in Appendix.)

Roberta Runningbear was a 32-year-old Ojibwa woman who visited Dr. Miller for a pregnancy test; she had missed her period, despite using oral contraceptives, and was afraid she might be pregnant. She had had two previous pregnancies. Her first infant was born at 36 weeks with induction because of pre-eclampsia and oligohydramnios; he was a low birthweight infant and had spent several weeks in the neonatal intensive care unit; now he was a small three-year-old boy. Her second infant was born prematurely at 28 weeks, and after two months in an intensive care nursery and multiple operations for necrotizing enterocolitis, he had died at home in her arms.

When the pregnancy test this time came back positive, Roberta was silent. Dr. Miller asked about her feelings about the pregnancy and waited for her reply.

Finally, she said, "I would love to have a healthy pregnancy and a healthy infant, but I am afraid of having another pregnancy with serious complications." She cried quietly for a while and then continued, "How come I have so many difficulties when I am pregnant? I don't drink alcohol or take drugs or even smoke cigarettes." She sighed, adding, "I have a good job and good health insurance and get my prenatal care. Why? I don't understand. . . . How can I keep this pregnancy and be able to face any problems that might arise?" After a few more minutes, she wondered out loud, "And if I had another premature baby? I don't know that I can cope with another long terrible intensive care stay . . . especially if the baby might die." (*See* full vignette in the Appendix.)

Preterm birth is a profound healthcare problem. Medical care systems recognize that preterm birth poses health risks for the infant, but preterm labor and delivery, its antecedent risks, its medical management, and the later responsibility for a high-risk infant also pose a subsequent and sometimes ongoing burden on the mother's emotional health, financial stability, and future functioning. Risk factors for preterm labor and delivery include a variety of medical and psychosocial conditions that disproportionately affect certain groups of women. No interventions have yet shown effective prevention of prematurity. Around the world socioeconomic influences are the major factor determining the rates of prematurity.[28]

Tonya's experience is part of the wider epidemiology in the USA of preterm births (births under 37 weeks' gestation), which contribute to over 36% of infant deaths annually and are the leading cause of death among African-American infants.[29] In 2004, the Centers for Disease Control and Prevention (CDC) reported an infant mortality rate of 13.6 deaths per 1000 live births among African-Americans, compared to 5.6 per 1000 live births for whites. Preterm birth is responsible for 46% of the excess deaths seen in this ethnic-racial group.[30] Poverty is certainly part of this disparity, even in countries like Canada with national health insurance.[31] In several other developed countries, although low socioeconomic status confounds the link between race and poor birth outcome, racial and/or ethnic disparities in preterm birth rates persist.[32-4] While such racial disparities have been long-standing, the mechanisms of disparity are poorly understood. A risk-based approach tends to hold the mother responsible, making a woman like Tonya feel blamed, even though she may be unable to change most of the factors that seem to put her at risk.

Problematically, the preterm birth rate is increasing among both blacks and whites in the USA with the rate for the whole population increasing to nearly 13% in 2005, the highest ever recorded, up 2% from 2003–4 and a rise of 20% since 1990.[35] About one of every eight babies in the USA, more than a half million infants per year, are born prematurely. Because prematurity accounts for as much as 36% of infant deaths,[29] the rate of preterm birth is directly linked to the infant mortality figures for developed nations. For Native Americans such as Roberta, their high infant mortality rate – 8.45 per 1000 live births – (next highest after African-American infants) is linked to preterm birth in only 22% of infant deaths; their rate relates more to their higher rate of congenital malformations, SIDS, and unintentional injuries compared to non-Hispanic whites.[29] Clearly, factors well beyond the control of either Dr. Miller, Tonya, or Roberta underlie these statistics. Statistics from England, Wales, Canada, the Netherlands, and Japan show increases in prematurity as well, partially explained by the increase in multiple births from assisted reproductive technologies such as in-vitro fertilization, but also by iatrogenic causes such as preterm induction and preterm elective cesarean section.[28]

Improvements in preterm delivery outcomes have been achieved predominantly on the neonatal rather than the obstetrical management side – treating the baby after birth rather than preventing preterm delivery in the first place. The development of centralized and regional neonatal intensive care units (NICUs), improved ventilation techniques, the use of surfactant, and the use of respiratory stimulants are examples of these neonatal advances. Obstetrical advances such as the use of antenatal steroids to promote lung maturity in the premature fetus, the use of standardized antibiotic regimens for preterm antenatal patients with high-risk conditions such as rupture of membranes, and the use of tocolytics to delay preterm delivery are examples of interventions that positively affect the outcome of the preterm infant; however, all these interventions represent medical responses to preterm labor rather than measures of prevention.

The epidemiology of disparities in preterm birth and infant mortality is intensely dynamic and increasingly reflects the interaction between social factors, public health, technical innovation, and the clinical capacity to intervene. The early initiation of prenatal care is one factor associated with fewer preterm births for both African-American and white women in the United States, as well as for women in other countries.[28] Thus, the rates of first-trimester prenatal care for black, Hispanic, or Native American US mothers – half the rate of white women – may explain part of the disparities in preterm birth.[36] Differing levels of education, too, may explain part, but not all, of the differences in prenatal care and birth outcomes among women by race and ethnicity, since racial and ethnic differences in outcomes still prevail among women with similar education who initiate prenatal care in the first trimester.[37] The potential explanatory factors for these persistent and disturbing findings include economic, cultural, educational and logistical barriers to prenatal, neonatal and postnatal care, unexplained by differences in maternal age, parity, marital status, or education.

So for Dr. Miller and his patients, Tonya and Roberta, what are the woman-centered issues around preterm birth and its consequences? Clearly, technological interventions have failed to achieve significant improvement in reducing preterm birth. Given that the risks associated with preterm birth include poverty, alcohol, tobacco and substance use, mental illness, domestic violence, and inadequately treated medical illness, Dr. Miller's woman-centered approach to preterm birth must first and foremost recognize these multifactorial risks and situate them in Tonya's and Roberta's individual social contexts. Dr. Miller's challenge will be to understand this wider context, working personally with each of them to acknowledge conditions and individual risks while at the same time avoiding blaming them for these risks. This approach strives to empower women to change or reduce their modifiable risks. Although not all these services will be needed to care specifically for Tonya and Roberta, Dr. Miller will need to have established professional referral networks with smoking cessation programs, substance use programs, counseling services, shelters, and a host of social support agencies. These networks then act to establish cohesive, defined relationships between women and needed community services. Modifiable risks will be more difficult to identify for Roberta, who does not have most of the strictly socioeconomic risks, and who already recognizes her own strengths as well as her vulnerability.

Second, given that early access to prenatal care may reduce preterm birth rates, Dr. Miller and his group have to maximize accessibility to prenatal care. Their practice needs to address the barriers and burdens that interfere with access to care. For example, they can offer flexibility in scheduling and local community-based access, with options for childcare during appointments and easy access to public transportation.

They can advocate for the office/center to provide the potential for "one-stop shopping" with preferably on-site links to medical insurance, programs offering nutrition supplements, and interpretation services.

Dr. Miller also needs to consider issues of racism and its resultant health disparities. All studies of preterm labor have acknowledged the causative role of "psychosocial factors." Stress in the broadest sense may ultimately be the best explanation. Racism is one form of stress experienced by women of color in the USA, like Tonya and Roberta, and by indigenous peoples all over the globe. The long-term and subtle yet pervasive effects of racism may explain why African-American women in the USA and native women in North America or Australia have worse outcomes.[34,38] Immigration stress that includes subtle racism may underlie disparities in outcomes even for women who get similar prenatal care.[39] White women have worse reproductive outcomes as teenagers that improve as they get into their twenties; in contrast, African-American women actually have deteriorating birth outcomes in their twenties. Geronimus proposes the "weathering" hypothesis to explain this unexpected outcome: that African-American women's bodies age faster and therefore have less reproductive reserve because of the additive burden of socioeconomic adversity as they get even a few years older.[40] Even improved economic conditions after a childhood in poverty do not ameliorate the tendency toward low birthweight infants among black women, while low birthweight deliveries among white women decrease when their economic situation improves.[41] Dr. Miller's woman-centered focus allows him to recognize that women of color continue to suffer from racism in many ways – in their neighborhoods, their access to goods and services, and their experiences with the medical care system. At some point in the process of prenatal care with Tonya and Roberta, Dr. Miller will need to investigate their experience of these issues.

CHAPTER 4

Women Giving Birth at Older Ages

Richard Long

Melissa was a 38-year-old married software engineer who was a team leader in a highly competitive company. She worked 12-hour days and had no time for exercise or relaxation. She and her husband, Kirk, also an engineer, had been trying to get pregnant for the last year and had proceeded through an infertility evaluation that found no specific cause. When she finally missed her period, Melissa did a home pregnancy test with Kirk in attendance reading the instructions. They called the on-call doctor for Woman-Centered Community Family Practice that night with several questions about what came next in the care plan. This doctor reassured them that they could make a first prenatal appointment with Larisa sometime in the next few weeks. They felt that they could not wait that long but needed some time to adjust both their work schedules to fit in the prenatal appointments. (*See* full vignette in Appendix.)

Prior to World War Two, 14% of pregnancies in the USA were to women 35 years of age or older. The percentage dropped to about 5% in the 1970s and, since the 1980s, rose again to about 14% in 2002.[42] The trend of women giving birth at older maternal ages is expected to continue for at least another decade as the last of the "baby boomers" enter menopause in the USA and other developed countries.[43] Mainstream approaches to maternity care emphasize the increased risk of "older" women for preterm delivery, spontaneous abortion, stillbirths, and birth defects, and for higher rates of complications such as hypertension, diabetes, cesarean delivery, and infertility.[43-6] However, some studies suggest that the age-related increased risk of cesarean delivery for older mothers cannot be explained by any increase in medical complications that predispose women to operative delivery.[47,48] Possibly the perception of an increased risk for older women underlies the higher operative rates,[48,49] or perhaps belief in the "precious baby syndrome"[50] increases providers' willingness to perform cesareans for older women. Unfortunately, the preoccupation with obstetrical risk for older mothers carries the potential to stigmatize and blame women for their delayed childbearing choices, represented by the label "Advanced Maternal Age" on their medical charts.

Larisa's woman-centered approach acknowledges the perinatal trend toward older motherhood by recognizing the wider cultural, educational, and reproductive choices now enabling women to postpone childbearing into their thirties and forties. The resulting delay relates to many factors: the increased number of women in this age bracket, later marriage, second marriage, more contraceptive options, opportunities for further education and career advancement for women, and the availability of assisted reproductive technologies (ART), not available to previous generations.[50,51]

Larisa reframes her perspective to see that older mothers like Melissa in fact also contribute substantial strengths to family. They are more often educated, financially stable, and emotionally mature; they are more likely to be concerned about safety and less often involved in higher risk behaviors than young women.[51] Teasing out the medical risks for healthy older women remains difficult due to a paucity of research that controls for other known risks.[50] Larisa's task in caring for women who are postponing pregnancy to an older age is to help them find the healthiest pathway to pregnancy. Larisa underscores Melissa's many strengths as well as her risks, and seizes the opportunity to recommend care and lifestyle changes that will lead to the fewest possible risks as she undertakes her first pregnancy in her late thirties. Larisa's woman-centered care addresses both benefit and risk, biological and psychosocial, including Melissa's worst fears – having an "abnormal" baby, losing control, feeling uncertain about her capacity to mother, combining motherhood and career. Over the course of this book, we will see Larisa working with Melissa around those issues from pre-conception wellness care through labor and delivery and the life changes thereafter.

CHAPTER 5

Obesity: An Epidemic But Where is the Woman?

Lucy M. Candib

Felicity began her third pregnancy more than 50 pounds heavier than her post-partum weight after the birth of her second child. Always heavy, she attributed this most recent weight gain to the use of hormonal contraception. However, she also admitted eating fast food several times a week with the children, doing no exercise apart from walking, and snacking late at night. Without a car, she found it difficult to get from the public housing project to a supermarket where she might buy cheaper fresh fruits and vegetables than were available at the corner store. Her mother, grandmother, and sisters were also all heavy. Felicity disliked how the staff at the community health center insisted on her getting weighed in the hallway. She felt criticized by the medical staff for her weight and found the word obese very demeaning. At her initial nurse visit for this pregnancy, the nurse reminded her that "obese women" have more risk of cesarean section and other complications. Felicity felt that this harping on her weight was particularly judgmental since she could not do anything about her weight at that moment. Apart from the negative experience of being publicly weighed at each prenatal visit, Felicity had actually felt less self-conscious about her weight during her prior pregnancies; pregnancy was a time when being "big" felt normal, and pregnancy gave her permission to eat "for two" without need for dieting or an expectation of weight loss. Felicity hoped that Harmony, the new obstetrical nurse practitioner who did her first prenatal exam, would continue to be her prenatal provider and would not nag her about her weight. Harmony Lott was an Afro-Caribbean woman who herself was overweight. (*See* full vignette for Felicity and biography for Harmony Lott in the Appendix.)

The epidemic of obesity in developed countries is accelerating out of control with the age of onset of obesity, and its frequent co-conspirator, diabetes, becoming younger and younger. Excess calories in the form of fatty foods, sweet foods, carbonated beverages, and fast foods, coupled with decreased physical activity and increased passive recreation (television and video/computer games), have rendered one-third of the US population overweight (body mass index (BMI) 25–30) and another one-third obese (BMI greater than 30).[52] Even in developing nations, multiple forces are pushing poorly nourished populations with previously low caloric intake into obesity with high-calorie diets relying on cheap fats and sweeteners.[53] In the USA, low-income women and particularly women of color appear to be especially at risk of obesity for both environmental and possibly genetic reasons. Low-cost foods are full of fats and dense with calories; healthy choices like fresh fruits and vegetables are more expensive and sometimes completely unavailable to exactly those sectors of the population most in need of a healthful diet. Discouragingly, fewer than 20% of adults effect significant long-term weight loss in the absence of bariatric surgery,[54] suggesting that obesity is deeply problematic and largely irreversible for the great majority of women.

A consequence of this epidemic of obesity is the increasing prevalence of over-weight and obese women in prenatal and obstetrical settings. Obesity affects perinatal health in multiple ways, including fertility rates,[55,56] prenatal medical complications such as diabetes or stillbirth,[57,58] and labor problems such as dysfunctional labor.[59] Even interval weight gain between pregnancies appears to predispose to more complications.[60] More recent studies underscore the increased rate of intrapartum complications such as more epidural failures[61] and more cesarean sections in obese women.[57,62]

One issue with many of these studies is that few actually control for other known risks for negative outcomes related to the risks of obesity. For instance, Weiss does not adjust the risk of cesarean in obese women for underlying diabetes, which is an independent risk factor for cesarean.[57] Obesity increases the risk of gestational dia-betes, and gestational diabetes in turn increases the risk of both macrosomia and cesarean, but for obese women who do not develop gestational diabetes or fetal macrosomia, the overall risk of cesarean may not be as high as reported without controlling for these complications.[62] Excess weight gain in pregnancy contributes to an increased risk of macrosomia and cesarean section but does not fully explain the rise in cesareans.[63]

Invisible in these recent discussions of obesity in pregnancy are the genetic, social, economic, psychological, media-related, and familial reasons why a woman might now be obese, and might have been programmed for such obesity for many years if not from birth or her own prenatal period.[53] Furthermore, a woman's weight is deeply connected with her body image and sexuality. The public and the obese woman herself see obesity as a character flaw, a weakness, a lack of self-control that is the responsibility of the individual, not a public health problem. Thus many obese women feel a deep sense of shame and stigma because of their size, having taken much of the society's blame onto themselves.

How can a woman-centered clinician care for women in this context? One significant issue is the difficulty for thin young professional healthcare providers to avoid stigmatizing or disdaining the legions of overweight and obese low-income women and women of color. Such providers need to recognize their own prejudice against people who are obese and set aside any value judgments to find a way to be woman-centered in approaching women like Felicity.

Medical awareness of increased intrapartum complications for obese women has the potential to cause a "labeling effect"[64] whereby providers, who assume that increased risk is at play for obese women, intervene more quickly for even minimal aberrations from a normal course, potentially creating a cascade of further technological interventions. Such intervention may include jumping sooner to the elective cesarean option in obese women. To be woman-centered, Harmony's clinical care throughout pregnancy and the other providers' intrapartum care needs to avoid letting obesity trump all other clinical indicators of perinatal risk and drive clinical decision-making into further intervention. Little evidence exists about successful perinatal care options for obese women. For instance, retrospective data suggests that morbidly obese women (with a BMI over 40) have a higher risk of stillbirth,[58,65] but whether serial antenatal testing for fetal well-being changes that risk is an unanswered question. Such testing has false-positive results that could potentially cascade into further invasive testing or induction of labor, which in itself may lead to a higher cesarean rate than would be expected from the woman's obesity alone. Such care perpetuates the obese woman's view of herself as pathological as well as the clinician's perception of her higher risk.

CHAPTER 6

Intrapartum Care: How is it Not Woman-Centered Right Now?

Sara G. Shields

Larisa trained at a family medicine program where her prenatal and obstetrical training took place at a large public tertiary hospital with over 3000 births a year, mostly attended by obstetricians, with a small group of family physicians including Larisa's residency program faculty also offering intrapartum care. Larisa's experience with the obstetricians involved a model of care in which most of the intrapartum care was done intermittently by busy nurses in an understaffed environment. The labor triage area had one room with several beds separated by curtains where women were assessed before admission. Virtually all laboring women received continuous electronic fetal monitoring once in active labor. The hospital offered around-the-clock anesthesia coverage with separate obstetric anesthesia staff and residents, and a 90% epidural rate. The overall cesarean rate for low-risk women was 25% and climbing. When Larisa entered her new practice after residency, she chose a community hospital known for its lower intervention rates, but was surprised there to learn that the hospital was about to stop offering a trial of labor after cesarean, due to risk-management concerns. Larisa consciously chooses to go back to basics and adopt a woman-centered approach to normal pregnancy. She hopes that choosing woman-centeredness as her principal value will enable her to develop the finest care for her patients.

When Larisa thinks about her maternity practice, she needs to especially consider how she is going to provide intrapartum care. In this era of escalating obstetric intervention and cesarean rates, Larisa will need woman-centered approaches to the following issues: labor support, continuous electronic fetal monitoring, strategies for pain relief during labor, induction of labor, and both "patient-choice cesarean" and the rising primary cesarean rate. Even though she may be a provider interested in a more "low-tech, high-touch" approach,[66] she may find that her work within a more interventionist hospital begins to reflect the institutional standards, rather than a more individualized approach.[67]

One of the critical ways that intrapartum care in many hospitals fails to be woman-centered is the lack of systematic doula support for women having their first baby. Estimates of the frequency of intrapartum doula support, derived from extensive surveys, range between 3% to 5%.[68,69] This kind of para-professional labor support provides a personalized care model that improves multiple perinatal outcomes, including lowering the risk of cesarean section.[70] Although hospitals appear to encourage lay support by allowing family members to attend women in labor, such family presence does not change obstetrical outcomes in the same way as formal doula support.[71] Furthermore, several studies suggest that even professional staff such as nurses do not provide the kind of emotional or continuous support that doulas can.[72,73] Nevertheless, public health attempts to address perinatal health issues like the rate of operative deliveries, depression, and breastfeeding, have neglected this key strategy.[74-7]

The emphasis on the technology of electronic fetal monitoring further diminishes the woman-centeredness of intrapartum care. As of 2003, the most recent year for which national birth data reported this procedure, about 85% of women delivering in the USA underwent this type of monitoring,[78] even though the effect of such monitoring on perinatal health outcomes remains controversial.[79,80] Canadian rates are similar.[81-3] In many hospitals, labor units have "central monitoring" (remote surveillance by fetal monitor) allowing nurses to watch fetal heart tracings from outside the laboring woman's room, thus requiring fewer staff. The result is that laboring women are left alone for even longer periods while still being "monitored." Given that intermittent labor support does not have the same effect on birth outcomes as continuous support, the ultimate effect of central monitoring is to further limit nurse presence with laboring women and thus reduce the potential for positive effects from such staff support. Furthermore, the central monitoring technology itself compared with bedside EFM has not improved delivery outcomes.[84] The structural and functional implications of technologies such as central fetal monitoring remain largely unexamined and certainly opaque to consumers unaware of the reduced staffing that follows from such technology. Finally, efforts in health technology assessment to examine such issues have faced industry opposition in court.[85]

While the increasing use of epidural analgesia for labor may seem woman-centered in that this technology clearly provides effective pain relief, the uncritical embrace of epidurals leads to a slippery slope of not providing other pain relief options and then not offering true informed consent about the risks of epidurals as well as their benefits. When epidurals are seen as the only valid pain-relief option, hospitals and their staff neglect to offer other less invasive choices for either early labor or more intense labor, such as hydrotherapy, doula support, or alternative positions in labor or for delivery.[68,69] In the USA, women have few choices for other pharmacologic pain care during labor; such as nitrous oxide, a method that allows more patient control and may have less impact on length of labor or operative delivery rate.[86] Without these options, women in the throes of labor in fact do not have real choice, and thus "choose" an epidural as their only way to cope. The issue of informed consent about the timing, dosing, and style of epidural will be discussed further in Part One, Chapter 10 on evidence-based maternity care.

Another significant intervention in North American obstetric care in the last few decades is the rise in labor induction[35] with up to one-third of women in the USA[87] and over one-quarter of women in Canada[88:30] having their labor started artificially rather than awaiting spontaneous labor. Larisa has learned in her training that for certain maternal or fetal health issues such as worsening pre-eclampsia or intrauterine growth retardation, inducing labor helps prevent morbidity or mortality. However, the increasing rates of induction do not parallel any increase in such medical indications,[89] and in fact up to 15% of these inductions may not have standard clinical indications.[87] While one purported reason for such "elective" inductions is prevention of stillbirth,[90] little evidence exists about how induction affects this outcome for otherwise healthy low-risk women. Other reasons for induction include provider-centered convenience issues, such as provider or hospital staffing logistics or perceived liability.[91,92] Even when the woman's own scheduling concerns lead to request for an induction, the woman-centered approach encourages scrutiny of such a choice that may reflect lack of cohesive home support and may provoke increased intervention in labor and delivery.

Furthermore, Larisa is aware that the different hospitals in her community have widely different induction rates even with similar populations, suggesting that multiple factors other than clinical indication or evidence drive these interventions.[89,93,94]

She knows about newer pharmacologic methods such as prostaglandins that help make induction more likely to lead to vaginal delivery than other methods of induction, yet is also aware of strong retrospective evidence that labor induction particularly for first-time mothers is linked to an increased risk of cesarean delivery even after such cervical ripening.[95-7] She has also heard about the strategy of "active management of risk at term" with liberal use of induction to prevent cesarean delivery,[98-100] and wants to consider woman-centered ways to incorporate these ideas with caution about cascades of interventions and operative risk.

CHAPTER 7

Cesarean Sections:
The Operative Epidemic

Sara G. Shields

Dr. Jonathan Rosen is a family doctor who decided after two years in practice to pursue an obstetrics fellowship so that he could perform cesarean sections, tubal ligations, dilation and curettage procedures, and abortions for the women in his care. He came to the community health center with the goal of joining a practice caring for under-served families and providing woman-centered care. His residency training and obstetrics fellowship also emphasized finding and applying evidence to his clinical care of patients. He teaches regularly in both the local community hospital family practice residency and in continuing education programs about how to read journal articles and how to stay on top of the latest evidence. (*See* full biography in the Appendix.)

Multiple factors contribute to the international epidemic of cesarean sections. Although the pendulum swing away from vaginal birth after cesarean is one factor in rising cesarean rates, primary cesarean rates are climbing rapidly as well. In the USA and elsewhere, attempts to tackle the escalating operative delivery rate have neglected to address the above-mentioned package of intrapartum care: early labor admission, elective induction, early epidural use with associated bedrest, continuous electronic monitoring, and lack of doula support.[77,101-3] Physician convenience and malpractice anxiety also foster increased cesareans. In developing countries, where rates of cesareans in private hospitals in major cities exceed 50%,[104] the physicians' motivation can be called into question. While many have attempted to say that it is women themselves, in countries like Brazil, who want cesarean sections, exploration of women's preferences have revealed that women feel pushed by the physicians to have an operative delivery.[105,106]

Cesarean sections done for no medical indication, also labeled "elective" cesarean or "cesarean on demand," have been a highly visible topic in recent maternity care and the subject of a recent National Institutes of Health (NIH) conference[77] as well as guidelines from both the American College of Obstetricians and Gynecologists (ACOG) and the International Federation of Gynecology and Obstetrics (FIGO).[107,108] The data on prevalence and etiology of this kind of cesarean (in multiple countries)[109] is, however, limited and confounded by multiple factors such as whether the indication is by obstetrician report or maternal description, and when and how during pregnancy this assessment of maternal request is made.[110-12] For instance, some studies assume that reports of postpartum maternal satisfaction with childbirth equate with maternal request for cesarean.[109,113] While birth certificate data shows that about 5% of live births in the USA result from cesareans done for "no apparent medical indication,"[114] this term does not translate to cesareans "done for maternal request." Providers should be cautious in using such "proxy" studies.[115] Such factors in data collection may cause over-reporting and aggravate the tendency to cite the rise in this type of cesarean as a primary driving force for the steep rise in overall cesareans.[112,114] Two large national surveys of US mothers report that fewer than 1 in 1000 women interviewed had a planned elective cesarean without other indication, suggesting a much lower rate than reported elsewhere, and 9% of respondents reported provider pressure to have a cesarean.[68,69] While one UK survey of women after childbirth suggests a slightly higher rate of maternal preference (3% for first-time mothers, and over 5% overall including women with prior cesarean),[116:100-1] data since 2004 in Canada suggest that less than 0.5% of first cesareans are done for maternal request.[117:6] More limited surveys in Australia also concluded that very few women request cesarean in the absence of a medical indication.[110,118] The purported rise in maternal request cesareans may be more due to a lower provider (and patient) threshold to do cesareans rather than any change in indication.[119-21]

What are the ostensible reasons for maternal request for cesarean that Jonathan should consider? Answering this means facing methodological challenges similar to those already mentioned, yet the question is critical to woman-centered care. When women are asked, early in pregnancy, about preferred mode of delivery, one finding is that their prior birth experiences may have been difficult enough that they now wish for more control over their subsequent birth.[122] Later in pregnancy, women may change their mind about elective cesarean.[123] They may ask for a specific date in order to schedule around work, home needs or provider availability if they have a particularly strong relationship with their primary maternity provider. Some studies suggest that women who report early in pregnancy a desire for an elective cesarean may have specific fears or anxieties about childbirth,[122,124] and may change their perception and their request after psychological counseling to address these feelings.[124]

Concerns about future pelvic floor dysfunction or fetal well-being may be a woman's primary concern about labor and may evolve throughout the pregnancy. Despite the familiarity of the public with cesarean sections, the adverse effects are less visible to consumers: women requesting elective cesarean sections are unaware of[69] or ill-informed about[110] the significant risks to mothers and infants posed by such intervention, both during the current pregnancy[125-9] and also the complications related to later pregnancies.

Jonathan's woman-centered response to these concerns will draw on his use of all aspects of the patient-centered clinical method: understanding the woman's fears, ideas, function, and expectations; finding common ground; promoting healthy outcomes; and understanding his clinical relationship with the woman and the health system. Clarifying the reasons for a woman's request for cesarean involves assessing possible residual post-traumatic stress disorder from a prior difficult birth, ambivalence about this pregnancy, or the woman's feelings of inadequacy about her own capabilities either in labor or postpartum. Jonathan's task is to address possible unmet psychological needs, review evidence about prenatal and intrapartum choices that may impact on pelvic floor function and fetal well-being, and discuss options for scheduling and home assistance. After careful exploration of such factors and appropriate consultation for psychological or other medical issues, woman-centered care will involve elective cesarean at term for some small number of women. However, woman-centered care avoids allowing this to spiral into ever-rising numbers of surgical deliveries. Resource availability, such as anesthesia capability, provider scheduling issues or time constraints, economic issues, or a woman's employment demands, should not be solved with the panacea of life-altering surgery. Nor should fear of various childbirth outcomes, in any manifestation, drive maternity providers or the healthcare system to "merely reach for the scalpel"[130] in a self-fulfilling process that normalizes operative delivery as the primary treatment of anxiety around childbirth.

The other issue in the discussion of patient-choice cesarean is the lack of women's choice about vaginal delivery for breech presentation or in trial of labor after cesarean. If maternity providers uphold the rights of autonomous women to choose a primary elective cesarean, what about a woman's right to choose a vaginal delivery?[131] With fewer obstetricians skilled in attending vaginal breech delivery, and fewer rural hospitals allowing trial of labor after cesarean section, women have fewer options for subsequent deliveries.[132] This situation creates a lack of choice and also drives up cesarean rates.

Indeed, the history of VBAC in the USA offers a lesson in how a woman-centered approach became overwhelmed by multiple, complex forces. Two decades ago, consumers in the USA demanded individualized care in re-examining the safety of a trial of labor after cesarean section. When national consensus statements finally supported the practice of a trial of labor, the rate of VBAC climbed, peaking in 1996.[133] At the same time the primary cesarean rate dipped slightly but not as dramatically. When studies began to suggest that a higher perinatal morbidity and even mortality might result from a trial of labor, however, the VBAC rate began to plummet,[134] and many rural and community hospitals stopped offering this option of care. Canadian rates of VBAC have similarly dropped, although not quite so far as in the USA.[101,102] Australian rates are also decreasing, with less than 20% of women with prior cesarean having VBAC.[103] However, re-examination of the safety data on VBAC suggests that careful application of policies toward selected women can minimize the risks associated with VBACs.[135-7] Perhaps in the rush to increase the VBAC rate in the 1990s, providers attempted trials of labor in some women who were not such "good" candidates – such as women who had had a particularly difficult first labor that had resulted in cesarean section or women who needed induction in the subsequent pregnancy. Hospitals and insurers may also have pushed for higher rates of trials of labor without looking more carefully at the potential risk issues. For women without such risk factors, a trial of labor may still be safe and successful. Women who wish to have a trial of labor after cesarean find fewer options for a provider and a hospital willing to offer this for them.[131] The same is true for women who wish to attempt a vaginal breech delivery, an issue that we will discuss later.

Now with the greatly reduced rate of VBACs, the primary cesarean rate portends the rate of future interventions since any woman with a first cesarean faces the likelihood of operative delivery in future pregnancies. The primary cesarean rate in the USA is now approaching 1 in 5, with the total cesarean rate at a record high of 1 in 3 women,[138] similar to Australia's total cesarean rate of nearly 31%.[103] In Canada, the primary cesarean rate in 2001 was over 18%.[102] The main reason for primary cesarean is dystocia, or difficult/stalled labor, a diagnosis most common for first-time mothers. Woman-centered intrapartum care demands a refocusing of cesarean prevention strategies. The small number of patient-choice cesareans is not the key problem. It is time to consider approaches to labor dystocia that do not focus solely on technology (such as high-dose oxytocin) but rather on systems and provider issues as well.[139,140]

CHAPTER 8

Postpartum Care: Breastfeeding and Mood Disorders

Colleen Fogarty

During her residency, Larisa structured her prenatal and postpartum care using standardized protocols in her residency clinic. These prompted her to give anticipatory guidance during the last few weeks of prenatal care about specific postpartum issues such as breastfeeding and postpartum depression. Her clinic's routine was to see newborns within one to two weeks of hospital discharge and to see mothers back for routine postpartum care at about six weeks after delivery. She became interested in finding ways to increase breastfeeding duration and in doing better screening for postpartum depression.

The epidemiology of two critical aspects of postpartum care, breastfeeding and postpartum mood issues, reflect the lack of woman-centered care in our current healthcare system and greater social culture. Both issues reveal the dearth of adequate social support for women and families facing the challenges of these immediate newborn weeks. Even in countries with plentiful social and nursing services for women postpartum, postpartum depression remains a challenging problem interrelated with women's situations in a variety of social, economic, and political environments.[141,142] In addition, although many developed countries meet or surpass the criteria for the World Health Organization's breastfeeding promotion program, the Baby-Friendly Initiative (*see* Part Five), this program emphasizes the baby rather than the mother.

BREASTFEEDING

How woman-centered is our social value on natural nutrition for neonates? The 1950s and 1960s marked the era of "modernization" of infant feeding by the development and entrenchment of the infant formula industry. Physicians and mothers in industrialized countries bought into this myth of the supposed superiority of breast milk substitutes with rates of breastfeeding in the 1960s below 30%.[143,144] By the latter years of the 1990s, breastfeeding regained its appropriate stature as the best way to nourish a human infant, with increasing numbers of women initiating breastfeeding.[143,145] The last two decades have seen a rise in biomedical knowledge about the many physiological and psychological benefits of breastfeeding, as well as a strong resurgence in lay support programs for breastfeeding, notably La Leche League.[146] These professional and lay acknowledgments of the benefits of breastfeeding clearly focus on the benefits to baby, and even society, by breastfeeding, but do little to acknowledge the woman herself, including her challenges, emotions, and social and family context.

Many societal structures place barriers in the way of most new mothers' successful breastfeeding experience. One such barrier is the prevalent cultural norm of seeing the breast primarily as a sexual object. For women who hold this belief, or whose partners or family members do, breastfeeding in public, or even in the home in the presence of another person, may be unacceptable. Teenage mothers may be particularly vulnerable around this issue as they and their partners are just learning about their emerging sexuality in the midst of childbearing. Another such barrier relates to issues of class and employment. Multiple studies document the income/social class gradient for breastfeeding with each month of life; upper-income women consistently breastfeed longer than lower-income women.[145] In the USA, many pressures exist for low-income working women, where many factory and service sector jobs provide only six weeks of maternity leave for uncomplicated births, often unpaid. Women may be the sole wage earner, and thus not have the option of taking off a longer maternity leave. In addition, these workplaces often do not provide either the time or the space to either breastfeed or express milk.[147] Even mothers in higher-income groups, or professional occupations, returning to the workplace after even a "generous" maternity leave of 12 weeks, face difficulties continuing to breastfeed. For any woman, the additional responsibility of continuing to breastfeed while upholding the responsibilities of wage earner, worker, life-partner/spouse, and possibly mother to other children can be overwhelming. Negative reactions, work overload and role overload all result in stress that may adversely affect her milk production and may even affect her self-image as nurturer to her neonate. Workplace colleagues, particularly men, may not understand these stresses and may expect "usual work performance."

The provision of breast milk substitutes in the hospital, both as supplements in the nursery and in the infamous "discharge packets," can undermine a woman's confidence in her own ability to produce and maintain a milk supply for her baby. Despite verbal support for breastfeeding and increased food coupons for mothers, those new mothers who receive Women, Infants, and Children (WIC), the supplemental food program for low-income individuals in the USA, actually have a much lower rate of breastfeeding than women who are not receiving WIC.[148] Thus despite the apparent promotion of breastfeeding in WIC policies, the provision of free formula to all babies under one-year-old probably undermines any positive message about lactation and acts as a major disincentive.[149]

UNICEF and the World Health Organization (WHO) collaborated in 1991 to develop a description of the "Baby-Friendly Hospital," which would adhere to a list of 10 key hospital policies to encourage breastfeeding, such as early initiation and no routine artificial supplements (*see* Part Five). However, notably absent on the list, and in the title of the program, is the mother. A more respectful woman-centered approach would incorporate the issues for the mother in increasing breastfeeding initiation and duration and would adopt "Mother-Friendly" language that would recognize women's centrality in successful breastfeeding.

POSTPARTUM MOOD DISORDERS

Women face similar system-based struggles in coping with the myriad emotional changes following childbirth. The spectrum of postpartum mood disorders ranges from postpartum blues, a self-limited and extremely common experience in the immediate postpartum period, to postpartum depression (PPD), up to and including psychosis. The magnitude of postpartum depression is difficult to grasp in our currently fragmented, non-woman-centered model of care. A postpartum mother may not see her obstetrical provider until six weeks postpartum. This provider may or may not be the one who cared for her during pregnancy or labor or even before pregnancy. Although a new mother may see the baby's healthcare provider prior to her own check-up, this clinician may not be prepared to inquire about, let alone treat, the mother's problems.

The days, weeks, and months following the birth of a baby represent a particularly vulnerable period for the mother's mental health. The birth of a baby, whether the first-born or a subsequent child, requires both the mother's and family's adjustment to the new infant, accommodating their life and routines to the new arrival. The stresses of this adjustment for managing even a healthy term baby in the home are difficult for almost all mothers and families. Despite widespread recognition of such stresses in the developmental and family systems literature, as well as in lay sources, much modern medical care does not acknowledge the dramatic changes affecting the woman and her significant others during pregnancy and afterwards. Postpartum care in the hospital usually focuses on the mother's initial physical recuperation, her plans for contraception, and a successful feeding plan for the baby. Various English-speaking countries (USA, Canada, Australia, and the UK) have moved toward shortened postpartum hospital stays, with research demonstrating no significant changes in the readmission rate for infants with jaundice or in the duration of breastfeeding.[150-2] These shortened stays, while perhaps "successful" from a "hard biomedical outcomes" perspective, often do not provide adequate support for the new mother and her significant others. Although some women may be more comfortable and empowered in their home environment,[153] most health systems have not created an adequate continuum of care from hospital to home for those who need additional support for either mother or baby.[154]

Thus, most new mothers are left relatively on their own, sometimes with a partner and extended family, sometimes not, to experience and cope with the dramatic changes of the postpartum period. A fortunate woman will have a nurse or lay home visitor, and some will locate a community group of other new mothers. Unfortunately, many women will muddle, unsupported, through the mood swings and crying spells, wondering about their own adequacy as mothers and as women. The popular literature and parenting magazines, depicting perfect postpartum mothers, fathers, and infants, deliver a subtle message of perfect bliss to the newly adjusting family. So at odds with the real stresses on the family, this idyllic media portrayal can undermine their postpartum adjustment.

Those women who consult a parenting book or postpartum leaflet may find reassuring words about the normalcy of this condition. Many others will be left to wonder where they have gone wrong in their mothering to feel so distressed. Not discussed in the literature on postpartum blues is the fact that healthy women with no particular predisposition to depression have real worries about their new and vulnerable babies. Clearly, a new mother's mental health and emotional state are not hers alone, but are intimately tied to the health, stability, and prognosis of her baby as well as of the supports around her. The specialty medical system is not at all set up to address the mother-baby unit as a dyad, nor to view pregnancy and the postpartum period as a continuum. Economic systems (such as in the USA) that lack adequate parental leave for both mothers and fathers fail to recognize the enormous responsibility and transition entailed in managing a home with an infant.

Even our raw epidemiologic data about PPD reflect a lack of woman-centeredness in our understanding of this common condition. We have trouble defining PPD, both in terms of its timing, and its differentiation from normative responses to the challenges of new motherhood. The effect of PPD on infant attachment and development remains unclear. We have only just begun to recognize the multifactorial causes of PPD with a predominance of psychosocial risk factors. The plethora of explanations and risks for PPD reveals how little the medical system understands this "disorder" and how devalued women feel as they face the realities of this difficult life transition.

Many cultures share a common notion of "a morbid state of unhappiness following childbirth,"[155] but not all cultures recognize PPD as a *medical* illness.[155-7] As with other mood disorders, the medical sector of developed and industrialized countries under-recognizes PPD.[74] Efforts to encourage practitioners to look for PPD have promoted the use of screening questionnaires to rate the frequency of a set of standard symptoms and to raise clinicians' awareness of the prevalence of PPD. However, questionnaires that essentially rely on a deficit approach to PPD are not the complete answer to the lack of detection. Many women may prefer to discuss their symptoms with a clinician;[158] still others may be uncomfortable or unwilling to address their symptoms with a healthcare provider whose approach may have been strictly biomedical.[159] Sole reliance on this screening approach misses the woman's story and potentially important details about her adjustment to the role of mother for the new person in her life.[160,161] Beyond detection, when providers do recognize PPD, they may not successfully refer patients to treatment.[162] The women themselves may experience multiple complex factors that interfere with their ability to receive appropriate services.[163] System barriers also contribute to under-treatment; many locales lack appropriate mental health facilities.[164]

Finally, the appropriate use and adequate availability of the full spectrum of current treatment options for PPD also fail to be woman-centered.[165] Increasing understanding of the potential harms from pharmacologic treatments gives conflicting messages to both women and their clinicians. The antidepressants (SSRIs) that often work well in non-pregnant depressed people have subtle effects on the newborn when given during pregnancy,[166–9] although the issues for infants exposed only during breastfeeding are less clear.[170,171] At the same time, untreated depression is problematic for both maternal and infant health.[172,173] A new mother may find it very confusing trying to sort out what is best for her and what is best for her infant and whether what is best is best for both. Although both pharmacologic and non-pharmacologic treatment options for PPD have been studied, research about their comparative efficacy is lacking.[174,175] Furthermore, while several studies demonstrate the efficacy of psychotherapy, including cognitive behavioral therapy, for treating PPD,[158,176] getting from the diagnosis to treatment has proven difficult. The majority of women in one study did not agree to follow-up contact, further assessment, or treatment, demonstrating that women are likely to prefer patient-centered care with a known clinician or team of clinicians to receive treatment and support for this condition.[177] Ultimately, a woman-centered practice for PPD would begin with the recognition of a woman's strengths and competencies and pursue an approach that matches her preferences for treatment.

CHAPTER 9

International Issues

Martha Carlough

Dr. Usha Rao is a second-generation Indian American whose parents were both obstetricians in India. They migrated to a rural area in Canada where they continue to practice obstetrics with a low-income population. Usha grew up hearing her parents' conversations about obstetrics and also absorbed their commitment to service. She had thought she would become an obstetrician as well, but when she got to medical school she decided that she liked taking care of children and teenagers as well, and chose family medicine with maternity care. She was eager to join Woman-Centered Community Family Practice with its supportive environment and woman-centered focus. She is married to a neurologist and is balancing her practice with raising two small children. (*See* full biography in the Appendix.)

Anjana was a 32-year-old Tamil-speaking woman from South India who was pregnant with her first child. Though she and her husband Ram, along with both sets of their parents, immigrated almost two years ago when Ram was offered a long-term job in computer engineering, Anjana continued to live a largely Indian lifestyle. She cooked and cleaned for her parents and in-laws, did not drive or go out alone, and had few friends outside of family contacts. Because of Ram's job, they had excellent insurance and chose Woman-Centered Community Family Practice because they saw Dr. Usha Rao's name on the list of potential maternity providers, and they hoped she would be able to speak Tamil. As it turned out, Usha spoke only a few words of Tamil as her family came from North India and spoke Hindi, Urdu, and English at home. For Tamil, Usha needed to rely on a telephone interpreter. At each office visit for prenatal care with Usha, Anjana's mother or her mother-in-law accompanied her, but Ram was not able to attend, as he was too busy to take time off from work.

Anjana's pregnancy was relatively uncomplicated, though Usha had difficulty getting her to talk about any specific issues, such as nutrition or plans for breastfeeding. Even with the telephone interpreter, Anjana did not volunteer much information. Her only request, at every visit, was that her blood be tested. Anjana's shyness reminded Usha of the recently immigrated Indians she had met through her family, and she was distressed that she could not communicate better with her.

At 36 weeks during a routine prenatal visit Anjana's blood pressure (BP) was 152/92. Usha rechecked the BP three times, with the same result. When she asked Anjana about any symptoms – including headache, blurry vision, or abdominal pain – Anjana reported none. Usha explained that increased blood pressure late in pregnancy might be a sign of pre-eclampsia and needed to be watched carefully. She recommended blood work, a 24-hour urine collection, and a return visit in three or four days for a recheck of her BP. To be certain that Anjana understood, Usha asked the telephone interpreter to have Anjana repeat back the instructions in Tamil to the interpreter. Anjana stayed in the waiting room until results of her stat blood work, which were all normal, were complete. Usha talked Anjana's care over with Greg, the obstetrician consultant, who thought her plan was appropriate. But Usha continued to worry and asked her parents on the phone long distance that night if they would have done anything differently.

Forty-eight hours later, when Usha checked the lab tests, the 24-hour urine results were not yet ready. When she tried to contact Anjana on the phone to follow up, an older man who spoke no English answered. The phone number given for Anjana's husband at work was also incorrect. Three days later, Usha received a phone call from University Hospital in the city 50 miles away letting her know that Anjana had presented to the Emergency Room with a severe headache earlier that day, after being taken there by ambulance from a suburban shopping mall. After waiting three hours to be seen, Anjana was transferred to the labor ward. There, while the nurse struggled with Anjana to get an IV started, she had an eclamptic seizure. Before her husband arrived at the hospital, and with no consent obtained, Anjana underwent an emergency cesarean section, which fortunately went smoothly. (*See* Appendix for full vignette.)

Caring for immigrant women from different countries allows Usha to situate her clinical work within a wider international reality and to look for less US-centric models of care to improve her care for immigrant women. Despite the dreaded complication of eclampsia, the outcome of this birth story was ultimately a healthy one for mother and child. In international settings with fewer resources, the outcome would no doubt have been far worse. Usha knows that in countries where girls and women are undervalued and where girls are less likely to go beyond primary education, reduced fertility and improvements in infant and child mortality are directly related to higher age at marriage and completion of secondary education.[178] The global tragedy of maternal mortality claims more than half a million women's lives each year;[179] 99% of these deaths are in low and middle-income countries. And in some areas, including many countries in Africa and South Asia, estimates are that at least 25–33% of all deaths to women of reproductive age (18–45 years of age) are due to pregnancy or childbirth.[180]

The global causes of maternal mortality are in general well known and relatively consistent. The major direct causes are hemorrhage, infection, eclampsia, prolonged/obstructed labor and complications of unsafe abortion.[179] Maternal deaths from unsafe abortions are one of the most preventable portions of maternal mortality. Legalization of abortion is essential to safe motherhood around the world.[18] Important indirect causes of maternal mortality include the complications of HIV/AIDS, anemia, tuberculosis, malaria, heart disease, violence, and trauma. Underlying these causes are women's devaluation and disempowerment through lack of education, lack of rights of property ownership, and vulnerability to domestic violence. In settings where women are so devalued, resources such as food and money for medical care are less likely to be dedicated to women's health.[181] In addition to the risk of maternal death, 25% of all adult women in the developing world suffer short or long-term disability related to pregnancy and childbirth, such as chronic anemia, obstetric fistula, infertility, pelvic inflammatory disease (PID), chronic pelvic pain, and uterine prolapse. Neonatal health is closely connected to maternal health, and up to two-thirds of the almost five million early neonatal deaths worldwide each year are due to maternal health problems during pregnancy and lack of skilled attendants at birth.

In framing her encounters with immigrant women such as Anjana in a more global perspective, Usha can look to the United Nations' Millennium Development Goals (MDGs, *see* Box 1.1), established in 2000 with multilateral, multinational support. Each of these goals has associated targets and indicators used to measure progress. The commitment to continue to focus energy on these vital areas of health and development remains firm in spite of pessimism about achieving the goals by 2015.[182] Three of these goals directly address the health and welfare of women in the world, and the rest do so indirectly through their farther-reaching sociologic impact on women's societal position (*see* Box 1.1). Usha's awareness of women's health around the world is high because of her exposure to her parents' experience of delivering obstetrical care in India. She knows that almost half of births in developing countries take place without the help of a skilled birth attendant,[183] and that a woman living in Sub-Saharan Africa has a 1 in 16 chance of dying in pregnancy.[179] This compares to a 1 in 4000 risk for a woman in North America.[179,184] Unfortunately, sexual and reproductive health, including access to safe abortion, was omitted from the framework of the MDGs for political reasons, although later assessments have acknowledged that this omission was a mistake.[185,186] Not surprisingly, international policy on this issue is often at the mercy of political forces whose interests are remote from women's lives and deaths.

BOX 1.1 The Millennium Development Goals[1]

1 Eradicate extreme hunger and poverty
2 Achieve universal primary education
3 Promote gender equality and empower women
4 Reduce child mortality
5 Improve maternal health
6 Combat HIV/AIDS, malaria and other diseases
7 Ensure environmental sustainability
8 Develop a global partnership for development

Understanding these international statistics helps Usha see that this risky backdrop of pregnancy and childbirth is the cultural and social reality for most of the world including Anjana's native village. Healthcare systems where maternity care is prohibitively costly, geographically and culturally inaccessible, and condescending to women, guarantee persistence of unacceptably high rates of maternal and infant mortality.[181] Although emergency obstetric care – including access to essential medications (antibiotics, antihypertensives, uterotonics), safe blood transfusion and surgical intervention – has been critical to improving maternal and neonatal mortality and morbidity in Western countries in the last century, many lessons remain to be learned from a global perspective on maternal health. Principles from models of care elaborated and used internationally can shed light on the practice of woman-centered care in the context of the developed world.

One such model for Usha to consider in her care of Anjana is the "Three Delay Model" from the international safe motherhood literature.[187] This model seeks to clarify the problems of how women access maternity care at all stages of pregnancy. Although designed for and applied in developing countries, this model can illuminate problems in the care of immigrant women in the developed world. The first delay is in the decision to seek care. For instance, this delay may be due to a lack of understanding of important symptoms, gender bias, or the low status of women with an accompanying lack of control over family decision-making. Alternatively, this delay may reflect either an individual woman's or a culture's acceptance of normal risk during pregnancy and childbirth, an acceptance that does not mandate medical intervention. The second delay is in reaching care. Though geographic barriers are less problematic in most Western contexts, many women cannot or do not have easy access to transport or, such as in Anjana's situation, do not have understandable information about where and when to seek care. The third delay is in receiving care. Clearly, Anjana now lives in a setting where emergency care such as magnesium sulfate and cesarean section are far more available than in rural areas of her native country, yet factors such as racial discrimination, linguistic and cultural barriers, financial constraints and poor coordination/cooperation within the healthcare system prevent her from promptly receiving necessary care in critical situations.

Anjana's is the story of three delays, with a disease outcome (eclampsia) that modern obstetrics has sought to prevent through a specific system of prenatal care focused on the third trimester – usually with weekly visits in the last month of pregnancy. Yet in the developing world, the schema of weekly visits at a well-equipped medical clinic for the last weeks of pregnancy does not fit into the life of a rural or traditional woman and is often not economically, geographically, or culturally feasible. Nevertheless, improvements in obstetrical outcome in developing countries can come about through other methods of care based on an alternative strategy of prevention. The Birth Preparedness model proposes a different focus of visits and providers.[188]

The Birth Preparedness Model largely grew out of the findings of the WHO's multi-center Antenatal Care randomized trial which demonstrated that for women who do not have evidence of pregnancy complications or known medical conditions exacerbated by pregnancy, a reduction in the number of antenatal visits (to a minimum of four visits), paired with an increase in health education during visits, resulted in:

➤ no significant difference in recognizing pre-eclampsia or preterm labor
➤ no significant difference in maternal complications due to: infection, obstructed labor, hemorrhage, or eclampsia
➤ no significant difference in low birth weight incidence
➤ decreased healthcare expenditure and improved quality of service provision.[189]

In addition, women's satisfaction was greater with midwife or GP/FP-managed care than with obstetrician-managed care (likely related to longer time spent with women and care provided closer to home communities).[189]

The principles of the Birth Preparedness Model and woman-centered care can overlap:
1 questioning standard practices that may not change desired outcomes[189]
2 emphasizing the community context of and multidisciplinary responsibility for maternity care[188]
3 increasing emphasis on self-education and self-empowerment during maternity care (with a deliberate shift of power from provider to woman as elaborated below).

Usha's Western obstetric training viewed prenatal care as a screening process to detect pre-clinical phases of disease in order to address and treat problems in a predominantly healthy population. This strategy has not been proven valid or cost-effective[189,190] as many prenatal problems are not predictable, screening tests are limited in sensitivity and specificity, and, for many problems, early treatment of a pre-clinical state does not provide significant benefit. This view of prenatal care is provider-centered and has resulted in a culture of maintaining control and limiting potential for a woman's empowerment and education.

Important components of the Birth Preparedness Model of prenatal care include the following elements:[188]

➤ use only of those lab examinations that serve an immediate purpose with proven benefit

➤ non-physician providers carry out interventions whenever possible

➤ and, most importantly, the power shifts from the care provider to the pregnant woman, with major emphasis on health education about warning signs of complications and birth preparedness.

This power shift is important, as many women "at risk" never develop complications, while a significant number of women who are "low risk" do. Pregnant women need to understand the implications of warning signs, such as Anjana's headache, and need to know how, when and where to seek medical care in an emergency.

The Birth Preparedness Model encourages women to make "birth plans" for a normal birth, including planning for place of delivery and presence of a skilled attendant at birth. The provider, pregnant woman, and her family also discuss complication readiness: appointing a designated and available decision-maker, planning for emergency finances and transport, and rapid referral if necessary. Many women who prepare for a normal birth will also need to be ready to deal with complications. Understanding this possibility before an event saves lives, but also reduces stress and panic, and gives the woman some control over what may otherwise be a devastating and frightening situation.[188] Birth plans are further discussed in Part Four.

As comprehensive woman-centered care becomes a key measure of the adequacy of healthcare systems globally, three issues become central requirements.

➤ Choice – a woman's right not only to make choices about her own health and healthcare but also her right to both education about these choices and real access to choices, all of which involves political, sociocultural, economic, and educational factors.

➤ Access – a woman's access to care is clearly determined by available and competent providers of care, but is also dependent on issues of travel distance, logistical or administrative barriers to services, and cultural issues, including issues of caste, race, and gender.

➤ Quality – the details of what defines quality healthcare differ enormously in different situations, but the elements of quality care informed by evidence, tailored to each woman's needs and voiced desires in an atmosphere of respect and privacy, are internationally recognized key components.

Evidence-based clinical standards have significantly evolved over the past two decades since the first publication of *Effective Care in Pregnancy and Childbirth* in 1989.[190] The

Collaborative Eclampsia Trial[191] and Magpie Trial[192], as well as numerous multi-center trials currently underway coordinated by WHO and The Cochrane Group, exemplify an international approach in evidence-based clinical care for resource-limited settings. Some of these trials will shape the delivery of maternity care in low and middle-income countries in the 21st century as international donors seek to apply their resources to making motherhood safer. Many of these research trials look at issues such as care-seeking behavior, adult health education methods, and balancing quality and cost of care. However, helping providers at all levels understand the limits of meta-analysis and reframe evidence-based care in woman-centered ways remains critical.

CHAPTER 10

Evidence-Based Practice in Maternity Care: Examining the Evidence

Michael C. Klein

Jonathan's residency and fellowship training emphasized evidence-based medicine. While reading the medical literature, he learned to look for ratings of a study's strength of evidence. In his office now, he can search quickly in the Cochrane Database of Systematic Reviews to find the latest meta-analysis of many common obstetric issues. He has learned to rely on such searches to make decisions on the spot in his busy clinical schedule. (*See* full biography in Appendix.)

Many contemporary obstetric interventions, while seemingly helpful to women and their newborns, also create inadvertent consequences. The debate about these interventions is also part of a larger discussion on the role of evidence-based medicine in a risk-aversive society.

In the early 1980s, obstetrical practice was evolving from an empirical, unscientific approach based on providers' personal experience to an approach more based on evidence. The publication of *Effective Care in Pregnancy and Childbirth* in 1989[190] set the stage for many studies that would potentially improve maternity care. One of the first practices to be systematically studied was episiotomy. Several randomized controlled trials (RCTs) in Europe[193,194] and one in Argentina,[195] all conducted by midwives, demonstrated that episiotomy did not confer benefit in preventing perineal trauma. Little change occurred in North America until a Canadian trial studied both the physician practice and the usual North American median technique of episiotomy.[196] This study demonstrated that median episiotomy was the principal cause of the very trauma that it was intended to prevent: the most severe perineal trauma, third and fourth-degree tears. Moreover those physicians who clung to the use of episiotomy within the trial were not only responsible for disproportionate amounts of perineal trauma but also for an increased use of many other procedures, including cesarean section in a population of "low-risk" women.[197]

This randomized controlled trial, as well as other studies before and after the trial, had a marked effect on practice. Between 1980 and 1998, episiotomy rates in the USA dropped from 65% to 39%, with Canada's rates similarly declining from 55% to 25%.[198-200] Most importantly, in the USA, the rate of severe perineal trauma fell during this time period from 4.2% to 1.5%.[198] The information from episiotomy trials finally became widely available and was used by both practitioners and women to initiate reciprocal discussion between women and with their caregivers, so that women could avoid a damaging procedure. This unusual and rapid change in practice demonstrates an ideal use for evidence. As well, the discovery of an association between physician beliefs and a constellation of attitudes and harmful practices opened the way for further questioning of previously uncontested assumptions in obstetrical care. Nonetheless, the ACOG bulletin recommending no routine episiotomy did not appear until 2006.[201]

OTHER RANDOMIZED CONTROLLED TRIALS IN MATERNITY CARE – DO THEY MAKE SENSE?

The publication of *Effective Care in Pregnancy and Childbirth* not only offered hope that maternity care would become evidence-based, but also, in the wake of the Cochrane Collaboration, provoked an avalanche of new studies on obstetrical topics. With RCTs acknowledged as the highest form of evidence, investigators launched and published many new trials. Unfortunately, unlike the episiotomy trials, these newer studies as outlined below have yet to fulfill the promise that EBM would be an effective tool to make childbirth safer and more woman-centered.

Epidural Anesthesia

As discussed earlier, one clinical area of contemporary obstetrics subject to both much study and controversy is epidural analgesia. The woman-centered approach to labor would require a prenatal discussion between a pregnant woman and her provider of the various options for pain relief in labor, leading to a good understanding of the pros and cons of the use of each intervention. In this context, when a woman requests epidural anesthesia, and the provider thinks the timing appropriate, her request should be honored and facilitated. In fact, some obstetrical caregivers believe that any delay in epidural analgesia, when a woman has requested it, is cruel and disrespectful.[202,203] A recent report from the Canadian Institute for Health

Information indicated that four out of five Canadian women received one or more major obstetrical interventions, with epidurals high on the list; rates approach 80% in various Canadian settings[102] and are likewise high in the United States (in 2005, 71% in whites, 65% in non-Hispanic blacks, and 58% in Hispanics).[204] About half of UK mothers, on the other hand, give birth without interventions.[205] As noted earlier, in some settings the nursing staffs have moved away from use of their personal skills and presence to support women in labor, perhaps because of the widespread availability of epidural anesthesia, defining their nursing roles increasingly around the need to conduct surveillance through continuous electronic monitoring.[81,206–11] Many women's magazines and some childbirth education classes now present epidurals as the principal method of dealing with the pain of labor. Nevertheless both consumers and maternity care providers are ambivalent about what epidurals do to normal labor. Professionals seem reluctant to acknowledge that the ready availability of epidural analgesia has created a complex change in the birthing environment, with both positive and negative consequences.[212]

Epidural analgesia is clearly the most effective form of pain relief.[213] But associated with its use come a variety of unwanted side effects, including longer labors, increased incidence of maternal fever (with associated increase in maternal/newborn antibiotic use), more malpositions, increased rates of operative vaginal delivery and increased perineal trauma.[214] Evidence-based, woman-centered, informed choice would require that pregnant women, in making their birth choices, have a good understanding of the unwanted effects of epidural anesthesia and other associated interventions.

Surprisingly, the Cochrane Collaboration, the most authoritative source of information on evidence-based medicine, **does not** report an increase in the cesarean section rate in association with epidural analgesia.[214] For many practitioners, this finding went against the common experience in everyday practice that epidural use, especially when used before the active phase of labor, *did* seem to increase the cesarean rate.[212] Earlier meta-analyses, both from Cochrane and other sources, had shown a modest increase in the cesarean rate when compared with other methods of analgesia,[215] and one trial showed such a major increase that it had to be stopped.[216] Klein's studies from Vancouver have shown a clear association between the overuse of epidurals and an increase in cesareans, and even an excess of newborn special care unit admissions among women cared for by practitioners whose patients had high rates of epidural use.[217,218]

Careful re-examination of the Cochrane meta-analysis of epidural anesthesia reveals that the methodology of this meta-analysis combined heterogeneous studies of both early and late use of epidurals. When Klein dissected the Cochrane studies comparing epidural analgesia to narcotic analgesia for labor pain relief, excluding studies that utilized epidurals only when labor was well established (greater than 4 to 5 cm cervical dilation), he found that cesarean section was 2.5 times more likely to occur if epidural analgesia was employed early in labor (before 4 to 5 cm of dilation).[212] Studies subsequent to those included in the Cochrane review continued to make the same methodological mistake,[202,219] and thus continued to conclude erroneously that epidural analgesia will not raise the frequency of cesarean section. In fact, no one has yet studied in a controlled trial the role of early epidurals in contributing to cesarean increase, although the results of the Klein dissection of the Cochrane meta-analysis suggest that they are implicated.

Collateral Damage

Inadvertently, the Cochrane meta-analysis of epidural analgesia has had the consequence of increasing epidural use. A cascade of further interventions and complications result: more continuous electronic fetal monitoring, more laboring women kept at bedrest, usually with an intravenous line, more instrumentation, higher rates of maternal fever and perineal trauma, an increase in the cesarean rate, and for many women, likely feelings of failure.[212] This unexpected collateral damage contributes to making childbirth appear even more at risk for complications leading some to suggest that, since childbirth is already so "unnatural," cesarean section on request is not such an unreasonable idea – a surgical solution for a non-surgical problem.[77] But an increase in the number of cesarean sections is not an innocent outcome, as noted in prior discussion of the cesarean epidemic.

Other Practices Affected by the use of EBM

Another example of unexpected outcomes in an RCT affecting beliefs about common intrapartum practices was a study that purportedly showed the apparent uselessness of "walking in labor" in altering such outcomes as cesarean delivery or length of labor.[220] Closer examination of the methods of this widely cited study reveals specific parameters that render its conclusions non-generalizable. First, the study was done in a hospital with an already enviably low baseline rate of cesarean section and a strong adherence to the principles of active management of labor, a method of intrapartum care that likely affects both length of labor and possibly cesarean rates.[221,222] Second, the study randomized laboring women in the labor evaluation unit, when they were already 3 to 5 cm dilated, and thus already in active labor, yet not officially admitted to the hospital. Most women do their walking before the active phase. Third, the rate of epidural anesthesia, which is known to affect length of labor, was strikingly low for women in the entire study, between 5% and 6%, and, finally, EFM was not routinely used, a care plan very different from most US hospitals. Given these parameters, the study was unlikely to be able to show any significant impact of walking on the progress of labor or delivery type. Alternate conclusions from this study could be that hospitals that do not admit women before active labor, do not use routine EFM, and keep their epidural rates low, can have remarkably low intervention rates unaltered by ambulation.[223]

Another study that transformed maternity care in recent years was the Canadian Post-Term Trial,[224] yet its methodology and conclusions bear further analysis to again underscore the need for cautious interpretation of evidence. This study randomized women who were 41 weeks of gestation to either induction or expectant management, with serial measurements of fetal well-being. The results demonstrated that early induction at 41 weeks or slightly thereafter actually lowered the cesarean rate compared to the expectant group. However, on closer analysis at least some of this difference may have been due to different induction methods for women in the expectant group who ended up needing induction for medical reasons.[90] The study furthermore reported a non-significant increase in stillbirth in the expectant management arm and no difference in neonatal morbidity between the two groups. In the wake of this study, both Canadian and US clinical guidelines suggested routine induction at 41 weeks or soon thereafter,[225] even though the absolute risk of stillbirth in the forty-first week remained very low and the number of women needing to be induced to prevent one stillbirth was estimated at 1000.[90] Unfortunately, under real world conditions in usual practice, women having their first births have higher rates of cesarean if their labor is induced rather than spontaneous, as described earlier.[89,92,95-7] The discrepancy in cesarean rates between the results of this trial and these other descriptive studies under ordinary conditions likely has multiple explanatory factors: the biological reality that individual women produce placentas of variable maturity at a given gestational age; gestational age calculations under real world conditions are not as precise as under trial conditions; inductions often take place when women's cervices are unready (unripe); or continuous EFM during induction keeps most women in bed leading to labor dystocia and subsequent cesarean. Thus, this routine induction at 41 weeks ostensibly to prevent fetal mortality creates, in the process, a range of excess maternal and fetal morbidities including increasing the risk of cesarean section in the first and subsequent pregnancies.

Woman-centered care needs to involve full discussion about these risks with a pregnant woman who is post-term.[226,227] Woman-centered maternity care cannot take place when women do not receive full disclosure of all the consequences of the interventions proposed to prevent stillbirth. For example, cesarean sections are associated with excess stillbirths in subsequent pregnancies. If maternity care providers do not present a full picture of the tradeoffs between early induction and expectant management, women may be coerced into making decisions that inappropriately place them in false conflict with their fetuses. The result is "throwing the mother out with the bathwater."

Another clinical strategy, cesarean section for all breech presentations, purports to be evidence-based while promoting significant interventions that on further study lead to debatable conclusions. First, one large randomized study, the Term-Breech Trial, compared women attempting a vaginal breech birth with those delivering by cesarean section.[228] The initial trial results showed less newborn mortality for breech babies born by elective cesarean and less incontinence at three months' postpartum for mothers delivering by cesarean. Even before the publication of these results, many fewer women in North America were having vaginal breech deliveries, in large part due to obstetricians losing skills in attending such births and feeling more comfortable with their cesarean skills; many European obstetricians, on the other hand, had maintained the needed skills and were reporting much better outcomes than found in this trial.[229] Systematic reviews rapidly integrated these initial trial results, strongly urging the abandonment of vaginal breech births. When subsequent follow-up showed no difference in either infant or maternal outcomes at two years,[230] this information was not widely disseminated nor used as an opportunity to retrain obstetricians with the necessary lost skills. Thus, with most obstetricians now feeling safer doing a cesarean section for breech presentation, an apparently objective EBM study foreclosed on another woman-centered maternal choice in the name of "safety."

Conclusion for this Chapter

Evidence-based medicine in the form of meta-analysis can be helpful and time-saving for busy practitioners, but faulty construction or interpretation of randomized controlled trials, considered the highest form of evidence, can also promulgate misleading information. We need to ask ourselves for each study whether the evidence makes **clinical** sense in our particular practice environment. Practitioners need to be vigilant about exactly what evidence is used to create the "evidence base" for contemporary recommendations and which studies are incorporated into the meta-analyses.

> Larisa finds that she can join an electronic discussion group (mcdg@list.cfpc.ca) that brings together hundreds of North American maternity care providers who are questioning the "evidence." With members of this group, she learns to re-examine the individual studies that make up the meta-analyses – in order to determine if study conditions match her clinical reality. Otherwise, she fears that uncritical incorporation of the results from meta-analyses will continue to push her clinical practice into increasingly technical interventions.

To present true woman-centered choices to the women under her care, Larisa needs to know if the evidence is clear and balanced. She will need to help women look at their plans for future pregnancies. Epidural analgesia and many other apparently harmless interventions have important consequences – positive ones like pain relief and negative ones like an increase in interventions and adverse perineal and other outcomes. Woman-centered care looks at all potential decisions and how each one fits into the woman's plans and hoped-for experience. Woman-centered care, in the largest sense, considers the consequences of all decisions – not only the ones that may be preferred by the institution or individual practitioner – and helps the woman negotiate this complex territory.

SUMMARY OF PART ONE

Larisa and her colleagues both in her community practice and at the local community health center face many challenges trying to deliver woman-centered care in a context where women have limitations on their control over their own fertility; where factors outside women's control (for instance, racism and poverty) conspire to cause more maternal complications; where women's specific situations (for instance, older age and obesity) result in high rates of interventions; where intrapartum care has traded high touch for high tech, away from woman-centeredness; where an increasingly technical labor and delivery environment results in a cascade of interventions for which the woman is not prepared; where postpartum care does not recognize or address women's challenges with depression and breastfeeding in any woman-focused way; where low-income and immigrant women in the USA face delays in care not so different from delays for women around the world, in direct relationship to the extent of their disempowerment; and where the evidence base of academic research guiding the current high-tech environment is vulnerable to misinterpretation and uncritical acceptance of increasing intervention. As she begins her practice, Larisa consciously chooses to go back to basics and adopt a woman-centered approach to normal pregnancy. She hopes that choosing woman-centeredness as her principal value will enable her to develop the finest care for her patients.

REFERENCES

1 United Nations Development Programme. Millennium Development Goals. 2008 [cited January 24, 2009]. Available from: www.undp.org/mdg/basics.shtml

2 Henshaw SK, Singh S, Haas T. The incidence of abortion worldwide. *Int Fam Plann Persp.* 1999; **25**: S30–8.

3 Finer LB, Henshaw SK. Disparities in rates of unintended pregnancy in the United States, 1994 and 2001. *Perspect Sex Reprod Health.* 2006: 90.

4 Espey E, Cosgrove E, Ogburn T. Family planning American style: why it's so hard to control birth in the US. *Obstet Gynecol Clin North Am.* 2007; **34**: 1.

5 DiCenso A, Guyatt G, Willan A, *et al.* Interventions to reduce unintended pregnancies among adolescents: systematic review of randomised controlled trials. *BMJ.* 2002; **324**: 1426.

6 Singh S, Darroch JE. Adolescent pregnancy and childbearing: levels and trends in developed countries. *Fam Plann Perspect.* 2000; **32**: 14–23.

7 Wilkinson P, French R, Kane R, *et al.* Teenage conceptions, abortions, and births in England, 1994–2003, and the national teenage pregnancy strategy. *Lancet.* 2006; **368**: 1879–86.

8 Information Services Division. Sexual health: teenage pregnancy. 2009 [cited January 23, 2009]. Available from: www.isdscotland.org/isd/information-and-statistics.jsp?pContentID=2071&p_applic=CCC&p_service=Content.show&#Teenage_pregnancy_key_points

9 Arthur J. Abortion in Canada: history, law and access. 1999 [cited October 8, 2008]. Available from: www.prochoiceactionnetwork-canada.org/articles/canada.shtml

10 Lyons B. Abortion: What's the provincial reality? 2008 [cited 11/8/08, 2008]. Available from: www.prochoiceactionnetwork-canada.org/articles/nb-reality.shtml

11 Sethna C, Doull M. Far from home? A pilot study tracking women's journeys to a Canadian abortion clinic. *J Obstet Gynaecol Can.* 2007; **29**: 640–7.

12 Frost J, Sonfield A, Gold R. *Estimating the Impact of Expanding Medicaid Eligibility for Family Planning Services.* Guttmacher Institute; 2006. Report No. 28.

13 Foster DG, Parvataneni R, de Bocanegra HT, *et al.* Number of oral contraceptive pill packages dispensed, method continuation, and costs. *Obstet Gynecol.* 2006; **108**: 1107–14.

14 Skinner SR, Hickey M. Current priorities for adolescent sexual and reproductive health in Australia. *Med J Aust.* 2003; **179**: 158–61.

15 Finer LB, Henshaw SK. Abortion incidence and services in the United States in 2000. *Perspect Sex Reprod Health.* 2003; **35**: 6–15.

16 Henshaw SK, Finer LB. The accessibility of abortion services in the United States, 2001. *Perspect Sex Reprod Health.* 2003; **35**: 16–24.

17 Calcutt C. Abortion services in Australia. *O and G Magazine*. 2007: 27–8.

18 Grimes DA, Benson J, Singh S, *et al.* Unsafe abortion: the preventable pandemic. *Lancet*. 2006; **368**: 1908–19.

19 IPAS. *Ensuring Women's Access to Safe Abortion: essential strategies for achieving the millennium development goals*. IPAS; 2005.

20 Burke AE, Shields WC. Millennium Development Goals: slow movement threatens women's health in developing countries. *Contraception*. 2005; **72**: 247.

21 Gold MA, Sucato GS, Conard LA, *et al.* Provision of emergency contraception to adolescents. *J Adolesc Health*. 2004; **35**: 67–70.

22 Raine TR, Harper CC, Rocca CH, *et al.* Direct access to emergency contraception through pharmacies and effect on unintended pregnancy and STIs: a randomized controlled trial. *JAMA*. 2005; **293**: 54–62.

23 Cantor J, Baum K. The limits of conscientious objection: may pharmacists refuse to fill prescriptions for emergency contraception? *N Engl J Med*. 2004; **351**: 2008–12.

24 Griggs SK, Brown CM. Texas community pharmacists' willingness to participate in pharmacist-initiated emergency contraception. *J Am Pharm Assoc*. 2007; **47**: 48–57.

25 Hellerstedt WL, Van Riper KK. Emergency contraceptive pills: dispensing practices, knowledge and attitudes of South Dakota pharmacists. *Perspect Sex Reprod Health*. 2005; **37**: 19–24.

26 Shacter HE, Gee RE, Long JA. Variation in availability of emergency contraception in pharmacies. *Contraception*. 2007; **75**: 214–17.

27 Jones RK, Zolna MR, Henshaw SK, *et al.* Abortion in the United States: incidence and access to services, 2005. *Perspect Sex Reprod Health*. 2008; **40**: 6–16.

28 Fox GF. Available statistics on premature birth. *Fetal Matern Med Rev*. 2002; **13**: 195–211.

29 Mathews TJ, MacDorman MF. Infant mortality statistics from the 2004 period linked birth/infant death data set. *Natl Vital Stat Rep*. 2007; **55**: 1–32.

30 Hamilton BE, Martin JA, Ventura SJ. *Births: Preliminary data for 2006*. National Center for Health Statistics 2007.

31 Katz SJ, Armstrong RW, LoGerfo JP. The adequacy of prenatal care and incidence of low birthweight among the poor in Washington State and British Columbia. *Am J Public Health*. 1994; **84**: 986–91.

32 Dejin-Karlsson E, Ostergren PO. Country of origin, social support and the risk of small for gestational age birth. *Scand J Public Health*. 2004; **32**: 442–9.

33 Kramer MS, Seguin L, Lydon J, *et al.* Socio-economic disparities in pregnancy outcome: why do the poor fare so poorly? *Paediatr Perinat Epidemiol*. 2000; **14**: 194–210.

34 Luo ZC, Kierans WJ, Wilkins R, *et al.* Infant mortality among First Nations versus non-First Nations in British Columbia: temporal trends in rural versus urban areas, 1981–2000. *Int J Epidemiol*. 2004; **33**: 1252–9.

35 Martin JA, Hamilton BE, Sutton PD, *et al.* Births: final data for 2005. *Natl Vital Stat Rep*. 2007; **56**: 1–103.

36 Martin JA, Kung H-C, Mathews TJ, *et al.* Annual summary of vital statistics: 2006. *Pediatrics*. 2008; **121**: 788–801.

37 Healthy Start National Evaluation 2006. Racial and ethnic disparities in infant mortality: evidence of trends, risk factors, and intervention strategies. 2006 [cited January 24, 2009]. Available from: http://mchb.hrsa.gov/healthystart/evaluation/benchmarkreport/riskfactors.htm

38 de Costa C, Child A. Pregnancy outcomes in urban Aboriginal women. *Med J Aust.* 1996; **164**: 523–6.

39 Alder J, Fink N, Lapaire O, *et al.* The effect of migration background on obstetric performance in Switzerland. *Eur J Contracept Reprod Health Care.* 2008; **13**: 103–8.

40 Geronimus AT. Black/white differences in the relationship of maternal age to birthweight: a population-based test of the weathering hypothesis. *Soc Sci Med.* 1996; **42**: 589–97.

41 Colen CG, Geronimus AT, Bound J, *et al.* Maternal upward socioeconomic mobility and black–white disparities in infant birthweight. *Am J Public Health.* 2006; **96**: 2032–9.

42 Resta RG. Changing demographics of advanced maternal age (AMA) and the impact on the predicted incidence of Down syndrome in the United States: implications for prenatal screening and genetic counseling. *Am J Med Genet A.* 2005; **133**: 31–6.

43 Jacobsson B, Ladfors L, Milsom I. Advanced maternal age and adverse perinatal outcome. *Obstet Gynecol.* 2004; **104**: 727–33.

44 Cleary-Goldman J, Malone FD, Vidaver J, *et al.* Impact of maternal age on obstetric outcome. *Obstet Gynecol.* 2005; **105**: 983–90.

45 Seoud MA, Nassar AH, Usta IM, *et al.* Impact of advanced maternal age on pregnancy outcome. *Am J Perinatol.* 2002; **19**: 1–8.

46 Rosenthal AN, Paterson-Brown S. Is there an incremental rise in the risk of obstetric intervention with increasing maternal age? *Br J Obstet Gynaecol.* 1998; **105**: 1064–9.

47 Bell JS, Campbell DM, Graham WJ, *et al.* Can obstetric complications explain the high levels of obstetric interventions and maternity service use among older women? A retrospective analysis of routinely collected data. *BJOG: An International Journal of Obstetrics and Gynaecology.* 2001; **108**: 910–18.

48 Weaver J. Complications, or fear of complications? *BMJ*: Rapid response. 2001 [cited October 11, 2009]. Available from: www.bmj.com./cgi/eletters/322/7291/894

49 Ezra Y, McParland P, Farine D. High delivery intervention rates in nulliparous women over age 35. *Eur J Obstet Gynecol Reprod Biol.* 1995; **62**: 203–7.

50 Carolan M, Nelson S. First mothering over 35 years: questioning the association of maternal age and pregnancy risk. *Health Care Women Int.* 2007; **28**: 534.

51 Viau PA, Padula CA, Eddy B. An exploration of health concerns and health-promotion behaviors in pregnant women over age 35. *Am J Matern Child Nurs.* 2002; **27**: 328–34.

52 Ogden CL, Carroll MD, Curtin LR, *et al.* Prevalence of overweight and obesity in the United States, 1999–2004. *JAMA.* 2006; **295**: 1549–55.

53 Candib LM. Obesity and diabetes in vulnerable populations: reflection on proximal and distal causes. *Ann Fam Med.* 2007; **5**: 547–56.

54 Wing RR, Phelan S. Long-term weight loss maintenance. *Am J Clin Nutr.* 2005; **82**(1 Suppl): 222S–225S.

55 Metwally M, Li TC, Ledger WL. The impact of obesity on female reproductive function. *Obes Rev.* 2007; **8**: 515–23.

56 van der Steeg JW, Steures P, Eijkemans MJC, *et al.* Obesity affects spontaneous pregnancy chances in subfertile, ovulatory women. *Hum Reprod.* 2008; **23**: 324–8.

57 Weiss JL, Malone FD, Emig D, *et al.* Obesity, obstetric complications and cesarean delivery rate – a population-based screening study. *Am J Obstet Gynecol.* 2004; **190**: 1091–7.

58 Chu SY, Kim SY, Lau J, *et al.* Maternal obesity and risk of stillbirth: a meta-analysis. *Am J Obstet Gynecol.* 2007; **197**: 223–8.

59 Vahratian A, Zhang J, Troendle JF, *et al.* Maternal pre-pregnancy overweight and obesity

and the pattern of labor progression in term nulliparous women. *Obstet Gynecol.* 2004; **104**: 943–51.

60 Villamor E, Cnattingius S. Interpregnancy weight change and risk of adverse pregnancy outcomes: a population-based study. *Lancet.* 2006; **368**: 1164–70.

61 Dresner M, Brocklesby J, Bamber J. Audit of the influence of body mass index on the performance of epidural analgesia in labour and the subsequent mode of delivery. *BJOG.* 2006; **113**: 1178–81.

62 Vahratian A, Siega-Riz AM, Savitz DA, *et al.* Maternal pre-pregnancy overweight and obesity and the risk of cesarean delivery in nulliparous women. *Ann Epidemiol.* 2005; **15**: 467.

63 Rhodes JC, Schoendorf KC, Parker JD. Contribution of excess weight gain during pregnancy and macrosomia to the cesarean delivery rate, 1990–2000. *Pediatrics.* 2003; **111**: 1181–5.

64 Crowther CA. Treatment of gestational diabetes mellitus (author reply). *N Engl J Med.* 2005; **353**: 1629–30.

65 Salihu HM, Dunlop A-L, Hedayatzadeh M, *et al.* Extreme obesity and risk of stillbirth among black and white gravidas. *Obstet Gynecol.* 2007; **110**: 552–7.

66 Larimore WL, Cline MK. Keeping normal labor normal. *Prim Care.* 2000; **27**: 221–36.

67 Carroll JC, Reid AJ, Ruderman J, *et al.* The influence of the high-risk care environment on the practice of low-risk obstetrics. *Fam Med.* 1991; **23**: 184–8.

68 Declercq E, Sakala C, Corry M, *et al. Listening to Mothers: report of the first national U.S. survey of women's childbearing experiences.* New York: Maternity Center Association; 2002 October.

69 Declercq E, Sakala C, Corry M, *et al. Listening to Mothers II: report of the second national U.S. survey of women's childbearing experiences.* New York: Childbirth Connection; 2006 October.

70 Hodnett ED, Gates S, Hofmeyr GJ, *et al.* Continuous support for women during childbirth. *Cochrane Database Syst Rev.* 2007: CD003766.

71 Madi BC, Sandall J, Bennett R, *et al.* Effects of female relative support in labor: a randomized controlled trial. *Birth.* 1999; **26**: 4–8.

72 Hodnett ED, Lowe NK, Hannah ME, *et al.* Effectiveness of nurses as providers of birth labor support in North American hospitals: a randomized controlled trial. *JAMA.* 2002; **288**: 1373–81.

73 McNiven P, Hodnett E, O'Brien-Pallas LL. Supporting women in labor: a work sampling study of the activities of labor and delivery nurses. *Birth.* 1992; **19**: 3–8.

74 Gaynes B, Gavin, N, Meltzer-Brody S, *et al.* Perinatal depression: prevalence, screening accuracy, and screening outcomes. *Evidence Report/Technology Assessment No. 119.* Publication No. 05-E006-2. Rockville, MD: Agency for Healthcare Research and Quality; 2005.

75 Chaillet N, Dube E, Dugas M, *et al.* Evidence-based strategies for implementing guidelines in obstetrics: a systematic review. *Obstet Gynecol.* 2006; **108**: 1234–45.

76 Clark SL, Belfort MA, Byrum SL, *et al.* Improved outcomes, fewer cesarean deliveries, and reduced litigation: results of a new paradigm in patient safety. *Am J Obstet Gynecol.* 2008; **199**: 105.e1–7.

77 Anonymous. National Institutes of Health state-of-the-science conference statement: cesarean delivery on maternal request. March 27–9, 2006. *Obstet Gynecol.* 2006; **107**: 1386–97.

78 Martin JA, Hamilton BE, Sutton PD, *et al.* Births: final data for 2003. *Natl Vital Stat Rep.* 2005; **54**: 1–116.

79 Alfirevic Z, Devane D, Gyte GM. Continuous cardiotocography (CTG) as a form of electronic fetal monitoring (EFM) for fetal assessment during labour. *Cochrane Database Syst Rev.* 2006; **3**: CD006066.

80 Thacker SB, Stroup DF. Revisiting the use of the electronic fetal monitor. *Lancet.* 2003; **361**: 445–6.

81 Davies B, Hodnett E, Hannah M, *et al.* Fetal health surveillance: a community-wide approach versus a tailored intervention for the implementation of clinical practice guidelines. *CMAJ.* 2002; **167**: 469–74.

82 Levitt C, Hanvey L, Avard D, *et al. Survey of Routine Maternity Care and Practices in Canadian Hospitals.* Ottawa, Ontario: Minister of Supply and Services Health Canada; 1995.

83 Davies BL, Niday PA, Nimrod CA, *et al.* Electronic fetal monitoring: a Canadian survey. *CMAJ.* 1993; **148**: 1737–42.

84 Withiam-Leitch M, Shelton J, Fleming E. Central fetal monitoring: effect on perinatal outcomes and cesarean section rate. *Birth.* 2006; **33**: 284–8.

85 Banta HD, Thacker SB. Electronic fetal monitoring. Lessons from a formative case of health technology assessment. *Int J Technol Assess Health Care.* 2002; **18**: 762–70.

86 Rosen MA. Nitrous oxide for relief of labor pain: a systematic review. *Am J Obstet Gynecol.* 2002; **186**: S110.

87 Lydon-Rochelle MT, Cardenas V, Nelson JC, *et al.* Induction of labor in the absence of standard medical indications: incidence and correlates. *Med Care.* 2007; **45**: 505–12.

88 Health Canada. *Canadian Perinatal Health Report.* Minister of Public Works and Government Services Canada, 2003.

89 Zhang J, Yancey MK, Henderson CE. U.S. National trends in labor induction, 1989–98. *J Reprod Med.* 2002; **47**: 120–4.

90 Menticoglou SM, Hall PF. Routine induction of labour at 41 weeks gestation: nonsensus consensus. *BJOG.* 2002; **109**: 485–91.

91 Rayburn WF, Zhang J. Rising rates of labor induction: present concerns and future strategies. *Obstet Gynecol.* 2002; **100**: 164–7.

92 Simpson KR, Thorman KE. Obstetric "conveniences": elective induction of labor, cesarean birth on demand, and other potentially unnecessary interventions. *J Perinat Neonatal Nurs.* 2005; **19**: 134–44.

93 Simpson KR, Atterbury J. Trends and issues in labor induction in the United States: implications for clinical practice. *J Obstet Gynecol Neonatal Nurs.* 2003; **32**: 767–79.

94 Zeitlin J, Blondel B, Alexander S, *et al.* Variation in rates of postterm birth in Europe: reality or artefact? *BJOG.* 2007; **114**: 1097–1103.

95 Luthy DA, Malmgren JA, Zingheim RW. Cesarean delivery after elective induction in nulliparous women: the physician effect. *Am J Obstet Gynecol.* 2004; **191**: 1511–15.

96 Seyb ST, Berka RJ, Socol ML, *et al.* Risk of cesarean delivery with elective induction of labor at term in nulliparous women. *Obstet Gynecol.* 1999; **94**: 600–7.

97 Vahratian A, Zhang J, Troendle JF, *et al.* Labor progression and risk of cesarean delivery in electively induced nulliparas. *Obstet Gynecol.* 2005; **105**: 698–704.

98 Caughey AB. Preventive induction of labor: potential benefits if proved effective. *Ann Fam Med.* 2007; **5**: 292–3.

99 Caughey AB, Nicholson JM, Cheng YW, *et al.* Induction of labor and cesarean delivery by gestational age. *Am J Obstet Gynecol.* 2006; **195**: 700–5.

100 Nicholson JM, Kellar LC, Cronholm PF, *et al.* Active management of risk in pregnancy at term in an urban population: an association between a higher induction of labor rate and a lower cesarean delivery rate. *Am J Obstet Gynecol.* 2004; **191**: 1516–28.

101 British Columbia Perinatal Health Program. *Caesarean Birth Task Force Report 2008.* British Columbia Perinatal Health Program; 2008.

102 CIHI. Giving birth in Canada: regional trends from 2001–2 to 2005–6. 2007 [cited January 10, 2009]. Available from: http://secure.cihi.ca/cihiweb/dispPage.jsp?cw_page=AR_1106_E

103 Laws P, Hilder L. Australia's mothers and babies 2006. National Perinatal Statistics Unit, editor. Australian Institute of Health and Welfare; 2008.

104 Villar J, Valladares E, Wojdyla D, *et al.* Caesarean delivery rates and pregnancy outcomes: the 2005 WHO global survey on maternal and perinatal health in Latin America. *Lancet.* 2006; **367**: 1819–29.

105 Potter JE, Berquo E, Perpetuo IH, *et al.* Unwanted caesarean sections among public and private patients in Brazil: prospective study. *BMJ.* 2001; **323**: 1155–8.

106 Potter JE, Hopkins K, Faundes A, *et al.* Women's autonomy and scheduled cesarean sections in Brazil: a cautionary tale. *Birth.* 2008; **35**: 33–40.

107 ACOG. Surgery and patient choice. *Ethics in Obstetrics and Gynecology.* 2nd ed. Washington, D.C.: The American College of Obstetricians and Gynecologists; 2004. p. 21.

108 FIGO Committee for the Ethical Aspects of Human Reproduction and Women's Health. Ethical aspects regarding caesarian delivery for non-medical reasons. *Ethical Issues in Obstetrics and Gynecology.* London: FIGO; 1999. pp. 55–6.

109 Gamble JA, Creedy DK. Women's request for a cesarean section: a critique of the literature. *Birth.* 2000; **27**: 256–63.

110 Gamble JA, Creedy DK. Women's preference for a cesarean section: incidence and associated factors. *Birth.* 2001; **28**: 101–10.

111 Kingdon C, Baker L, Lavender T. Systematic review of nulliparous women's views of planned cesarean birth: the missing component in the debate about a term cephalic trial. *Birth.* 2006; **33**: 229–37.

112 McCourt C, Weaver J, Statham H, *et al.* Elective cesarean section and decision making: a critical review of the literature. *Birth.* 2007; **34**: 65–79.

113 Teijlingen ER, Hundley V, Rennie A-M, *et al.* Maternity satisfaction studies and their limitations: "What is, must still be best". *Birth.* 2003; **30**: 75–82.

114 Menacker F, Declercq E, Macdorman MF. Cesarean delivery: background, trends, and epidemiology. *Semin Perinatol.* 2006; **30**: 235–41.

115 Young D. "Cesarean delivery on maternal request": was the NIH conference based on a faulty premise? *Birth.* 2006; **33**: 171–4.

116 Thomas J, Paranjothy S. *National Sentinel Caesarean Section Audit Report.* London: RCOG Press; 2001.

117 South Community Birth Program. *The South Community Birth Program Final Report: 2003–6.* Vancouver, BC; 2006.

118 Walker R, Turnbull D, Wilkinson C. Increasing cesarean section rates: exploring the role of culture in an Australian community. *Birth.* 2004; **31**: 117–24.

119 Leitch CR, Walker JJ. The rise in caesarean section rate: the same indications but a lower threshold. *Br J Obstet Gynaecol.* 1998; **105**: 621–6.

120 Robson MS. Can we reduce the caesarean section rate? *Best Pract Res Clin Obstet Gynaecol.* 2001; **15**: 179–94.

121 Schindl M, Birner P, Reingrabner M, *et al.* Elective cesarean section vs. spontaneous delivery: a comparative study of birth experience. *Acta Obstet Gynecol Scand.* 2003; **82**: 834–40.

122 Hildingsson I, Radestad I, Rubertsson C, *et al.* Few women wish to be delivered by caesarean section. *BJOG.* 2002; **109**: 618–23.

123 Pang MW, Lee TS, Leung AK, *et al.* A longitudinal observational study of preference for elective caesarean section among nulliparous Hong Kong Chinese women. *BJOG: An International Journal of Obstetrics and Gynaecology.* 2007; **114**: 623–9.

124 Nerum H, Halvorsen L, Sorlie T, *et al.* Maternal request for cesarean section due to fear of birth: can it be changed through crisis-oriented counseling? *Birth.* 2006; **33**: 221–8.

125 Fogelson NS, Menard MK, Hulsey T, *et al.* Neonatal impact of elective repeat cesarean delivery at term: a comment on patient choice cesarean delivery. *Am J Obstet Gynecol.* 2005; **192**: 1433–6.

126 Hansen AK, Wisborg K, Uldbjerg N, *et al.* Elective caesarean section and respiratory morbidity in the term and near-term neonate. *Acta Obstet Gynecol Scand.* 2007; **86**: 389–94.

127 MacDorman MF, Declercq E, Menacker F, *et al.* Infant and neonatal mortality for primary cesarean and vaginal births to women with "No indicated risk," United States, 1998–2001 birth cohorts. *Birth.* 2006; **33**: 175–82.

128 Villar J, Carroli G, Zavaleta N, *et al.* Maternal and neonatal individual risks and benefits associated with caesarean delivery: multicentre prospective study. *BMJ.* 2007; **335**: 1025–9.

129 Tita ATN, Landon MB, Spong CY, *et al.* Timing of elective repeat cesarean delivery at term and neonatal outcomes. *N Engl J Med.* 2009; **360**: 111–20.

130 Bewley S, Cockburn J. Responding to fear of childbirth. *Lancet.* 2002; **359**: 2128–9.

131 Leeman LM, Plante LA. Patient-choice vaginal delivery? *Ann Fam Med.* 2006; **4**: 265–8.

132 Roberts RG, Deutchman M, King VJ, *et al.* Changing policies on vaginal birth after cesarean: impact on access. *Birth.* 2007; **34**: 316–22.

133 Guise J-M, McDonagh, M, Hashima J, *et al.* Vaginal births after cesarean (VBAC). *Evidence Report/Technology Assessment No. 71.* Rockville, MD: Agency for Healthcare Research and Quality; 2003.

134 Martin JA, Hamilton BE, Sutton PD, *et al.* Births: Final data for 2004. *Natl Vital Stat Rep.* 2006; **55**: 1–101.

135 Cahill AG, Stamilio DM, Odibo AO, *et al.* Is vaginal birth after cesarean (VBAC) or elective repeat cesarean safer in women with a prior vaginal delivery? *Am J Obstet Gynecol.* 2006; **195**: 1143–47.

136 Grobman WA, Gilbert S, Landon MB, *et al.* Outcomes of induction of labor after one prior cesarean. *Obstet Gynecol.* 2007; **109**: 262–9.

137 Waldman R, Mielcarski E. Vaginal delivery after cesarean section: is the risk acceptable? *J Midwifery Womens Health.* 2001; **46**: 272–3.

138 Hamilton B, Martin J, Ventura S. Births: preliminary data for 2007. *Natl Vital Stat Rep.* 2009; **57**(12): 1–23.

139 McCarthy FP, Rigg L, Cady L, *et al.* A new way of looking at caesarean section births. *Aust N Z J Obstet Gynaecol.* 2007; **47**: 316–20.

140 Shields SG, Ratcliffe SD, Fontaine P, *et al.* Dystocia in nulliparous women. *Am Fam Physician.* 2007; **75**: 1671–8.

141 MacArthur C, Winter HR, Bick DE, *et al.* Effects of redesigned community postnatal care

on women's health 4 months after birth: A cluster randomised controlled trial. *Lancet.* 2002; **359**: 378–85.

142 Morrell CJ, Spiby H, Stewart P, *et al.* Costs and effectiveness of community postnatal support workers: randomised controlled trial. *BMJ.* 2000; **321**: 593–8.

143 Ryan AS. The resurgence of breastfeeding in the United States. *Pediatrics.* 1997; **99**: e12.

144 Ryan AS, Rush D, Krieger FW, *et al.* Recent declines in breast-feeding in the United States, 1984 through 1989. *Pediatrics.* 1991; **88**: 719–27.

145 Center for Disease Control. Breastfeeding practices – results from the national immunization survey. 2007 [cited April 21, 2008]. Available from: www.cdc.gov/breastfeeding/data/NIS_data/data_2004.htm

146 Section on Breastfeeding. Breastfeeding and the use of human milk. *Pediatrics.* 2005; **115**: 496–506.

147 Witters-Green R. Increasing breastfeeding rates in working mothers. *Fam Syst Health.* 2003; **21**: 415.

148 Oliveira V. *WIC and Breastfeeding Rates.* Economic Research Service, United States Department of Agriculture; July 20, 2003.

149 Kent G. WIC's promotion of infant formula in the United States. *Int Breastfeed J.* 2006; **1**: 8.

150 Radmacher P, Massey C, Adamkin D. Hidden morbidity with "successful" early discharge. *J Perinatol.* 2002; **22**: 15–20.

151 Scrivens L, Summers AD. Home too soon? A comment on the early discharge of women from hospital after childbirth. *Aust J Midwifery.* 2001; **14**: 28–31.

152 Yanicki S, Hasselback P, Sandilands M, *et al.* The safety of Canadian early discharge guidelines. Effects of discharge timing on readmission in the first year post-discharge and exclusive breastfeeding to four months. *Can J Public Health.* 2002; **93**: 26–30.

153 Lock LR, Gibb HJ. The power of place. *Midwifery.* 2003; **19**: 132–9.

154 Emmanuel E, Creedy D, Fraser J. What mothers want: a postnatal survey. *Aust J Midwifery.* 2001; **14**: 16–20.

155 Oates MR, Cox JL, Neema S, *et al.* Postnatal depression across countries and cultures: a qualitative study. *Brit J Psychiatry Suppl.* 2004; **46**: S10–16.

156 Posmontier B, Horowitz JA. Postpartum practices and depression prevalences: technocentric and ethnokinship cultural perspectives. *J Transcult Nurs.* 2004; **15**: 34–43.

157 Rodrigues M, Patel V, Jaswal S, *et al.* Listening to mothers: qualitative studies on motherhood and depression from Goa, India. *Soc Sci Med.* 2003; **57**: 1797–1806.

158 Clark R, Tluczek A, Wenzel A. Psychotherapy for postpartum depression: a preliminary report. *Am J Orthopsychiatry.* 2003; **73**: 441–54.

159 Chaudron LH, Kitzman HJ, Peifer KL, *et al.* Self-recognition of and provider response to maternal depressive symptoms in low-income Hispanic women. *J Women Health (Larchmt).* 2005; **14**: 331–8.

160 Edhborg M, Friberg M, Lundh W, *et al.* "Struggling with life:" narratives from women with signs of postpartum depression. *Scand J Public Health.* 2005; **33**: 261–7.

161 Ussher JM. Depression in the postnatal period: a normal response to motherhood. In: Stewart M, editor. *Pregnancy, Birth and Maternity Care: feminist perspectives.* Edinburgh: Elsevier; 2004. pp. 105–20.

162 Downie J, Wynaden D, McGowan S, *et al.* Using the Edinburgh postnatal depression scale to achieve best practice standards. *Nurs Health Sci.* 2003; **5**: 283–7.

163 Templeton L, Velleman R, Persaud A, *et al.* The experiences of postnatal depression in

women from black and minority ethnic communities in Wiltshire, UK. *Ethn Health.* 2003; **8**: 207–21.

164 Chisholm D, Conroy S, Glangeaud-Freudenthal N, *et al.* Health services research into postnatal depression: results from a preliminary cross-cultural study. *Brit J Psychiatry Suppl.* 2004; **46**: S45–52.

165 Einarson A, Koren G. Prescribing antidepressants to pregnant women: what is a family physician to do? *Can Fam Physician.* 2007; **53**: 1412–14, 23–5.

166 Chambers CD, Hernandez-Diaz S, Van Marter LJ, *et al.* Selective serotonin-reuptake inhibitors and risk of persistent pulmonary hypertension of the newborn. *N Engl J Med.* 2006; **354**: 579–87.

167 FDA. FDA public health advisory: Paroxetine. 2005 [cited December 8, 2005]. Available from: www.fda.gov/cder/drug/advisory/paroxetine200512.htm

168 Levinson-Castiel R, Merlob P, Linder N, *et al.* Neonatal abstinence syndrome after in utero exposure to selective serotonin reuptake inhibitors in term infants. *Arch Pediatr Adolesc Med.* 2006; **160**: 173–6.

169 Moses-Kolko EL, Bogen D, Perel J, *et al.* Neonatal signs after late in utero exposure to serotonin reuptake inhibitors: literature review and implications for clinical applications. *JAMA.* 2005; **293**: 2372–83.

170 Eberhard-Gran M, Eskild A, Opjordsmoen S. Use of psychotropic medications in treating mood disorders during lactation: practical recommendations. *CNS Drugs.* 2006; **20**: 187–98.

171 Weissman AM, Levy BT, Hartz AJ, *et al.* Pooled analysis of antidepressant levels in lactating mothers, breast milk, and nursing infants. *Am J Psychiatry.* 2004; **161**: 1066–78.

172 Bonari L, Bennett H, Einarson A, *et al.* Risks of untreated depression during pregnancy. *Can Fam Physician.* 2004; **50**: 37–9.

173 Mian AI. Depression in pregnancy and the postpartum period: balancing adverse effects of untreated illness with treatment risks. *J Psychiatr Pract.* 2005; **11**: 389–96.

174 Dennis CL. Treatment of postpartum depression, part 2: a critical review of nonbiological interventions. *J Clin Psychiatry.* 2004; **65**: 1252–65.

175 Dennis CL, Stewart DE. Treatment of postpartum depression, part 1: a critical review of biological interventions. *J Clin Psychiatry.* 2004; **65**: 1242–51.

176 Spinelli MG, Endicott J. Controlled clinical trial of interpersonal psychotherapy versus parenting education program for depressed pregnant women. *Am J Psychiatry.* 2003; **160**: 555–62.

177 Thoppil J, Riutcel TL, Nalesnik SW. Early intervention for perinatal depression. *Am J Obstet Gynecol.* 2005; **192**: 1446–8.

178 Grown C, Gupta GR, Pande R. Taking action to improve women's health through gender equality and women's empowerment. *Lancet.* 2005; **365**: 541–3.

179 Ronsmans C, Graham WJ. Maternal mortality: who, when, where, and why. *Lancet.* 2006; **368**: 1189–1200.

180 Campbell O, Foster L. A brief history of safe motherhood. 2007 [cited January 24, 2009]. Available from: www.maternal-mortality-measurement.org/MMMResource_Background_History.html

181 Freedman LP, Waldman RJ, de Pinho H, *et al.* Transforming health systems to improve the lives of women and children. *Lancet.* 2005; **365**: 997–1000.

182 Sachs JD, McArthur JW. The Millennium Project: a plan for meeting the Millennium Development Goals. *Lancet.* 2005; **365**: 347.

183 Department of Reproductive Health and Research. Proportion of births attended by a skilled health worker: 2008 updates. 2008 [cited January 23, 2009]. Available from: www.who.int/reproductive-health/global_monitoring/skilled_attendant_at_birth2008.pdf

184 Rosenfield A, Min CJ, Freedman LP. Making motherhood safe in developing countries. *New Eng J Med.* 2007; **356**: 1395–7.

185 Glasier A, Gulmezoglu AM, Schmid GP, *et al.* Sexual and reproductive health: a matter of life and death. *Lancet.* 2006; **368**: 1595–1607.

186 Glasier A, Gulmezoglu AM. Putting sexual and reproductive health on the agenda. *Lancet.* 2006; **368**: 1550–1.

187 Thaddeus S, Maine D. Too far to walk: maternal mortality in context. *Soc Sci Med.* 1994; **38**: 1091–1110.

188 JHPIEGO. *Monitoring Birth Preparedness and Complication Readiness.* Baltimore, MD: JHPIEGO; 2004.

189 Villar J, Ba'aqeel H, Piaggio G, *et al.* WHO antenatal care randomised trial for the evaluation of a new model of routine antenatal care. *Lancet.* 2001; **357**: 1551–64.

190 Chalmers I, Enkin M, Keirse M, eds. *Effective care in pregnancy and childbirth, volume I: Pregnancy; Volume II: Childbirth.* New York: Oxford University Press; 1989.

191 Eclampsia Trial Collaborative Group. Which anticonvulsant for women with eclampsia? Evidence from the Collaborative Eclampsia Trial. *Lancet.* 1995; **345**: 1455.

192 Anonymous. Do women with pre-eclampsia, and their babies, benefit from magnesium sulphate? The Magpie trial: a randomised placebo-controlled trial. *Lancet.* 2002; **359**: 1877.

193 Harrison RF, Brennan M, North PM, *et al.* Is routine episiotomy necessary? *Br Med J (Clin Res Ed).* 1984; **288**: 1971–5.

194 Sleep J, Grant A, Garcia J, *et al.* West Berkshire perineal management trial. *Br Med J (Clin Res Ed).* 1984; **289**: 587–90.

195 Argentine Episiotomy Trial Collaborative Group. Routine vs selective episiotomy: a randomised controlled trial. *Lancet.* 1993; **342**: 1517–18.

196 Klein MC, Gauthier RJ, Jorgensen SH, *et al.* Does episiotomy prevent perineal trauma and pelvic floor relaxation? *Online J Curr Clin Trials.* 1992; Doc No 10.

197 Klein MC, Kaczorowski J, Robbins JM, *et al.* Physicians' beliefs and behaviour during a randomized controlled trial of episiotomy: consequences for women in their care. *CMAJ.* 1995; **153**: 769–79.

198 Klein MC. Use of episiotomy in the United States. *Birth.* 2002; **29**: 74–6.

199 Kozak LJ, Weeks JD. U.S. Trends in obstetric procedures, 1990–2000. *Birth.* 2002; **29**: 157–61.

200 Weeks JD, Kozak LJ. Trends in the use of episiotomy in the United States: 1980–98. *Birth.* 2001; **28**: 152–60.

201 ACOG. ACOG Practice Bulletin No. 71. Episiotomy. Clinical management guidelines for obstetrician-gynecologists. *Obstet Gynecol.* 2006; **107**: 957–62.

202 Camann W. Pain relief during labor. *N Engl J Med.* 2005; **352**: 718–20.

203 ACOG. ACOG Committee Opinion No. 295: Pain relief during labor. *Obstet Gynecol.* 2004; **104**: 213.

204 Menacker F, Martin J. *Expanded Health Data from the New Birth Certificate, 2005. Nat Vit Stat Rep.* 2008; **56**(13): 1–24.

205 National Health Services. NHS maternity statistics, England: 2006–7. 2008 [cited January

16, 2009]. Available from: www.ic.nhs.uk/statistics-and-data-collections/hospital-care/maternity/nhs-maternity-statistics-england:-2006-2007

206 Gagnon AJ, Waghorn K. Supportive care by maternity nurses: a work sampling study in an intrapartum unit. *Birth*. 1996; **23**: 1–6.

207 Gale J, Fothergill-Bourbonnais F, Chamberlain M. Measuring nursing support during childbirth. *MCN: Am J Matern Child Nurs*. 2001; **26**: 264–71.

208 Goldberg L. Rethinking the birthing body: Cartesian dualism and perinatal nursing. *J Adv Nurs*. 2002; **37**: 446–51.

209 Graham ID, Logan J, Davies B, *et al*. Changing the use of electronic fetal monitoring and labor support: a case study of barriers and facilitators. *Birth*. 2004; **31**: 293–301.

210 Sleutel M, Schultz S, Wyble K. Nurses' views of factors that help and hinder their intrapartum care. *J Obstet Gynecol Neonatal Nurs*. 2007; **36**: 203–11.

211 Miltner RS. Identifying labor support actions of intrapartum nurses. *J Obstet Gynecol Neonatal Nurs*. 2000; **29**: 491–9.

212 Klein MC. Does epidural analgesia increase rate of cesarean section? *Can Fam Physician*. 2006; **52**: 419–21, 26–8.

213 Leeman L, Fontaine P, King V, Klein MC, Ratcliffe S. The nature and management of labor pain: part II. Pharmacologic pain relief. *Am Fam Physician* 2003; **68**: 1115–20.

214 Anim-Somuah M, Smyth R, Howell C. Epidural versus non-epidural or no analgesia in labour. *Cochrane Database Syst Rev* 2005: CD000331.

215 Morton SC, Williams MS, Keeler EB, *et al*. Effect of epidural analgesia for labor on the cesarean delivery rate. *Obstet Gynecol*. 1994; **83**: 1045–52.

216 Thorp JA, Hu DH, Albin RM, *et al*. The effect of intrapartum epidural analgesia on nulliparous labor: a randomized, controlled, prospective trial. *Am J Obstet Gynecol*. 1993; **169**: 851–8.

217 Janssen PA, Klein MC, Soolsma JH. Differences in institutional cesarean delivery rates: the role of pain management. *J Fam Pract*. 2001; **50**: 217–23.

218 Klein MC, Grzybowski S, Harris S, *et al*. Epidural analgesia use as a marker for physician approach to birth: implications for maternal and newborn outcomes. *Birth*. 2001; **28**: 243–8.

219 Wong CA, Scavone BM, Peaceman AM, *et al*. The risk of cesarean delivery with neuraxial analgesia given early versus late in labor. *N Engl J Med*. 2005; **352**: 655–65.

220 Bloom SL, McIntire DD, Kelly MA, *et al*. Lack of effect of walking on labor and delivery. *N Engl J Med*. 1998; **339**: 76–9.

221 Frigoletto FD, Jr., Lieberman E, Lang JM, *et al*. A clinical trial of active management of labor. *N Engl J Med*. 1995; **333**: 745–50.

222 O'Driscoll K, Meagher D, Robson M. *Active Management of Labour: the Dublin experience*. 4th ed. Edinburgh; New York: Mosby; 2003.

223 Klein MC. Walking in labor. *J Fam Pract*. 1999; **48**: 229.

224 Hannah ME, Hannah WJ, Hellmann J, *et al*. Induction of labor as compared with serial antenatal monitoring in post-term pregnancy. A randomized controlled trial. The Canadian multicenter post-term pregnancy trial group. *N Engl J Med*. 1992; **326**: 1587–92.

225 ACOG Committee on Practice Bulletins – Obstetrics. ACOG Practice Bulletin No. 55: Management of postterm pregnancy. *Obstet Gynecol*. 2004; **104**: 639–46.

226 Gulmezoglu AM, Crowther CA, Middleton P. Induction of labour for improving birth outcomes for women at or beyond term. *Cochrane Database Syst Rev*. 2006: CD004945.

227 Heimstad R, Skogvoll E, Mattsson LA, *et al*. Induction of labor or serial antenatal fetal

monitoring in postterm pregnancy: a randomized controlled trial. *Obstet Gynecol.* 2007; **109**: 609–17.

228 Hannah ME, Hannah WJ, Hewson SA, *et al.* Planned caesarean section versus planned vaginal birth for breech presentation at term: a randomised multicentre trial. Term breech trial collaborative group. *Lancet.* 2000; **356**: 1375–83.

229 Kotaska A. Inappropriate use of randomised trials to evaluate complex phenomena: case study of vaginal breech delivery. *BMJ.* 2004; **329**: 1039–42.

230 Hannah ME, Whyte H, Hannah WJ, *et al.* Maternal outcomes at 2 years after planned cesarean section versus planned vaginal birth for breech presentation at term: the international randomized term breech trial. *Am J Obstet Gynecol.* 2004; **191**: 917–27.

PART TWO

Understanding the Experience of Pregnancy and Childbirth

CHAPTER 1

The Experience of Normal Pregnancy: an Overview

Stacy Potts and Sara G. Shields

The patient-centered clinical method, as described by Stewart et al.,[1] asks us first to explore both the disease and the illness experience. Disease is a theoretical construct, a diagnosis based on medicine's attempt to categorize, explain, and generalize about objective physiologic and anatomic dysfunction. Illness is the unique personal experience of feeling sick, sometimes but not always indicating a disease process in an individual. Woman-centered care views normal pregnancy not as a disease state but rather as a normal life process. However, some women experience part or much of pregnancy as an illness. While pregnancy follows similar physiologic courses among women, each woman has her own pregnancy experiences, and different pregnancies for the same woman will be different. A woman-centered provider identifies this uniqueness, seeks to understand the woman's personal experience of pregnancy, and sees the woman, not just her medical risks. The goal of woman-centered care is a balance of attention to both the common physiologic changes of pregnancy and the subjective experiences of the individual pregnant woman, as well as appropriate clinical care for problems if and when they arise.

Modern obstetric care views pregnancy as a medical event at best, a medical crisis at worst. With the risks of pregnancy and childbirth at the forefront, clinicians expect to focus on preventing complications. Contemporary prenatal care, which is doctor-centered, protocol-centered, and risk-centered rather than woman-centered, looks for the worst that can happen and overlooks the preparation for the journey of a normal pregnancy and childbirth. This disease focus interferes with the freedom of a woman (and those who care for her) to experience pregnancy and childbirth in her own unique way, as a normal life event. The focus on pathology and not on the woman herself may explain some aspects of patient dissatisfaction with some obstetrical providers.

Despite the risk-centered approach of modern obstetrics, the World Health Organization (WHO) has designated fostering of a woman's experience of pregnancy and birth as a positive life experience to be one of the primary aims of antenatal care. The WHO Europe Health Evidence Network recognizes four main and equal goals of antenatal care (*see* Box 2.1).[2] Woman-centered maternity care, through eliciting the woman's experience during the processes of achieving the other goals, encompasses all the WHO aims.

BOX 2.1 **World Health Organization Primary Aims of Antenatal Care (adapted from Banta, 2003)[2]**

- Detect early factors that might heighten the perinatal risk of both individual pregnancies and members of vulnerable groups.
- Intervene to improve outcomes.
- Educate all who provide or receive care
- Help make pregnancy and birth a positive life experience.

Mishler[3] explores the disease and illness dichotomy through two contrasting voices: the voice of medicine and the voice of the lifeworld. Physicians in their verbal and non-verbal dominance of the traditional medical interview often ignore, deflect, or devalue the patient's lifeworld voice in order to remain in control of the interview.[3] This tendency to ignore the life contexts of patients is especially significant when layered on top of the tendency for a woman's voice of life experience to be devalued or ignored in traditional male-dominated arenas such as medicine. Furthermore, the tendency of patients as well to devalue their own voice[4] exacerbates this dominance of the voice of medicine over the voice of the lifeworld. Actively listening for and inquiring about the voice of the lifeworld offers woman-centered providers an opportunity to explore how the pregnancy experience affects the woman in her entire context. Through this window into the pregnant woman's lifeworld, the woman-centered provider stays open to unexpected or surprising responses, remaining respectful and engendering trust while seeking insight and reflecting on the meaning of the woman's experience.[5]

Medical inquiry and lifeworld inquiry are different. Essential "medical" questions include: "When was your last menstrual period? Were you using any birth control at the time of conception? Are you having any cramping or bleeding?" Typical "lifeworld" questions might include: "What are you most concerned about? How has the pregnancy changed your life? Have you found any limitations affecting you or your relationships? Are there particular ways that you think I can help you?" Throughout the pregnancy, such "lifeworld" questions enable the providers to see beyond the physical dimensions of the woman's pregnancy and come closer to understanding all dimensions of her pregnancy experience.

Thus, woman-centered care in normal pregnancy involves a shift of focus from clinician to woman, from risk-based assessment to self-discovered health resources, from a language of disease to one of health.[6,7] The woman-centered clinician expects, encourages, and listens for the woman's self-assessment of her situation; after hearing this, the clinician supports the woman in utilizing her self-identified strengths as resources for answers. A carefully crafted key question[6,7] permits the woman-centered maternity provider to reframe his or her approach to look for the woman's specific strengths and resources as tools in her perinatal care. Examples of such questions might be, "What have you tried so far that helps you with the nausea (back pain, heartburn, etc.)?" "What are you thinking might be the cause of this symptom that has been bothering you?" "How will you handle the changes that a baby will bring?" There is no one question for every woman. Clinicians can use individualized versions of such questions to structure the clinical interview but must develop the particular questions within the context of the woman's own situation.

Pregnant women articulate their hopes that their prenatal care will manifest a confident relationship, competent protection, and continuous participation.[8] Woman-centered clinicians strengthen this bond and relationship through investigation of the four dimensions of patient-centered care that Stewart *et al.*[1] describe: feelings, ideas, function, and expectations. In the journey of each of her pregnancies, a woman will experience the described dimensions uniquely, and each dimension changes during the dynamic course of pregnancy.

CHAPTER 2

Pregnancy Diagnosis

Sara G. Shields

Kerry was a 23-year-old preschool teacher who had just missed her period. She and her husband Ron, 24, a contractor, had been eagerly awaiting their first pregnancy, having postponed it until Ron finished building their first house. Kerry was the oldest of four children – she had always entertained her younger sisters and brother and often looked after the neighborhood children, as well. No one was surprised when she majored in early childhood education and took a job right away after college as a preschool teacher. Kerry and Ron lived in the same community near both sets of parents who were all awaiting their first grandchild. Kerry was excited when her period was late. She bought a home pregnancy test and waited until she and Ron were both home to do the test. They were ecstatic when it came out positive. He picked her up and swung her around. They could hardly wait to phone their parents, but decided to wait until they had a chance to celebrate alone by going out to dinner. Kerry carefully avoided any alcohol because now she knew she was pregnant. (*See* full vignette in Appendix.)

Pat, age 17, was in her last year of high school; her mother had died earlier that year after a long battle with cancer. Pat's relationship with her boyfriend deteriorated over the course of her mother's illness and during her mourning; they broke up just before graduation. Pat's period had always been irregular, so she did not think much about its delay later that month. When she could not keep food or drink down all one hot summer weekend, even after trying some of the anti-nausea medicine still in the house from her mother's chemotherapy, she called her family doctor's office where the on-call doctor recommended remedies for gastroenteritis and an appointment the next day if she had not improved. At that appointment Pat was stunned when the doctor suggested a pregnancy test and then burst into tears when the results came back confirming that she was indeed pregnant. (*See* full vignette in Appendix.)

Melissa (whom we met in Part One) and her husband, Kirk, also an engineer, had been trying to get pregnant for the last eight months. They had been having scheduled intercourse on the thirteenth and fifteenth days of her regular cycle without success. Melissa read online about infertility and lifestyle issues and had been careful to cut down on caffeine and alcohol. She was only a bit overweight. She did not smoke and had always tried to eat a healthy diet. . . . One month her period did not come, and both she and Kirk hoped that this meant she was pregnant, but the home pregnancy test they used after five weeks was negative. Still hoping at six weeks, they visited her doctor, Larisa Foster, and requested the most sensitive test available but again had their dreams dashed when it, too, was negative. The next day Melissa's period started.

FEELINGS

The moment when a woman learns she is pregnant is a watershed moment for most women, even when the pregnancy is planned. Modern technology enables women to know they are pregnant through home pregnancy tests long before any medical appointment. Nevertheless, many women with delayed or missed periods suspect they are pregnant well before taking a test either at home or in a medical setting. Modern medical care assumes that the "diagnosis" with chemical "testing" is essential and necessary to "prove" pregnancy, but such reliance can disempower a woman and keep her from understanding her body's physiology and function. For Kerry and Melissa, home testing is more woman-centered than laboratory testing; the simplicity of the kits and the privacy of the process empower each woman at this crucial moment. For women with fewer resources or in less technically oriented societies, the self-diagnosis of pregnancy will still rest on subjective symptoms: the nausea, missed period, breast tingling and sensitivity, and often overwhelming fatigue. The woman-centered provider teaches each woman to attend to such individual, internal signals and thus honor her body's messages.

Knowing that a woman is already likely to have an idea about the result, before reporting pregnancy test results to a woman, a woman-centered provider asks what the woman thinks and how she will feel about the results. Indeed, given the significance of the life change involved in the news of a new pregnancy, practitioners of woman-centered care need to rethink not only how to give the results but also how to suggest a pregnancy test in the first place. These results, whether positive or negative, are not the same as discussing an abnormal potassium level. Some women, like Kerry or Melissa who are trying to become pregnant, intentionally seek either home or clinic testing for confirmation. For others like Pat with unintended, accidental pregnancies, the provider – as part of the clinical evaluation of a seemingly unrelated problem – must find a way to put into words the real possibility of pregnancy.

The woman-centered clinician is open to hearing about the whole range of human emotions that may arise with pregnancy diagnosis. For a woman like Melissa, negative results disappoint and distress, releasing a multitude of emotions about her ability to become pregnant or to fulfill long-held dreams and expectations about motherhood. Positive results for Kerry similarly unleash multiple and potentially conflicting emotions – excitement, joy, anticipation, along with fear and anxiety about what comes next. For Pat, for whom even doing a pregnancy test is shocking, positive results upset and overwhelm her. Because of this wide range of possible responses to any pregnancy test result, a woman-centered provider explores these feelings at the moment of requesting a pregnancy test: "So one of the possibilities is that you are pregnant. I suggest that we have you do a pregnancy test. What do you think about that?" The clinician follows up with, "How will you feel if the result shows that you are pregnant?" or ". . . if the result shows that you are *not* pregnant?" depending on the woman's mindset.

In addition to inquiring about a woman's own feelings about this news of pregnancy, a woman-centered clinician needs to know something about her plans to share news with others in her life. Some of the most important moments in a woman's experience of pregnancy occur with this sharing. Regardless of her own feelings or plans about pregnancy, the woman may struggle with telling her family or friends, particularly with an unplanned or unexpected pregnancy, or if she is a single woman or a teenager. Sharing news about an unexpected pregnancy forces a teenager to reveal that she has been sexually active, something she may have hidden until now from her parents or other family. News of a pregnancy can come at an unexpected time for family members. Even when a woman welcomes a pregnancy, others in her life may have had different plans for her or for their own role. A pregnancy represents a lifelong commitment to a new life, not only for the individual, but also for the entire family. The reaction to the news by the woman's partner and other significant support systems may strongly affect the woman and her own feelings toward the pregnancy. A woman-centered provider can discover much of the context of her feelings by asking the newly pregnant woman how she will tell others and whom she will tell first.

> Pat's family doctor, knowing about the recent death of her mother, touched her hand gently as she reacted to the pregnancy test results. "Pat, I know this is a tough time for you, and this is unexpected news."
>
> As Pat began to suppress her tears, she blurted out, "I can't tell my father about this. He would be so devastated."
>
> The doctor responded, "Is there someone in your life right now who might be able to help you think through this? When you leave here, who do you think you'll be able to call to talk this over with?"
>
> "I guess I could tell my aunt. She got pregnant in college. She could help me without my father having to know."

IDEAS

A woman's ideas about pregnancy depend greatly on her personal situation, family context and family birth stories, and occupational and cultural location. A pregnancy diagnosis for 17-year-old Pat is a personal crisis coming after her mother's death, an unexpected, almost unthinkable disaster. She cannot imagine it. Pregnancy for Kerry is the fulfillment of her vision of herself as a woman, of her marriage and of her role in her extended family. The meaning of pregnancy for Melissa is as yet unclear, but not getting pregnant is clearly a failure to her, a process in her life that she is unable to manage through hard work and perseverance. Planned or unexpected, accident or fulfillment, interruption or unfolding, the pregnancy carries implicit and explicit meanings for every woman. Inquiring about what a pregnancy would mean to a woman before having the answer to the pregnancy test enables the provider to prepare for her responses afterwards.

FUNCTION

A woman's functioning in her life may not appear to change immediately upon pregnancy diagnosis. However, for most women, regardless of how the pregnancy proceeds, these early weeks after diagnosis involve suddenly increased contact with the health system, necessitating juggling of work and home needs and schedules. For women such as Pat who are considering pregnancy termination options, finding privacy to schedule appointments may be difficult. Women's thinking about their function in the world may change immediately upon pregnancy diagnosis; for example, even before her first prenatal visit, Kerry chooses to avoid alcohol right away, listening to the messages women receive everywhere about avoiding risky behaviors. Women with jobs that involve handling chemicals may worry from the start about potential exposure and options for job modification. Melissa, trying to get pregnant but having yet another negative pregnancy test, may wonder about reducing stressful job demands. A woman-centered provider telling a woman about the results of a pregnancy test can inquire briefly about such home and work contexts and make a plan for further education and discussion in subsequent care.

EXPECTATIONS

At the moment of pregnancy diagnosis, a newly pregnant woman's expectations of the healthcare system are influenced by her feelings, ideas, and function as described above. With a known patient, the woman-centered clinician may already have some sense of how this pregnancy fits into this woman's life cycle and family system. With new patients a full exploration may not be practical or realistic in a brief test-oriented visit. However, the clinician can ask about the woman's initial expectations around communication with the system and providers simply in preparing for the moment of reporting the test results: "How do you want me to tell you the results – do you want to wait here until we know for sure, or do you want me to call you later?" Even these small choices show the woman that the provider believes in putting control into her hands. Once the woman knows the results, the next steps of woman-centered care include knowing enough about the woman's feelings about pregnancy to be prepared to meet her expectations for an appropriate referral – for prenatal care or for pregnancy termination, if that is the woman's choice, or for further pregnancy counseling if she is unsure at the time of the positive test of which direction she wants to take. (*See* Part Five for further discussion of a woman-centered approach to options counseling.)

Kerry's, Pat's, and Melissa's stories illustrate a few examples of the vast range of complex feelings, ideas, function and expectations that pregnancy test results can evoke. Woman-centered care allows time and place for this experience, and understands that a negative pregnancy test is more than an opportunity for pre-conception care, but rather a time to reflect on the full meaning of being pregnant or not being pregnant for this woman at this moment in her life, and to empower women even in seemingly small ways.

CHAPTER 3

Early Pregnancy

Stacy Potts and Sara G. Shields

As happy as she was to be pregnant, Kerry at her first prenatal visit with Larisa looked and felt tired and wan. Kerry reported multiple episodes of vomiting for the last week and was only holding down small amounts of liquids. She had expected to feel nauseated but was unprepared for the vomiting. She also felt fatigued, arriving home after work feeling she needed to go to bed right away. She had tried to go to work, but had had to leave the classroom several times to vomit. Although she had not wanted to take any medications during her pregnancy, she was now willing to "do anything" not to feel so sick. Usually, Kerry did most of the cooking as she got home earlier than Ron, but this week, she was too nauseated and tired, so Ron stepped in to do the cooking. Kerry left the office visit with multiple suggestions: vitamin B6, ginger capsules, ginger ale, nausea bands, morning crackers, and a word of caution to call if she was not urinating in normal amounts or if she felt weak and dehydrated.

FEELINGS

Pregnancy is a time of lost control. A woman who has previously been in charge of her life may become very anxious when she realizes she has no control over what might happen. This feeling can surface as early as the first trimester when the common physical symptoms of early pregnancy can overwhelm women who have previously felt physically well. Even for women with planned, wanted pregnancies who feel joyful, hopeful, or fulfilled by finally being pregnant, emotions can vacillate widely in the first trimester exacerbated by the physical changes and emotional power of her new state on her and on those close to her. Along with happiness and wonder may come fear of complications or life role changes, or annoyance at changing bodily symptoms such as urinary frequency or nausea. Women who feel unwell during the first trimester may fear that the entire pregnancy will be overwhelmingly difficult, or may recognize such symptoms as part of the expected discomforts of pregnancy rather than as an illness experience.[9] In contrast, women who do not feel the typical first trimester nausea or fatigue may worry that something might be wrong with the pregnancy, particularly if they have had previous complications.

This sense of lack of control can be even more important to address for women continuing their pregnancies with initially unintended pregnancies or without partner or family support. As a woman comes to terms with the ramifications of pregnancy for her life, she may experience complex feelings. These can include guilt about getting pregnant or about considering termination, or resignation and disempowerment about something that feels "out of control" for her. Single women in a culture that emphasizes being part of a couple during pregnancy may feel especially isolated and alone in the early weeks as they come to terms with multiple absences and losses – of partner support, of family support, of their prior expectations of their life's trajectory.[10]

The woman-centered clinician makes no assumptions about positive or negative emotions. Instead, the clinician needs to be open and attuned to the whole range of negative emotions for women struggling with single motherhood or with unplanned pregnancies. The clinician explores these feelings non-judgmentally with active listening skills, using open-ended comments such as "Some women who get pregnant have a lot of different feelings in the early weeks. How has this time been for you?" These feelings evolve over the course of the pregnancy, potentially exacerbating the normal fears and anxieties of all women as labor and parenthood approach. (*See* later discussion about the third trimester.) Woman-centered care thus continues this conversation throughout pregnancy.

One moment when clinicians can ascertain much about a woman's feelings and ideas in the first trimester comes when she hears the fetal heartbeat for the first time. This external technical validation of the reality of the pregnancy usually occurs before she has any perception of fetal movement; the moment may be definitive for the woman in acknowledging the reality of the pregnancy. Cognizant of the wide array of possible emotions, particularly for women with unintended pregnancies, the woman-centered clinician watches the woman's face for non-verbal cues as she hears the heartbeat. The clinician's role is to remain silent but attentive, allowing the moment to belong to the woman while learning from her cues.

Women with a history of infertility, previous miscarriages, or other complications may have particular need for reassurance in these early weeks. However, at times the very tests needed for reassurance will raise anxiety from previous frightening experiences. A clinician may be surprised that a woman asks for an ultrasound for reassurance but then cancels or misses the appointment. Her fear of getting bad news may overwhelm her desire for reassurance.

IDEAS

A woman-centered discussion of a woman's ideas about the first trimester follows Bondas' three central themes of a woman's experience of pregnancy: the wish for a healthy baby, the sense of an altered "mode of being," and the wish for family connection.[9] The early months of pregnancy force a woman into a heightened focus on both her own health and its effects on the baby's health. Even at these early visits, women are likely to have heard many messages about healthy pregnancy behaviors, from nutrition to exposures to suggestions for alleviating the common symptoms of early pregnancy. The woman-centered clinician inquires, "Tell me a bit about your diet now, and what changes you have made because you are pregnant. How have you learned about these changes so far?" While such messages reflect that pregnancy makes women no longer take their health for granted, part of the clinician's task in early pregnancy is to educate and provide knowledge and information in an individualized way that avoids overwhelming the woman with anxiety-generating information and empowers her to make healthy choices.[9]

Much of a pregnant woman's information is likely to come from books, the media, or her family and friends.[11] This barrage of health messages often proscribes very authoritatively certain behaviors, intakes, or exposures in ways that neglect to individualize the woman's context or capacity to follow these demands. The woman-centered provider can help contextualize potential risks and reframe them in self-empowering ways. For example, when Kerry worries about her potential exposure to childhood illnesses as a teacher, Larisa responds, "You are already taking the first steps that all new parents need to, by educating yourself proactively about the health issues that you and your baby might face. What do you know about the risks for pregnant preschool teachers?" Larisa then corrects any misinformation while making a plan for preventive measures or further evaluation if necessary. She alters the message from "You must eat this or take this or do this" to "Let's talk about how you can fit these changes better into your life now and for the rest of the pregnancy, without blaming yourself if one day you eat something or take something you have been told not to."

Without oversimplifying or ignoring risky behavior, woman-centered clinicians seek any opportunity to build on positive choices that women have made as examples of their inner strengths and resources. Sometimes a positive action can be as basic as keeping an appointment after several missed ones. Rather than accusing or blaming the woman even with subtle non-verbal cues, the woman-centered clinician says, "I'm really glad you made it to this appointment today, so that we have time to talk more about other ways you can have the healthiest pregnancy and child possible."

First-trimester symptoms and early bodily changes can cause much discomfort to women, with a variety of reactions. Women's bodies begin to change shape and function very early in pregnancy, for example with urinary frequency or breast tenderness. Without underestimating or diminishing how exhausted and nauseated women can feel in these early weeks, the woman-centered clinician listens actively to how women describe their symptoms and tries empathetically to reframe the illness symptoms as a sign of a healthy pregnancy. Kerry may wonder, "Are my symptoms normal? Why am I so tired? Do I feel this sick because my mother had awful morning sickness throughout pregnancy? Will my pregnancy be just like hers?" Larisa explores such ideas simply by asking, "What do you know or what have you heard about nausea in pregnancy? How have other people suggested that you handle your symptoms?" Women with difficult physical symptoms at the beginning of an unwanted pregnancy may think that such symptoms are retribution for their accidental pregnancy. One question to get at this idea is, "Some women struggling with such tough symptoms wonder 'why me?' and think of different causes for their symptoms. It's helpful for me to know what you think about why you feel this way."

With these sorts of experiences, women in the first trimester begin to take on the new life role or identity of motherhood. This new role (or expanded role, in the case of multiparous women) can have multiple different meanings. Depending on her life stage, a newly pregnant woman will consider a variety of ideas about how she will be different as a woman because of this pregnancy and this child. For some women, having to attend to healthy behaviors and symptoms more closely because of the baby challenges their independence and sense of control. The woman-centered clinician reframes this as part of a life stage and helps the woman identify ways to ask for help without feeling demeaned or disempowered (for example, Kerry and Ron change who is doing the cooking).

> Rosa was a 22-year-old undocumented Guatemalan immigrant with a third-grade education who lived with her husband José and several other friends and family in a small apartment. She had her first baby at home with a midwife in her village when she was 16 and left that child in her native country with his father's family to come to the United States with José. She worked on an assembly line at a plastics company.
>
> During her first prenatal visit, Dr. Jonathan Rosen took a brief family history and learned that Rosa's mother had been ill. Watching Rosa's quiet, respectful demeanor answering his questions, he paused and asked through the interpreter, "How is that for you being here and thinking about your mother and your new child?" Rosa looked very sad as she acknowledged how torn she felt but knew that she would put herself and her fetus at risk if she went home and then tried to make the arduous and uncertain migration journey over again. (*See* full vignette in Appendix.)

Understanding the woman's relationship with her own mother or other maternal figures in her life is also an important part of a woman-centered exploration of these meanings. A woman often feels a renewed connection with her mother and even a need for her approval during pregnancy.[9] Having a positive connection with her mother predicts positive parenting adjustment for a pregnant woman.[12] Women want their partners and families to share the experience of pregnancy and share their feelings for the developing child.[9] However, for women whose mothers are deceased or whose mothers are not supportive of an unexpected pregnancy, the woman-centered clinician needs to be extra sensitive to the feelings and ideas about motherhood that such loss or disconnection bring. Immigrant women such as Rosa who are very distant from their mothers and their homeland may feel particularly sad or lonely.

Part Three will address further how this new life stage fits into a pregnant woman's life cycle, the ways that her partner and her family will change with this new baby, and the impact of her cultural context upon these ideas.

FUNCTION

How a woman functions during early pregnancy reflects her unique situation and shares common themes with other pregnant women. Even in the first trimester, clinicians should consider a woman's ideas about her own functioning. Although most women expect to be healthy enough to work up until late pregnancy or when they go into labor, limitations in certain work activities may be necessary to maintain health and well-being for a woman during pregnancy. A woman defines herself in many functions daily – in jobs, household responsibilities, relationships, and lifestyle. Early pregnancy changes may affect all of these. For instance, the fatigue and nausea of the first trimester may affect early on how a woman feels about her functioning and ability to maintain her lifeworld unaltered.

> The following week Ron called Larisa's office saying that Kerry seemed more nauseated than ever, and he thought she might be dehydrated. Indeed Kerry had ketones in her urine when she got to the office, and readily accepted the offer of hospitalization for hydration and medication to try to control her nausea. Ron confided to Larisa while Kerry was at the lab that he wondered if he had done anything wrong to make Kerry so nauseated – that maybe she was really upset about something, although he did not know what. Later when Kerry was alone with Larisa, she revealed that she hated the nausea so much that if it were just up to her, she would just have an abortion. She also felt terribly guilty that she felt this way, since she and Ron really wanted a baby, and she knew that Ron was going to be a great father, but she was hating the process so much, she would like to "get rid of it." She hated herself, as well, for these feelings.
>
> After five days in the hospital, with intravenous hydration and metoclopramide, Kerry was finally able to tolerate some small frequent bland meals. Ron agreed to continue doing all the cooking until the nausea resolved, and Kerry took off a few weeks from work. Larisa assured Kerry and Ron that the nausea did not have emotional origins, and would usually improve with the treatment and with time. Over the course of the five days and nights, Kerry had a chance to talk frequently with the nurses on the prenatal floor who assured Kerry that such bad feelings about oneself and the baby were temporary reactions to the nausea and did not

have anything to do with how competent a mother she will be. Kerry hoped they were right, but was not convinced.

Kerry finally left the hospital able to keep down very small amounts of a very bland diet although she was still pretty nauseated.

Although Kerry has multiple supports, her early symptoms limit her functioning significantly. These difficulties bring up many unexpected feelings that influence her confidence in her ability to manage the challenges ahead. Sensitive nursing care helps Kerry explore these issues in the wake of her overwhelming nausea.

Rosa worked on an assembly line at a plastics company. When Rosa learned she was pregnant, her friend who worked there too told her that the fumes from the plastics might affect the baby. She asked her community advocate Lupe about this, who interpreted her question for Dr. Rosen.

Occupational exposure is another common concern about functioning in the first trimester of otherwise normal pregnancies. Maternity clinicians are often asked by both women and their employers about exposure risks in early pregnancy. Women in low-paying employment, such as housekeeping or hairdressing, with potential job-related chemical exposures, may have few if any resources for either sick time or job modification. Employers may struggle to balance their legal need to meet occupational hazard standards with their limited options for job reassignment. Women may be unfairly excluded from certain employment due to overzealous concern for potential reproductive hazards. Women in highly competitive environments or in specialized teams may worry about job discrimination because of their pregnancies or about colleagues' annoyance with their withdrawal from job responsibilities. A woman may be passed over for promotion because her supervisor thinks she will be less committed to work as she enters motherhood. The woman-centered clinician remains sensitive to these potential restrictions on a woman's function in early pregnancy.

EXPECTATIONS

Most women expect early prenatal care to evaluate the baby's health first and foremost, with evaluation of their own health a close second expectation.[13] Women expect a schedule of frequent antenatal visits, with variation depending on their birth experience, parity, or pregnancy intendedness. Women with prior miscarriages, stillbirths, or prior negative birth experiences, may anticipate more frequent visits, while women with unintended pregnancies or multiparous women without prior complications may want fewer visits.[13] Whatever the number of visits, women expect each visit to include the routines of listening to the fetal heartbeat and measuring the fundal height, anticipating that these are ways to assess for fetal well-being and that the provider will reassure that "everything is fine."[9] The woman-centered clinician's communication in the first trimester about the numerous blood tests and other evaluations can focus on confirming the woman's dignity, alleviating her suffering, and empowering her in her own context. While emphasizing education for empowered decision-making, the provider nonetheless remains sensitive to the possibility of overwhelming women with too much information; more and more knowledge may not always alleviate fears and may even exacerbate them.[9]

For many previously healthy women, particularly in their first pregnancies, the frequent and intimate contact with a health provider is a new experience. The woman-centered clinician acknowledges the importance of this relationship and explores with the woman how these appointments will fit around her other life demands, how she expects to hear about test results, how she contacts the provider between visits if needed. Some women expect and value continuity of care prenatally, so that early in pregnancy women may expect to see the same provider for most visits. Part Six will further discuss both the complexities of continuity and the clinical relationship between the pregnant woman and her provider.

> Ruth and Lewis were recent college graduates who lived in a commune and worked in community development programs. They were pregnant with their first baby and had decided to have a home birth with a midwife. Lewis' father was a psychiatrist in another state and his mother had been a midwife many years ago; Ruth's mother was a counselor. Ruth and Lewis did not want technological interventions in the pregnancy (use of Doppler, ultrasound or specific genetic screening such as quadruple screen), but they did want standard laboratory monitoring (blood and urine tests). They were aware of the small but real risk of an obstetrical emergency with the potential for a bad outcome for either mother or baby but preferred that risk to what they perceived as the risk of unnecessary technological intervention and early separation from the newborn in the hospital environment. (*See* full vignette in Appendix.)

Some low-risk women such as Ruth may opt for less medical testing, expecting that pregnancy and birth will be a healthy event for them and that being out of the hospital environment will allow them to have a more natural experience. Clarifying such expectations about testing and technology early in the pregnancy facilitates further discussion throughout pregnancy, whether or not any abnormalities arise.

Besides having specific expectations of the medical system during prenatal care, women may expect specific involvement from their partners or family. Their engagement can range from expectations about logistics such as attending prenatal visits or childbirth classes, or assisting with supplies for the baby or chores at home, to more emotionally significant expectations about shared anticipation of the new baby and the new life roles ahead for the whole family.

CHAPTER 4

Second Trimester

Stacy Potts and Sara G. Shields

FEELINGS

As the pregnancy continues, women often have a relative feeling of well-being, both emotionally and physically. For women who were struggling with an unplanned pregnancy, they may have grown in acceptance of the pregnancy. Poole suggests that women's perception of pregnancy as unwanted or mistimed changes between the first and third trimesters with about one-quarter of women who initially reported such feelings about pregnancy becoming more positive later in pregnancy.[14] For women who were excited about the pregnancy in the first trimester, further delight may characterize the second trimester with new joy and energy, feeling the baby's movements for the first time and starting to plan for the upcoming birth. For other women new fears may emerge about the baby, their ability to be a mother, or their own health. With the medical details of the first trimester mostly clarified, prenatal visits with a woman during her second trimester afford more time for exploration of a woman's feelings about the pregnancy and upcoming birth, as well as about her support systems and her new maternal role.

Women's feelings in the second trimester also reflect continuing physical changes. Although morning sickness may be resolving, more obvious physical changes necessitate being more open with others about the pregnancy. Women may feel differently about now having to share the news with co-workers, neighbors, and even strangers. In this trimester, women may feel more in the public eye, with a resultant lack of privacy and control. Some women may feel embarrassed or annoyed when other people touch their growing pregnant bellies.[9] A woman-centered clinician explores all these feelings about acceptance in her community, workplace, and relationships with the newly showing pregnancy: "How does it feel when other people notice you're pregnant?"

A woman usually notices fetal movement for the first time during the second trimester, confirming the reality of the new being inside her. This sensation may bring about many emotions: pleasure and anticipation as she learns about the fetal response to her daily activities, but also awareness and fears of the responsibility she is undertaking. Clinicians can ask, "What do you think about or feel when you notice the baby move?"

IDEAS

Kerry's nausea finally dissipated as she neared 16 weeks' gestation. Her fellow teachers who were already parents offered her frequent advice about what to eat during lunch breaks, and her mother-in-law hearing of Kerry's new craving for certain foods remembered her own pregnancy cravings with Ron and was convinced this meant that the baby would be a boy.

A woman in this mid-trimester often wonders if her experiences are normal or whether any given symptom represents a possible warning sign for a complication. Cultures invent many mechanisms to try to predict and understand unpredictable events. Common myths still abound: reaching overhead during pregnancy causes a breech presentation; seeing a rabbit causes a cleft palate; heartburn means a baby with lots of hair, etc. Asking a woman, "What does your family say about this symptom?" or "What have you read or heard about this symptom?" allows the woman-centered clinician to start exploring these ideas and then providing any needed reassurance.

The woman's growing awareness of fetal movement and size also brings new ideas about the baby and its identity and personality. As the reality of the baby becomes more obvious, the woman having her first baby develops further changes in self-identity as a mother. Multiparous women often compare this pregnancy's physical changes and fetal activity with prior pregnancies and attribute either gender differences or specific traits to this fetus. The clinician asks, "What is different this time? What do you think that means about this baby compared with your other(s)?" The response can lead later into a discussion about parenting more than one child.

FUNCTION

Susan was a 36-year-old nurse practitioner and athlete who ran 40 miles a week and regularly competed in half-marathons and triathlons. In the first few weeks of her pregnancy she felt tired enough that she cut down on her running, but continued to run shorter distances several days a week and to do yoga to stay flexible. By the time she was 16 weeks pregnant, however, she was slowing down a bit, noticing her growing uterus now halfway up to her umbilicus, and feeling somewhat uncomfortable with pelvic pressure while running. Her provider, Dr. Judith Peters, at this visit asked about exercise and encouraged Susan to continue with whatever level felt comfortable to her. (*See* full vignette in Appendix.)

In the second trimester, women often notice an improvement in function when fatigue and morning sickness resolve. However, some women face employment problems as their pregnancy progresses. Some may perceive resentment from co-workers and find that their role at work is different even though they are still doing the same activities. Others may face restrictions on what they may do at work. For instance, women who work on airlines are restricted from regular travel starting as early as 20 weeks' gestation. With very limited data available about definitive risk from workplace exposures, fetocentric employers may insist on other limitations out of fear of reprisal if the woman has a pregnancy complication. Likewise, women may need to restrict some leisure activities such as contact sports, although most other exercise that a woman engaged in regularly prior to pregnancy continues to be safe including distance running. Woman-centered questions can explore the dynamic changes of pregnancy on a woman's function as the trimester passes.

EXPECTATIONS

Women bring a variety of expectations to the second trimester usually centered on a growing physical reality of the fetal presence, the woman's body changes and accompanying discomforts, and ongoing interactions with the healthcare system.

> Finally past the unrelenting nausea of the first trimester, Kerry began slowly to put on weight and feel renewed energy. She enjoyed sharing stories with the other teachers at work about their prenatal experiences. As she entered her fourth month, her friends asked, "Do you know what you're having?" and "When is your ultrasound?" They showed her their baby books with the first pictures of ultrasounds prominently displayed. Kerry and Ron went together after work to their scheduled ultrasound. Ron was allowed into the room, but the screen faced away from them until the sonographer had finished all the measurements and then took time to show them a few views. Kerry, who had not yet felt any fetal movement, was surprised by how much the fetus was moving on the ultrasound screen.

Ultrasound is one of the common expectations of the second trimester, even for women who have already had first trimester ultrasonography. In many developed countries, pregnant women routinely receive second-trimester ultrasounds, regardless of their risks for any of the potential anomalies that ultrasound may detect. Because ultrasound is so common in prenatal care, many women expect an enjoyable, bonding experience with the fetus, not a screening or diagnostic test. The ultrasound is a chance to meet the baby, visualize the reality of the pregnancy, and be reassured about fetal well-being.[15] For many women, sharing the experience of the ultrasound with their partner is important in feeling that their partner can be more connected with both the fetus and with them as the mother. The woman-centered clinician in scheduling the ultrasound asks who if anyone will accompany the woman.

As ultrasound technology allows more detailed fetal imaging, however, more women are likely to have ultrasounds with unexpected abnormal findings that have unclear long-term significance, creating a gulf between the expected pleasure of the baby's first photo and the shock of hearing of possible problems. As part of scheduling or performing a routine ultrasound, the woman-centered clinician educates the pregnant woman ahead of time about the potential for both false-negative and false-positive outcomes. Thus Larisa asks Kerry, "What have you heard about prenatal ultrasounds?" and "Have you ever heard of anyone having a difficult experience related to an ultrasound, such as a wrong diagnosis?" She adds, "Most ultrasounds are normal, but even with as much as we know about ultrasound and the details you can see, ultrasounds are not perfect. Sometimes there are parts that look unusual and need further views or pictures, and sometimes even after that we are not sure just what they mean." Further issues surrounding a woman's experience of abnormal findings on routine ultrasounds will be detailed in the fourth chapter of Section Two.

The woman-centered clinician also clarifies certain procedures or policies about ultrasounds in his or her system; for instance, who is allowed to accompany the pregnant woman in the ultrasound room, the potential for certain physical discomforts such as a full bladder or a darkened, cold exam room, and whether the sonographer will give a full report or wait for a radiologist or perinatologist to review the films.

In countries with routine screening ultrasound at 16 to 18 weeks, women may want to know the sex of the baby, and may be very disappointed if the ultrasound is inconclusive. This uncertainty may lead parents to insist on a later ultrasound even with no medical indication. In countries with a strong preference for male infants, women with prior girl children may experience great pressure to abort a female infant, and may themselves prefer an abortion to the stigma and castigation they may experience for bearing another girl. These expectations persist despite the illegality of performing ultrasounds for gender determination in those countries. Neither the American College of Obstetricians and Gynecologists nor the International Federation of Gynecology and Obstetrics consider ethical any method of sex selection for non-medical reasons, including ultrasound.[16,17] Nevertheless, immigrants from countries where gender selection is practiced may beg practitioners for ultrasound screening if they face family pressure not to bear another girl child. The moral and cross-cultural complexities of responding to such requests require an individually tailored approach. (*See* Part Three for further details of cross-cultural issues in general.)

Women in developed countries, especially those in their thirties, will expect genetic screening even though their understandings of the results are often inaccurate, and providers explain the results poorly.[18] While genetic screening offers some statistical probabilities of normality, it cannot provide the reassurance that every woman wants – that her baby is perfectly normal. Some women think that a normal serum genetic marker screen and ultrasound guarantee such normality, and do not realize that such tests only identify a portion of the problems that babies might have at birth. The complexities of these issues are discussed in Part Five.

Many women expect the second trimester to be a time of relative physical well-being, past the nausea and fatigue of first trimester and before the possible awkwardness of the third trimester. When the nausea or fatigue persist or feel more overwhelming, accompanied by the increasing bodily changes of the second trimester, a woman may be troubled by unrealistic expectations for herself, for the pregnancy, and even for her healthcare.

> At about five months of pregnancy Jackie, a multiparous African-American woman, was not tolerating many foods as "everything" gave her right-sided abdominal pain, and she was having a lot of back pain. Although she wanted the baby very much, she was angry about feeling sick all the time, and kept pushing her doctor, Judith Peters, to "do something." She called the office regularly with symptoms and was often given a squeeze-in appointment so that Judith could assess her in person. (*See* full vignette in Appendix.)

Jackie's provider, Judith, seeks to clarify with her just what "doing something" might mean in this mid-trimester with medical issues that are unlikely to become less symptomatic as the pregnancy progresses but that also need to be assessed as potential signs of more serious illness. During these frequent visits, Judith repeatedly assesses Jackie's feelings, ideas, function, and expectations. This empathetic strategy helps Jackie to weather the rest of her pregnancy.

CHAPTER 5

Third Trimester

Stacy Potts and Sara G. Shields

> A decade after her first pregnancy, Pat was living with her partner Mike and unexpectedly became pregnant again. That pregnancy ended with an early miscarriage, but Pat and Mike decided to get married and soon conceived again. Now in the third trimester of this pregnancy, they brought to each visit a long list of questions and concerns about possible exposures, illnesses, and symptoms. They worried about all the unusual outcomes mentioned in the popular books on pregnancy and childbirth. One of these books also mentioned writing a birth plan. They came to their 32-week visit to discuss this further with their provider, Dr. Simon Miller. One part of the plan they felt strongly about was having their own provider for visits as much as possible, and meeting ahead of time anyone who might be on call when Pat actually started labor. Dr. Miller was curious about why Pat and Mike, two otherwise healthy adults, had so many medical anxieties. He uncovered in

Pat's genogram the history of her mother's death from cancer that the family felt the doctors did not diagnose on time. Mike also felt distrustful in medical settings because of some high school sports injuries that he felt never healed properly.

As a woman enters the last few months of pregnancy, her feelings, ideas, function, and expectations evolve with the increasing physical reality of the baby's presence, the intensifying of prenatal visits, and the looming labor and delivery. Woman-centered clinicians remain flexible in eliciting these changing issues and in responding to them. Specifically, the woman-centered clinician alleviates fears, corrects misconceptions, encourages the woman in taking on decision-making, and simply is present for her.[1] Woman-centered care is flexible enough to allow more time for questions and concerns during the course of routine care in this trimester.

FEELINGS

For Pat, the third trimester means increasing anxiety about many of the normal physical discomforts and symptoms of this time. Indeed even if Pat were not vocalizing her fears overtly, her clinician needs to inquire about them, given how common such feelings are.[19,20] Instead of dismissing her frequent symptoms and worries, Dr. Miller validates her, first by acknowledging how common such fears are for pregnant women. He then compliments Pat on her attempts to self-educate, to attend to details of her body's sensations, and to advocate for her needs within the medical system – all skills she will need in her future as a parent.

Some of the key questions for a woman-centered clinician to ask include: "What worries you most about the labor and delivery, besides medical complications? What helps the most to relieve your worrying? You've done so many things to stay healthy and have a healthy baby during this pregnancy – now it is time for you to just let it happen. What would help you most to let this process unfold now?" The clinician here can suggest common unspoken worries such as being in pain, being undressed, making a fool of herself, or not feeling listened to. The answers to these questions can help Pat and Dr. Miller plan together for the remaining part of pregnancy and the beginning of parenthood. The clinician also stays attuned to deeper unspoken issues underlying the overt anxiety.

Fear of labor and delivery may dominate a pregnant woman's fears in the third trimester, primarily fear of pain and fear for the baby's health.[19,20] Some of Pat's anxiety about symptoms may in fact be related to such underlying fears of labor, leading the astute clinician to probe further and to inquire about past experiences of fear or anxiety that may explain her coping style. Women also worry about their "performance" in labor, about staff issues in labor, and about technology, as well as about the specific outcomes.[9] These worries may underlie more overt anxiety and need to be explored even if women do not voice them initially.

Normal physical changes evoke many feelings in the late trimester. As a woman's body grows, her emotions about her body size can fluctuate from enjoyment to disgust.[9] She may feel clumsy and awkward, the antithesis of the femininity that the idea of motherhood stereotypically invokes. Her size may make her feel fat, burdening her with all the negative connotations of excess weight in Western culture. She may need help with basic daily tasks and either dislike the feeling of dependency or welcome the respite from household chores, gladly relinquishing these duties to others. The clinician can inquire, "How is it for you to be dependent on others for certain daily tasks such as carrying loads or tying your shoes?" The insomnia and interrupted sleep typical of the third trimester may sap her energy and erode her enthusiasm. Even more now than in the second trimester, she is at risk for other people touching her abdomen without invitation, which may feel invasive or embarrassing.[9] Alternatively, the attention to her abdomen and to her baby may be a welcome connection, for instance with her partner or other family members.

The anticipation of the upcoming birth can make these weeks very exciting. The provider might ask, "Sometimes women wish labor and delivery would hurry up and come, and sometimes women want this to last for a while longer because they don't feel quite ready for a new baby yet – how are you feeling about that?"

IDEAS

As the woman's own motherhood becomes more and more of a reality, an important part of exploring her ideas in the third trimester involves understanding her relationships with mother figures in her own life. The process of doing a simple genogram offers ample opportunity to ask about those in the woman's life who have given her ideas about pregnancy, birth, and becoming a mother. For Dr. Miller, knowing about the loss of Pat's mother, an expanded genogram includes discussion of other possible mother figures for her. This discussion is important not only for first-time mothers but also for multiparous women who face the issue of handling a growing family.

To further elicit a woman's ideas in the third trimester, the woman-centered clinician asks questions such as: "What was your mother's/sister's/other important maternal figure's experience of birth? How do you think your pregnancy and birth will compare to that woman's experience? What do you want to remember later about this stage of your pregnancy? What is your idea of the ideal birth experience?" Again, no single question fits every woman – the woman-centered clinician selectively chooses the phrasing depending on the particular woman's unique life context.

> Susan the runner had always been lean and fit, and found the late trimester weight gain and other physical changes of pregnancy especially hard to tolerate. The stretch marks made her feel ugly, and she worried that she would not be able to lose the weight after the baby was born. She liked that Judith did not overemphasize her weight at each visit, encouraged her overall healthy eating habits, and referred her to a pregnancy-related yoga class. But when her feet started to swell at 36 weeks, so that her favorite shoes no longer fit, she wondered if she would ever see her ankles again.

Ideas about nutrition and body image can be a part of any trimester of pregnancy but can become more significant for women during the third trimester's increasingly obvious uterine and fetal growth. This sensitive issue may come up specifically at the ritual weigh-in during prenatal visits. The thoughtful clinician recognizes and responds to women for whom this ritual can be problematic, such as women who have previously struggled with weight-control issues. Many women feel that there is greater social acceptability of obesity during pregnancy,[21] and they relax their usual restrictions, leading some habitual dieters to relish the chance to "eat for two" without being hassled by family and friends about their weight or their food intake. The woman-centered clinician acknowledges in a non-judgmental way the additional nutritional needs of pregnancy while providing accurate information about adequate intake. Other women like Susan struggle with the bigness of their pregnant body, even feeling disgust or anger at these changes.[9] Judith needs to normalize this preoccupation with size and reframe these ideas as part of the continuum of a new mother's healthy choices and expected postpartum weight differences. Finally, some women may fear that a big baby will lead to a difficult labor or even a cesarean section, and therefore attempt to limit the baby's growth by eating less. The woman-centered clinician can address this fear by asking about what size baby the woman thinks is best for her, and by normalizing expected weight gain in pregnancy.

FUNCTION

Later in the pregnancy, Rosa's fundal height started to lag behind her pregnancy's gestational age, so Dr. Rosen ordered sequential ultrasounds to confirm that the baby was growing normally. When her due date neared, Dr. Rosen and her advocate Lupe spent much of each visit describing the various hospital routines such as electronic monitoring and the options for pain medication during labor. Rosa tried to follow all the providers' prenatal recommendations, but did not really understand much about the tests that Dr. Rosen ordered. Rosa was concerned about all the appointments she needed since she had to take time off from work for these and did not get any paid sick time. She missed a couple of appointments as a result.

In the early third trimester Kerry's weight increased a bit faster than expected, and she suddenly felt big and immobile. She was having more trouble sleeping. She headed into the final two months of pregnancy with more frequent symptoms such as heartburn, urinary frequency, and back pain. Ron was working extra hours now in order to have some financial cushion to be able to take time off after the baby's birth. He was not around home much to help with some of the chores that were becoming harder for Kerry to do, such as laundry, or even to help when by 36 weeks she had trouble putting on her shoes.

The third trimester is also a time when women face changes in their ability to function in the arenas of work, whether this be employment outside the home or housework. The woman-centered clinician stays attuned to the competing demands on a pregnant woman's responsibilities in the third trimester. The increasing frequency of prenatal visits in this trimester affects a woman's life schedule in these penultimate months before the biggest schedule change of all: labor, birth, and parenting. Woman-centered care requires flexibility in arranging appointments to meet women's work hours or childcare needs.

Depending on national insurance and maternity leave policies, women employed outside the home will need to review and finalize details of maternity leave, which may or may not be paid; sometimes these programs demand the maternity provider's input to verify pregnancy status or date of delivery for such leave. (*See* Part Three for more discussion about pregnancy and work roles.) Some women with normal discomforts in the third trimester feel that these symptoms require them to alter or stop their work before maternity leave might usually begin – e.g. back pain, leg swelling, increasing fatigue from interrupted sleep due to more nocturia. Others feel it important to prove that they can continue to carry a full load despite the pregnancy. (The latter group has more difficulties when complications of late pregnancy require that they cut back or stop working.) The woman-centered clinician responds sensitively to these issues and understands the wider context of these competing demands.

Such competing roles can be part of a woman's life at home as well as at work in the late trimester. The needs of other children or the tasks of running a household such as laundry and meal preparation can exhaust a pregnant woman at this stage. Particularly if medical risks such as preterm labor, bleeding, or hypertension occur, the woman-centered clinician, understanding these demands, may need to encourage a woman to ask for help with such daily needs in this trimester. For some women the ability to keep on doing many of these tasks throughout pregnancy is essential to their self-esteem. Others who might welcome relief from these chores may not have adequate home support and might not feel empowered enough in their relationships with partner or extended family to insist on such help, and may need the clinician to voice this for them.

The normal physical changes of late pregnancy bring about general function changes, too. With an enlarging abdomen and changing pelvic laxity, women often walk differently, move more slowly, and bend over or rise out of a chair or bed with less agility. The woman-centered clinician inquires about these changes, understanding that such limitations may contribute to discrimination (such as unwanted job reassignment) or benefits (such as being offered a seat on an otherwise crowded bus).

As labor nears, the woman-centered provider also attends to the wider needs of this woman for organizing her life to get ready for the pending birth and for transporting herself if needed to the intended delivery site. For a multiparous woman such as Jackie, these issues include arranging for childcare for her older children during labor. Dr. Rosen, knowing that Rosa lacks a car and does not understand English, discusses how they can communicate with each other when labor starts about when and how to come to the hospital.

EXPECTATIONS

> Pat had several visits between 34 and 36 weeks because of frequent contractions, vaginal discharge, and leg swelling, all of which made her panic about preterm labor, ruptured membranes, or pre-eclampsia – all problems she had read about. Dr. Miller tried to reassure her but also wanted her to report any danger symptoms. The office nurse triaged most of her calls and squeezed her in for visits if Pat reported anything concerning, such as decreased fetal movement or leaking of water. Pat insisted on these visits being as much as possible with Dr. Miller, even if it meant waiting longer to see him because he was already overbooked. At one of these visits, both she and Mike asked about getting another ultrasound "just to make sure the baby is okay." At her 38-week visit, both she and Mike were stressed to hear that her Group B Streptococcus screening test was positive. They had lots of questions about what this meant about the baby's risk of infection.

In the third trimester, a woman has many changing expectations – of the healthcare system, of the doctor, of her family/support, of medical technologies, of herself – as labor nears. As the frequency of prenatal visits intensifies at this time, women have even more exposure to the healthcare system and to health providers, affording clinicians more opportunity to engage in discussion of these expectations. More pregnancy discomforts may stimulate more questions, either at prenatal visits (thus lengthening them) or by phone between visits – women may expect 24-hour access to any provider, or to their own specifically. The woman-centered clinician anticipates such expectations, encourages the woman to voice them, and then overtly addresses them.

The increasing use of medical testing in the last trimester, especially as delivery nears, means that some women expect additional ultrasounds or other fetal monitoring. Although many women (and many clinicians) assume that such non-invasive testing is harmless, the woman-centered clinician needs both to explore the anxieties behind such requests and to discuss the potential for unnecessary invasive testing should these initial tests mistakenly show abnormalities. Without patronizing or dismissing the woman's worries, the clinician can offer reassurance coupled with some understandable explanation of false-positive test results. For instance, reframing Pat's frequent calls, Dr. Miller says, "You have learned a lot from your reading and your health providers that there are some symptoms late in pregnancy that can be signs of something more serious. This kind of self-education is great preparation for being a new parent." Dr. Miller can also acknowledge that the health system does not always allow the continuous or longitudinal care the way Pat requests, but can validate that this is an important need for her.

Although in some studies women indicate preferences for intrapartum care styles that match what their local system provides,[22] in other studies women mention wanting not only excellent healthcare but personalized, trusting, communicative providers who view each woman "as a unique person and not as an object, a womb."[9] Clinicians who have had the opportunity throughout prenatal care to elicit all dimensions of a woman's experience are in the best position to fulfill this expectation.

Childbirth classes or some form of childbirth education are often part of the third trimester, especially for nulliparous women. Hospital-based childbirth classes may present only the style of labor and delivery typical of that setting, without offering a range of birthing options,[23] so women who attend these classes may not learn about less interventionist birth practices. Most contemporary childbirth education classes include partner involvement. Women without a supportive partner may feel excluded from such classes, or have increased anxiety about coping strategies in labor without such support.

As a woman's due date nears, many women, particularly those having their first baby, anticipate that they will give birth just before or right on their due date. Starting at these last few prenatal visits, to begin the discussion of the unpredictability of labor's beginning, the woman-centered provider asks in an open-ended way about such expectations. "As we get close to the due date, what are you expecting about when you will go into labor?" With each visit closer to the due date, a woman's anticipation may build and evolve, so this question is worth repeating at each visit in the last month.

Women may expect labor to begin dramatically and ensue rapidly, as in hospital television shows or movies that depict sudden spontaneous rupture of membranes followed immediately by rapid delivery. Inquiring in late pregnancy about a woman's sense of such media portrayals of birth can help a woman-centered provider clarify each woman's birth expectations. These media images of societal expectations may strongly influence a pregnant woman's sense of appropriate labor and delivery behavior,[24] particularly if she ends up comparing her performance negatively to these depictions.

Multiparous women with a prior "straightforward birth" may have high expectations for a subsequent labor and birth. Other multiparous women report feeling more prepared for the "realities of giving birth" with less sense of the unknown and perhaps more sense of being able to cope.[25;260-1] Some women with difficult prior experiences do report feeling "cheated" from a natural labor experience and either expect a better experience with the next labor, postpone subsequent pregnancies out of fear of the same experience, or have lowered their expectations for subsequent labors.[25] Thus exploring the woman's prior experiences can help a provider better understand her current expectations.

Pain is central to women's expectations as they approach active labor. Pain can engender fear – of being overwhelmed, of labor or birth complications, of dying – even for women in developed countries where maternal mortality is rare. Women with extreme fear in anticipation of childbirth may have particularly unrealistic expectations of either an epidural with their first contraction or a primary cesarean.[26] Acknowledging the existence of such fears during pregnancy, rather than waiting until labor ensues, is critical to developing a woman-centered care plan.

Most women hope for a short labor and manageable pain.[27] As part of exploring what a woman thinks about labor pain, the woman-centered provider ascertains how a woman has coped with pain, either emotional or physical, at other times in her life. The provider asks the woman, "What helped you get through these other tough situations in your life?" In considering the coping strategies she used previously, the provider helps her see parallels to strategies she may be able to use during labor, focusing on positive strategies and seeking alternatives to less helpful strategies.[28] Focusing on what to expect through coping strategies also emphasizes that the goal of labor care is relief of suffering and not solely removal of physiologic pain. (*See* pain discussion in Part Four.)

Any anticipatory discussion of labor pain includes asking what women expect for pharmacologic pain relief and when they expect to receive it, if at all. When a woman reveals that she expects an automatic, early epidural "as soon as I get to the hospital," the provider can then engage her in an ongoing, evolving discussion of this hope. (*See* Part Four for further elaboration.) A similar collaborative exploration of options can happen for a woman with expectations at the other end of the spectrum, such as Ruth hoping for a home birth without technological interventions or for a woman anticipating a hospital delivery but wanting to avoid electronic monitoring.

Many women have unrealistic expectations about prenatal care, not realizing that even mothers who "do it all right" can have unforeseen negative outcomes. This inherent uncertainty in pregnancy is anathema to society's craving for certainty and for black-and-white answers. The woman-centered provider's task is thus a balancing of three expectations: optimism that most pregnancies are healthy and do not need a lot of interventions or testing, empowerment for women to avoid unnecessary blame or guilt about every possible action they take, and realism that occasionally even with the most careful prenatal care, unexpected difficulties occur. Although this discussion begins early in pregnancy, the woman-centered provider returns to the issue in the third trimester when expectations run particularly high.

As her due date approaches, the pregnant woman may alternate rapidly between excitement about meeting her child and concerns about how her labor will progress. Every day she wakes and wonders: "Will today be the day?" The woman-centered provider has set the stage since early pregnancy for the great uncertainty and unpredictability about the actual labor and delivery, normalizing and reassuring the woman. Reframing the woman's concerns from a lifeworld perspective and affirming her own strengths in self-care throughout pregnancy can also set the stage for strength-based care as labor begins. For first-time mothers, this time around the due date can be especially challenging.

CHAPTER 6

Woman-Centered Normal Labor and Delivery

Clara Keegan

Kerry planned to work up until she went into labor, but as her due date came and went, she was deluged by calls and inquiries about "when will this baby come?" At her baby shower, several friends told their birth stories, most of which revolved around long labors or dramatic deliveries.

At just past 41 weeks, Kerry woke up with painful contractions just after midnight. Ron called the on-call provider, who suggested that they wait at home as long as they could. Within a couple of hours, however, Kerry found the contractions too uncomfortable, and Ron called again. They decided to go to the hospital, where the night nurse examined Kerry and found her only 1 cm dilated. After discussion with the on-call provider over the phone, they opted to return home and contact the office once the contractions were stronger. At home, Kerry took a warm bath and tried to sleep, but by breakfast time she again felt too uncomfortable, and Ron drove her to the office for the first morning appointment. Larisa had a full schedule already but evaluated Kerry quickly and reported that she was still just 2 cm dilated and not yet effaced much. She and Ron felt discouraged and tired but agreed to return home to try to sleep. Finally, at supper time Kerry was feeling exhausted and unable to cope, but she did not want to go back to the hospital only to find out that she was still not dilating. Ron felt helpless and finally called the answering service again at around 10 p.m. Just as they were deciding that maybe Kerry should return now, she reported from the other room that she thought her waters had broken, so they again went to labor and delivery. There, about 24 hours after Kerry first woke with contractions, the night nurse checked and found that Kerry's cervix was now 3 cm dilated and 90% effaced.

FEELINGS

As labor begins, first-time mothers may oscillate between excitement and anxiety or fear. Anxiety about the unpredictability of the timing and the course of labor may be one of the strongest feelings for some women entering early labor. The woman-centered provider through the course of pregnancy will have set the stage for strategies to deal with this anxiety and to celebrate the uncertainties rather than be paralyzed by them. ("This is all part of preparing you for parenting.") Although anxiety and fear may predominate especially for first-time mothers entering labor, other possible emotions include anticipation of finally seeing, touching, and knowing the new baby; eagerness to get the pregnancy over with; and power in anticipating the physical challenge of labor. The woman-centered clinician can reframe the fears and anxieties of labor by helping the woman and her partner to focus on these positive emotions also, saying for instance, "Let's keep in mind the baby at the end of all of this! Your baby is going to be as glad to see you as you will be to greet him or her finally."

Early contractions can be strong enough to prevent much rest, with exhaustion thus exacerbating other intense feelings. For Kerry, having come to the hospital and later the office assuming that she is in active labor, the triage process that quickly defines the process as "false" or prodromal labor feels particularly frustrating or even distressing. Appropriately not admitted to the hospital at this early stage, Kerry returns home already exhausted, confused about misreading her painful symptoms, and becoming terrified about how much discomfort she will feel in true labor. She begins to doubt her ability to interpret her body's signals or to tolerate the rest of labor. Larisa will need to recognize the role that fear and self-doubt can play in long early labors and validate these feelings.

Because these fears can be multifactorial, one of the tasks of the provider is to avoid assumptions about an individual woman's fears as labor begins. For instance, many women fear not only pain, but also fear making a fool of themselves, or "not being able to do it" somehow, or "losing it," all fears that can interrupt the progress of normal labor. Women with a past history of sexual abuse may be particularly frightened of birth as another painful event, out of their control, involving the sexual parts of their bodies. (*See* Part Three and Four.) Other possible fears include the fear of disappointing her spouse/partner, the fear of hospital systems, the fear of technology/drugs, the fear of loss of privacy or nakedness in front of men or strangers. Even in the developed world where maternal mortality is exceedingly rare, some women anticipating labor fear their own death.[29]

Other women, especially multiparas, may experience early labor as similar to menstrual cramps, or may be unaware of contractions until they are in active labor. Some women notice signs that labor may be approaching, such as loss of the mucus plug or bloody show, or more subtle changes like a waddling gait or nesting behaviors. The woman-centered provider takes these signs seriously and provides reassurance, reminders on labor signs and the practice's call system, and if appropriate and with the woman's agreement, a cervical exam.

Particularly when the on-call provider is a stranger, attention to the woman's sense of privacy may alleviate some of her fears during labor. When preparing for an exam or an intervention, the woman-centered provider first asks the laboring woman whom she would like in the room, who should stand behind a curtain, and who could consider taking a coffee break off the floor during this time. Using a sheet to cover her during the exam can further protect the woman's modesty.

> Kerry was finally admitted to the hospital when her waters broke when she was 3 cm dilated. Although glad to be making progress, she was still exhausted after 24 hours of prodromal labor and discouraged that labor still had so far to go. The nurses encouraged her to walk and take a shower; finally, Kerry requested an epidural around 3 a.m. when she was at last 4 cm dilated. Once she had this anesthesia, she slept briefly and so did Ron, after taking phone calls from the eagerly waiting grandparents.

> Samantha, a teenager, at the end of her pregnancy was still not reconciled with her mother but glad to have the support of her cousin Alice and boyfriend Jack. She started having painful contractions and had several visits where she was not quite in labor and was sent home. Finally, on her fifth trip to the hospital, she was 4 cm dilated and quite uncomfortable. Her labor nurse convinced Samantha to get into the shower for a while to help with the pain, and when she got out, she was already 7 cm dilated but starting to panic with the intensity of the contractions. Samantha's caregivers encouraged her: "You've been able to get this far in labor. You don't need to feel scared of how it is going to happen or that it will never end. You just need to keep doing what you are doing." (*See* full vignette in the Appendix.)

Active labor brings intense physical feelings as contractions increase in frequency and intensity. Especially late in labor, women often experience powerful involuntary sensations and reactions such as vomiting and large muscle shaking.[24] Fear and anticipation build with these physical symptoms and the contraction pattern. Women have a variety of other feelings during active labor and delivery.[30] Although not ignoring the negative feelings – overwhelmed, weak, frightened, agitated, groggy, helpless – the woman-centered provider keeps the laboring woman focused on positive feelings: alert, capable, calm, unafraid, competent, powerful. Women may also feel panicked in late labor, overwhelmed with a fear that labor will never end. In the midst of this intensity of physical and emotional symptoms, the laboring woman often cannot clearly express all of these feelings. The woman-centered provider stays attuned to the woman's non-verbal expressions and checks in regularly about possible feelings. "This is a very intense time. You look like you might be feeling overwhelmed and even afraid. Is that right? What else are you feeling?" To address panic, the provider can encourage her, "You may be feeling scared that this will never end. But you are progressing normally. Here is what is going to happen. You just need to keep doing what you are doing."

As the cervix nears full dilation, many women exhibit behavior like yelling or cursing, which may take them and their partners by surprise. Fear of this behavior may even contribute to a woman's overall fears of labor, especially if she hears another woman in transition through the wall or down the corridor. The woman-centered provider watches for and addresses such points of tension.

> For Samantha at 9 cm, the pushing urge was overwhelming, but being in the hands–knees position helped that sensation, and she eventually started pushing in that position even though it felt unusual and was not what she remembered her friends talking about for this part of labor. After 20 minutes the baby's head was crowning, and Samantha resisted pushing because of the overwhelming burning sensation. She began to panic again and was about to scream. Dr. Epps quietly asked her to focus right on the doctor's voice and coached the teen through easing the baby's head out with gentle short pushes so that her perineum did not tear. The baby boy Kyle was vigorous and went straight into Samantha's arms while Jack cut the umbilical cord.

Finally, cervical dilation is complete, and the second stage of labor begins. For many women the chance to take control and push is a welcome change from the overwhelming, out-of-control feelings of the end of the first stage of labor. The unanesthetized woman will need little coaching; her body will tell her what to do, and she will be overcome by the need to push. For some subset of women, however, pushing is uncomfortable enough to prevent this pushing urge, especially at first, and later, women may be afraid of pushing for fear of perineal tearing. Birth attendants need to remain sensitive to how these fears may impede the second stage. In addition, the increasingly available option of epidural anesthesia significantly diminishes these sensations.

As the fetus descends into the birth canal, many women will become aware of rectal pressure. This sensation might be the only way a woman knows she is having a contraction. Especially at the end of a long first stage of labor, exhaustion may be the woman's primary emotion. The woman-centered clinician reframes this in a strength-based way: "You have made it to this point. You may feel tired, but your body still knows what to do and still has strength. Add to that as much as you can."

IDEAS

Over the course of seven months of prenatal visits and anticipation, a pregnant woman has heard more and more birth stories from family, friends, and strangers. For Kerry, for instance, every time she turns on the television, she finds a program depicting a real or fictional delivery. She sees movie character after movie character turn to her husband and say, "Honey, it's time," or break her water in dramatic fashion. These scenes are inevitably followed by a frantic drive to the hospital, then a few minutes of excited pushing before a chubby, clean newborn is passed into the new mother's arms. Many of the stories and images seem to focus on fear or pain. At her baby shower, she hears more stories about women who spend a brutal 48 hours in labor, and others who arrive at the hospital so far into labor that they are denied analgesia when they request it.

However, as is more typical for a first-time mother, Kerry has a slow progression into active labor, plenty of time to get to the hospital, and a couple hours of pushing before her baby is born. As part of childbirth education, the woman-centered provider teaches these ideas before labor starts and throughout the prodromal time. Such teaching can use empowering, positive language to reaffirm the woman's strengths and capacity. For example, rather than telling Kerry she is "only 1 cm" or "still just 2 cm", Larisa can emphasize the change in cervical effacement, validate how hard Kerry has worked to get to that stage, and further explore what Kerry's ideas are about her labor as it is happening.

> Ruth started having contractions one afternoon while at work. Later that evening, she checked in with the midwife, calling her again just after midnight when her waters broke. As the contractions quickly intensified, she alternated between the rocking chair and the shower, with Lewis and the midwife nearby offering massage and frequent sips of water and juice. By noon she entered transition with the peak of each contraction almost overwhelming her. "I'm never doing this again!" she told Lewis. "I can't do this!" The midwife reassured her, and reminded both of them that this was what they had talked about ahead of time, of what hard work this stage of labor would be and how these feelings of hopelessness and endlessness were common. She suggested staying focused on each contraction one at a time, and described different options for coping. Ruth wanted to stay mostly in the shower until she felt like pushing. The midwife also reminded Ruth how healthy she had been throughout her pregnancy, and reiterated, "This baby is doing great, thanks to all your hard work keeping yourself so healthy."

When elucidating women's ideas about labor, providers want to assess how women feel about a sense of being in control. Active labor is about letting go and relinquishing control, but not becoming passive or helpless. Ideally, the astute provider prepares a woman for this before active labor, but can remind her during labor, too. "You're at that point in labor that we talked about, where we need to help you figure out how to let labor happen and not fight it." One of the prenatal tasks thus is to talk over with a woman what she thinks will be helpful for her when the experience of intense labor pain may overwhelm rational thought.

> At the end of Siobhan's second pregnancy, she received care from Dr. Miller, a new provider to her. With her first birth, she had not met the delivering doctor until just before Danny Jr. was born. With this labor, her waters broke about a week before her due date, and Dr. Miller over the phone advised her to come to the hospital. Shortly after settling in to her room, Siobhan began having regular contractions. Dr. Miller arrived and examined her to confirm that her water had broken, but she had not yet dilated. They talked about a care plan, including intermittent monitoring and pain-management choices. Siobhan, at ease with this familiar doctor, joked, "I thought the baby would come right now, since you're already here!" She talked about how awful the pain had been for her with her first labor and was emphatic

that this time she wanted more help with that, no matter how fast the labor progressed. Dr. Miller asked her to guide him and the nurse specifically about what to do to help her cope.

After a few hours of alternately resting, walking, or rocking, with the doctor in and out of the room offering encouragement, Siobhan thus asked for pain medication as she was more uncomfortable and now 3 cm dilated. Dr. Miller spent time between contractions reviewing again her choices. Siobhan got brief relief from a parenteral narcotic, and two hours later asked for an epidural. She had dilated another 2 cm. After the anesthetic took effect, Siobhan was so comfortable that she slept for an hour. Stronger contractions and an urge to push awakened her, and Dr. Miller checked to see that she was fully dilated. Siobhan gradually pushed out baby Katie with gentle pushes guided by Dr. Miller, who passed the baby directly to Siobhan's belly while Danny Sr. cut the cord. Siobhan, smiling and laughing throughout the delivery, felt amazed by the difference between her two labor experiences less than one year apart. (*See* full vignette in the Appendix.)

Multiparous women may have specific ideas about labor in comparison to their previous experiences. If their prior deliveries felt difficult they may have certain assumptions about how this labor will go and their own coping capacity.[25;260-1] Reminding the woman that each baby is different, the provider asks, "How is this labor going compared to your last labor? What helped you in that labor? What do you think would be helpful for you now? How would you like this labor to be different?" Given the panoply of hospital and provider styles, if she gave birth previously in a different setting or with another provider, a multiparous woman may be surprised by dissimilar practices such as monitoring or provider presence.

Helen, the midwife in Judith's practice, came in to the hospital on her day off when she got the call that Alexandra was in labor. Alexandra's pregnancy had been uncomplicated, and she was at term. Helen was somewhat skeptical about her teen's specific request for natural childbirth and no epidural. Although she was 19, Alexandra had always seemed to be very "young" to Helen, but she had asked very good questions. She came to every prenatal appointment and participated in the school-aged pregnancy program. Alexandra was actively laboring at 6 cm when Helen arrived. The midwife was pleased to meet Alexandra's two older sisters in the labor room. Alexandra's labor flourished beautifully under her sisters' ministrations, and she proceeded without anesthesia or pain medication to full dilation and delivery of a healthy baby girl, Jasmine, within a few hours. (*See* full vignette of Alexandra and Helen's biography in the Appendix.)

Women have a variety of ideas about the role of pain and their response to it in labor. For some women such as Ruth, keeping the process of labor unmedicated is critical. Her choice of provider and birth site emphasize the importance of this for her. Other women like Alexandra may say, "I want to go natural," but the meaning of that is less obvious. The provider explores both prenatally and again during labor what ideas the woman has about this. "What does go natural mean to you? What do you need from me and the rest of us here to feel like you've done that?" For some women, "going natural" may mean no medication, or no epidural. For others, even if they have an epidural, the experience of working to push their baby out may make them feel that they had a "natural" birth. Goals vary widely: some women want to prove something, and others want to avoid something (e.g. pain, shame, or intervention). Some want just to "get it over with," and still others enter the experience with an open mind, ready to embrace whatever comes as they move closer to holding their baby in their arms. Women may have many different ideas about ways to help relieve labor pain, from physical support such as massage, or a hot shower, or emotional support including the choice to have extra people with them during active labor. Supporting a woman in her choice, adapting to her needs as labor progresses, and emphasizing her crucial and powerful role in the birth are evolving tasks during woman-centered labor.

> At around 8 a.m., Kerry felt like she needed to have a bowel movement, so the nurse checked and found that Kerry was indeed fully dilated. Larisa, Ron and the nurse worked together to help Kerry with different pushing positions. At first Kerry did not want to push much with everyone watching her because she did not like the idea of defecating in front of the nurse. She was also embarrassed about the grunting noises she made with the pushes that the nurse said were the best ones. With reassurance that this was normal, the nurse cleaned the bed frequently, and she and Larisa encouraged Kerry's efforts. Finally, after two hours of pushing in different positions, Kerry gave birth to baby Erika.

For Kerry, concerns about modesty and behavior come into play during the actual delivery. Having explored earlier her worst possible fears in labor, including her fear of "not doing it right," Larisa can also inquire about what the woman thinks about permissible behavior in active labor. Ideally, this occurs prior to the intensity of active labor when focusing on a provider's questions may be difficult. The nurse also attends to Kerry's concerns that pushing well includes passing stool, with resulting embarrassment inhibiting her ability to push effectively. Kerry's nurse responds to this sensitive issue by helping to interpret the sensations, by reassuring about the normality of the process, and less overtly by changing bed linens as needed.

> When labor ensued, Rosa came to the hospital well along in her labor. She had already had ultrasounds and fetal monitoring antenatally, but had not been expecting to have to stay attached to a monitor during active labor. She worried that even though the labor felt a lot like her first labors at home in her country, this baby must have something wrong with it to need all this monitoring. José, having accompanied her to the hospital where he had never been before, was not quite sure where he was supposed to go while the nurses were settling Rosa into a room. He spoke a bit of English but was uncomfortable watching Rosa in pain and remembered to ask the nurse to call Rosa's advocate Lupe to come in to help with translation.

A woman and her partner may be familiar with the hospital birthing environment after an antenatal tour, or from visiting friends or family members there, but many women enter labor with minimal knowledge of typical hospital procedures or technology. The hospital setting can be particularly foreign for women needing language interpretation or coming from cultures or countries without these technologies, an issue discussed further in Part Three.

FUNCTION

As we have seen, some women like Kerry and Samantha are incapacitated by early labor and are unable to do more than seek relief from the pain of contractions. However, for other women the ability to ignore early contractions and continue their life activities in early labor is important.

> Ruth's contractions started one afternoon a few days before her due date, but she continued working at her job to finish up details of an important project before calling the midwife when she arrived home about the increasingly strong contractions.

> When labor finally began just after supper one night, Felicity (see Part One) wanted to finish cleaning the kitchen, putting her older kids to bed, and folding up some new baby laundry before deciding to go to the hospital.

Clinicians help women to remain vigilant to the unpredictability of just how long their labor might take – setting the groundwork earlier in pregnancy for how to handle early symptoms and preparing the woman with her first pregnancy not to arrive too soon at the birth place nor the parous woman too late. For hospital births, the primary provider is not often in person with the woman in early labor but can nonetheless provide telephone advice during this time if need be. Those in attendance can encourage the woman to eat and drink lightly but sufficiently and can suggest rest, bathing or showering, as well as whatever possible relaxation techniques she and her home support can do. Emphasizing rest whenever possible for both the woman and her support people is also important especially for primigravid women with potentially longer labors: "You're feeling excited, which can make it hard to sleep or rest. What do you think might help you to use the time between contractions to rest as much as you can?"

A woman's function during labor depends both on her desires and on the amount of monitoring performed in her labor setting. Unmedicated women have few barriers on their movement at home and should have few barriers in the hospital setting, where ideally they should be able to move at will to find positions that allow labor to progress as comfortably as possible. Narcotic pain medication and epidural anesthesia limit a woman's movement, as she is largely confined to the bed by fetal and maternal monitors as well as by the sleepiness or leg numbness that accompany these interventions. Some women may feel inhibited about assuming certain labor positions because of cultural or family ideas about appropriate modesty. Some women have difficulty asking for help because they believe they should be self-sufficient, and others do not know what to ask for.

While the birth attendant will use many different support methods, the presence of a non-medical support person other than the laboring woman's partner, such as a doula, is associated with a higher rate of vaginal delivery.[31,32] Doulas can be especially important in the hospital system where birth attendants and labor nurses often are unable to stay with a woman throughout her labor because of other responsibilities. The doula can help her client express feelings and expectations as they evolve through labor, then communicate these to the provider. The doula also can provide physical support such as massage or assistance with finding a comfortable labor position. Part Four has further discussion of doula strategies.

The rest time between contractions may lengthen during the second stage. The provider can use this extra time to assess what coaching and support techniques are helpful and which are not, if the woman has not expressed this herself in the moment. Some women respond well to counting during each push, but the woman-centered provider avoids overemphasizing a certain number, rate, or loudness to the counting and relies on the woman's innate pushing urges (assuming that anesthesia has not ablated them), emphasizing empowering positive statements such as "what a strong push!" rather than phrases with negative connotations such as "Get mad at it!" Other women appreciate the tactile sensation of the clinician giving digital pressure against the posterior vaginal wall and perineum in directing efforts, but this area can be very sensitive because of the increased blood flow during labor. Some women want to push constantly as the fetus descends and need help relaxing between contractions and pushing only with contractions. The woman-centered provider remains attuned to the woman's verbal and non-verbal responses, and reflects energy back into the process.

An extended second stage may benefit from position changes or techniques such as pulling on opposite ends of a towel or sheet to help move the fetus down through the pelvis. The second stage is an ideal time to involve various family members in active ways such as holding the woman's leg, supporting her shoulders, helping her squat, or providing cool cloths or hot compresses. A woman having a physiologic delivery (i.e. without an epidural) can test out a variety of positions and identify the pushing position that works best for her; this ability to choose means that she becomes more in charge of her labor and less the passive parturient who follows instructions.

EXPECTATIONS

Women's expectations in latent labor include support, comfort, and reassurance, ready contact with a known provider and system, and steady progress in labor. The task of the woman-centered provider is to encourage women to find in their own personal support systems methods of self-coping and comfort, such as showers or ways to rest as much as possible, preferably in their own environment. Having an empathic professional address increasing symptoms or additional coping strategies during this time can further help women like Kerry with protracted prodromal labor. Since many women think labor is a concrete event, not a process, an astute clinician will educate women during the last few weeks of pregnancy about the likelihood of on-again, off-again contractions as part of the entire preparation for early labor. Reminding Kerry of the normality and uncertainty of prodromal labor can help her refocus on this process.

Birth plans are one way to explore expectations for labor and delivery. In concert with their providers, women are able to consider different scenarios of birth and make decisions about their priorities. This opportunity to make decisions and understand the process of care during pregnancy and childbirth helps ground in reality a woman's expectations, yet still gives her a sense of control. By actively eliciting any unrealistic expectations about labor, especially around pain, the woman-centered provider can offer ways to anticipate a variety of self-care strategies during labor. Control, information, choices, and taking part in decisions have all been linked to positive experiences in childbirth (*see* discussion below). Part Four explores the metaphor of a "birth plan" for perinatal care focusing on the relationship between the provider and the woman as a means to understand expectations.

> When Samantha began to panic at 7 cm dilation, Alice, remembering her own natural labors, helped her with back massages and cool facecloths and nodded reassuringly when Dr. Epps started discussing options including anesthesia and amniotomy. Dr. Epps asked Alice and Jack about their prior experiences with labor and reassured them about Samantha's normal progress so far. They all worked with her with breathing and massage and position changes, and she tried the shower again before her water broke spontaneously when she was 9 cm dilated.

Having already articulated with the woman a birth plan with specifics about the delivery itself, the woman-centered provider reviews this care plan with the woman and her partner and any other family members during breaks between contractions earlier in labor. Some partners may be excited to cut the cord, while others may have no interest. If a partner is sensitive to blood, the provider can make sure a chair and perhaps an ammonia packet are readily available. The new mother may want to see her infant immediately and may appreciate delivery directly on to her abdomen; the provider can facilitate this by preparing the nursing staff so warm blankets can be available and positioned appropriately. If the circumstances warrant immediate evaluation of the newborn (i.e. in the event of an infant who does not breathe spontaneously), the woman-centered provider can anticipate many of the fears the new parents may experience when the infant is immediately brought to the warmer for resuscitative measures.

Many women expect support from a partner during active labor. The woman-centered clinician watches during labor how the pregnant woman interacts with her partner. Although the well-functioning healthcare team works to incorporate the partner and other family members into care strategies during active labor, the professionals need to remember both not to abdicate all emotional and physical support to the partner and also not to neglect his or her need for support, as well. Tensions in the woman's relationship with her partner may flare during the intensity of active labor or may be subsumed in the excitement of the arrival of a new family member. The task of the woman-centered clinician in coping with such tensions is to refocus all involved to the needs of the laboring woman and yet to remain sensitive to how such tension can impact on her anxiety, labor progress, and postpartum outcomes. Part Six will discuss further how to incorporate a partner into woman-centered care.

What do women expect from nursing staff during active labor? In one prospective study of primigravid women in childbirth classes, they expected nurses to offer physical support to keep the laboring woman as comfortable as possible, emotional support to stay calm, informational support to help with breathing and relaxation, and specific direct clinical care activities such as monitoring, assisting the physician, and dealing with any medications. The vast majority of women expected the nurse to be in the room most of the time during labor.[33] Samantha's nurse fulfills all these roles in supporting her through an unmedicated delivery.

The work of MacKinnon *et al.* further elucidates this expectation of nursing presence: "Women wanted the nurse to be available, to be emotionally involved, to help create a special moment, to hear and respond to their concerns, to share the responsibility for keeping them safe, and to act as a 'go-between' for their family and the medical institution."[34;32] Even the simple statement, "You're doing a good job", can help women feel empowered.[35] "You are so strong" is another empowering phrase. In settings where midwives provide primary labor and delivery care, women expect support from them.[27] In North America where physicians provide most labor and delivery care, women may not expect as much time or support from the doctor during labor. What women do hope for is some sense of feeling known and understood as a unique person.[34,36] This kind of individualized relationship establishes trust for the woman experiencing labor's physical intensity, a trust in her caregiver that permits her to focus on her own coping and not worry about her safety or that of her baby.[34]

How this hope for an individualized relationship relates to a woman's expectation of continuity during labor and delivery is complex. Most studies of continuity have been done in environments where midwives rather than physicians provide intrapartum care. Prospective studies of what women expect in labor[27] may give more weight to the importance of continuity than retrospective studies of what women actually experience during labor. (*See* further discussion of continuity in Part Six.) While women may expect that nursing and medical staff may change, particularly during a long labor, they remain aware of shift changes even in the throes of labor and can find these disruptive.[24] In the USA, for up to a third of women, the provider attending their delivery will be someone not well known to them or even someone they have never met before.[30] For a provider who is meeting a woman in labor for the first time, a few simple inquiries about the woman's past feelings, ideas, and expectations can help foster her feeling of uniqueness and trust. (*See* Sidebar: "Strategies to be Woman-Centered.")

Providers often do not recognize that during the course of a woman's labor they are participating in the construction of a birth narrative. Fortunate women may be able to realize the birth experience they hope for; others must make compromises as they discover the realities of labor or as the physiology of their own labor develops. Today, because so many births occur in highly technical environments with constant fetal monitoring, early epidural anesthesia, frequent induction, and predisposition to intervention, many birth experiences turn into surgical emergencies. Emergency cesarean section often redefines what happens into what *had to happen*. The woman's own agency disappears in the narrative of crisis. Nevertheless, whether the woman receives some or no medication, chooses an epidural, or undergoes an operative delivery, the goal of the woman-centered provider is still to render the birth narrative as an experience of empowerment. Usually, this task involves underscoring with words and actions the woman's strength and power during the labor and birth, however the baby emerges.

No two women have the same labor, and no woman has the same labor twice. The woman-centered provider perceives the laboring woman's anxieties and needs through observation, asks questions and listens carefully to the answers to estimate her thought process, then advocates for her as necessary. A labor suite can be a hectic, stressful place even during low-risk labor and delivery. Through all of this, using the model of assessing the woman's feelings, ideas, function, and expectations can provide a framework for staying woman-centered while maintaining the ultimate goal of a healthy mother and healthy baby. The woman-centered provider is optimally positioned to achieve this goal with the greatest satisfaction on all sides.

Strategies to be Woman-Centered when Meeting a Woman in Labor for the First Time

Feelings:

- What are you feeling right now when you have a contraction? (Don't take "pain" for an answer.)
- Tell me more about what you mean by that. Where do you feel it? What have you tried so far for that and how did it go? (The provider explains the physiology causing the feeling.)
- Some women are afraid. How about you? What part frightens you the most? (The provider describes ways to make that part less scary.)
- What hard or painful things have you done in the past? You can do this, too!

Ideas:

- Where does your mind go during contractions? (The provider can help her refocus if need be.)
- How did you hope your labor would be? Apart from a healthy baby, what is really important to you?

For primigravidas:

- Have you been at any deliveries? Seen movies? What was your dream about how your labor and delivery would be? Are there special things you know about that you want to happen at your delivery? (Offer support for her choices and encouragement for the hard work she is doing to try to make it happen.)

For multigravidas:

- How did your last delivery go?
- Are there things you'd like to be the same or different from that delivery? Are there things your doctor/midwife did/did not do that you would like me to do/ not do today?

Function: (In general, women can become more in charge if they are more upright or more in charge of position changes.)

- How would you like to try a change in position?
- How would you like to get up to the bathroom? The shower? The rocking chair?
- Let's see how your partner/labor coach can help you do something to feel stronger and more on top of this part of labor.
- Who is here with you and what is their relationship to you? (Learn the first names and relationship to the woman of everyone in the room and likely to come before delivery. When there is time, find out the maternity experiences of the other women present. For multiparous women, learn about other children and who is taking care of them.)
- How will you feed the baby? Would you like to breastfeed right away after delivery?
- (If woman is comfortable, inquire about work, school, plans for maternity leave, support after going home, planned contraception.)

Expectations:

- When you talked with your primary provider (use his or her name) about labor, what kinds of plans did you make? What were you thinking about pain control? Are there certain things that you definitely want or do not want to happen? (Address how realistic those expectations are given the clinical situation or setting.)
- Whom do you want to cut the cord?
- What do you know about what happens after the delivery? (Describe usual hospital routines that might apply in her situation.)

CHAPTER 7

Understanding the Normal Postpartum Experience

Sara G. Shields

THE FOURTH TRIMESTER

After a couple of hours of squatting, lunging, and kneeling, Ruth gave birth, with the midwife placing the baby right onto Ruth's chest so she and Lewis could greet the baby and then be the first to see that it was a boy. After a few minutes, Lewis cut the umbilical cord, and Ruth put Zachary to the breast right away. The placenta delivered easily, and the midwife prepared to suture Ruth's second-degree perineal laceration. It was not bleeding much, so the midwife offered Ruth the option of waiting until she was done nursing. The midwife reminded the new parents about their desire to take some early photos, and then Lewis held Zachary while the midwife repaired Ruth's tear, helped clean up the various supplies, showed them the placenta, and then examined the baby now back in his mother's arms.

When Pat had her cesarean delivery, Mike accompanied her into the operating room (OR) and was able to help Pat hold baby Madeline skin-to-skin right away while the doctors were finishing her surgery. Pat immediately felt a bond but was also quite nauseated and uncomfortable while still in the OR. In the recovery room, she felt that all the various tubing for intravenous lines and blood pressure monitors made it hard to move around, let alone hold Madeline comfortably. Her sore incision also made it hard to get comfortable breastfeeding. Moving around in the bed and later trying to get out of bed for the first time were difficult even with Mike's help and encouragement.

After an uncomplicated hospital stay, Kerry, Ron, and Erika went home with both their families visiting and helping out. Kerry had planned to take three months off and to return only to substitute teaching, to stay home longer with the baby. She found, however, that she missed both the classroom and the adult companionship of her fellow teachers, and by six weeks negotiated a half-day position at her old school where she could still be home in the afternoon with Erika. Ron's mother had offered to help with childcare. Ron, proud of his wife and baby, accompanied Kerry to her postpartum visit to help with Erika while Kerry had her pelvic exam. They mentioned to Larisa that Ron's new business had finally taken off, however, and he was incredibly busy, leaving before dawn and arriving home exhausted at dark, with little energy left for Kerry or Erika. Ron was feeling guilty but did not remember his own father doing much of the work of fathering the small child, and did not really know how to be different. Larisa, remembering their prenatal conversation, reminded Ron what he had been able to do to help out before his work got so busy, and suggested that maybe they could figure out a way to work around Erika's sleeping and feeding schedule and Ron's morning hours. They decided that Ron could take the baby after her morning nursing, dress her and prepare her for the day before he left; Kerry could take her to Ron's mother's house on the way to work, with Ron then picking Erika up on his late lunch break to bring her to Kerry at the end of her day. Both liked the feel of this plan. Ron lagged a minute after Kerry went out with the baby to thank Larisa. "You make me feel like a real dad."

Woman-centered postpartum care primarily addresses a woman's physical and emotional transition to motherhood. The challenge for all providers caring for women in this time is to balance focusing on the newborn infant's needs with empowering women in their new role as responsible caregivers. The interdependence of the mother–infant dyad in these first few weeks after birth means that addressing the infant's health and well-being necessarily includes incorporating the mother's issues, so that even pediatric providers need to be woman-centered. The other main challenge of this transition time is for woman-centered providers to recognize both how common physical and psychological difficulties are for postpartum women, and how little women discuss all their symptoms with their providers.[30] Staying woman-centered means acknowledging the full range of possible experiences for a new mother through thoughtful inquiry about her feelings, ideas, function, and expectations.

The postpartum experience has a clear beginning but a less well-defined ending; this time of major transition therefore becomes a continuum with individualized endpoints. The traditional definition of a six-week postpartum period involves medical belief about return to a non-pregnant physiologic state (i.e. complete uterine involution occurs at about this time), with a focus on recovery of reproductive organs rather than the successful psychological transitions of new motherhood.[37] Interestingly, many cultures use a similar time frame for defining this transition of about 40 days (*la cuarentena* for instance, in many Spanish-speaking countries).[38,39] In general the major aspects of a woman's postpartum adjustment initially involve learning to care for the newborn including breastfeeding demands, fitting the newborn into the rest of the family, undergoing physical changes including sleep deprivation and sexuality issues, and at some point a "return to normal" that includes a new lifelong self-definition as a mother.[40]

FEELINGS

Just as during prenatal care and delivery, the postpartum task of the woman-centered provider is to be open to hearing the individual woman's expression of the many often conflicting emotions that surface postpartum. Media portrayals of new mothers' contented spiritual fulfillment notwithstanding, many women around the world (up to 25% of postpartum women in the United States) experience negative feelings after giving birth, including feeling tired, messy, unsure, isolated, sad, discouraged, or confused.[30] Providers should avoid assumptions about either positive or negative feelings and inquire with open-ended, normalizing, non-directive statements such as "Many women normally feel lots of different emotions in these first few weeks, as if they are on a roller-coaster. What sorts of feelings have you been having?" Larisa can encourage Kerry to express not just her joy in Erika's birth and development but also her unexpected feelings of needing ongoing adult companionship and more shared responsibility for the demands of newborn care. "It's sometimes hard to talk about unexpected feelings in these first few weeks. There are a lot of 'shoulds' about how new mothers feel about the baby or about the other people and tasks still in their lives. How are you doing with this?"

Normalizing negative postpartum emotions includes discussion of postpartum blues, a transient mood change that occurs within the first week of delivery for the majority of women. "Baby blues" symptoms include overwhelming feelings, mood swings, fatigue, irritability, anxiety, and crying spells; none of this affects the mother's ability to care for her infant. Anticipating these feelings, the woman-centered provider reviews the basics of baby blues with the new mother and her family. Framing the normalcy of these symptoms as part of the continuum of a new mother's transition, the provider recognizes how these negative emotions can surprise women and also undermine their self-definition as a mother: "You may think there is something wrong with you because everyone around you thinks you should be always blissfully happy with a beautiful newborn baby. But this is a challenging time with a lot of different emotions, and normal worries about your baby's health. Feeling unhappy or frustrated does not mean you are a bad mother." A woman-centered approach to postpartum depression will be discussed further in Chapter 10 of Section Two.

While remaining open to negative emotions, woman-centered providers also seek every opportunity in postpartum care to boost whatever feelings of competence most new mothers begin to have.[30] For instance, given the predominance of postpartum sleep deprivation for new parents, with resultant feelings of disorganization or slowed function, Larisa can say to Kerry, "Having a newborn can make new parents really tired so they don't feel like they think straight. In spite of that, you've been able to get you and the baby here today on time, with everything you know you need for a newborn. You're doing a great job learning to be a mother!"

IDEAS

> After phone calls to family, Ruth was ready to eat, surprised by how hungry and thirsty she felt. While Zachary rested in the bassinette they had prepared, Lewis prepared a light meal, and the midwife helped Ruth to the bathroom. She felt a lot of symptoms suddenly: her legs were wobbly, her stitches stung, her uterus was cramping, and she wondered if her vaginal bleeding was heavier than it should have been.

> Pat and Mike were both anxious about Madeline's breathing and skin in spite of reassurance from the nursing staff and Dr. Miller.

Exploring a new mother's ideas about the postpartum time again requires that the woman-centered provider refocus on the mother, not just the infant, while still respecting the primacy of the dyad. While many of the mother's ideas may relate to the infant's health and symptoms, the mother nonetheless needs to have a way to express her explanations and thoughts about common postpartum issues such as fatigue, bleeding, nutrition needs, and contraception. Given the cultural roots of most postpartum rituals and explanations, these concepts are discussed further in Part Three's discussion of woman-centered care exploring the cultural context of this period.

Women may have many unmet informational needs after childbirth, whether or not they had any prenatal education about postpartum issues. These gaps can include obvious physiologic issues such as the expected duration of lochia (vaginal discharge), the changes in breast milk over the first few days, or perineal care methods, but women also want discussion about often overlooked topics such as diet, exercise, and fatigue.[41] Multiparous women may want more information about dealing with older children and may feel more comfortable with baby care so ask more about self-care. New mothers and fathers both wish for more information about sexuality in the later postpartum period.[41] For the initial postpartum time, the woman-centered clinician develops a flexible but comprehensive "postpartum talk" to review the individual woman's needs, using the FIFE method (*see* Sidebar: "Postpartum Discharge Talk"). This discussion includes the infant care for those providers who will continue providing care to the baby as well as the mother.

Postpartum Discharge Talk (using FIFE)

Before you go home, I would like to discuss several issues with you about your care and your baby's care. Before I start, I wonder if there are any specific questions that you have about yourself or the baby. Also, please remind me of your baby's name.

Those are great questions. There are a few other topics I'd just like to review with you. You may have heard about some of this from other people, too. You also may not remember everything I'm going to say, and that's okay. We'll talk about other ways for you to get your questions answered once you go home. Many women have lots more questions once they're home that they didn't remember to ask or didn't realize they needed to ask.

One of your jobs as a new mom is to figure out when and how to get advice about yourself or the baby if you have questions, and when is something worrisome enough to call the doctor. How do you think you'll figure that out?

Feelings: Many women feel a lot of different emotions – excitement yet fatigue, happiness about the new baby, yet worry about how everyone's doing. It can even be normal to feel sad and cry some. We call that "baby blues," and most women get that in the first week or so. But if those feelings stay on, or if you're feeling so sad that you can't take care of yourself or the baby, or you want to hurt yourself, then this may be more of a postpartum depression. Let us know if you are feeling that way.

In terms of feelings, you'll learn about your baby's different feelings. Pay attention to his or her different cries. Sometimes s/he is hungry, sometimes s/he is cold or wet or has a dirty diaper, sometimes s/he wants to be held or wrapped snugly.

Ideas: Is there anything about the birth that you are wondering about or that you didn't understand?

Tell me some about what you know about how to take care of yourself in these first few weeks.

What are your ideas right now about contraception?

There is lots of information about taking care of your son/daughter. You've probably heard certain things from the nurses, and from the baby videos. You'll probably hear more from family and friends after you go home. Are you reading any books about baby care? Sometimes people say different things about baby care, so one of your jobs as a parent is to learn and to choose what makes sense for you and your baby.

Here are a few basic safety issues to think about: sleeping, car seat, fever, shaken baby.

Here are a few things I'd like you to call us about if you're experiencing them: too much bleeding, sore breasts, fever.

Function: Let's talk about diet and activity. What have you heard? What have people told you, or what have you read? (Expand to support and recommend depending on clinical situation. Encourage rest, support, time for self).

Let's talk about breastfeeding and sexual function. What have you heard? What have people told you, or what have you read? (Elaborate based on understanding and information for the clinical situation. Support knowledge base when accurate).

Expectations: Who will be helping you out at home? When are you expecting to return to work/school?

Many people expect the baby to sleep a lot. But right now the baby is getting used to a new world and has a very small stomach. So s/he needs to eat regularly, more often than you think, and also needs contact with you through the night. That's pretty tiring for moms and dads.

Do you know how to reach your baby's healthcare provider if you need to after you go home? Do you know when your baby's first appointment is?

Even though Dr. Miller had maximized Pat's and Mike's control over the decision-making that led to her cesarean, he still thought she might be disappointed not to have had a vaginal delivery and might feel that she herself had somehow been inadequate to the challenge. He thought hard about how best to address these emotions and decided to talk through with her on the first day postpartum how she felt about the whole labor and delivery experience.

Postpartum debriefing is one method of exploring a woman's ideas. The idea behind structured retelling of birth stories comes from strategies in the psychiatric literature for trauma or disaster survivors to undergo formal crisis counseling in hopes of abating long-term mental health effects. The few randomized trials of postnatal debriefing provide conflicting results about its benefit, with one study suggesting less short-term anxiety and depression[42] and others showing no benefit and possibly increased depression rates in women who had debriefing.[43–5] However, women's subjective experience in one study was that the chance to discuss their birth story was helpful.[45] Thus, the woman-centered approach suggests that at least some women may benefit from telling their birth stories to a trained provider. At a minimum, the postpartum provider may want to clarify at various points in the postpartum period (immediately in the first few days after birth, again at the early newborn or well woman visits, and again later in the woman's first postpartum year) whether there was any part of the delivery experience that the woman did not understand or would like explained further. One suggested structure for empathic inquiry about birth narratives is shown in Box 2.2.[46]

BOX 2.2 Ground rules for reviewing birth experiences with new mothers (Adapted from Callister, 2004)[46]

- Start with open-ended questions such as "Tell me about your experience."
- Respond by asking the mother to elaborate with questions such as "How was that for you?" or "Can you give me an example?"
- Listen for expressions of frustration, sadness, or confusion. Allow the mother to express such feelings, affirming them and not just focusing on the "facts" of her birth experience, and then clarify why an intervention or action may have been necessary.

- If the mother expresses any sense of personal failure, help her identify strengths, endurance, and coping ability.
- Learn what the mother would want to do differently with birth experiences in the future.

FUNCTION

Susan the runner chose to go home on her first postpartum day, feeling confident about breastfeeding and about home support. She was surprised to find that climbing the stairs to her bedroom the first day home was more tiring than she expected, and she spent most of the first few days letting her partner bring her meals and getting out of bed just to rock the baby or use the bathroom. Every time she coughed, sneezed, or even lifted the baby, she involuntarily leaked urine; the leaking made her feel particularly desperate since it had been her main preoccupation about vaginal birth to begin with. The visiting nurse who came to check her and the baby recommended that Susan start doing Kegel exercises right away. She continued to feel stiff and sore with stair climbing but was anxious to get back to some physical exercise so by one week postpartum tried to go out for a short walk with the baby briefly each day.

Clearly, a new mother's function changes in dramatic ways in both the immediate postpartum period as well as throughout the early months with a new child. In spite of these obvious changes, new mothers often do not report the quantity or quality of their physical or psychological changes to their providers.[11,30] Furthermore, functional status postpartum has not been well-defined or well-studied.[37] One possible definition for postpartum function involves the mother's integration of her new maternal role with her other household and work duties and her resumption of self-care activities.[47] Woman-centered care routinely addresses these dimensions of postpartum function. While it is easy to jump straight to questions about physical, sexual, and work function, the woman-centered provider remembers to assess the new mother's feelings and ideas in order to provide a framework for understanding her function.

The most obvious physical changes for a postpartum woman relate to genitourinary issues such as temporary incontinence or perineal pain, but other physical symptoms such as backache, hemorrhoids or other bowel concerns, and even upper respiratory infection are common, too.[48] Judith asks Susan, "How are you getting around? What physical activities would you like to resume but have not felt able to?"

Melissa worried about baby Martin's cephalohematoma when she first held him. Larisa reassured her and commented on how eagerly Martin rooted at Melissa's breast in spite of his difficult start. Melissa was surprised how tender her nipples felt at first and had to work with the nurses over the first few days on different breastfeeding positions and other nipple-care routines.

> After Danny Jr. was born, Siobhan did not get to hold him for a little while but was so tired that she did not mind getting some rest and asked the nurse to give him a bottle. She tried to breastfeed for a few days but stopped when she became frustrated over her inverted nipples and apparent lack of milk. She had thought she could adjust to breastfeeding in front of others, but when she had to add the nipple shield (and then the additional tubing), it became too much for her.

> When Rosa and Eva came to the baby's one-month visit, Eva was thriving, but Dr. Rosen noticed that Rosa was giving a bottle in spite of her leaking breasts. When he inquired about this, Rosa said that she was planning to return to work the next day. He mentioned that Rosa could pump milk for the baby, but Rosa looked at him blankly. He called Lupe to help him understand, and she reminded him that Rosa worked in a setting where there were no facilities for privacy to pump, and that (as an undocumented immigrant) her limited insurance coverage for the pregnancy and delivery did not cover the cost of a breast pump or rental.

Breastfeeding is the physical function most unique to the postpartum period and is emblematic of the biological dyad of mother and infant. Whether the provider is primarily caring for the mother or for the newborn or both, supporting breastfeeding with accurate information and skilled assistance is critical to a woman-centered approach. Ideally, both the maternity and pediatric providers have had opportunities during the prenatal process to encourage and educate about breastfeeding. For Siobhan's provider, this role includes recognizing her inverted nipples and beginning discussion about a postpartum plan to facilitate latching on in spite of this physical challenge.

To be truly woman-centered, this facilitation process has to continue into the crucial immediate postpartum period and beyond. Both Ruth's midwife and Larisa assist each new mother with getting her son to the breast as soon as possible, even during the perineal repair if the mother desires that. This early nursing not only emphasizes ideal health for the babies but also in Melissa's case can help alleviate some of her disappointment about needing a vacuum-assisted delivery. Larisa can emphasize, "You have the perfect milk that Martin needs right now, and look how the two of you can get this going right away together."

For Rosa who must return to work in employment that does not facilitate breastfeeding, Dr. Rosen can help her think through options other than complete weaning; ideally, such a discussion happens well before her return to work. At every pediatric or adult medical contact during a woman's first postpartum year, the woman-centered approach routinely asks about breastfeeding in relation to issues like sleep or medications.

A woman-centered approach to breastfeeding addresses more than the medical aspects of latching, timing, duration, and milk quantity, however. Applying the FIFE method to the complexities of this postpartum function enables the provider to both normalize a woman's breastfeeding experience as well empower her about lactation within her life context. Ideally, the clinician begins this discussion prenatally and then continues it during the critical immediate postpartum period when so many women struggle with initiating lactation. Throughout, the provider goes beyond simply asking, "Are you planning to breast or bottle feed your baby?" or "How often and for how long are you nursing? Is the baby gaining weight?" Using empowering, encouraging language to explore various aspects of the breastfeeding experience,[49,50] the provider seeks to understand the entire process of breastfeeding, not just its outcomes.[51] Woman-centered breastfeeding care takes time,[52] but even a busy provider can address common feelings, ideas, function, and expectations with a few key questions integrated with observation of breastfeeding.

Women may have strong feelings positively or negatively about breastfeeding, with some viewing the experience as the ultimate in motherly bonding and others finding it too demanding, distasteful, or too sexual. For many a new mother, how she nourishes her newborn touches deeply-held feelings of success or failure as a woman. When breastfeeding initiation goes well, the new mother can feel a sense of harmony, balance and rhythm with her body and her infant, and feel satisfied with being able to comfort and nourish her growing infant.[53] Any perceived "failure," however, whether in the newborn's response or the mother's milk production, may elicit disappointment, guilt, or even feelings of rejection.[54]

When Siobhan struggles with complicated methods to supplement, she may feel confused and overwhelmed, questioning, "Am I doing this right? Am I good enough at this?" She may fear that somehow she is "starving" her baby or that "the baby doesn't like me." Given how maternal tension potentially affects hormonal letdown and other lactation physiology, the provider needs to elicit, validate, and then problem-solve around these negative emotions. Siobhan's provider can thus reframe her self-doubt and frustrations by emphasizing her strengths and her capacity to make healthy choices: "You're working so hard to do the best for your baby in a way that will work for you also – what a great mother you are!"

> Mariana was a Brazilian first-time mother who had just given birth to Veronica after induction for mild pre-eclampsia and gestational diabetes. The first few times Mariana tried to nurse baby Veronica, she struggled to position the baby comfortably, and found that the initial suckling was intensely painful. Her nipples felt cracked and dry after the first couple of feedings. She worried that Veronica was not satisfied and wondered how else to comfort her. When Dr. Miller visited on the first postpartum day, Mariana asked about supplementing, saying she was not sure she could handle the nipple soreness and that she thought the baby needed more milk. (*See* full vignette in Appendix.)

The link between a breastfeeding woman's physical feelings and emotions is also a critical aspect of understanding her experience. For many women, the physical closeness with the newborn during breastfeeding symbolizes the unique intensity of maternal bonding. The physiologic hormonal changes of letdown can cause physical relaxation or calming. When the initial moments and days of breastfeeding cause physical pain, however, with cracked nipples or engorgement, coping with these unexpected sensations may again invoke anxiety that then interferes with letdown.

> Dr. Miller discussed lactation physiology with Mariana briefly on the first post-partum day, and on the day of discharge arrived to see Mariana when both her mother and her mother-in-law were there waiting to take her home. He invited questions from the grandmothers about how both Mariana and Veronica were doing and learned that neither grandmother had breastfed her children. Dr. Miller with the interpreter's assistance reviewed lactation and addressed the grandmothers' questions.

Particularly in the first few days of breastfeeding, a woman hears multiple messages from family and support people about how to feed her newborn. Key questions from her provider address these sources of information: "Who in your family or among your friends has breastfed before? How did it go for them? What are they saying to you now about breastfeeding?" Women whose mothers and grandmothers did not breastfeed may have mistaken ideas about how lactation occurs or what the benefits are. They may hear different strongly held beliefs about the symbolic meaning of breastfeeding, either romanticizing the nurturing and bonding aspects or emphasizing the potential restriction that "no one else can feed the baby."

> Melissa also struggled at first with sore nipples during breastfeeding. Kirk helped her find extra pillows to prop herself more comfortably, and took on the diaper changing after each feeding. He listened carefully when the nurses worked with Melissa over the first few days on different breastfeeding positions and other nipple-care routines.

The woman's perception of support from the baby's father strongly affects her ideas about breastfeeding.[55-7] (*See* Part Six for further discussion.) Women may want the baby's father to take on more responsibility in feeding the baby and thus wonder how that can happen with breastfeeding. Women may have specific worries about temporary or permanent changes in their breasts after breastfeeding, and how that will affect their sexual image or their partner's perception of their sexuality. The provider can correct misinformation and also emphasize the other ways that support people can assist a breastfeeding mother, such as bringing her what she needs to get comfortable while breastfeeding, diaper changing, or watching older siblings while she focuses on the newborn.

Even women who have read extensively about breastfeeding may find the reality of lactation challenging. Melissa, with all her book knowledge about different positions and latching strategies, struggles with how hard it is to get the full areola into Martin's mouth. In these early postpartum days, women may need different strategies of teaching: some women may do well with written information, while others may feel too busy or in too much pain to read.[52] Consistent messages about technique or supplementing can avoid confusion for the new mother when multiple staff members are providing breastfeeding education and assistance.

> On the first postpartum day, Dr. Miller suggested that Mariana try breastfeeding while the nurse was there so that he could observe and help problem-solve. While Mariana was working to position Veronica, the nurse asked, "OK if I help with getting her to latch by touching your breasts? I'll try to be gentle. Let me know if it's too uncomfortable."

Ideas about body privacy or modesty may influence a woman's decision to breastfeed or her comfort with breastfeeding.[54] Women who feel modest about their breasts may feel embarrassed both about exposure during breastfeeding but also about milk leakage or draining.[49,50,54] Staff trying to assist women with the physical aspects of breastfeeding by positioning the breast need to be sensitive to women's modesty or discomfort about physical touch – some women perceive a nurse's assistance as "grabbing" their breast or being rough with the newborn.[54] Nonetheless, mothers need to practice the positioning and holding of the newborn after the nurse demonstrates; otherwise they may not feel comfortable in doing it themselves after discharge.[52]

Women also may have specific ideas about duration of breastfeeding and when to start supplementing, particularly as they think ahead about integrating lactation into their daily functions.[49,50] New mothers who anticipate returning to employment or school may feel daunted by pumping and storing breast milk. As noted above, others may want family members to participate more in feeding the infant in order to allow the mother more sleep or respite from the demands of newborn care. However, support people may feel ill-equipped to help with a nursing infant because they feel uncertain about how to comfort a hungry infant.[49,50]

> Because Samantha was an adolescent mother, she received maternity care coordination with Shereen, a postpartum case worker. Shereen visited Samantha while she was still staying at her cousin Alice's house one week after Kyle was born to check on them. Samantha was tired, but doing well and still seemed on a "high" about having a new baby. She had wanted to breastfeed, but did not feel that she had enough milk, and Alice had suggested that she give the baby formula, too, which she had been doing. Samantha believed this was helping Kyle sleep better and be less hungry and fussy.
>
> Shereen asked Samantha if she felt that Kyle was happy and healthy. Samantha replied, "I think he may be too skinny." She wondered if this might have been her fault because she had not gained much weight and had smoked throughout pregnancy. She added, "I don't think my milk is 'rich' enough for him." She also admitted that at this point she was doing pretty much what Alice told her to do because she had been so helpful through the pregnancy.

Finally, the woman-centered provider uncovers and addresses any unrealistic expectations about breastfeeding. One common myth relates to how much milk is available right at birth, with new mothers anxious about the infant's apparent hunger and their own apparent lack of supply. This anxiety couples with the need that many women (or support people) have to know precisely the amount of the infant's intake.[54]

Inadequacy of milk supply is one of the most common reasons given for early cessation of breastfeeding.[58-60] Sometimes the mother's perception of inadequate supply leads her to begin supplementing with formula, leading into the physiological cycle of decreased milk production once the infant becomes accustomed to artificial nipples and formula and suckles less from the mother. Even for women who continue exclusively breastfeeding beyond the initial newborn period, the times of predictable infant growth spurts (at about three weeks, six weeks, and three months of age, for example) when babies seem insatiable again, are also vulnerable times for women to stop breastfeeding or supplement because they feel they cannot keep up or are "starving" their infants. The woman-centered provider can correct misperceptions about how much volume of milk a newborn actually needs, can offer reassurance that the exact quantity is less important than how the infant responds in terms of hydration and growth, and can anticipate growth spurts with suggestions for how to cope and information about the expected duration of such frequent feedings.

Other unrealistic expectations derive from some women's belief that breastfeeding should not hurt, nor take a long time, nor be difficult for a newborn who has innate suckling reflexes since lactation is "natural" or "automatic." Women may not expect the reality of fussy, irritable infants or the unpredictability or the "relative insecurity of breastfeeding."[54] Women may not expect how time-consuming or physically challenging breastfeeding is.[61] For some mothers "sleeping through the night" may be the major marker of a successful feeding regimen,[51] leading to formula supplementation in hopes of achieving this goal.

With multiparous women, the provider needs to find out about their prior lactation experiences and how they would like to change or keep the same aspects for this newborn. Again, the questions go beyond only "Have you breastfed before?" to include also, "How did that go for you? What made it easy or hard for you? What are you planning this time that might be different or the same?" Some breastfeeding advice has changed over the years, such as the use of vitamin supplementation or nipple shields, so that multiparous women may need updated information. They may also have concerns about older siblings' reactions and needs when the newborn is nursing.

> When Dr. Miller met with Pat and Mike for discharge planning on the third postpartum day, he reviewed what they had discussed prenatally about postpartum birth control options. He nodded when Pat and Mike both said, "Wow, after all we just went through, having sex again seems a long way off." He asked, "What are your thoughts about when you want to be ready to have sex again?" As they discussed this, he also inquired, "What do you expect from each other about this? What do you think about birth control that will work for you?"

The woman-centered provider also asks about postpartum sexual function within the context of changes in the woman's relationship. (*See* Part Six.) While such a topic needs to include advice about contraception, a woman-centered discussion moves beyond birth control methods into more detailed inquiry exploring the common issues of relationship changes, the new mother's body image, and changes in sexual desire. Such alterations are common and under-reported, with up to half of women in the first three months postpartum reporting dyspareunia and decreased libido,[37] often lasting throughout the first year postpartum.[62] Traditional postpartum advice about resuming vaginal intercourse has been to wait six weeks, which corresponds with the *cuarentena* or other culturally based rules about abstinence for new mothers.[38,39] Woman-centered providers individualize advice in this area, knowing that many couples may not wait six weeks to resume sexual relations; that late pregnancy and postpartum can be times when male partners have other partners; and finally that women need to feel empowered to decide when and how to have sex for the first time after delivery.

Employment issues for women after childbirth are another important functional issue that woman-centered providers confront in various ways in the postpartum period. The woman-centered provider is aware that the moment when the woman's partner or other support returns to outside work can be challenging for a new mother, now coping with primary responsibility for an infant with minimal assistance. Larisa openly discusses such role changes and balances with both Kerry and Ron, in order to empower each of them. The return to employment and the subsequent balancing act may increase women's stress and subsequent physical and mental symptoms more in the later postpartum period.[37] Providers need to remember to inquire about such stress throughout these postpartum months. This topic will be further discussed in Part Three.

> Mariana's family went home with plans for a home visit by a nurse the next day and an office visit five days later. The home nurse's written report arrived at Dr. Miller's office on that appointment day, and noted that breastfeeding was going well with mother pumping for one bottle a day. At the office visit, with Roberto and both grandmothers present, along with Mariana, Veronica was alert and vigorous and had regained her birth weight. Mariana's mother was holding the baby, and Roberto's mother had packed the diaper bag and knew where to find everything.

Finally, a new mother's function changes in terms of her life-cycle stage and role. First-time mothers change generations with the birth of their first child, and multiparous women with subsequent births take on the role of parenting more than one child and juggling sibling relationships. For the woman-centered provider who has seen the woman through pregnancy, understanding this aspect of family function postpartum will follow having explored prenatally expectations of such change. After delivery, the provider might ask, "How are you doing with all these tasks of motherhood?"

EXPECTATIONS

What do women expect in both the first few days and the first few months postpartum? Again, the task of the woman-centered provider is to link the new mother's expectations about the infant with those about herself, and not neglect attention to the latter. Thus the provider needs to ask not only "Is your son or daughter what you expected?" but also, "How is being a new mother [or the mother of two, three, etc.] so far? What about it were you expecting? What seems most surprising to you about being a mother?"

After the intensity of the last few weeks of prenatal care, the focus on the new mother in the prenatal period and the attention that everyone places on the life-changing experience of the birth itself, women may not expect the redirected focus on the infant rather than themselves. Suddenly, their contact with the medical system goes from weekly visits with a known provider to one or two visits in the next six to eight weeks. While studies of the benefits of intensive home visiting or formal postpartum support have had mixed results in terms of preventing postpartum depression, much of the research has been done in the UK, where regular visits from a nurse or midwife in the immediate postpartum period are standard. For low-income women in the USA, support in the form of consistent home visiting by a single nurse beginning during pregnancy and continuing until the child is three years old has shown unequivocal benefits well beyond the postpartum period. A continuous caring relationship with a home-visiting nurse correlates with improved outcomes in employment, child spacing, psychological functioning, and child health and behavior outcomes.[63-6] To alleviate feelings of isolation or loneliness, prenatal providers can make referrals for home visits by nurses when available and encourage women to seek out postpartum support groups or new mothers' groups, including offering specific linkages and reiterating during immediate postpartum care the potential benefit of such peer support.

Women may have unrealistic expectations about their own physical recovery from childbirth. Even women with normal vaginal deliveries may not expect the extent of their muscle soreness, breast discomfort, exhaustion or fatigue, or genitourinary morbidity such as incontinence. These unanticipated symptoms may surface even more for women with assisted vaginal deliveries or even uncomplicated cesareans.[37] For women like Pat who have never had major surgery, recovery from a cesarean brings many unanticipated feelings and symptoms. With the increasing frequency of operative deliveries, the woman-centered provider stays attuned to the discordance between expectations and experience postpartum for such mothers: "I know that you were not expecting a cesarean section. What do you expect in your recovery?" While recognizing the limitations of standardized checklists, providers can inquire specifically about a woman's self-perceived readiness for discharge using a structured format that assesses multiple domains of her experience including pain, strength, energy, mood, functional ability, and self and baby care knowledge.[67-8]

Women have multiple diverse expectations about newborn care. Depending on an individual woman's prior experience with infants, these expectations may be more or less realistic. Sleep is a major issue. The clinician can begin to address prenatally the normal range of newborn sleep habits and encourage each woman to anticipate how she might cope with interrupted sleep. The clinician can avoid the common trap of asking new mothers first, "Is the baby sleeping through the night yet?" or defining babies as "good" if they sleep longer, which can lead women to wonder about their parenting adequacy and blame themselves for "bad" habits that are in fact normal newborn waking cycles. An alternate question that avoids implying maternal or infant "failure" is to ask, "How is the baby sleeping? How is that going for you?"

> At Mariana's office visit with baby Veronica, everyone had lots of questions about her mild facial rash, her yellow stools, and her sneezing. Dr. Miller, observing how Mariana cradled her daughter closely and cooed back at the baby's wide awake eyes, commented, "Veronica seems to know how lucky she is to have all of you caring for her. You are already an expert at comforting her, Mariana." He reviewed normal newborn issues and added, "Moms and dads often have lots of worries and concerns about the baby in these first few days and weeks. Let's talk about some of the ways Veronica can communicate with you, even at this age, and about how you can figure out when to call to get more help."

Rather than setting themselves up as the authority on all newborn care or intimidating vulnerable mothers with their professional expertise, providers can guide new mothers in reading their newborns' cues and developing their own parenting strategies. Throughout discussion of what to expect in the newborn period, the clinician can emphasize the normalcy of the range of emotions and of the likelihood of unexpected issues. Anticipating and reviewing coping strategies in advance can empower her later even in moments when she might feel inadequate as a mother.[69]

Women often internalize the extent to which society expects a mother to assume without difficulty the primary burden of newborn care, so that when such care becomes overwhelming, the new mother feels she has failed to meet such expectations. Providers thus need to understand both the woman's own expectations of this responsibility as well as the social context in order to more fully assess potential feelings such as powerlessness, inadequacy, guilt, loss, exhaustion, ambivalence, anger, and resentment.[40] The woman's life context significantly influences the degree of dissonance between expectation and reality, as noted by this physician's personal experience:

> After a short and uncomplicated labor and delivery in a birth center, with our daughter vigorous and healthy, my husband and I chose to go home after just six hours because a longer stay would have meant separation from my husband. He had to return to work within two days due to sudden work crises demanding his presence, and I was left alone with this tiny, hungry, crying creature.
>
> Even as a professional working with pregnant and postpartum women, even as someone used to frequent sleep deprivation, I had not anticipated the incredible personal challenges of the unrelenting constancy and immediacy of care necessary in the first few weeks with a newborn. Furthermore, after years of deriving my self-definition from my work setting and from my work colleagues, I abruptly had almost no contact with them (they were all working full time!) or with others since I had had little time to develop a social network in this new town. Struggling with a colicky baby, minimal support, and my own high self-expectations about

what new motherhood was supposed to involve (wasn't this supposed to be joyful and thrilling and priceless time home with my baby?), I felt lonely and isolated. I sought various social contacts: I found the La Leche League in my town, but did not connect with their "stay-at-home-mom" message and knew I was moving soon; I went to a few drop-in "mom and baby" sessions at the birth center to meet other new moms, but again knew that I would soon be more than an hour away from that site.

Isolation of the new mother in the postpartum period is all too common in Western developed countries where many couples live far away from either side of grandparents or any siblings. Addressing the loneliness and isolation experienced by the new mother is an often-unmentioned task of the woman-centered clinician. If familial support is available, women may have high expectations of partner and family support in these first days to months postpartum. Parts Three and Six will explore these relationship issues further.

Problems in Pregnancy

Each of the dimensions of the subjective experience of pregnancy becomes especially critical to consider when medical problems occur. When women experience infertility or abnormal or complicated pregnancies involving miscarriage, the diagnosis of fetal anomalies, preterm labor and delivery, prolonged labor, emergency cesarean section, or postpartum depression, the woman-centered clinician needs to elicit each woman's feelings, ideas, function, and expectations. The clinician in these complex and often urgent moments helps a woman cope with the uncertainties and unpredictabilities of the clinical course by being empathic and taking additional time both to allow verbal and non-verbal expressions of feelings, and to repeat or clarify complicated information. Throughout, woman-centeredness means empowering a woman through these problematic experiences in ways that add to her self-confidence and self-esteem, so that "a healthy mother [can] be born."[36:28]

One key issue in addressing a woman's feelings about complicated pregnancy is to recognize the potential for self-blame or guilt when pregnancy goes awry. The emphasis in contemporary obstetric care on possibly modifiable risk factors (*see* Part Five) can covertly or overtly blame women who do not change potentially risky behaviors, particularly when untoward outcomes occur. The woman-centered clinician inquires non-judgmentally about this emotion with the goal of defusing the woman's likely self-blame. Acknowledging the fear and uncertainty about sudden, unpredictable complications is also essential in woman-centered care at this time. The intensity of fear and anxiety may overwhelm the woman's capacity to make urgent decisions, so that the challenge for her provider becomes not only permitting her to express such emotions but also allowing time to revisit decisions and information-sharing when possible. When a complication and especially a loss occur, women and their partners may blame the medical care system and their providers especially since they often receive unclear, indirect, and conflicting messages in the course of the diagnosis; for instance, of a threatened abortion that becomes an inevitable abortion.

Inquiring about a woman's explanatory models for pregnancy complications includes understanding the assumptions of normalcy that many women have about pregnancy. These assumptions involve not only medical normalcy but also psychological normalcy in terms of a woman's ideas about her innate capacity for healthy motherhood.

Many complications of pregnancy directly impact on a woman's functioning in both home and work spheres. Hospitalization or recommendations for bedrest or curtailing of activities can significantly affect both women's employment security and women's caretaking roles within families. The woman-centered clinician incorporates a knowledge of these roles into the woman's care plan during complicated pregnancies.

Finally, women experiencing pregnancy complications have a wide range of expectations of the healthcare system during their care. Some women may expect their medical providers to "do all you can," while others may favor "letting nature take its course," and others may change their expectations as the dynamic clinical situation unfolds. When things go wrong or do not turn out well, dashed expectations may lead to anger at the system and specific individuals within it, and may result in the choice to litigate. The woman-centered clinician's task is to ask about expectations not only initially but also throughout the care, revisiting issues during any clinical changes.

CHAPTER 1

The Experience of Pregnancy and Chronic Disease

Sara G. Shields

Ann was a 26-year-old woman married for a year and wanting to get pregnant. However, she developed perplexing symptoms of joint pains, facial rashes and fatigue, and eventually, after multiple medical visits and tests, was diagnosed with lupus, with kidney complications. As she and her husband Joe struggled with adjusting to this chronic illness, they wondered about their plans for pregnancy and parenting. The nephrologist was worried about how active her disease seemed to be and recommended that before conceiving she meet with a perinatologist in consultation to discuss the risks in pregnancy and the potential fetal risks of her various medications. Ann herself felt guilty that she could not be the wife and mother that Joe had hoped for, and became quite depressed; their primary care internist recommended both individual and couples' counseling with Joe to address the strain on their marriage that such issues caused. When Ann's symptoms finally abated on treatment, she felt strong enough to cope with parenting, but she was worried about having to stop her medication because of fetal risk while trying to get pregnant. She had also heard about a significant rate of miscarriage and fetal demise during pregnancy, and a risk of worsening disease for her post-partum. She and Joe decided not to risk pregnancy and began considering their other choices. (*See* full vignette in Appendix.)

Even young women of reproductive age have serious chronic medical illnesses, like congenital heart disease, diabetes, rheumatoid arthritis, lupus, multiple sclerosis, and others. Just like all other women facing pregnancy, women with chronic diseases need discussions about sexuality, contraception, fertility, and childbearing, but often their potential for pregnancy may get lost among their other medical needs. They may find themselves pregnant while taking a panoply of powerful medications. These women have real concerns about many interwoven issues: their ability to conceive, carry a pregnancy to term, and deliver without complications; the impact of their illness on the pregnancy; and the impact of any pregnancies on both short and long term health. Women with chronic medical illness may face real conflicts when their own health requires premature intervention in the pregnancy. Such women may also feel very guilty about the possibility of transmitting their illness to the fetus or of harming a fetus through medications for their illness. While primary care clinicians may not see such women very often during pregnancy, and while they may often end up in high-risk care programs, women with chronic illness are nevertheless part of general medical practice; their potential for pregnancy, their concerns, and their complex needs require a woman-centered approach.

> Sabrina was a 26-year-old Haitian woman pregnant with her first child, who entered prenatal care at nine weeks of gestation. She lived with her husband, father-in-law, aunt, and younger sister. Her parents had both died in Haiti after she had emigrated three years ago. Her husband worked full-time while Sabrina stayed home with her family who "helped take care of her." Over time and multiple visits, it emerged that Sabrina had diabetes, and had had it for some years. She and her husband very much wanted this pregnancy, even though they had heard that diabetes was bad for babies and that women with diabetes could get even sicker in pregnancy. (*See* full vignette in Appendix.)

Part Five examines the complexity of risks that Sabrina faces in carrying this pregnancy. Providers caring for women like Sabrina or Ann either pre-conception or during pregnancy need the support of a multidisciplinary team and the constant reminder to keep the focus on the woman and not on her disease. This team includes not only medical specialists and high-risk obstetricians but also psychologists and others to address the ongoing emotional struggles that many women go through when serious illness overlaps the maternity experience.

CHAPTER 2

The Experience of Infertility

Rachel Wheeler

Some women intending to get pregnant find themselves in the midst of the unwanted illness experience of infertility. Infertility causes profound adjustments in a couple, changing their views of themselves as women and men, spouses, and family members. Once-confident young couples face fears of possible outcomes they had not imagined and grief over lost expectations. Ideas that current or past life choices could cause or contribute to infertility can cause feelings of guilt. Sexual function may be affected both by these complex feelings and by the impact of timed tests on a couple's choices about when to have sex. Women experience their once familiar bodies as imperfect, often with a powerful impact on any future pregnancy experiences. Couples may have unrealistic expectations that modern medicine can fix any newly discovered problem. Melissa and Kirk, whom we met earlier, are frustrated by their initial inability to get pregnant.

> For Melissa, sex now seemed like work and she just wanted to get it over with. When she married five years earlier, she had felt that her sex life was satisfactory without difficulty with interest or orgasm. . . . She had made some lifestyle changes to be healthier as part of trying to get pregnant, and she was very frustrated that none of this effort seemed to help, and found herself in tears each time her period began. She was particularly frustrated with the frequent advice that stress could cause infertility and should be avoided, as this seemed impossible to her, and also made her feel as if she were the cause of the problem.
>
> After eliciting this history, Larisa took a few minutes to express her empathy for these feelings of fear and frustration. She also explained that half of all couples who have not conceived in the first six months of trying will conceive in the following six months. Melissa was skeptical that these statistics applied to her, as she had been so careful in tracking her ovulation. Furthermore, a 50:50 chance of conception without intervention was unacceptable to Melissa and Kirk. They had read that fertility declines with age and were anxious to find what they assumed was a problem and to fix it right away.

Infertility often comes as a highly unwelcome surprise to couples. The emotional reaction to infertility is commonly stronger for the woman than for the man, and families assume that the infertility is a female problem. In almost all cultures, motherhood is viewed as a central aspect of a woman's identity and shapes her role in both family and community. (*See* example of Mai Yer in Part Three.) Language used to describe infertile women as "barren" or "sterile" is laden with negativity. Inability to bear children may be sufficient reason in some cultural communities for a woman to be rejected by a husband or for the husband to take another partner.

In addition to feeling a great sense of loss of the imagined child, the woman experiencing infertility may feel assaulted in her self-concept as a future mother. She may experience strong feelings of guilt. The degree to which a woman believes that she is responsible for her own infertility will depend on her previous choices regarding reproduction, the strength of her self-concept as a healthy person, and on her secular and religious ideas about causation. Young professionals like Melissa and Kirk who have delayed childbearing will often interpret failure to conceive as a result of "waiting too long." Feelings of guilt will be magnified if one spouse perceives that the ability to produce and parent children was one of the important reasons that the partner entered into the marriage. In a modern, secular society, the intensity of these feelings may come as a surprise to women and their partners. Couples accustomed to being in control confront a new challenge that requires a different set of skills and responses compared with challenges they had faced previously; often, such couples and will require support to adjust to this loss of control.

Exploration of feelings and ideas about infertility with both members of a couple is usually helpful and revealing. In the face of a woman's diminished self-esteem and feelings of guilt, the healing professional can offer a realistic assessment of the possibility that prior choices or personal characteristics are the cause of current problems. She or he can also offer prognostic information, and affirm that until a full evaluation is complete it is premature to assume that pregnancy will not occur. A couple can explore together the extent to which they jointly made decisions about when to try to conceive. The clinician can also help them to begin the discussion of what alternatives are acceptable if a biologic child carrying both their genes is ultimately not possible. Feelings of anxiety will often diminish as worst-case scenarios are confronted jointly. A partner may also offer reassurance about the relative importance of fertility in the context of all the other reasons for committing to this relationship. Likewise the clinician can gently help the partner to hear and acknowledge the feelings a woman is experiencing rather than minimizing the significance or the possibility of the potential loss.

> While Melissa and Kirk had not really considered the possibility of male infertility, they readily agreed to semen analysis. This was scheduled and was normal. Kirk expressed some relief at this. They next bought an ovulation test kit and began using it. The next two cycles showed a definite luteinizing hormone (LH) surge on day 13, but did not result in pregnancy. Blood tests for thyroid hormones and prolactin were normal, and a mid-luteal phase progesterone level confirmed ovulation.

At their next office visit, Larisa discussed options for further evaluation. They agreed that a hysterosalpingogram and hysteroscopy to evaluate for tubal infertility factors were important, and Larisa arranged a referral to a gynecologist who could perform these tests. Melissa and Kirk were also unhappy to learn that many infertility tests such as post-coital examination of cervical mucus and timed endometrial biopsy were quite limited at predicting eventual success or at pointing toward a clear treatment strategy. Larisa, hearing the expressions of anger and frustration, asked about what it was like to live with so much uncertainty, and Melissa began to cry.

Larisa asked Melissa about her fears and encouraged her to think through the worst-case scenarios. As they talked, it became clear that Melissa was confident that even if she did not succeed in having a baby, she and Kirk would become parents through adoption. She did not believe that Kirk would in any way reject her, but she did believe that lack of a biological child would be a deep disappointment to both Kirk and to her family, and that she would feel responsible and guilty. She saw her body as defective. She felt responsible for having made things worse by delaying childbearing. She certainly could have tried to have a baby before she got to this age. Kirk could have chosen a different wife. This prompted reassurance from Kirk that this situation was not her fault. While he was also very disappointed by the infertility, he did not see Melissa as a vessel for his babies and wanted to be with her no matter what. They were both able to say that it was very hard to give up the hopes that they had talked about – that their baby would have his musical talents, her brown eyes, and the genetic components of their intelligence that had been so important to both of them.

For a particular couple, many personal and contextual factors will determine the illness experience of the infertility evaluation and treatment. The medical system will often act intrusively in their lives in a wide variety of ways. In the USA, some women will not have any insurance coverage for infertility; for others private insurance companies may dictate access to technologies. Tests will involve repeated exposure and examination of a woman's body and may be painful. Specialists will ask the couple to time sexual relations to a testing schedule. None of the treatments offer certainty of success. Perhaps the couple, the extended family, or the community will easily accept an adopted child, or a child who is the biologic child of only one member of the couple – or not. Family members may hold the same or conflicting values and beliefs about adoption, nature versus nurture, the importance of early infancy care, and the importance of physical resemblance or of racial or ethnic origin. Some couples will want to share the story of their infertility journey with extended family and friends, while others may find it necessary to be completely secretive. Well-meaning friends and relatives who have no close experience with infertility may find it hard to understand a woman who experiences every menstrual period as a major loss and is in tears about it. A woman may feel very isolated from her usual sources of support at a time when her feelings soar to heights of hope then plummet to despair and then back up again. Encouraging women and their partners to join local or national support groups for infertility such as Resolve (www.resolve.org/site/PageServer) can establish support from people outside her usual network who share the same experience. Understanding the personal and cultural context for the woman and couple involved will help the woman-centered clinician to serve as a guide both to the technology and to the emotional landscape, and will facilitate finding common ground in the choice of technology to employ.

> Eventually, the hysteroscopy and hysterosalpingogram were normal, although Melissa found the experience of undergoing these tests in a room full of strangers and big machines exceedingly unpleasant. Melissa and Kirk found themselves coping with "unexplained infertility" – something they had thought did not exist in the high-tech medical system. When they learned that clomiphene could sometimes help as a treatment for unexplained fertility, they talked over the risk of multiple gestation and agreed to go ahead. They were action-oriented people and felt relieved to be finally doing something that might help.
>
> It worked! When she finally missed her period, Melissa did a home pregnancy test with Kirk in attendance reading the instructions. Elated about the positive results, they called the doctor that night with several questions about what would come next in the care plan. The on-call doctor reassured them that they could make a first prenatal appointment with Larisa in the next few weeks. They felt that they could not wait so long but also needed some time to adjust both their work schedules to fit in the prenatal appointments.

If and when pregnancy occurs for a woman experiencing infertility, not surprisingly, both the woman and her physician are likely to feel a heightened anxiety about the pregnancy. Pregnancies after infertility treatment do have a higher rate of pregnancy complications and adverse outcomes, even with a single fetus.[70] Moreover, the woman's confidence and her partner's confidence in her body are very likely to have been badly damaged. They are likely to worry that if the pregnancy results in miscarriage, a second prolonged and painful period of infertility will follow. Anticipating and addressing these fears openly helps to keep them in perspective. Larisa, working with Melissa during the rest of her pregnancy (*see* Part Four), can review many normal test results and remind her and Kirk about the resilience they have already shown in coping with the first difficult experience. Staying sensitive to issues even into the postpartum period is essential, too; for example, at her postpartum follow-up, Melissa may need Larisa's permission to talk about any possible disappointment with labor and delivery and later her ambivalence about returning to work. Acknowledging this disappointment is part of the continuum of both understanding Melissa's past feelings and experiences and reframing her new challenges and strengths in her role as a mother.

Sometimes, couples choose to adopt, sometimes due to infertility, sometimes due to significant genetic or medical illness, or sometimes because of personal choice. Some women with otherwise normal pregnancies and births may choose to release the infant for adoption. While a full discussion of the complexities of the adoption experience from both the birth mother's and adoptive mother's perspective is beyond the scope of this book, clinicians can nonetheless adopt a woman-centered strategy in caring for such women (*see* Box 2.3).

BOX 2.3 Adoption

Questions to consider with women considering releasing an infant for adoption:

- What are your ideas about adoption? How are they reflected in the language you might choose to use as you consider this option? What does it mean to say "give up" a baby? Is there other language that is more positive?
- What are your feelings about adoption, and what do you anticipate they will be in the future? How can you cope with ambivalence, anxiety, or sadness that you may feel? How will your family and people you are close to feel about your decision? Who will you tell now? Who will you want to know about your decision in the future? Who will be able to support and help you with both the grief and pride you may feel?
- Are there particular ideas you have about adoptive parents? Is it important to you to have some choice about who they are? Are religion, age, race, or culture of adoptive parents important to you? Is it important to you whether or not there is a period of foster care before final placement? Do you want to find adoptive parents who will be open to some ongoing contact or relationship with you (open adoption)? Which local agencies will support your values and wishes?
- How does the plan for adoption influence birth plans? How much contact do you want with the baby in the hospital? Do you want to breastfeed while you are with the infant? Do you want the adoptive parents to be present for the birth, later in the hospital, or not at all?
- What legal issues are important? Will the birth father support your plan emotionally? Legally?
- What plans do you need to make for the postpartum period? Will you return to school or work? What will you do about contraception?

Questions to consider in the care of a woman who is adopting an infant through an agency:

- What ideas do you have about adoption and how are they reflected in the language you use with your friends and family? What ideas do friends, family members, and strangers have about adoption? What does it mean to be a "real" mother? What will you plan to tell your child about why the birth mother did not raise the child? Does it matter to you if you and your child look alike? What do you think it will mean to your child, and how might you address this? If your child was born in another country, will it be important to share the culture of the country of origin with the child?
- What information do you need about how infants may experience separation from the birth mother? What may your child need to know in the future about biologic parents? What potential infant health issues do you need to be aware of, both for international adoptions and for infants whose birth parents may not

have been healthy? If it is possible, will you want to have contact with the birth parents? What are your hopes and fears about this?

■ Sometimes adoptions that are anticipated fall through. In the face of this uncertainty, how can you prepare, physically and mentally, for the change of becoming a parent? Adoption often proceeds on a far less predictable schedule than pregnancy. How can you plan for maternity and paternity leaves? What will this mean for your job? What will you, your partner, and the infant need? Remember that you may feel fatigue, uncertainty, and insecurity after your initial excitement; these feelings are normal.

CHAPTER 3

The Experience of Pregnancy Loss

Lori DiLorenzo

While the experience of pregnancy is often a joyous occasion, at some point in their lives anywhere from 12% to 31% of women will experience a spontaneous loss or miscarriage.[71] This life-changing event can cause women to feel a range of emotions from grief, guilt, and isolation, to incompetence and inadequacy. The traditional medical model of care teaches clinicians how to medically diagnose and treat a miscarriage, but women also need individualized emotional assessment and treatment during this loss.

> Pat, a decade after her high school abortion, was newly pregnant. She and her current partner, Mike, had been together for two years. Although they had not planned to start a family right now, the pregnancy news was welcome and crystallized their decision to marry. Pat had a few friends who were mothers and called them for advice when the initial excitement of the positive pregnancy test passed and she started feeling nauseated and tired. She called the health center and got an appointment in a couple of weeks for her first prenatal visit. At her first visit with Dr. Miller, Pat had lots of questions about treatment and about possibly dangerous exposures she might have had before she knew she was pregnant. She called a few times before the first visit to ask about additional concerns about her pregnancy's progress; the office nurse reassured her.

> At about seven weeks, Pat had some vaginal spotting in the middle of one night and panicked, calling the on-call doctor who tried to reassure her that this was a relatively common symptom, but after she hung up the phone, she and Mike decided to go to the emergency room anyway. There she waited several hours to be seen but eventually had an ultrasound that showed a pregnancy too early to definitely see a heartbeat, and her blood work showed a level of human chorionic gonadotropin (HCG) that was compatible with the early gestation. She was told to follow up with her primary provider. Pat called later that morning when the office opened and insisted on being seen that day, accompanied by Mike. The covering doctor, Dr. Rosen, was rushed due to the added visit and quickly reviewed her chart but did not yet have the final ultrasound result. He told her, "Don't worry, almost one-third of women have some early bleeding and more than half of them go on to have a normal pregnancy," and left the room.

The woman-centered method of care proposes that by eliciting the feelings, ideas, function, and expectations surrounding the miscarriage, the clinician will have a better understanding of what the miscarriage means to this particular woman, and therefore will be more able to tailor a personal treatment plan. The experience of miscarriage is different from other losses because of societal secrecy about the experience, the negative connotations of the language used to talk about miscarriage, the strong cultural emphasis on reproduction as a self-defining event for women, and the uncertainties around the clinical course of early pregnancy loss.

In North American culture, miscarriage is still often viewed as a shameful event that should be kept secret, not to be talked about in public. Women may continue grieving the loss for months after the event, well after the time that others think appropriate for grieving. Others may not know how to respond to a woman's miscarriage; one cannot simply purchase a greeting card to acknowledge a miscarriage or stillbirth, because none exist.[72] Consequently, many women hide their emotions surrounding their miscarriage in order to avoid alienating or even offending others. This cultural attitude is also evident in the language used to define miscarriage. The word *miscarriage* itself implies failure, while the word *abortion*, even preceded by the words *spontaneous* or *missed*, conveys the implication of intent to terminate a pregnancy, when often the woman is trying to come to terms with a devastating loss.

Miscarriage often elicits feelings that are bound to the very heart of a woman's identity. Pregnancy is a critical moment, often a "rite of passage."[72] Despite increased social acceptance of the choice not to parent, many women do not feel complete until they have borne a child. As a result, the loss of a wanted pregnancy carries far more weight than clinicians and outsiders might imagine.

Pat's story is a common scenario – a woman undergoing a potentially devastating event sees a clinician new to her who is already overwhelmed by a busy day. How could the clinician use the woman-centered model during a time-pressured situation in order to treat the woman effectively? First, the woman-centered clinician tries to elicit the woman's feelings surrounding this event. These feelings are often dependent upon prior experiences. Pertinent medical history should be available to the treating clinician before she or he walks into the exam room. For example, a woman who has had multiple miscarriages or who has received infertility treatment may have a different experience of vaginal bleeding during pregnancy from that of a woman who is pregnant for the first time, or a woman who has had multiple healthy prior pregnancies. When the treating clinician does not already know the woman, she or he might try, when feasible, to speak with the primary care physician to get a sense of the woman's personal history and previous experiences. A quick chart review to get the details of pregnancy history, possible prior losses, and prior visits and phone calls may also be helpful. For instance, if Dr. Rosen can briefly review Pat's chart, he will discover some clues about her concerns regarding possible prior exposures, and some suggestion that she may be anxious about the pregnancy, given that she has called several times even before the bleeding started.

Aided by this history, the clinician can inquire about the woman's feelings first, with open-ended questions, such as "Tell me what you are most worried about just now." Without making assumptions about the woman's current emotional state, the clinician needs to be aware of the myriad possible emotions that she might have about miscarriage, including uncertainty, dread, guilt, emptiness, grief, lack of control, and fear and vulnerability around future childbearing.[73] Acknowledging early in the process both the lack of control and the inherent uncertainty and unpredictability of the clinical course is also important.

> Pat was convinced that she was going to miscarry because of her exposures early in pregnancy. She took a few sick days off of work and rested at home, without any further spotting until a week later, when she awoke in the middle of the night with some vague lower abdominal cramping and again noted some blood on her underwear. She woke Mike in a panic, and they decided again to call the on-call doctor, who advised them to stay at home and come in to the office in the morning. Pat had a nervous few hours and again called promptly when the office opened. The same doctor, Dr. Rosen, saw her early in the day, knew that she had called earlier, and after reading in her chart about her prior calls, took time during the exam to ask more about how Pat was handling all of this. He initially reassured her that her cervix was closed, but offered to arrange an emergent ultrasound later that day. He asked her to have another HCG level done. He also checked his office schedule for the rest of the day and asked if Pat and Mike could return directly from the ultrasound, explaining that he preferred to review the results in person with them, whatever it showed.
>
> Later, with the report of the ultrasound showing a gestational sac but no embryonic development, also known as a blighted ovum, Dr. Rosen patiently and gently explained this to Pat and Mike, who looked stunned. He asked before proceeding if they were okay with further discussion right away or wanted some time together. They asked for more information, and he explained the likely natural course of the non-developing pregnancy, and the choices of expectant care, medication to induce miscarriage, or surgical evacuation.

Receiving this type of news is often emotionally overwhelming, shocking, and traumatic for a pregnant woman. Knowing the power of message, the woman-centered clinician delivers the information as compassionately yet as clearly as possible: "I'm very sorry to have to tell you this. You've had a miscarriage." For pregnant women hearing this news, immediate reactions often mirror a typical response to any stressful or bad-news situation: numbness, devastation, surprise, disbelief, denial. Clinicians should keep in mind that the miscarrying woman may not hear or process much beyond the initial news of the miscarriage and may not be able to express her own feelings immediately.

Surveys of women post-miscarriage reveal several underlying themes regarding their expectations of clinicians when delivering life-altering news. They hope for simplicity of information, compassion and empathy. Women generally prefer to hear the news in person, and not over the telephone, even if it means that the primary doctor is not the one telling them the results. A simple, "I'm sorry for your loss" is appropriate; depending upon the relationship with the patient, a gentle touch on the arm or even a hug can effectively communicate sympathy.

Besides eliciting feelings, the woman-centered clinician also addresses what ideas the woman may bring to explain the cause and the course of the miscarriage. Research among Swedish women suggests that women having a miscarriage seek meaning or reasons even if the provider has not given one, and often that includes self-blame.[74] The clinician can ask, "Women often have ideas about what might have caused this to happen. What are your thoughts about this?" Gentle reassurance is appropriate that nothing she has done put her pregnancy at risk; nevertheless, the clinician must keep in mind the pervasive and persistent nature of a woman's self-blame, especially within the cultural context that proscribes so much about pregnant women's behavior, food intake, etc. If Dr. Rosen had known about Pat's prior abortion, he might have been able to explore her feelings further: "Sometimes a miscarriage can bring up thoughts and feelings about a prior termination of pregnancy. Has that happened for you?" Women who understand that their pregnancies failed for medical reasons have less self-blame and anxiety post-miscarriage.[75]

Women may also have specific ideas about the expected course of miscarriage. To lead into discussion of this, the woman-centered clinician asks, "You may have heard about different treatment options at this point. Tell me about what you already know or are thinking about." Establishing the woman's ideas about possible treatments can help the clinician correct misconceptions and lay the groundwork for the woman to begin regaining some sense of control at this time of great uncertainty. A simple discussion of options is appropriate and necessary, with the understanding that she may get home and have to call with questions because the information did not sink in the first time. Allowing her to choose the type of treatment, if medically possible, is important in reaffirming a sense of control in a situation that feels very out of control. Women enabled to choose their own treatment have improved quality of life in the months after a miscarriage.[76]

Given the uncertain clinical course and the likelihood of pain and bleeding leading to further interactions with the medical system, the clinician also needs to find out basic information related to the woman's functioning during this time of uncertainty. Questions to ask include, "What are your job or home needs over the next few days as your symptoms evolve? What will happen at your home or job if you have a lot of bleeding or pain? You may need to take some time off for additional tests or medical visits. How will that affect you at home or at work?"

The woman having a miscarriage may not know what she wants to do and may not initially have clearly defined expectations. Thus she will need concrete follow-up plans and some level of continuity of communication with trusted providers during this time. The woman-centered clinician can help facilitate these plans by exploring what the woman expects from the medical system. One simple example is to ask whether she has a preference for telephone or face-to-face follow-up. "When and how would you like to check in with me or one of our group to see how things are going?" As part of the follow-up plan, clinicians also need to know what the woman expects from ultrasounds and blood tests, and how she wants to learn the results. In this process, a provider can clarify office or clinic routines, such as whether the ultrasound technicians will give the woman any specific results, as discussed in the next chapter.

Finally, the clinician should consider the woman's partner's reaction to the news. Even though the partner is not experiencing physical symptoms, the loss is likely similarly devastating, augmented by concern over what the woman is going through both physically and spiritually. Research on fathers' experiences of pregnancy and perinatal loss shows that the intensity of loss was greater than the fathers had anticipated, and that the impact was greatest for those who had seen ultrasound pictures or heard the heartbeat and thus formed a bond with the baby.[77]

Once he realized that the pregnancy was no longer viable, Mike wanted to get everything over with as soon as possible, but Pat was too shocked to decide, and was not sure she wanted any kind of surgery. Mike was nervous about her choice but agreed to go home with careful instructions about warning signs. He felt torn between leaving her at home and returning to work where his boss had been warning him about missing too much time. Mike wondered about asking the doctor for a note for work. Later that day Pat had more cramping and heavier bleeding, and called Mike at his office. Her symptoms frightened Mike, who insisted that they go back to the emergency room, where Pat passed several clots and tissue while waiting to be seen. By the time the doctor was ready to see her, her cramping was better and the bleeding had diminished. She declined further testing or ultrasounds, feeling like she had reached her limit. The emergency room physician gave her a prescription for pain medication that she did not fill, and a plan for follow-up with her primary provider, Dr. Miller. Mike returned to his office but had a hard time concentrating on his work.

Pat and Mike came together to see Dr. Miller two weeks later. Her pain and bleeding were gone, and she reported that her spirits were fine. They were moving ahead on their plans to get married. They felt ready to have a baby and showered the doctor with questions about when they could try again to conceive.

The initial follow-up visit for a woman who has just had a miscarriage can further focus on feelings, ideas, function, and expectations. Reactions may range from guilt and anger to positive thinking. Anger and blame toward the provider about how events unfolded can sometimes lead the woman to sever the relationship and seek care elsewhere even though the provider was in no way responsible for the loss. The woman-centered clinician thus needs to be fully present and empathetic. Even when Pat describes "fine" spirits, this visit is still a good time to discuss the stages of normal grief. Dr. Miller can counsel Pat and Mike that they may feel grief at divergent times and for differing lengths of time. Women after miscarriage cope in a variety of ways, ranging from being with children to avoiding children and other pregnant women. The clinician can help a woman explore how her experience may affect her functioning in her relationships and daily life. The emotions of the experience can also affect a woman's close relationships, including those with other children, her own siblings, and her parents. Because women who miscarry often lack social support,[78] the provider can offer additional support and ask about others whom she might lean on. Clinicians should avoid underestimating the amount of psychological distress that a miscarriage may cause. In addition to depression, women may experience post-traumatic stress disorder and anxiety following a pregnancy loss.[79-81] In contrast, women who receive counseling over time in a woman-centered manner show lower anger scores at one year after the miscarriage.[73]

> Six months later, when Pat's home pregnancy test was positive, she and Mike were both delighted and scared. They decided not to tell anyone right away, but called Dr. Miller begging for an ultrasound as soon as possible to be able to see that the baby was okay. He explained that it was still too early to tell, and offered a visit in a couple of weeks for blood work and physical exam. At that visit, because of her anxiety, he agreed to an early ultrasound. Pat wanted to book it at a time that Mike could be there, too. In the waiting room of the ultrasound office, she suddenly felt sweaty with palpitations and a dry throat. Going into the darkened room with the somber technician made her even more nauseated, and waiting for the silent technician to show them any of the images caused Pat's head to pound. Finally, the technician turned the screen to show them the tiny embryo and its heartbeat. Although reassured for the moment, both Pat and Mike continued to be anxious about a variety of symptoms, including vaginal discharge and palpitations, with frequent calls to the health center.

A miscarriage affects a woman's sense of herself and her expectations and feelings in a subsequent pregnancy, often leading to a higher anxiety level. Fathers also demonstrate increased concern and a need for more vigilance during a subsequent pregnancy.[77] A woman-centered perspective leads the clinician to consider each woman's individual situation. Does she have other children at home? Was she undergoing treatment for infertility prior to the miscarriage? How much time has elapsed since her miscarriage? All of these factors influence how she will relate to a pregnancy after miscarriage. Women compare their current pregnancy to the one that was lost and mark significant milestones such as getting past the gestational age of the loss, the first ultrasound, and getting to the point of viability.[82] They may, like Pat and Mike, delay telling family about the pregnancy and may not allow themselves to get excited until its normalcy is confirmed. As with Pat, clinicians should expect that during a subsequent pregnancy the woman and her partner will be more anxious and may exhibit changes in the way they relate to their healthcare provider.

Because miscarriage is a common event in maternity care, clinicians often use a set of stock phrases to talk with women and their partners: "It wasn't meant to be," "Nature's way of taking care of things," "It wasn't a complete embryo," etc. Women at this time are exquisitely sensitive to the words and tone of the language used. For instance, the term "blighted ovum" may sound unduly negative to the ears of a woman who has just miscarried a wanted pregnancy. Before entering into standard explanations and potentially inscribing indelible painful memories, the clinician would do well first to explore a woman's feelings and ideas about her miscarriage, and subsequently to address how she is doing and what she expects. When the clinician centers his or her words about the miscarriage within an awareness of the woman's reality, she will have the best opportunity to heal from her loss, and the provider is more likely to be an effective caregiver.

CHAPTER 4

The Experience of Abnormal Ultrasound

Sara G. Shields

As noted earlier, routine antenatal ultrasound is a part of most women's pregnancies in the developed world, and even in parts of the developing world. While clinicians primarily use these ultrasounds as screening tools, women usually anticipate them for their non-medical views of the fetus or for reassurance about fetal health.[83] When unexpected abnormalities appear during such routine ultrasound, the woman-centered clinician in the midst of the medical crisis seeks to fully understand the woman's experience of such unanticipated findings.

Feelings crash at the moment of diagnosis. Having anticipated a "fun, enjoyable" time for this "first photo" of the baby, a woman and her family may experience even more shock than when an ultrasound follows abnormal serum screening or other diagnostic reason. Those clinicians who do ultrasounds on their own patients can discuss abnormal findings immediately and in person, but for many women, the ultrasonographer contacts the ordering provider who then delivers the news.

> Felicity, whom we met in Part One, Chapter 5, was 20 years old and pregnant with her third child. Harmony, her prenatal nurse practitioner, ordered a routine ultrasound at 16 weeks to help confirm her due date since Felicity was not sure when her menses were and due to her irregular periods did not realize she was pregnant until nearly 12 weeks along. Rafael, her boyfriend and the father of her daughter, accompanied her to the ultrasound office, eager to see a picture and learn if this time it would be a boy. The technician silently did the ultrasound and then told them that she would be calling in the ultrasound doctor to discuss the results further with them. Felicity, seeing her solemn face, felt her heart sink, and asked worriedly, "What's wrong?" but the sonographer without looking her in the eye replied only, "I need to talk to the doctor who can then talk with you." Rafael, not having been with Felicity for their daughter's ultrasound, was puzzled, thinking this was the routine, but Felicity said, "This didn't happen before," and gripped his hand nervously while they waited. Finally, the radiologist arrived and told them that the fetus appeared to have a "space in the heart," which was sometimes a marker for Down syndrome. She mentioned the term, "echogenic cardiac focus."

In the moment of hearing unexpected news, a woman can place particular significance on the sonographer's or provider's specific words and on non-verbal behaviors such as not making eye contact. The woman-centered sonographer, detecting a problem, can acknowledge non-verbal issues by saying, "I'm going to be quiet while I finish the exam, and then I'll get the doctor to talk to you."[83:233] The policy of many ultrasound units not to have sonographers give any diagnoses can complicate a woman's experience of abnormal results, especially if she leaves the unit assuming everything is normal or if she knows something is wrong but has to wait any length of time for further discussion with her provider.[83] Even in the throes of distressing news, many women understand that a sonographer may not be qualified to fully interpret the results, but do want to hear some kind of diagnosis and follow-up plan before they leave.[84]

Even the physical environment of the ultrasound room may exacerbate the potential for profound shock at bad news: such rooms are usually darkened, with women passively lying on a cold table half undressed, and the ultrasound screen turned away from them initially.[83,84] The dashed expectations of a happy experience may initially prevent a woman from hearing any other information. Thus the woman-centered clinician's task is to acknowledge the emotional significance, and wait for the woman to be ready to hear about next steps in sharing information. At times bringing another family member or support person into the room may be necessary before going into further plans.

> Felicity asked, "What do you mean? Is the baby's heart okay? Oh my god . . ." The doctor answered, "I'm sorry. You didn't expect to hear this. It's supposed to be such a happy time to see your baby, and now I'm telling you something is a bit out of the ordinary. There's a lot of complicated information to share about what all this means for you and your baby. Would you like a minute to gather yourself? Then you can either get dressed and come out into the office to talk more comfortably, or we can stay in here to look at the ultrasound together."

The woman-centered clinician also inquires both about a woman's ideas about what the abnormality means and about options for gathering more information and making any needed decisions. Exploring these dimensions becomes particularly important if termination is an option, given the time-sensitive nature of such choices.

> The ultrasound doctor asked what Felicity and Rafael already knew about both her own risk of Down syndrome and the further options for diagnosing it, and then offered written information and Internet resources for them to explore further. The doctor also told Felicity that she would notify her primary provider at the health center so that Felicity could have an appointment promptly there to review options, including an appointment with the genetic counselor to have more time to discuss the option of amniocentesis.

Another issue in assessing the woman's experience of unexpected fetal anomalies on ultrasound is when and how to show the woman the actual abnormality on the screen. Preferring to keep their own image of a healthy baby, some women may fear at first seeing anything "monstrous" or may want more focus on what is normal about their baby rather than the sonographer's focus on technical interpretation. Some women learning of fetal impairment may benefit from seeing the normal aspects of the fetus and its movement.[83] Interpreting medical terminology such as cystic hygroma or hydronephrosis while showing a specific image may help some women to begin to understand the diagnosis. Aiding women and families in coping with unexpected fetal abnormalities challenges even the most skilled woman-centered clinician. Yet the time spent doing this early on in the process allows for collaborative development of a care plan in the midst of the potential tragedy and need for technical intervention in such pregnancies.

> Lisa was a 28-year-old married Anglo woman expecting her second child. Her first child, Abigail, now three years old, had been healthy after an uncomplicated pregnancy and birth, so Lisa was not anticipating any problems with this planned pregnancy. She had left her job as an administrative assistant when Abigail was born and had done part-time home-based sales work since then to allow her to spend more time at home. Wanting to know this baby's sex, Lisa looked forward to the routine ultrasound that Dr. Usha Rao, her primary provider ordered. However, the ultrasound showed likely gastroschisis, an abnormal formation of the fetal

abdominal wall. Lisa and her husband Randy reeled with this news as the perinatologist briefly discussed what it meant. (*See* full vignette in the Appendix.)

Some women may have a feeling that something is not quite right with their pregnancy even before standard medical tests suggest the possibility of abnormalities. The clinician listens to such feelings and explores the woman's fears and anxieties about the pregnancy, especially at this time of uncertainty, while awaiting confirmatory testing. Having some sense of the woman's daily function can help the clinician identify up front how best to report final results, whether via phone or follow-up appointment. The common practice of calling "only if there's a problem" may work for normal results but creates problems if the clinician ignores how that phone call might affect the woman's other life roles. At times, even though subsequent testing is normal, women remain convinced that "something" is wrong after an initial abnormal quadruple screen or ultrasound finding.[85,86]

Felicity's initial feelings of shock and dismay about her baby's potential cardiac issue were tempered as she learned more about the prognostic significance of the finding, and she opted not to take the risk of amniocentesis. However, knowing that something about her baby was "different" stayed with her for the rest of the pregnancy. She found herself worrying privately about the baby's health and about each minor pregnancy symptom, but even though both quadruple screening and subsequent ultrasounds turned out to be normal, she doubted their accuracy, convinced that something would be wrong when the baby was born. At each prenatal visit she outwardly joked with Harmony about how well she was doing and how this strongly kicking baby kept her up all night, but inwardly she found herself even more focused than with the other pregnancies on whether the heartbeat sounded normal when Harmony listened during office visits. When labor finally came, Felicity was torn between going to the hospital right away to hear the fetal monitoring and staying at home as long as possible to avoid learning any bad news from the monitoring. When baby Omar was finally in her arms looking healthy and normal, Felicity at last felt relieved.

CHAPTER 5

The Experience of Fetal Anomaly

Sara G. Shields

When confirmatory tests reveal significant fetal abnormalities, urgent face-to-face appointments with the woman and whomever she designates as support people are usually essential to allow further exploration of not only the medical issues but also her expectations of the provider and the systems of care that now become necessary. After the initial diagnosis of an unexpected fetal anomaly, women face multiple possible experiences for the remainder of their pregnancy: further workup to confirm the diagnosis, possible multiple hospitalizations or consultations with specialists both obstetric and neonatal, and either pregnancy termination or continuation. Depending on the nature of the anomaly, some women may expect and indeed demand high levels of technological intervention with a "do everything you can" attitude, while others may prefer to "let nature take its course" and avoid invasive treatments. Woman-centered care throughout this process involves non-judgmental, supportive, and ongoing dialogue with the woman, helping her and her family manage the uncertainty and unpredictability[87] and remaining attuned to the dynamics of her feelings, ideas, functioning and decision-making, and expectations.

For the woman who continues her pregnancy with a fetal anomaly, the clinician acknowledges and validates her attachment to the fetus regardless of the complications and ascertains how she is navigating the complex terrain of information about delivery and treatment options, such as advice from friends and family as well as from the Internet. The intensity and complexity of such information coupled with the emotional stresses can exacerbate the difficulty of decision-making. If a woman in preparation for a newborn with significant anomalies has the option of specialized neonatal care at a referral facility, the woman-centered clinician asks how such a plan may disrupt a woman's home functioning and social support systems. Such systems are likely to be more complex for women with disabilities – hearing impaired, visually impaired, or limited in ambulation, for example – who may need specific additional supports at the referral center.

Lisa and Randy, after their initial brief meeting with the local perinatologists following the abnormal ultrasound, juggled their schedules and childcare for Abigail to go to the regional high-risk perinatal center to meet with the obstetrical and neonatal specialists. The doctors discussed with them a plan for both prenatal care and immediate newborn surgery.

After the initial grief at the diagnosis at 20 weeks, Lisa struggled with worrying about the baby's prognosis and yet feeling so healthy herself and noticing all the normal symptoms and fetal movements she remembered from her first pregnancy. She was not sure she wanted to name the baby now as they had done at six months with Abigail's pregnancy, but Randy in his worry wanted that connection with his unborn son. Lisa told her friends from a mothers' group about the baby's problem; several offered immediately to do whatever they could for childcare and other home support. One of her closest friends was also expecting a second child due around the same time. Lisa used to want to get together with her frequently to share their experiences, but now found it awkward to talk about things like delivery plans and sibling adjustment. When she encountered strangers at the supermarket who would smile at her obvious pregnancy and ask how she was, Lisa was never quite sure how to answer as she thought about her son's problem. She now had to go to the regional center for prenatal appointments every other week, and decided after one round trip with her daughter that taking Abigail along was too much to handle so left her with one of these friends.

The perinatologist at the regional center noticed that she appeared anxious and tired and asked her about plans for support. When her tears welled up, he made a call to the perinatal social worker, Reina, who spent the next half hour with Lisa. Reina suggested that both Lisa and Randy come to the next appointment so that they could talk to her as a couple.

The perinatologist was hopeful that Lisa would make it to term, but at 34 weeks while at her appointment in the regional center, her waters broke. Randy was back home with Abigail and quickly arranged for their neighbor to stay with her so that he could get to the hospital in time. Just after he arrived, Lisa was taken to the operating room for a cesarean because of fetal distress. She barely got to see baby Anthony before he was taken for emergency neonatal surgery.

Randy went to the pediatric operating room waiting area while Anthony was undergoing surgery. The surgeon promised to come out and talk to him immediately after the surgery. During those few hours, Reina came up to the delivery floor to spend a little while with Lisa. She asked her if she would be interested in talking with another mother whose child had a gastroschisis. Lisa took the woman's phone number and hoped to call her within a few days.

The range of a woman's emotions throughout this process obviously relates to the medical significance of the anomaly. Regardless of the woman's choices for testing or terminating, grief for the loss of the perfect healthy child remains. Women facing fetal anomalies may also feel sorrow for the loss of a healthy pregnancy experience for themselves, and may find it stressful to attend routine prenatal visits with other pregnant women or healthy children in the provider's waiting room.[88] Other emotions include continued guilt and anger. The challenge for the woman-centered clinician is to recognize that sometimes these emotions surface within the patient-provider relationship and to allow the woman to vent these feelings with empathic support.[88]

A woman pregnant with a fetus with a non-lethal anomaly, such as Trisomy 21 (Down syndrome), if identified in the second trimester, has choices about continuing the pregnancy or opting for abortion. The decisions she and her partner make will strongly depend on their family history, class and cultural positioning, religion, and very personal reactions to raising a child who will always be visibly "different," with mental retardation, social stigma, and many potential medical problems. Support for either decision from family, friends, and the medical profession is not necessarily guaranteed. Martha Beck writes eloquently in her book, *Expecting Adam*, of the disbelief, disapproval, and stigma she encountered when she chose to continue her pregnancy with her son with known Down syndrome.[89]

Conversely, obtaining a second-trimester abortion, even for a recognized anomaly, may be very difficult and expensive to arrange, especially in the USA, and some women making this choice also face opposition and rejection (including excommunication from the Catholic Church) for their decision, and know that some elements of society will regard them as "murderers."[90] For a woman who opts to terminate, the social stigma of abortion and the need to travel to find later-gestation abortion services may significantly affect how she can access support and also how she arranges job and home needs. Eliciting and incorporating the woman's feelings, expectations, and ideas into a care plan for anomalies is a dynamic process that needs to be repeated empathically throughout the process given the emotional distress in such crises.

Women carrying a fetus with a lethal anomaly such as Trisomy 18 or anencephaly, usually detected in the second trimester, most often choose to terminate the pregnancy.[90] Because of religious beliefs, or if the anomaly is not detected until late in pregnancy, some women may choose to carry the pregnancy to term. (Consideration of their anencephalic infants as potential organ donors is a significant possibility for women whose pregnancies bring this dilemma.) Louise Acheson, a family physician, gives a first-hand account of her experience with such an anomaly.

DELIVERING A FETUS WITH TRISOMY 18

> In my first intended pregnancy I was 33 years old, not officially at the age to be a candidate for prenatal diagnosis. Yet I sought amniocentesis on my own "gut feeling." At 16 weeks, the sonographer told me there was not a large enough pocket of fluid to accomplish amniocentesis, "but you MUST come back at 18 weeks, because something is not right – it looks like this fetus may have hydrops." I admired her ability to perceive such things. On the return visit, everything went smoothly. I was surprised by how warm the fluid felt as it was withdrawn. The sonographer said nothing more about anomalies.

I was examining a patient when I was paged. The midwife had the report of the fetal chromosome analysis: a female with Trisomy 18. It was a business-like exchange; I wish she had asked me to come across the street to her office instead of giving this information by phone. I didn't tell anyone but finished the afternoon of patient care. Then I sat alone in my house and realized, "It's after 20 weeks, but I have never felt this fetus move. I should have suspected that something was wrong." My heart raced as I thought how difficult this decision would be if the abnormality had been Trisomy 21 rather than a lethal one such as Trisomy 18. I wanted to get it over with soon, as by the time results came, I was almost 22 weeks along.

I arrived at the labor and delivery ward where I knew the nurses and had attended many births as a physician. My clothes were replaced with a hospital gown. Everyone was somber and compassionate. The nurse gave me a consent form to sign. "What's this?" They wanted my consent to give not only the injection into the amniotic fluid that would induce abortion, but also to inject something to kill the fetus in utero. I wept: "It isn't necessary. I've never felt this fetus move. I was thinking that maybe I would see her move a little, and I would hold her until she dies. It's bad enough to have an abortion; don't deprive me of the opportunity to experience whatever there is here of birth and the chance to fully grieve." The doctor had to come in. She and the nurses explained that it was a medicolegal issue: they could not avoid attempting to resuscitate a fetus born with any signs of life. "This is absurd!" I was angry. I explained that since I had chosen to abort a 22-week fetus because of lethal congenital anomalies, I would not permit resuscitation. It was not up to me; I had to consent to a lethal injection or no abortion. This small absurdity, I realize, was the channel for my sadness and anger at the whole situation – but seemed cruel and senseless nonetheless.

That evening, after painful contractions, I suddenly felt something slip down into my vagina, and the pains stopped. I told the nurse that I was delivering and asked her to call the doctor. The doctor had already gone home, and had told the nurse after a recent digital exam that my cervix was only 1 cm dilated. The nurse told me I must be mistaken and not to bother the doctor until morning. On morning rounds, the physician extracted the tiny malformed fetus – macerated, limp, meat-red – and arranged to perform a D&C for the retained placenta. How could I have been so naïve as to imagine holding this half-developed fetus as it died?! One couldn't even discern that she was female. The hospital routine involved collecting memorabilia and a Polaroid photograph, but the labor experience was my catharsis. I have never again examined the items in that shoe-box on my top shelf. I do remember the compassionate support of my family and colleagues. Even the ones who were fundamentally opposed to abortion understood that it involved suffering, and expressed their personal support of me, for which they have my appreciation even many years later. (*Louise Acheson contributed this personal story.*)

Louise Acheson's experience reveals that medical providers, and sometimes the entire medical system, do not consistently work in a woman-centered way even when a woman is facing the impending birth of an abnormal fetus and the associated grief and loss. Providers must examine themselves, their routine practices, and the policies of their institutions, to promote thoughtful changes that will make these most difficult pregnancy and birth experiences into encounters of care and compassion centered in the woman herself.

CHAPTER 6

The Experience of Hospitalization in Pregnancy

Sara G. Shields

When pregnancy complications necessitate prolonged hospitalization, the clinician again explores the woman's feelings, ideas, function, and expectations fully as part of putting her care into an individual context. A woman-centered understanding includes assessing feelings such as guilt, sadness, and fear, but also boredom and frustration with uncertainty and unpredictability. Eliciting the multiple dimensions of the experience allows the clinician to appreciate more fully the profound impact of changing an able-bodied, healthy person with multiple life functions into a bed-bound woman dependent on others or on technology for basic daily tasks.

> Jackie had developed gestational diabetes. At about 33 weeks, with her blood sugars just under control, her blood pressure was high. Judith Peters, her provider, evaluated her for other signs and symptoms of pre-eclampsia, and all was normal, but she asked Jackie to return in three days to recheck her blood pressure. At that visit it was even higher, and Judith recommended hospitalization to evaluate Jackie more closely, given Jackie's diabetes and preterm status. Jackie had to find childcare overnight but agreed reluctantly to come to the hospital "as long as you're the one in charge of my care." She stayed overnight for monitoring and testing. With her BP normalizing, Judith discharged Jackie the next day, but recommended further close follow-up and modified bedrest. Jackie asked for a note for her employer to confirm her need for sick time, and wondered how she was going to handle her foster children's needs.

Evelyn was a 29-year-old G2P1 who had a young toddler at home and also worked as a night shift nurses' aide in order to supplement her spouse's income as a taxi driver. The night after her 27-week mark, Evelyn was at work and noticed a gush of fluid. She found herself feeling nauseated and dizzy. She called Dr. Rosen's answering service and was told to come to the hospital. Evaluation there revealed that she had in fact ruptured membranes but did not appear to be dilated or contracting yet. Dr. Rosen and the perinatologists recommended hospitalization for medical treatment to prevent infection, promote fetal lung maturity, and attempt to prevent such a preterm delivery. For the next 10 days, Evelyn remained in the hospital at bedrest. Her husband Ed brought their toddler Marilyn to visit after work, and then left her with Evelyn's mother overnight. Evelyn worried about how they were coping and about what would happen to her job. She also worried about the baby's prematurity and was willing to do whatever the doctors said might help, even though she was uncomfortable lying in bed for a long time. During the daily testing with the fetal monitor, she found it reassuring to hear the baby's healthy heartbeat and hear from the doctors that all seemed well for now. (*See* full vignette in Appendix.)

During these hospitalizations, Judith and Dr. Rosen focus on how to empower each woman through these illness experiences. They need to ask about each woman's experience, affirm the significance and validity of her responses, and respect her individuality and her decision-making capacity.[36] Each clinician inquires about the woman's ideas about her now high-risk pregnancy, in hopes of helping her shift toward realistic expectations and better coping.[91] Frequent sharing of information in a way that includes anticipatory guidance about potential complications can also allow women both to feel more involved in decision-making and to feel more control over an experience that often feels so out of control.[36] Finding ways to acknowledge her motherhood within the emergency setting also validates each woman's overall life experience. Judith and Dr. Rosen can acknowledge how Jackie's and Evelyn's maternal strengths are so apparent in their efforts to care for their other children while coping with the hospitalization.

CHAPTER 7

The Experience of Preterm Labor and Newborn Illness

Sara G. Shields

Caring for women with preterm labor especially demands a woman-centered approach in the midst of the usually fetus-centered medical focus of evaluation. Shock and fear may be the initial emotions for a woman facing unexpected preterm labor, quickly followed by self-blame as women themselves seek to understand possible causes. For some women, this explanatory model of owning responsibility may in fact work to give them back some control over an unexplained event and thus help them find a solution.[92]

In discussing the likelihood of preterm labor resulting from her preterm ruptured membranes, Dr. Rosen can inquire non-judgmentally of Evelyn, "Lots of women in your situation wonder about why this is happening. It helps me take better care of you if I understand what ideas you might have about this. What do you think is causing this preterm issue?" Some women may view preterm labor as a natural process, and consider the early symptoms to be the "usual aches and pains of pregnancy," thus not seeking or expecting medical intervention, or devaluing their own feelings in the throes of their juggling roles between work and home. Others associate preterm contractions or labor with physical or mental stress and report of an intuitive sense that "something is wrong," leading them to get medical care earlier.[92]

After the diagnosis of premature rupture of membranes and discussion of her risk of preterm delivery, Dr. Rosen continues to assess Evelyn's experience of the treatment plan. Although she does not yet have contractions or labor progress, he can anticipate such complications ahead of time and discuss treatment such as possible medications, especially since treatment frequently involves urgent care once contractions start. Even in the midst of rapid treatment decisions, the woman-centered clinician works to keep the focus on the mother's experience. Given the likelihood that once contractions begin for Evelyn, stopping labor will be difficult, Dr. Rosen also needs to help Evelyn have realistic expectations about her hospital course and the likelihood of preterm delivery even with any further treatments.

Treatment for preterm labor and subsequent care of the often-premature infant will have drastic effects on the woman's functioning. Recommendations often include bedrest and significant activity restrictions. The clinician acknowledges the reality of most women's domestic responsibilities and the likely difficulties in achieving recommended rest. Particularly if a woman has very traditional role division with her male partner, addressing different juggling of household tasks during preterm labor treatment is challenging. In the woman's function outside the home, for young women still in school or women in low-paid work without benefits, lost hours from hospitalization can lead to educational delay or job loss.

When pregnancy complications result in an ill infant, woman-centered care remains important in promoting the new mother's challenging transitions.

> After 10 days of hospitalization, one night Evelyn got up to use the bathroom, noticed cramping and more fluid leaking, and then realized the umbilical cord was coming out of her vagina. She had an emergency cesarean under general anesthesia and awoke in the recovery room with Ed at her side, telling her about their newborn son, 1100 g David. Although he had done well at first given the emergent nature of his delivery, breathing spontaneously, he soon developed respiratory distress and needed intubation so was already in the intensive care nursery. Evelyn, exhausted and astonished by all that just happened, and in pain from her unexpected surgery, was too tired and uncomfortable to visit David or to start pumping her milk in the first day.

Dr. Rosen recognizes that the sudden experience of preterm labor and neonatal intensive care brings a multitude of negative feelings generated by the unexpected outcome. Initially, fear and shock can overwhelm the new mother's transition to motherhood and overshadow other feelings.[93] Acknowledging the normality and intensity of these swift changes in feelings, Dr. Rosen checks in regularly over the first few days to revisit how Evelyn is feeling and coping. Throughout, he stays attuned to how the intensity of emotions may interfere with Evelyn's understanding of medical information about her son, and thus with her decision-making processes.

While, on the surface, fear for the infant's well-being can feel uppermost, woman-centered care means exploring further other feelings such as guilt. Part of the guilt may also be a sense of shame, that one was unable to give birth to a healthy baby and thus fulfill societal or spousal expectations of motherhood.[94] Grief over the loss of a normal pregnancy, birth, and newborn experience can also be a part of a new mother's experience of complicated birth or ill newborns. Dr. Rosen would do well to reframe the usual focus on Evelyn's biomedical risk factors for premature rupture of membranes, since such emphasis can covertly blame the mother. Evelyn in particular may already fault herself for working too hard, not eating regular meals, needing treatment for depression, or lifting her toddler. Dr. Rosen thus needs to explore not only her feelings but also her ideas about the causes of prematurity and gently correct her misperceptions.

The experience of unexpected premature delivery often includes prolonged newborn hospitalization, with unanticipated demands on parents and families to juggle work and home needs, such as job schedules and care for other children. At the same time, the mother is trying to recover from any delivery complications and address the more complicated postpartum issues such as pumping milk and breast-feeding a premature infant. When the woman is ready to discuss such function, the provider inquires about these responsibilities and anticipates how they might evolve over the course of prolonged hospitalization. Some women may be relieved to no longer be hospitalized themselves, but be overwhelmed by the complexities of going back and forth to the hospital for visits, particularly if they have other children at home or are struggling with postpartum exhaustion or breast-pumping.

> Once she had recovered enough to be discharged herself, Evelyn tried to spend as much time as possible at the hospital with David, continuing to rely on her mother to help with Marilyn. At first when he was still on the ventilator Evelyn was nervous about all the machinery and about touching him, and fearful that he might die. The day nurses, while kind and obviously competent, were busy, and Evelyn was shy about interrupting their work or the doctors on rounds to ask for more information. She still felt tired and sore after walking much or climbing any stairs, and she wondered how she would ever feel capable of caring for David when he got well enough to come home. She preferred visiting in the evenings when she did not have to worry so much about Marilyn and when she felt more included in David's moment-to-moment care by the nurses.

Supporting Evelyn during this early postpartum stage when the normal processes of attachment and bonding are lost to the technology of intensive care means asking about her anxiety and fears, her ideas about how she can still connect with her son, her struggles with the logistics of visiting regularly and continuing to care for her older child, and her expectations of the hospital staff and the care plan. Woman-centered care is sensitive to the complexities of emotions and the unfamiliar hospital environment, and seeks ways to empower Evelyn's mothering at every interaction.[94] For women like Evelyn with low-wage jobs without sick leave, the infant's extended hospitalization exacerbates financial stresses as well as the possibility of further maternal guilt, self-blame, and relationship difficulties.[95,96] Infants such as David often require extra care during the first few months of life, limiting Evelyn's ability to use her previous childcare provider, and further compromising their family income. She wonders if he will have some kind of long-term disability from being so premature, and whether he or their family might qualify for some increased benefits to cover his additional medical visits.

CHAPTER 8

The Experience of Prolonged Labor

Sara G. Shields

Caring for women having prolonged labor is another common challenge for maternity providers. A prolonged labor or assisted delivery may further suggest inadequacy to a woman who is predisposed to blame herself, or may lead to anger at the providers involved who, she feels, may "not know what they are doing." Exploring the dimensions of a woman's experience of difficult labor incorporates the basic tenets of the woman-centered model: eliciting and addressing common feelings such as fatigue and despair, inquiring about the woman's own explanatory models for such long labor, understanding her decision-making capacity during this challenge, and helping her find more realistic expectations about her labor. The provider's goal in this task is to remain positive and empowering and to find ways to give back to the woman some semblance of control and choice. The dynamic, ever-changing process of a long labor necessitates flexibility and frequent re-evaluation of each dimension.

Jackie's induction began with cervical ripening, but everyone in her family anticipated that the process would not take long, given that this was Jackie's fourth baby and her other labors had been relatively quick. Her best friend and her mother were in the labor room with her. The ripening drug set off uncomfortable, frequent contractions but did not cause much cervical change, and by the next day Jackie was exhausted and frustrated that her cervix was still only 2 cm dilated and not effaced in spite of frequent, tiring contractions. Judith suggested a brief rest but then continuing with an induction, given her blood pressure. The labor progressed arduously – Jackie's blood pressure edged up enough that Judith recommended magnesium therapy to prevent eclampsia, which made Jackie feel miserable. She eventually insisted on an epidural, even though her other children's births had been medication-free. Finally, she was fully dilated, but pushed for two hours without much descent even after trying position changes. As she neared the two-hour mark, the baby's heart rate started to become abnormal, and Judith decided a cesarean was likely imminent. She asked the consultant to see Jackie in case there was a possible chance of an assisted delivery. The consultant evaluated

Jackie and agreed that the baby was posterior and too high to safely attempt an assisted vaginal delivery and recommended a cesarean section.

Melissa worked full-time until 40 weeks when her membranes ruptured without her going into labor. She and Kirk dutifully walked around the hospital for several hours trying to get contractions going, but ultimately she needed to be induced. She did well until about 6 cm with Kirk's support, but at that point "lost it" and asked for an epidural. She reached full dilation and pushed for four hours with her dense epidural but ultimately required Larisa to perform a vacuum assist to deliver a healthy boy, Martin, who weighed 3.5 kg (7 pounds 12 ounces) with Apgars of 8 and 9, which Kirk was very certain to ascertain.

The experience of prolonged labor can include strong, even extreme, emotions that may overwhelm the laboring woman: feeling possessed by pain and the inability to manage it; feeling powerless, helpless or inadequate; feeling out of control; being dependent on others; falling into despair.[97] The strength of these feelings can even lead some women to thoughts of dying, with fear becoming the dominant emotion: fear for their own life, fear for the baby's condition, fear that labor will never end. These fears can then engender either panic and anxiety or despair and resignation, with exhaustion overwhelming any remaining sense of control or decision-making. For other women with long labor, particularly in second stage, feelings of ambivalence about motherhood or fear of letting go may impede progress.[98]

One way to begin inquiry about a woman's feelings during non-progressing labor is to ask after a contraction, "What was going through your head during that contraction?"[99:191] This phrasing emphasizes the emotional component of a woman's feelings more than the question, "What did you feel with that contraction?" Women may respond to the latter question, "Pain!" because the physical pain, as the most intense part of labor, is more easily verbalized than the other feelings noted above. The woman-centered provider responds to this answer by asking for more specifics in various ways: "Tell me more about that. What was the hardest part about the pain for you? Anything else?" Thus woman-centered inquiry about pain during prolonged labor, as during any labor, needs to evaluate more than physical pain but also coping emotions (*see* discussion of pain scales in Part Four, Chapter 7). Attending to a woman's varied feelings with inquiry such as this helps decrease her sense of vulnerability during difficult labors.[90]

After assessing the full spectrum of a woman's emotions during slowly progressing labor, the clinician asks what ideas the woman has about causes or effects of her slow labor. "What do you think is slowing your labor right now?" She may in the throes of arduous labor develop various explanations that fit within her life context. Jackie, having had normal spontaneous births with her other children without medical complications during pregnancy, may view induction as the cause of her dysfunctional labor, or question how her blood pressure and the medication affect her labor course. She may begin to think her earlier mistrust of doctors and consultants was in fact justified. As we will see in Part Three, Melissa has a history of childhood sexual abuse, which may affect how she handles a prolonged labor, especially in second stage. Melissa, pushing harder than she could have imagined possible and trying many different positions, in her frustration at the seeming endlessness of second stage, may worry that such prolonged pushing may permanently damage her body in a place that she feels has already been damaged.[99] Some women with ineffective pushing efforts may feel embarrassed about involuntary defecation or feel suddenly anxious about the realities of their impending motherhood.[98] Asking about ideas such as these, Judith and Larisa can correct misperceptions in ways that affirm each woman's underlying strength.

> Before evaluating Jackie's cervix and the baby's descent, Judith watched her through a contraction and asked, "You look like you're working really hard with that contraction. Tell me what you were feeling with that." Jackie shook her head in frustration, "Man, this baby was supposed to come easy, like his sisters did! Everyone's right that these contractions hurt more than regular labor, but they're not working the same." Judith nodded her head. "Yes, other women who have had both spontaneous and induced labors talk about that. It is frustrating that this labor has not been as smooth as your other labors were. We were assuming your strong body would do the same this time. . . . With all that you juggle so well in your life with work and being such an experienced parent, you know both that each child is different from the beginning, and that sometimes things do not go just as planned."

> Larisa observed Melissa push as she entered the second hour of second stage. As the contraction ended, Melissa groaned and closed her eyes, saying, "He's just not coming!" Larisa asked, "From what I see, you are working really hard with some good pushes. Why do you think the baby is not coming?" Melissa replied, "I just don't know. Maybe he won't fit. I really don't want to tear, either." Larisa reminded her, "Holding the baby in won't help that." She also reminded Melissa of the normal length of second stage with a first baby, and described how her perineal tissues would begin to stretch out as the baby's head descended further. After the next contraction, Larisa also reminded her that they had discussed in prenatal care different options for preventing perineal lacerations. (*See* Part Four for more on working with survivors in labor.)

The woman-centered clinician needs to not only acknowledge this cycle of negative emotions and mistaken explanations but also understand how much powerlessness, vulnerability, and self-blame impinge on a woman's decision-making during labor. Interestingly, women with long labors ending in cesarean or assisted delivery may end up feeling a sense of relief and gratitude rather than one of disappointment or failure.[97] Caught up in pain and powerlessness, unable to cope, women might ultimately feel relief in relinquishing control and decision-making to their care providers. (Fear of this powerlessness may also partially explain why women may prefer repeat cesareans over trials of labor with subsequent pregnancies.) Ideally, the clinician discusses during prenatal care the possibility that a woman during even a normal labor may change her mind about what she wants and how much control she wants, and then can refer to this discussion during intrapartum care.

The last dimension of understanding the experience of prolonged labor involves both ascertaining then reframing the laboring woman's expectations of the healthcare team and of herself, and of the natural course of labor. The clinician who has used this model in prenatal care has already set the stage for helping the woman cope with unexpected issues in labor. Having discussed the pros and cons of induction with Jackie prenatally, Judith can inquire again at the beginning of the induction what Jackie expects in this early stage, a time in her prior labors when she was at home but now is facing hospitalization and medication for pre-eclampsia. "What are you thinking will be different about this labor since we are inducing it? What are some of the ways we can help you cope with it? How often do you want me to examine you to see how your cervix is progressing?" For Melissa, each vaginal examination is difficult, even with her epidural. Larisa says as Melissa enters her second hour of pushing, "It will help me get a sense of how the pushing is going if I can examine you with one or two contractions. What can I do to help make that more comfortable for you?" The provider can also discuss expectations around the potentially conflicting needs for support or privacy during prolonged first or second stage. "Some women find long labor easier if they are by themselves without a lot of noise or people, and other women want to be distracted by their support folks or by television. What do you think will help you most?"

Women (and their families) do not necessarily expect prolonged labor; thus, in the midst of an unexpectedly long course, they may then request cesarean section, perceiving operative delivery as the only way to cope. When a woman is begging for surgery that is not medically indicated, the woman-centered clinician needs to explore the feelings behind such a request and find common ground as discussed in Part Four.

CHAPTER 9

The Experience of Difficult Breastfeeding

Sara G. Shields

With Danny Jr., Siobhan had stopped breastfeeding within a few days due to issues with inverted nipples and milk supply. With her second pregnancy, even though she was late to care, she considered again her breastfeeding options and wanted to try again, especially once she connected with Dr. Miller. He encouraged her at each of her late prenatal visits, discussing a care plan to help with the inverted nipple issue. Within minutes of baby Kate's birth, Siobhan put her to breast, with the nurse and Dr. Miller offering suggestions about her nipples. Over the first 24 hours, Siobhan's postpartum nurses taught her to use breast shells between feedings and other techniques to evert her nipples. Katie's vigorous suckling was still more painful than Siobhan expected, and she really did not want to end up with all the tubing and gadgets that she had briefly tried with Danny Jr. Using the pump hurt, too. Her first night at home with Katie, Siobhan was in tears each time she tried to nurse, and Danny Sr. tried to reassure her but wondered along with her if this just was not going to work. They ended up trying a bottle so that Siobhan could sleep. Two days later, at the early office newborn visit, Dr. Miller's nurse noted both Siobhan's tears and Katie's loss of weight and pointed this out to the doctor just before he entered the room. He reviewed what Siobhan had tried and how Katie was otherwise thriving. Siobhan was ashamed to admit that they had already supplemented with a bottle, feeling that she had let down herself and the doctor. As he re-examined her breasts and watched the stress of feeding, Dr. Miller commented, "You've worked really hard another time to make this work. That's one of your strengths as a mom, that you don't give up easily in situations where many women would give up sooner. One of your other strengths is to recognize when things aren't going well, and other options are needed. You're not a failure if you switch to formula."

With her other children, Felicity had chosen formula feeding from the beginning and liked that someone else could feed the baby at night or when she was at school. She thought her breasts were too big and did not like to expose them either in public or around anyone in her family. During this pregnancy, worrying about the baby due to the abnormal ultrasound, she decided with Harmony's encouragement to at least try breastfeeding. She remembered that her milk had come in with her other babies a day or two after her discharge from the hospital, and expected that to happen this time, too, so she envisioned no real issues with breastfeeding. But baby Omar, while healthy, was not that interested in breastfeeding at first. Felicity attended the hospital's daily breastfeeding class and got help with positioning from the daytime nurse. She had a hard time imagining that the few drops of colostrum that seemed to come out were really enough for the baby and asked lots of questions about how to tell the amount of breast milk that he was receiving, especially when he suckled only a few minutes at a time. While her postpartum nurses were kind and concerned, they had responsibility for caring for several women at a time, and once they got Omar positioned at the breast could not stay to help further. When Omar fell asleep yet again at the breast his first evening, and the evening nurse verbalized concern about whether he had had enough wet diapers, Felicity decided to give him a bottle, which he readily took. She then agreed that the next time he was hungry that night, he could get a bottle, and she would try nursing again the next day. She left the hospital doing both, with Rafael eager to help however he could. Two days later, she became so engorged that she could not figure out how to get Omar to latch on, and they both were frustrated. It felt a lot easier to satisfy Omar with a bottle. Within a few days, Omar was mostly bottle-feeding, and by the time of his two-week visit in the office, Felicity's milk supply had dried up. She reported matter-of-factly to Harmony, "I didn't have enough milk again. He was too hungry, and I couldn't keep up."

Lisa had breastfed Abigail for nearly a year and expected to breastfeed with this second pregnancy even with the anticipated complications of gastroschisis. After her preterm cesarean, however, she was groggy and in pain. Once she got a breast pump, all the parts felt awkward to put together, the cold plastic was uncomfortable, and she had forgotten how sore her nipples and breasts would feel at first, especially with using a machine. Lisa got discouraged early on by only getting a few drops of colostrum at a time. Meanwhile after surgery, Anthony remained intubated in intensive care, unable to eat. Even after he had been slowly weaned from the respirator, he remained unable to have anything by mouth until his intestines were more healed. After her own discharge at four days, Lisa juggled her surgical recovery with caring for Abigail, traveling to visit Anthony and continuing to pump and store milk. She tried various herbal remedies and medications in hopes of increasing her milk supply, but to no avail. Randy and her visiting mother, trying to be helpful, thought Lisa was not getting enough rest in order to pump and encouraged her to sleep through the night rather than wake to pump. Lisa felt that they did not understand how important it was for her to make milk for Anthony. The lactation consultant from the intensive care nursery worked with Lisa several times, both in the hospital and after discharge when she was able to come back to see Anthony. Finally, Anthony could eat, but between his prematurity and the long intubation, he suckled too weakly to get much milk directly from her breasts and gave up quickly while gulping readily from a bottle. Lisa tried a tubing device attached to her nipple to give Anthony the sense that he was getting some milk but found this also quite awkward and time-consuming. She was exhausted and saddened that she could not fulfill what she saw as her most important motherly role.

Although in the 21st century both professionals and laypeople acknowledge the benefits of breastfeeding, the usual focus is on the benefits to the baby, and even society, often with little attention to the woman's challenges, emotions, and social and family context. As noted previously, a new mother may have a wide range of feelings, ideas, function, and expectations around breastfeeding. For a woman who strongly desires to breastfeed and considers her success at this as a measure of her mothering ability, any perceived "failure," whether in her baby's response or her own milk production, may elicit disappointment, guilt, or even feelings of rejection.[54] Woman-centered providers working with women for whom breastfeeding does not go well need to attend to the complexities of these feelings.

Breastfeeding may not work for a variety of reasons. Sometimes newborn medical issues prevent early initiation or adequate suckling, as with Lisa and Anthony. Sometimes the mother's anatomy is an issue, as with Siobhan's inverted nipples. And sometimes, as with Felicity, an unfortunate mix of common issues, each potentially resolvable, coincide, such as perceived inadequate milk supply, a sleepy newborn, lack of individual attention, and the ease of using a bottle. Some women who have undergone childhood sexual abuse may unexpectedly experience breastfeeding an infant as yet another person making intimate demands on their body, thus causing confusion and ambivalence.[100] When birth complications affect the initiation of breastfeeding, as in Lisa's case, the provider needs to be especially attentive to all the dimensions of the woman's experience about lactation. For some women coping with complex postpartum or newborn illness, encouraging and facilitating their unique ability to breastfeed may help both to normalize and to validate their evolving individual maternal experiences in a tangible way. For women such as Lisa, bringing her milk to the neonatal intensive care unit is a unique act that ties her physiologically and emotionally to her infant. For others, such as Siobhan, when either physical anatomy or the overwhelming challenges of their personal reality interfere with their expectations about breastfeeding, the woman-centered clinician may need simply to hear and validate their sense of loss and help them find other ways of fulfilling their maternal role.

CHAPTER 10

The Experience of Postpartum Depression

Colleen Fogarty

Given the overlap of physical and emotional symptoms of a normal postpartum course with that of postpartum depression, a woman-centered approach to the latter necessitates careful, contextual assessment of the woman's experience. The clinician creates in each postpartum encounter a willingness to hear the full range of a woman's potentially conflicting feelings and negative thoughts during the postpartum transition. This can include not only normalizing such reactions but also being alert to more severe symptoms that may signify the need for more aggressive treatment. Even women with uncomplicated birth experiences, excellent postpartum support, and satisfying work can experience the disturbing depths of postpartum depression, as one physician describes:

> My second son's birth was beautiful and uncomplicated, and breastfeeding while never exclusive went better than with my older child. I was tired, as expected, but quickly got back on my feet after such a routine delivery. Leo's mellowness and help from my husband allowed me to spend time reading to and otherwise paying attention to my toddler, Aidan. I had arranged a 12-week maternity leave from my work with a subsequent four weeks at half my usual schedule. During this time I reconnected with other neighborhood women with babies. I had returned to work after 12 weeks with my first son, so I knew what to expect from my job, my commute, and the transition between home and work. I remembered well that awful feeling, "How can I ever leave my baby?" right before I returned to work after my first birth. With my husband staying home to care for the children, I was fortunate not to have major worries about childcare. However, once I resumed my full-time academic medical work, I was exhausted almost all the time. Although Leo was a great baby, he still awoke at least once during the night. I was often irritable, and almost always felt frustrated with my inability to stay on top of my professional work and finish any task at home. I had had plenty of guilty thoughts after returning

to work from Aidan, and these returned after my return to work from Leo. I worried the children would not know who their mother was, and fretted about the developmental milestones I'd miss.

About a month after I resumed full-time work, I began to worry about what would happen to my family after I died. Soon, those thoughts transformed into a strong conviction that my two young children and husband would be far better off if I were dead. I did not have any plan to kill myself, but could imagine the bus being crashed into, or terrorists infiltrating the subway system with lethal chemicals.

After several days of these frightening thoughts, I got a grip on myself. Within several days, I had an appointment with my family doctor, who had treated me with both of my pregnancies and attended both births. She immediately diagnosed postpartum depression, and we discussed risks and benefits of pharmacotherapy. We settled on sertraline as an initial choice. Within six weeks, I began to feel better, still tired and overwhelmed with work, but coping better with life. Most importantly, the frightening and uncontrolled thoughts of death had dissipated.

Understanding the experience of postpartum depression in a woman-centered way involves dynamic, flexible attention to subtleties and individual needs, recognizing that not all women will disclose the same symptoms to all providers at all times. Successful screening models serve clinicians in obstetrics,[101] general practice,[102] and pediatrics.[103] Providers in any discipline who interact with women postpartum should ask the new mother about the presence of depressive symptoms, her overall coping with the pregnancy and the infant, and her support systems in her family and community. Quantitative symptom checklists or written scoring screens have clinical utility but are imperfect and not tailored to individual profiles.

At Martin's two-month well-baby visit with Larisa, Melissa was tearful and upset, and within a few moments broke down into tears. She said, "There's no way I could possibly return to work as soon as they want me to. I cry every night nursing him, thinking about it." She was also exhausted from trying to "do it all" at home with more of the housework and traditional gender roles than she had expected. Kirk's job demands had escalated so that he could not take time off to come to this visit but had sent a list of questions along with Melissa and had agreed to be available by phone at the time of the visit. Larisa remembered how involved Kirk had been at prenatal visits, and after seeing the list, had Melissa phone him from the exam room. In discussing one of Kirk's concerns about Martin's stool patterns, Larisa learned that Kirk did most of the diaper changes and was willing to do the nighttime ones so that Melissa could get a bit more sleep. Larisa asked Kirk to come to Melissa's postpartum visit in a few weeks so that they could talk about the current parenting roles more fully.

While Larisa finished examining Martin, she asked Melissa a few screening questions specifically about postpartum depression. The screen that Larisa usually used scored Melissa as moderately depressed. They talked more about her work choices, and about counseling options or medication. Melissa thought the issues mostly were about her return to work, and did not think depression treatment was needed. Aware of her past history of sexual abuse, her harsh criticism of herself for needing a vacuum-assisted delivery, and her strong need for being in control, Larisa thought the postpartum conflicts might push her into a more significant clinical depression. She asked Melissa to call in about a week to discuss what was happening and to review her symptoms further.

While discussing possible symptoms, the clinician acknowledges both that "normal" stress without frank depression occurs for many women following childbirth and that given the societal stigma of mental illness, women may choose to not reveal the full magnitude of their symptoms for fear of being labeled "crazy" or losing custody of their children. Women may resist categorizing themselves as ill, and rather see themselves struggling to cope with the burdens of fatigue, isolation, and role change that permeate so much of this postpartum transition.[104] While asking what depression means for a woman in her particular life context, the woman-centered provider frames this inquiry in positive, strength-based language that acknowledges these coping strategies.

During her pregnancy, before her preterm labor, Evelyn had been overwhelmed by her schedule. She was sleeping poorly during the day while her toddler, Marilyn, was with her mother. Ed was working longer hours to keep up with their financial needs. They had been arguing about childcare and household chores. Evelyn found herself crying easily and being easily distracted, forgetting what tasks she had to do each day. She was feeling guilty that the baby might be affected by her stress and that she was not enjoying her pregnancy but rather dreading having to juggle even more duties with a newborn at home. At her 20-week visit she had lost a few pounds and looked noticeably tired; when Dr. Rosen mentioned this, Evelyn burst into tears, saying, "I'm really having a hard time."

Dr. Rosen, pausing, offered her tissues and gently touched her arm in sympathy. "I'm really glad you're able to let me know this. You're brave to share this. Let's talk through a few other possible symptoms." He asked about Evelyn's sleep patterns and used a depression screening tool that took about five minutes to complete. Evelyn revealed that in her late teens she was in treatment for major depression, and her mother had also been treated for anxiety and depression. Dr. Rosen commented, "It's really helpful that you can make a connection between depression in your family and in your teenage years with the way you feel now. I'm impressed by how well you've done since then and the strengths that you have had along the way." He wondered if there were any way for Evelyn and her extended family to consider additional help so that Evelyn could get a bit more rest. They discussed the options of cutting back her work hours and considering some brief counseling, as well as the possibility of medication. Evelyn did not want to take anything that would hurt the baby, but was willing to try some counseling if the scheduling could work around her childcare, work, and sleep issues. Dr. Rosen congratulated her, "It's great that you're being so thoughtful about your options. I can see that you already know that treatment for you is going to be helpful for your baby in the long run, too."

Evelyn began weekly visits with a social worker whose office was near her house. She arranged for her sister to take her toddler one afternoon a week so that Evelyn could sleep a bit longer on that day. Her husband continued to work long shifts but had also asked his sister to help out with one meal a week. Evelyn's mood stabilized, and by 26 weeks she had fewer depressive symptoms and was starting to look forward to the baby's arrival and her maternity leave, which she planned to start with the baby's birth, working up until her due date.

At 27 weeks, however, her waters broke, and eventually David was born prematurely by emergency cesarean section, requiring several weeks of hospitalization until he was stable enough to be discharged. In the course of recovering from surgery and juggling her toddler's needs, her return to work, and her husband's work schedule, Evelyn's depression symptoms flared again. She continued to have frequent crying spells, including tears at Dr. Rosen's office for her postpartum check-up.

In Evelyn's case, her prenatal provider recognizes signs of depression early in prenatal care and elicits her personal history and her family history of mood disorders. These factors, coupled with the demands of a toddler and three entry-level jobs shared between the couple, and with the stresses of a premature newborn with a prolonged hospital course, appropriately alert the clinician to Evelyn's increased risk for postpartum depression. The awareness of Evelyn's life context as well as her risks facilitates Dr. Rosen's subsequent diagnosis of postpartum depression. Her context is also relevant to her treatment plans. Like many women, Evelyn articulates a desire to avoid medications in the interest of "not hurting the baby." Yet counseling would need to fit into her multiple obligations and tight scheduling needs. After David's early arrival and difficult start, his pediatric provider needs to stay alert to any signs of postpartum depression when Evelyn brings him in for well-child care or acute illnesses. Dr. Rosen helps Evelyn reconsider her choices for treatment of her depression in the new family context. Throughout, eliciting Evelyn's experience through the FIFE method enables her clinician to find the best care plan for her, collaborating with her baby's provider and other health professionals to optimize care for Evelyn, her new baby, and the other members of her family.

CONCLUSION

The foundation of woman-centered maternity care is thus a careful exploration of each individual woman's life context, starting with the clinician eliciting and addressing the multiple dimensions of her current experience as described in this part of the book. Keeping the focus on the whole woman, not just her pregnancy or her potential risks, grounds the process of prenatal care in health and wellness rather than disease as much as possible. In the event of serious medical problems in maternity care, such a focus on understanding the woman's experience is especially critical to prevent the medical issues from overwhelming every interaction with caregivers and diverting attention away from the woman herself. Maintaining the woman-centered approach, the clinician can then widen his or her understanding of the woman's experience by situating her within both her unique developmental and life-cycle stage, as well as the broader social context of childbirth and motherhood. Part Three will elaborate further on this aspect of woman-centered care.

REFERENCES

1 Stewart M, Brown JB, Weston WW, *et al.*, eds. *Patient-centered Medicine: transforming the clinical method.* 2nd ed. Oxford: Radcliffe Medical Press; 2003.

2 Banta D. What is the efficacy/effectiveness of antenatal care and the financial and organizational implications? Copenhagen: WHO Regional Office for Europe; 2003. [Cited July 26, 2009]. Available from: www.euro.who.int/Document/E82996.pdf

3 Mishler EG. *The Discourse of Medicine: dialectics of medical interviews.* Norwood, NJ: Ablex; 1984.

4 Barry CA, Stevenson FA, Britten N, *et al.* Giving voice to the lifeworld. More humane, more effective medical care? A qualitative study of doctor–patient communication in general practice. *Soc Sci Med.* 2001; **53**: 487–505.

5 Dahlberg K, Drew N. A lifeworld paradigm for nursing research. *J Holist Nurs.* 1997; **15**: 303–17.

6 Malterud K, Hollnagel H. Talking with women about personal health resources in general practice: key questions about salutogenesis. *Scand J Prim Health Care.* 1998; **16**: 66–71.

7 Malterud K, Hollnagel H. Women's self-assessed personal health resources. *Scand J Prim Health Care.* 1997; **15**: 163–8.

8 Bondas T. Finnish women's experiences of antenatal care. *Midwifery.* 2002; **18**: 61–71.

9 Bondas T, Eriksson K. Women's lived experiences of pregnancy: a tapestry of joy and suffering. *Qual Health Res.* 2001; **11**: 824–40.

10 Keating-Lefler R, Wilson ME. The experience of becoming a mother for single, unpartnered, Medicaid-eligible, first-time mothers. *J Nurs Scholarsh.* 2004; **36**: 23–9.

11 Declercq E, Sakala C, Corry M, *et al. Listening to Mothers II: Report of the Second National U.S. Survey of Women's Childbearing Experiences.* New York: Childbirth Connection; 2006 October.

12 Zachariah R. Mother–daughter and husband–wife attachment as predictors of psychological well-being during pregnancy. *Clin Nurs Res.* 1994; **3**: 371–92.

13 Hildingsson I, Waldenstrom U, Radestad I. Women's expectations on antenatal care as assessed in early pregnancy: number of visits, continuity of caregiver and general content. *Acta Obstet Gynecol Scand.* 2002; **81**: 118–25.

14 Poole VL, Flowers JS, Goldenberg RL, *et al.* Changes in intendedness during pregnancy in a high-risk multiparous population. *Matern Child Health J.* 2000; **4**: 179–82.

15 Clement S, Wilson J, Sikorski J. Women's experiences of antenatal ultrasound scans. In: Clement S, ed. *Psychological Perspectives on Pregnancy and Childbirth.* Edinburgh: Churchill Livingstone; 1998. pp. 7–24.

16 ACOG. ACOG Committee Opinion No. 360: Sex selection. *Obstet Gynecol.* 2007; **109**: 475–8.

17 Serour GI. Ethical guidelines on sex selection for non-medical purposes: FIGO committee

for the ethical aspects of human reproduction and women's health. *Int J Gynaecol Obstet.* 2006; **92**: 329.

18 Bramwell R, Carter D. An exploration of midwives' and obstetricians' knowledge of genetic screening in pregnancy and their perception of appropriate counselling. *Midwifery.* 2001; **17**: 133–41.

19 Melender HL. Experiences of fears associated with pregnancy and childbirth: a study of 329 pregnant women. *Birth.* 2002; **29**: 101–11.

20 Melender HL, Lauri S. Fears associated with pregnancy and childbirth – experiences of women who have recently given birth. *Midwifery.* 1999; **15**: 177–82.

21 Wiles R. "I'm not fat, I'm pregnant." The impact of pregnancy on fat women's body image. In: Wilkinson S, Kitzinger C, editors. *Women and Health: feminist perspectives.* London: Taylor & Francis; 1994. pp. 33–48.

22 Hundley V, Ryan M. Are women's expectations and preferences for intrapartum care affected by the model of care on offer? *BJOG.* 2004; **111**: 550–60.

23 Monto MA. Lamaze and Bradley childbirth classes: contrasting perspectives toward the medical model of birth. *Birth.* 1996; **23**: 193–201.

24 VandeVusse L. The essential forces of labor revisited: 13 Ps reported in women's stories. *MCN: Am J Matern Child Nurs.* 1999; **24**: 176–84.

25 Green JM, Coupland VA, Kitzinger JV. *Great Expectations: a prospective study of women's expectations and experiences of childbirth.* 2nd ed. Cheshire, England: Books for Midwives Press; 1998. pp. 260–1.

26 Waldenstrom U, Hildingsson I, Ryding EL. Antenatal fear of childbirth and its association with subsequent caesarean section and experience of childbirth. *BJOG.* 2006; **113**: 638–46.

27 Gibbins J, Thomson AM. Women's expectations and experiences of childbirth. *Midwifery.* 2001; **17**: 302–13.

28 Escott D, Spiby H, Slade P, *et al.* The range of coping strategies women use to manage pain and anxiety prior to and during first experience of labour. *Midwifery.* 2004; **20**: 144.

29 Sjogren B. Reasons for anxiety about childbirth in 100 pregnant women. *J Psychosom Obstet Gynaecol.* 1997; **18**: 266–72.

30 Declercq E, Sakala C, Corry M, *et al. Listening to Mothers: Report of the First National U.S. Survey of Women's Childbearing Experiences.* New York: Maternity Center Association; 2002 October.

31 Hodnett ED, Gates S, Hofmeyr GJ, *et al.* Continuous support for women during childbirth. *Cochrane Database Syst Rev.* 2007: CD003766.

32 McGrath SK, Kennell JH. A randomized controlled trial of continuous labor support for middle-class couples: effect on cesarean delivery rates. *Birth.* 2008; **35**: 92–7.

33 Tumblin A, Simkin P. Pregnant women's perceptions of their nurse's role during labor and delivery. *Birth.* 2001; **28**: 52–6.

34 MacKinnon K, McIntyre M, Quance M. The meaning of the nurse's presence during childbirth. *J Obstet Gynecol Neonatal Nurs.* 2005; **34**: 28–36.

35 Matthews R, Callister LC. Childbearing women's perceptions of nursing care that promotes dignity. *J Obstet Gynecol Neonatal Nurs.* 2004; **33**: 498–507.

36 Berg M, Dahlberg K. A phenomenological study of women's experiences of complicated childbirth. *Midwifery.* 1998; **14**: 23–9.

37 Borders N. After the afterbirth: a critical review of postpartum health relative to method of delivery. *J Midwifery Womens Health.* 2006; **51**: 242–8.

38 Niska K, Snyder M, Lia-Hoagberg B. Family ritual facilitates adaptation to parenthood. *Public Health Nurs.* 1998; **15**: 329–37.

39 Zepeda M. Selected maternal-infant care practices of Spanish-speaking women. *J Obstet Gynecol Neonatal Nurs.* 1982; **11**: 371–4.

40 Mercer RT, Walker LO. A review of nursing interventions to foster becoming a mother. *J Obstet Gynecol Neonatal Nurs.* 2006; **35**: 568–82.

41 Moran CF, Holt VL, Martin DP. What do women want to know after childbirth? *Birth.* 1997; **24**: 27–34.

42 Lavender T, Walkinshaw SA. Can midwives reduce postpartum psychological morbidity? A randomized trial. *Birth.* 1998; **25**: 215–19.

43 Small R, Lumley J, Donohue L, *et al.* Randomised controlled trial of midwife led debriefing to reduce maternal depression after operative childbirth. *BMJ.* 2000; **321**(7268): 1043–7.

44 Small R, Lumley J, Toomey L. Midwife-led debriefing after operative birth: four to six year follow-up of a randomised trial [ISRCTN24648614]. *BMC Med.* 2006; **4**: 3.

45 Priest SR, Henderson J, Evans SF, *et al.* Stress debriefing after childbirth: a randomised controlled trial. *Med J Aust.* 2003; **178**: 542–5.

46 Callister LC. Making meaning: women's birth narratives. *J Obstet Gynecol Neonatal Nurs.* 2004; **33**: 508–18.

47 Tulman L, Fawcett J, Groblewski L, *et al.* Changes in functional status after childbirth. *Nurs Res.* 1990; **39**: 70–5.

48 Brown S, Lumley J. Maternal health after childbirth: results of an Australian population based survey. *Br J Obstet Gynaecol.* 1998; **105**: 156–61.

49 Raisler J. Against the odds: breastfeeding experiences of low income mothers. *J Midwifery Womens Health.* 2000; **45**: 253.

50 Raisler J. Midwives helping mothers to breastfeed: food for thought and action. *J Midwifery Womens Health.* 2000; **45**: 202.

51 Marchand L, Morrow MH. Infant feeding practices: understanding the decision-making process. *Fam Med.* 1994; **26**: 319–24.

52 Gill SL. The little things: perceptions of breastfeeding support. *J Obstet Gynecol Neonatal Nurs.* 2001; **30**: 401–9.

53 Leff EW, Gagne MP, Jefferis SC. Maternal perceptions of successful breastfeeding. *J Hum Lact.* 1994; **10**: 99–104.

54 Mozingo JN, Davis MW, Droppleman PG, *et al.* "It wasn't working." Women's experiences with short-term breastfeeding. *MCN: Am J Matern Child Nurs.* 2000; **25**: 120–6.

55 Pisacane A, Continisio GI, Aldinucci M, *et al.* A controlled trial of the father's role in breastfeeding promotion. *Pediatrics.* 2005; **116**: e494–8.

56 Stremler J, Lovera D. Insight from a breastfeeding peer support pilot program for husbands and fathers of Texas WIC participants. *J Hum Lact.* 2004; **20**: 417–22.

57 Bar-Yam NB, Darby L. Fathers and breastfeeding: a review of the literature. *J Hum Lact.* 1997; **13**: 45–50.

58 Blyth R, Creedy DK, Dennis CL, *et al.* Effect of maternal confidence on breastfeeding duration: an application of breastfeeding self-efficacy theory. *Birth.* 2002; **29**: 278–84.

59 Hill PD. The enigma of insufficient milk supply. *MCN Am J Matern Child Nurs.* 1991; **16**: 312–16.

60 Quinn AO, Koepsell D, Haller S. Breastfeeding incidence after early discharge and factors influencing breastfeeding cessation. *J Obstet Gynecol Neonatal Nurs.* 1997; **26**: 289–94.

61 Kelleher CM. The physical challenges of early breastfeeding. *Soc Sci Med.* 2006; **63**: 2727–38.

62 Pastore LM, Owens A, Raymond C. Postpartum sexuality concerns among first-time parents from one U.S. academic hospital. *J Sex Med.* 2007; **4**: 115–23.

63 Olds DL, Robinson J, O'Brien R, *et al.* Home visiting by paraprofessionals and by nurses: a randomized, controlled trial. *Pediatrics.* 2002; **110**: 486–96.

64 Olds DL, Kitzman H, Cole R, *et al.* Effects of nurse home-visiting on maternal life course and child development: age 6 follow-up results of a randomized trial. *Pediatrics.* 2004; **114**: 1550–9.

65 Olds DL, Robinson J, Pettitt L, *et al.* Effects of home visits by paraprofessionals and by nurses: age 4 follow-up results of a randomized trial. *Pediatrics.* 2004; **114**: 1560–8.

66 Olds DL, Kitzman H, Hanks C, *et al.* Effects of nurse home visiting on maternal and child functioning: age 9 follow-up of a randomized trial. *Pediatrics.* 2007; **120**: e832–45.

67 Weiss M, Ryan P, Lokken L, *et al.* Length of stay after vaginal birth: Sociodemographic and readiness-for-discharge factors. *Birth.* 2004; **31**: 93–101

68 Weiss ME, Ryan P, Lokken L. Validity and reliability of the perceived readiness for discharge after birth scale. *J Obstet Gynecol Neonatal Nurs.* 2006; **35**: 34–45.

69 Nelson AM. Transition to motherhood. *J Obstet Gynecol Neonatal Nurs.* 2003; **32**: 465–77.

70 Reddy UM, Wapner RJ, Rebar RW, *et al.* Infertility, assisted reproductive technology, and adverse pregnancy outcomes: executive summary of a National Institute of Child Health and Human Development workshop. *Obstet Gynecol.* 2007; **109**: 967–77.

71 Freda MC, Devine KS, Semelsberger C. The lived experience of miscarriage after infertility. *MCN: Am J Matern Child Nurs.* 2003; **28**: 16–23.

72 Layne LL. Motherhood lost: Cultural dimensions of miscarriage and stillbirth in America. *Women Health.* 1990; **16**: 69–98.

73 Swanson KM. Effects of caring, measurement, and time on miscarriage impact and women's well-being. *Nurs Res.* 1999; **48**: 288–98.

74 Adolfsson A, Larsson PG, Wijma B, *et al.* Guilt and emptiness: women's experiences of miscarriage. *Health Care Women Int.* 2004; **25**: 543–60.

75 Nikcevic AV, Tunkel SA, Kuczmierczyk AR, *et al.* Investigation of the cause of miscarriage and its influence on women's psychological distress. *Br J Obstet Gynaecol.* 1999; **106**: 808–13.

76 Wieringa-De Waard M, Hartman EE, Ankum WM, *et al.* Expectant management versus surgical evacuation in first trimester miscarriage: health-related quality of life in randomized and non-randomized patients. *Hum Reprod.* 2002; **17**: 1638–42.

77 Armstrong D. Exploring fathers' experiences of pregnancy after a prior perinatal loss. *MCN: Am J Matern Child Nurs.* 2001; **26**: 147–53.

78 Bansen SS, Stevens HA. Women's experiences of miscarriage in early pregnancy. *J Nurse Midwifery.* 1992; **37**: 84–90.

79 Bowles SV, James LC, Solursh DS, *et al.* Acute and post-traumatic stress disorder after spontaneous abortion. *Am Fam Physician.* 2000; **61**: 1689–96.

80 Frost M, Condon JT. The psychological sequelae of miscarriage: a critical review of the literature. *Aust N Z J Psychiatry.* 1996; **30**: 54–62.

81 Lee C, Slade P. Miscarriage as a traumatic event: a review of the literature and new implications for intervention. *J Psychosom Res.* 1996; **40**: 235–44.

82 Cote-Arsenault D, Mahlangu N. Impact of perinatal loss on the subsequent pregnancy and self: women's experiences. *J Obstet Gynecol Neonatal Nurs.* 1999; **28**: 274–82.

83 Mitchell LM. Women's experiences of unexpected ultrasound findings. *J Midwifery Womens Health*. 2004; **49**: 228–34.

84 Van der Zalm JE, Byrne PJ. Seeing baby: women's experience of prenatal ultrasound examination and unexpected fetal diagnosis. *J Perinatol*. 2006; **26**: 403–8.

85 Cristofalo EA, Dipietro JA, Costigan KA, *et al.* Women's response to fetal choroid plexus cysts detected by prenatal ultrasound. *J Perinatol*. 2006; **26**: 215–23.

86 Weinans MJ, Huijssoon AM, Tymstra T, *et al.* How women deal with the results of serum screening for Down syndrome in the second trimester of pregnancy. *Prenat Diagn*. 2000; **20**: 705–8.

87 Howard ED. Family-centered care in the context of fetal abnormality. *J Perinat Neonatal Nurs*. 2006; **20**: 237–42.

88 Chitty LS. Ultrasound screening for fetal abnormalities. *Prenat Diagn*. 1995; **15**: 1241–57.

89 Beck M. *Expecting Adam: a true story of birth, rebirth and everyday magic.* New York: Berkley Books; 1999.

90 Sandelowski M, Jones LC. "Healing fictions": stories of choosing in the aftermath of the detection of fetal anomalies. *Soc Sci Med*. 1996; **42**: 353–61.

91 Heaman M, Beaton J, Gupton A, *et al.* A comparison of childbirth expectations in high-risk and low-risk pregnant women. *Clin Nurs Res*. 1992; **1**: 252–65.

92 Williams SC, Mackey MC. Women's experiences of preterm labor: a feminist critique. *Health Care Women Int*. 1999; **20**: 29–48.

93 Jackson K, Ternestedt BM, Schollin J. From alienation to familiarity: experiences of mothers and fathers of preterm infants. *J Adv Nurs*. 2003; **43**: 120–9.

94 Wigert H, Johansson R, Berg M, *et al.* Mothers' experiences of having their newborn child in a neonatal intensive care unit. *Scand J Caring Sci*. 2006; **20**: 35–41.

95 Holditch-Davis D, Bartlett TR, Blickman AL, *et al.* Posttraumatic stress symptoms in mothers of premature infants. *J Obstet Gynecol Neonatal Nurs*. 2003; **32**: 161–71.

96 Singer LT, Salvator A, Guo S, *et al.* Maternal psychological distress and parenting stress after the birth of a very low-birth-weight infant. *JAMA*. 1999; **281**: 799–805.

97 Nystedt A, Hogberg U, Lundman B. Some Swedish women's experiences of prolonged labour. *Midwifery*. 2006; **22**: 56.

98 McKay S, Barrows T. Holding back: maternal readiness to give birth. *MCN: Am J Matern Child Nurs*. 1991; **16**: 250–4.

99 Simkin P. *The Labor Progress Handbook: early interventions to prevent and treat dystocia.* 2nd ed. New York: Blackwell; 2005.

100 Coles J. Qualitative study of breastfeeding after childhood sexual assault. 2009 [cited July 26, 2009]. Available from: http://jhl.sagepub.com/cgi/content/abstract/08903 34409334926v1

101 Thoppil J, Riutcel TL, Nalesnik SW. Early intervention for perinatal depression. *Am J Obstet Gynecol*. 2005; **192**: 1446–8.

102 Gunn J, Southern D, Chondros P, *et al.* Guidelines for assessing postnatal problems: introducing evidence-based guidelines in Australian general practice. *Fam Pract*. 2003; **20**: 382–9.

103 Downie J, Wynaden D, McGowan S, *et al.* Using the Edinburgh postnatal depression scale to achieve best practice standards. *Nurs Health Sci*. 2003; **5**: 283–7.

104 Small R, Astbury J, Brown S, *et al.* Depression after childbirth. Does social context matter? *Med J Aust*. 1994; **161**: 473–7.

PART THREE

Understanding the Woman in Context

Pregnancies occur in the context of the woman's own development across the reproductive years as well as within the context of her family and relationships. These relationships are critical for the woman's well-being and for her success as a parent. Pregnancy, birth, and parenting are nested within the larger framework of personal and social expectations of gender roles, for both the woman and her partner. When a woman chooses an alternative pathway, such as lesbian parenting, she must confront the sometimes-hostile expectations and values of her family, her workplace, and other social institutions while still cherishing the experiences of motherhood. Unfortunately, many women face violence in their lives from girlhood through adulthood, with the ensuing fear, despair, and hopelessness often constricting their potential development as women and as mothers. Sexual and physical abuse are frequent precursors to women's entry into substance abuse, a pathway harmful for herself and dangerous for her pregnancy. These problems, particularly the use of illegal substances, may land a woman in the penal system where her options as a pregnant woman are highly restricted. Providing woman-centered care across this broad range of women's experience requires a panoply of skills and understandings that we will describe in detail in the first section on the proximal context of a woman's pregnancy. The second section will address the distal context: the larger cultural community, with its social and economic factors, in which the woman and her family experience and interpret the experience of pregnancy, birth, and parenting.

Understanding the Whole Woman in the Context of Her Adult Development and Her Family

Lucy M. Candib

Woman-centered care recognizes that the timing of the first pregnancy makes an irreversible change in a woman's individual development. Her life has changed. She is defined as a sexual being to the world. For a woman who chooses to continue her pregnancy, whether it be planned or unplanned, whether she is single or has a partner of the same or different gender, pregnancy is a fundamental directional choice in her adult development, changing forever her relationship to her family of origin, her connection with current and future partners, and her participation in work or career. She will have to decide what kind of mother she wants to be in the context of the family she came from and in the context of the world she lives and works in today.

At the biological level, pregnancy and birth cause irrevocable changes in a woman's body. She experiences her body as capable of creating and sustaining another person. A successful experience – of pregnancy, labor, and delivery, and the provision of nourishment to her baby – constitutes a major life accomplishment for many women. At the same time, a pregnant woman may undergo both temporary discomforts as well as permanent changes, all of which imply relinquishing her body to forces outside her control – whether these changes be the ordinary changes of early-pregnancy nausea, stretch marks, weight gain, droopy breasts, or lack of lubrication during postpartum sexual intercourse, or other changes following complications such as an unpredictable delivery, an unexpected cesarean, or difficulties in breastfeeding. In sum, no one can become a biological mother without undergoing major physiological and body changes.

INTENDED OR UNINTENDED?

Whether a pregnancy is intended (wanted for some time or wanted at the moment) or unintended (not wanted now and perhaps not ever) is probably the most salient fact for the clinician approaching the newly pregnant woman. A woman may be clear that the pregnancy was unintended: her birth control method failed (broken condom, missed birth control pill, IUD out of place, etc.) and now she must decide what to do. She may not have intended to have sex, or she had sex in a situation out of her control; her boyfriend may have broken off with her after he found out she was pregnant, and her circumstances have changed. Whatever the context, she has to make a decision. For these women, careful options counseling is essential for them to make a decision that recognizes their agency, their life situation, and their future. (*See* discussion in Parts One, Two and Five). Some women may choose to keep a pregnancy but plan to release a baby for adoption; this complex choice requires a comprehensive plan involving adoption services that counsel about multiple possibilities, including open adoption. (*See* discussion of adoption in Part Two).

Some women may be ambivalent in their use of contraception not only because of uncertainty about the methods, cost, accessibility, etc., but also because they are truly ambivalent about whether or not to have a baby. They use getting pregnant itself as the way to resolve current uncertainty in their lives, adopting the viewpoint, "If it happens, it happens." Such a woman is opting *not* to take charge of the timing of a key moment in her adult development. The relationship with her current partner may be at stake: perhaps she thinks a pregnancy would cement the relationship. Her current work may be unfulfilling, or she may be looking for a way to leave her parents' home.

Once she has decided to keep a pregnancy, her "routine" prenatal care begins, but the uncertainties in her life, ambivalence about her future, and questions about her partner will continue to surface as her pregnancy advances and after the birth of her child(ren). Her provider may realize how ambivalence about major life issues is both a "risk factor" for decision-making throughout pregnancy and parenting but also an opportunity to work with the woman as she grows into her new roles. As noted in Parts Two and Four, the clinician aware of the circumstances and factors around a woman's initial decision about pregnancy will be much better suited to guide her subsequent plans when she must again decide about contraception and about these ongoing life issues.

TIMING

Despite the fact that around the world many pregnancies are unplanned (*see* Part One), the timing of pregnancy in a woman's life is critical. This section will first address pregnancy in adolescence, the cause of irreversible changes in a young woman's life, and then pregnancies occurring in older women, which also inevitably interact with the other events unfolding in women's life cycles.

Pregnancy in adolescence is an indicator that sexual activity has begun. In the absence of an obvious sexual partner, unexpected adolescent pregnancy may signal rape or incest.[1] Families may try to hide such pregnancies themselves, and the pregnant teen often comes late to medical attention, or not at all.[2] Sometimes a teen woman may arrive at the emergency room in labor, or may try to abandon the newborn.

Teen pregnancies are often outside of marriage.[3] While much of Western society has become accepting of this, in many cultures and in small closed communities a pregnancy outside of marriage may still be a source of stigma. At times the woman herself is accepting of the pregnancy, but her family is overwhelmed by shame. Rejection and isolation of the pregnant woman may be the result. The availability of confidential, safe, legal, and accessible termination of pregnancy can obviate such dire circumstances; however, at times, even women with the opportunity to choose will still choose pregnancy. Samantha, the teen mother we met in Part Two, decides to keep her pregnancy despite her mother's predictable anger:

> Samantha's mother was furious (about her pregnancy) as expected, and told Samantha not to come home. Samantha called her 25-year-old cousin Alice, who had two children herself but who offered to let Samantha stay with them for a while. The school nurse arranged for Samantha to get prenatal care through a school-mothers program and its connection to a prenatal clinic at the hospital. The doctors there were busy and harried, and Samantha did not like going there or talking to them about her family or the baby's father. She had a hard time figuring out the bus schedule from Alice's apartment to the clinic and thus missed a few appointments. As an alternative strategy, the school nurse arranged for her to transfer her care to the community health center where she would have one main provider, Dr. Adelle Epps. There, Samantha worked with the social worker to get some baby supplies and to attend some childbirth classes with other teen mothers. She started dating Jack, the older brother of one of these new friends, who promised to support her through the labor and postpartum period. The nurse and social worker tried unsuccessfully to encourage Samantha to reconcile with her mother. (*See* full vignette and provider biography in Appendix.)

Teen pregnancy can be one of the most demanding yet one of the most enjoyable aspects of providing prenatal care. Teenage women who feel respected and listened to can be open, energetic, articulate, and committed participants in making their pregnancies a chance to "do everything right." Unfortunately, doctors often underestimate how interested teen mothers will be in healthy pregnancy and parenting activities.[4]

In addition to regular prenatal care, maternity care for adolescents involves integration of their nuclear family or support structure (including sometimes their partner's family); attention to schooling, so easily interrupted by pregnancy and child-rearing; respectful inclusion and recognition of the young woman's partner, often a teenage man who may be very uncomfortable in the medical setting; and detailed focus on the teen mother's habits – diet, exercise, and smoking – critical issues for teen health. Although adolescents may face a higher risk of pregnancy complications near term, their earlier prenatal courses may not be medically complicated, but are emotionally tumultuous and socially problematic. Such social and emotional problems are associated with a higher risk of medical complications at term.[5-7]

Optimal care for pregnant teens requires an integrated team of clinicians, advocates, social workers, nutritionists, and educators. This team can promote a healthy outlook for the pregnant young woman and provide a reliable source of support for the clinician himself or herself when facing the complex social and emotional challenges of the teen's care. The clinician who also cares for the pregnant adolescent's mother may or may not be the right person to look after the young woman's pregnancy, depending on how the teen and her mother are getting along. Sometimes the young woman needs a clinician other than her mother's provider to emphasize that she is now an emerging adult who needs separate medical attention; sometimes the young woman can see her mother's clinician (at times her own family doctor) and benefit from a supportive and familiar clinical relationship during a time when her relationships at home may be rocky. Group prenatal visits may work particularly well for pregnant teens (*see* Part Five). Adolescents like Samantha and Alexandra (whom we will meet later) who participate in teen pregnancy programs in their schools and have childbirth education integrated into their regular curriculum, with ongoing daily attention to nutrition and education, are less likely to deliver low-birth-weight infants than teens who attend hospital-based clinics.[8] They may have the most considered labor plans and the best information about what is actually going on in their bodies. Graduates of teen pregnancy programs often become excellent mothers and thoughtful participants in their later healthcare.

Women entering desired or planned first pregnancies in their thirties and forties face a different set of challenges than teens have. While "older" primigravidas often have the advantage of a stable partner relationship, good family income, professional skills, and advanced education, they also face increased medical risks such as a higher rate of genetic abnormalities and greater likelihood of prenatal complications such as hypertension and pre-eclampsia. In addition to these risks, women who unintentionally become pregnant at the end of their reproductive life also often, like teenagers, feel ashamed; "change of life" babies reveal that a woman is still sexually active and that she did not take adequate "precautions." For reasons that have more to do with timing and socially accepted patterns of family life, a midlife pregnancy may represent a crisis equivalent to adolescent pregnancy and, even for healthy women, a source of substantial social and emotional challenge. Additionally, the mature woman having her first baby may be less tolerant of the physical discomforts of pregnancy and the uncertainties regarding the meaning and outcome of tests and the inherent unpredictability of what is to come. The professional woman, after planning her education, her career decisions, her wedding, the purchase of a home, etc., may be anxious to plan similar certainty about her delivery date and her maternity leave. In contrast to the teenager, "rolling with the punches" may not be a skill the older mother has had to develop; pregnancy may be the first time in her life when events in her life truly became unpredictable and out of her control. Here are Melissa and her husband Kirk, the software engineers we met previously, at the beginning of pregnancy:

> At the first and subsequent prenatal visits, Kirk peppered Larisa with many questions about what might happen and what the possible consequences were. Each visit was longer than average, as Melissa and Kirk found the waits and the unpredictable part of pregnancy very problematic and always had long lists of questions and concerns. Larisa felt frustrated with their need for certainty and schedules, and tried to explain that this was just the beginning of unpredictability in their lives, but they did not hear that.
>
> At the 10-week visit, Melissa and Kirk pulled out the brochure in their standard prenatal packet that discussed the pros and cons of the various methods for maternal serum screening for neural tube defects and chromosomal disorders. They had researched this question extensively on the Internet and were ready to talk about the decision.

Early prenatal visits with the "older" pregnant woman and sometimes her partner must address the possibility of a genetic abnormality: what will be the couple's approach? Because of their educational background, many such women are well-informed and have already made decisions about how they consider the eventuality of an abnormality. However, the reality of the pregnancy and of having a fetus inside may make a woman or a couple rethink that decision.[9] Deciding about any kind of genetic screening including amniocentesis and what to do about the results may make the early months of a pregnancy for an "older" woman a complex period for which only time can provide the answers. Learning to wait may be the hardest task of all (*see* further discussion in Part Five). Women and their partners may also make different decisions at different moments in their lives.

> Michelle, 39, and her husband George, 45, were both university professors. They had an amniocentesis with their first pregnancy because of their fears about an abnormal child. When they became pregnant with a much-desired second child, they mutually decided not to have another amniocentesis. They felt that if there were a genetic abnormality such as Down syndrome, they would still keep the pregnancy. When asked what had changed since their first pregnancy that led them to this decision despite an actual increase in risk, they answered that if their first child had been abnormal, they felt the defect would have been a huge assault on their "ego." Now that they were accomplished parents of their first child, they felt they could "handle" the potential impact of an abnormal baby. (*See* full vignette in Appendix.)

Pregnancies following a period of primary or secondary infertility are particularly tense. Anxieties for the couple about miscarriage may be particularly high in the wake of infertility treatment. In facing the anxiety and uncertainty of pregnancies in the wake of infertility, the woman-centered clinician's best strategies for couples like Melissa and Kirk are recognition of their worries and hopeful optimism in the face of each passing milestone (*see* discussion of infertility in Part Two).

PARITY

Each pregnancy is a milestone in the woman's own development. While first pregnancies redefine a woman as a mother, subsequent pregnancies exert their strongest effects on the woman within the context of the family she is creating. The next child permanently alters a woman's relation to her firstborn and intensifies issues of childcare, career interruption, and a woman's need for time as an adult, with her partner if she has one, or with other adults. Subsequent pregnancies with a new partner require renegotiation of relationships with the father(s) of prior children, and integration of the father of the current pregnancy into domestic arrangements and other children's understandings.

For the woman with one or more children in a stable relationship, a desired new pregnancy can be the source of great joy. Less frightened by the events to come, less intimidated by the medical system, more confident in her ability to handle uncertainty, more certain of her partner's capacity for support, she is more able to enjoy the process and even the unpredictability. The clinician can appreciate her engagement in her role as she delights in teaching her older child or children about the new brother or sister when they attend prenatal visits to hear the heartbeat. The birth of a subsequent child raises the issue of how best to encourage a loving and protective relation of the older sibling(s) toward the new baby and how best to discourage jealousy and rivalry. While toddlers and young children may have little realistic understanding of pregnancy and birth, the woman-centered clinician can make the office setting comfortable for them with toys, integrate them into the visit by letting them touch and hold the Doptone, and with older children count the heartbeat together. A teaching doll used in childbirth education classes (a fetus-doll attached by an umbilical cord to a placenta inside a net bag) makes an ideal "toy" to have available in the exam room when older children attend. When the clinician appreciates the woman's children and makes the visit fun for them, the pregnant woman can feel more at ease, and the medical setting becomes more comfortable should her children themselves need medical attention.

While the woman having subsequent children may already define herself as a mother, each child transforms the practical reality of what this means. Sometimes the mother asks the clinician for advice – how should she bring the baby home from the hospital to reduce jealousy? Should the older child be moved to a bed so the baby can go in the crib? If she is working outside the home, she will have to address the adequacy of her maternity leave options and whether she returns to work in the same capacity at the end of that leave. She will also now have to negotiate daycare for two or more children at the same or different settings. Women with adequate support and resources may choose to reduce their work hours with subsequent children, while women who are economically disadvantaged in countries without mandated maternity leave may have to return to low-paying jobs and leave their infant children in childcare settings much earlier than they would prefer.

> Felicity's first pregnancy occurred at age 16 with Tony, her first serious boyfriend. She hoped to have a lasting relationship with him and named the baby after him. However, Tony left Felicity during her pregnancy for another girlfriend, also pregnant, and had since remained only peripherally involved in parenting his namesake via court-mandated assistance. Since that first pregnancy, Felicity lived in turn with her mother, aunt, two friends, and most recently her boyfriend Rafael, the father of her daughter and now of the third child she was expecting.

Blended families are increasingly common. Both the mother and the father may have children by previous partners. Together they may raise the child of their current relationship as well as her older children and sometimes his. The clinician caring for the woman in this situation will want to inquire into the stability of the relationship. If her partner has prior children, what is his relationship to those children and to his previous partners? If their relationship is of recent duration, is the woman confident of her partner's fidelity? If not, she may be at risk for sexually acquired infections during the pregnancy and later. If he is involved with his previous children, will she be integrating them into her household occasionally or even permanently? If he is not involved with his previous children, what is the implication for his fathering for the baby to come? Likewise, if she has children from prior relationships, does she have contact with the fathers of those children? Is there any history of physical or sexual abuse by those partners? Is she at any further risk from them? Subsequent sections will further explore these abuse issues. As with other times, safety concerns extend to the care of her children. Since pregnancy and delivery may require that her children spend time in other households when she is unavailable, their well-being must be assured. Do her children ever spend any time with their biological fathers or paternal grandparents, and are they safe in those settings? All of these questions are relevant to health and safety of the woman and her children during the current pregnancy.

> Rosa (*see* Part Two and full vignette in Appendix) had had her first baby at home with a midwife in her Guatemalan village when she was 16 and had left that child in her native country with her husband José's father's family to come north with him. She had not seen her son since he was an infant, and appeared sad when Dr. Rosen asked for details of her first birth.

For an immigrant woman who has left older children in their homeland, a subsequent birth in the new country can be the source of much joy but also renewed sadness at the separation from her older children. The woman-centered clinician encourages such a woman to maintain contact with her family of origin in her home country during the pregnancy and after the birth. A phone card with discounted rates to call her homeland is a present she can request from her friends and an essential item to be packed in her suitcase for the hospital.

FAMILY OF ORIGIN

While the meaning of pregnancy is centered in the woman's life and current nuclear family situation (single, partnered, married, etc.), her pregnancy is also an event within the larger family systems of both the woman and her partner. The birth of a first grandchild on both sides is a unique generational moment; a pregnancy when a parent or grandparent is dying may have special relevance. When a woman's family does not approve of her partner or his family, they may be less welcoming and enthusiastic in the event of pregnancy, despite its generational implications. In very conservative settings, a woman's pregnancy may provoke a crisis such that when a woman gets pregnant "out of wedlock," she may be forced to marry or may be cut off from the family, as with Samantha, or with Jen, whom we will meet later in this chapter. The woman-centered clinician will want to situate the pregnant woman as a daughter and sister within the generational schema of her family of origin and explore the role of this pregnancy to best understand how it "fits." Sibling order may be an important factor in understanding how a woman views herself. An oldest daughter may feel confident and accomplished in her maternal role even though she is having her first pregnancy; a younger sibling may be less certain of herself; the youngest may have a unique role in the family, as with Alexandra from Part Two:

> Helen the midwife was pleased to meet in the labor room Alexandra's two older sisters, both of whom worked as medical assistants in a local medical office. . . . Her mother and another older sister soon joined them to celebrate the arrival of baby Jasmine. Helen began to appreciate Alexandra's role as the "baby sister" who was especially treasured in her family.

During pregnancy, women turn to women support figures, or confidantes, for advice, support, and reassurance.[10] For most women, their mothers, sisters, or other women family members play this central role. Occasionally, women in her partner's family may provide this support. However, for immigrant women whose mothers live in another country, or for women who are estranged from their mothers, this crucial linkage may be missing. An absent or remote mother may also raise issues for the pregnant woman about how she herself will parent and whom she will turn to as a role model.

Exploration of the woman's family system early in pregnancy using a genogram can help identify when loss and isolation are likely to become important issues in the pregnancy. A pregnant woman whose own mother has died may experience a unique sense of sadness and loss during pregnancy as she longs to ask her own mother about her experience of pregnancy or birth. Being woman-centered in this instance means exploring the family genogram with the woman, acknowledging the loss, and allowing the sadness its special position during pregnancy. Certain phrases ("she would have loved to share this with you" or "she would have been very proud of you") can make legitimate the woman's sadness even if her mother died many years previously.

For women whose mother is absent or remote, the identification of a woman friend or relative who can serve as support and confidante is crucial. If a woman is unable to name a support person within her family, ethnic community, or church, the woman-centered clinician will need to address the reason for her isolation. Such isolation may be an indicator that the woman's partner is abusive and controlling and has cut her off from such external contact. Even in the absence of abuse, prenatal anxiety is increased in the absence of social support,[11] making it critical that clinicians identify when such help is missing. The provision of individually based postpartum support may reduce the risk of postpartum depression in such women.[12]

Other family-of-origin issues also play a role during the intense role adjustment of the postpartum period. Grandparents on both sides may weigh in with their opinions about how babies should be fed and cared for. New mothers and fathers adjusting to their new roles may find themselves consciously or unconsciously mimicking the roles their parents played in their childhood families. Incorporating outside employment into these roles may prove especially challenging. We will address more of the workplace issues later in Section One of this Part.

PREGNANCY, LABOR AND BIRTH AS ACCOMPLISHMENTS IN ADULT DEVELOPMENT

For most women, pregnancy is an event that takes place only a few times in their lives and represents a key period in their self-definition. Pregnancy affords the opportunity for a woman to begin to take on the skills of motherhood and dedicate herself to her child's welfare. Pregnant women take seriously all the medical advice they get during pregnancy. Although women themselves may have little control over the onset of complications of pregnancy, they can take pride in "taking good care" of themselves, getting timely prenatal care, and "following doctors' orders." Walking more, eating less junk food, taking vitamins, cutting down or quitting smoking, avoiding alcohol and drugs, coming for appointments (however inconvenient), are all examples of women demonstrating commitment to becoming good mothers. Smokers may or may not be able to give up cigarettes on medical advice, but often they have discussed this choice with confidantes, and have decided that doctors do not have a realistic understanding of their situation.[10] Thus, "following doctor's orders" itself can be a problem when either these orders conflict with a woman's sense of what is right or what she hears from family members, or if the doctor's "orders" are too dogmatic or doctor-centered. Conversely, women may shoulder the blame for not taking good care of themselves if something goes awry.

The developmental tasks facing all women in pregnancy and especially in labor include letting go, trust in one's partner or support person, and trust in caregivers to provide the woman-centered care that she desires. The role of labor in a woman's adult development is a very individual matter and depends significantly on how the woman views herself – about her fear of pain and of how she might act, about whether she will be or become the woman she hopes to be during labor. (*See* Part Four for various ways that the clinician may foster these goals through woman-centered labor care). Inquiring into and addressing women's varying hopes and fears, as described in Part Two, enables the woman-centered clinician to tailor, as much as possible, the course of maternity care to each woman's needs as she engages in becoming a mother to this particular child.

Women with a past history of abuse, particularly sexual abuse, may have specific issues about their sense of adequacy and may be particularly vulnerable to a sense of shame, especially in a setting where they are again (during labor) out of control of a sexual part of their body. Fear, anxiety, and shame will all work to inhibit labor and contribute to a negative experience. The clinician aware of the woman's past experience works actively to thwart such negative dynamics (*see* Section Two, Chapter 2 in this Part and also Section Two Chapter 3 in Part Four). When the woman has difficulty with these tasks, she is less likely to have a sense of accomplishment about her labor. The woman-centered practitioner recognizes that how a woman handles labor is deeply connected to her sense of herself as a woman, both her strengths and her vulnerabilities.

In woman-centered maternity care, the birth event is a central moment in the drama of a woman's adult development, making it crucial that all involved in the birth process exert every effort to make the experience empowering and affirming. The labor and birth story is one of the key narratives of a woman's adult life. Because of its centrality in her personal history and sometimes in her self-definition, she will tell it many times. What from the outside may appear to be mundane details (e.g. when and where her water broke; what the doctor said about the baby's head; how many pushes she made) to the woman are pivotal moments in the story.[13,14] Professionals who witness and participate in births many times a day lose sight of the fact that they are part of what for the woman is a drama that will occur only once or a few times in her life. Thus the clinician's imperative from the onset of labor is to begin identifying, underlining and supporting the woman's strengths as part of the process of helping create her birth story: she is smart, she asks good questions, she is patient, she has had good prenatal care, she has stopped smoking, she plans for arrangements for her other children, she works many hours to support her family, she has made a long and arduous voyage to this country, she has left an abusive partner – and so on. Even when a woman eventually requires assistance, for instance, with a vacuum device or forceps, or a cesarean section, providers can emphasize how strong her work was to get to that point.

The tasks of the teenager in labor will be different from the tasks of an older woman having her first baby or a multigravid woman. Nevertheless, the goal with each is to affirm this woman as strong, powerful, and able. For every woman, because of the high likelihood that she may interpret any problems in the birth process as her personal failings, clinicians should continuously affirm her strengths, her endurance, her commitment, and should look for and address any expressions of guilt or failure on her part.

Sylvie was a 25-year-old Albanian woman pregnant for the second time. She and her husband Viktor had been devastated by her first pregnancy's miscarriage. Her self-esteem also suffered because Viktor's family had made it clear that they did not think she was good enough for him. She carried her healthy second pregnancy to term, but progressed slowly when she went into labor. Despite analgesia, oxytocin, epidural anesthesia, and adequate contractions, the baby did not descend. Sylvie was exhausted, and Viktor was fearful. He wanted his wife safe, and he wanted the doctors to do something. Her family doctor, Dr. Mercedes Burman, recommended a cesarean section, and Dr. Diamond, the obstetrician consultant, agreed. The surgery was uncomplicated, and a healthy baby girl, Elisabeth, was delivered with Viktor in the delivery room. . . . Sylvie quickly established a good breastfeeding pattern and recovered from the surgery without incident. On the day of discharge, Dr. Burman emphasized her strength and resilience in labor, her excellent lactation, and her good healing. She commented to Viktor in Sylvie's earshot, "What a strong and powerful wife you chose!" They both beamed. (*See* full vignette in Appendix.)

For many women, including immigrants like Sylvie, breastfeeding is a crucial competency that solidifies their sense of themselves as mothers. The woman-centered clinician can emphasize the strengths and knowledge about her baby that a woman gains by choosing to breastfeed, even when her delivery experience might have felt discouraging about her maternal abilities. For other women, breastfeeding is less central and the switch to bottle-feeding comes easily when they face any initial challenge in lactation. The clinician's role is to understand the underlying elements in the woman's choices around lactation and support her through the problems that arise. As described in Part Two, the woman-centered clinician must choose ways to disentangle the lactation problem from the woman's ability and identity as a mother, and continue to support her in her new role as a mother regardless of her baby's method of nutrition.

The clinicians caring for a pregnant woman can support her healthy choices, and movements toward these choices, as examples of her *competence*, of her ability as mother-to-be. For instance, in the example above, although Alexandra was "the baby," her careful prenatal care, successful natural childbirth with her sisters' support, and healthy postpartum course establish her competency as a mother, which the midwife Helen acknowledges at each prenatal and postpartum visit. Yet apart from "coaching" during labor, many prenatal caregivers while attending carefully to medical issues lose track of the woman's need to hear that she is doing a good job. The inherent disempowering nature of medical care almost inevitably blames problems and complications directly or indirectly on the woman herself (regardless of whether she actually has any control over the circumstances). Women themselves – already personally and socially vulnerable to feelings of inadequacy – are also highly likely to blame themselves for any pregnancy loss or complication. Thus, the woman-centered clinician must look for and underline the areas of the pregnant woman's life where she is doing things well. Identifying factors for health, salutogenesis[15] (*see* Part Five on risk and prevention), is an unfamiliar step for risk-focused prenatal caregivers. Moving toward a strength-based approach to healthcare (as opposed to a risk-based approach) will support women's empowerment as women and as mothers-to-be.

CHAPTER 2

Supports and Relationships in Pregnancy and Parenting

Katharine Barnard

Pregnancy and the transition to parenting are necessarily seated within the context of relationships. Partners, family, prior children, and friends all form part of this transformational life event. A woman's supporters, whether partner or friend, contribute to her ability to transition to mothering and her self-concept as parent. Certainly, the individual context of each woman differs according to her age, prior children, partner status, and plans for work or school; this social context influences a woman's expectations for pregnancy and parenting.

Given that women's situations differ so widely, women experience the transitions of pregnancy and parenting in a multitude of ways. For some, pregnancy may feel like the fulfillment of a marital relationship, either by growing a family or by cementing a new partnership. As noted earlier, a woman who finds herself in a failing relationship with a partner or family may hope that a pregnancy will heal that relationship. For a teen with low school success or poor financial resources, pregnancy provides one means of achieving some definition of success, an alternative to school or career success.[16] Around the world, societal norms, ethnic and cultural values, institutional practices (i.e. school, workplace, and government policies), and the experiences of friends and family all influence a woman's expectations of the pregnancy and subsequent parenting. For instance, Felicity, whom we met earlier, comes from a context that shapes her experience:

> Felicity was a 20-year-old in her next-to-last year of vocational high school when she became pregnant with her third child. She had grown up in a home with her mother, four siblings – all of whom had different fathers – and the father of her youngest sister, whom her mother recently married. Her grandmother, mother,

aunts, and two sisters all became pregnant as teenagers. During this third pregnancy, Felicity transferred from vocational high school to the school-age mothers program. School attendance was quite difficult for her, not only due to demands of pregnancy care and maternity absences, but also due to her other chronic medical conditions (low back pain exacerbated by obesity, depression and anxiety, and almost-daily migraine headaches). Despite difficulties with attendance, Felicity had maintained the goal of high school graduation. Although in the short term she planned to focus on parenting, she occasionally spoke of resuming vocational training to become a beautician. She now had stable housing with her current boyfriend Rafael and her two children. Help with childcare came mostly from Felicity's mother and older sister (herself with four children). Rafael, though present, struggled with his own chronic medical issues; within the relationship, Felicity took the majority of the responsibility for parenting as well as caretaking for Rafael.

Felicity's position as a parent is typical of the women around her from whom she gets most of her support. As a teen mother with three children already, her educational future is likely to be limited, and her occupational options restricted. Her situation contrasts with that of Michelle, whom we met earlier, who also faces occupational, marital, and parenting challenges:

Michelle and George had no close family nearby; George's parents had both died years ago, and Michelle's elderly parents lived at a great distance. However, in their university town, they had a rich social network and many friends, mostly other university couples who already had children. They felt very fortunate to have had excellent family daycare for their first baby, Nathan. Michelle and George both worked full-time after Nathan's birth, allowing them each to continue their full teaching schedules and academic work. They both believed strongly in sharing all the household roles and split the cooking, cleaning, childcare and household maintenance equitably with a minimum of gender-stereotyped activities. With the birth of their second child, Michaela, four years later, they jointly decided that one of them would need to work part-time at least for a few years. Michelle thought that the first year she should be the more at-home parent to be more available for breastfeeding; George agreed and worked on a plan for him to be part-time the second year. To save on childcare costs, they planned part-time nursery school for Nathan and part-time daycare for Michaela.

After Michelle had been home with both children on maternity leave for two months after the birth of Michaela, she found herself doing almost all the cooking and cleaning, as well as most of the childcare and child transportation. George "helped out" in the evening by doing the evening dishes and bathing Nathan and putting him to bed. Michelle became increasingly irritable and worried that her brain was "shriveling." She knew that George was a "great father" and that he would keep up his end of the bargain for Year Two, but she could not see beyond the next 24 hours. She had a month left before the end of her formal maternity leave, but was too tired to prepare any of her work for the part-time schedule coming up, much less do the reading to keep up in her field. After stewing about her increased assumption of parenting and "housewife" roles while George remained the "breadwinner," Michelle finally confronted him with the way their roles had become gender-stereotyped. She became very tearful; George wondered about postpartum depression. After talking half the night, they decided to make some changes in their plans: Michelle would remain part-time this year, but they would resume full-time childcare to enable her to continue her academic work.

Family itself creates a "culture" with norms for pregnancy and parenting. For women from different educational and economic situations, wide differences may exist between the expected, or more acceptable, age for first gestation or number of children, and for measures of successful parenting. In Felicity's family, women "do it all": they act as primary heads of households with men as transient participants, they support each other through pregnancy and labor, and they help each other with childcare. Felicity succeeds in her world model by becoming a caretaker. She enters adulthood by taking on responsibility for her own children. She has had some family support along the way, but in her daily life now she functions independently. Michelle, in contrast, completed her education and led a full professional life before having children in her late thirties. With elderly parents far away, she gets most of her day-to-day support from her spouse and from friends, with a strong sense of her professional identity and her egalitarian values providing the background to her roles as a mother and a spouse. Her ideal vision is one of shared parenting and gender roles between her and her stable partner. Nevertheless, despite her more comfortable economic position and advanced education, she, too, faces challenges in trying to integrate a new baby into her family life. The birth of her second child provokes changes in previous gender and occupational roles within the family and will require ongoing negotiation and flexibility.

What happens to the woman who "does it all"? For Felicity, although she strongly advocates for her children's needs, she often neglects her own health, and over her teen years has deferred her educational and professional goals. While she does not see many options, she still hangs on to her dream of finishing school and working in her chosen trade. Michelle, too, finds that she must postpone some of her career plans with the birth of her second child, but finds the alteration in her gender roles at home to be unacceptable. She does not believe in "doing it all" but does not have any extended support structure beyond formal childcare and a supportive spouse. She must take the lead to renegotiate their marital arrangement for her to combine her parenting with her professional role. Felicity and Michelle are not alone: women often take a lead role in maintaining family function across time and through life transitions.[17]

Felicity's family of origin clearly shapes her career as a mother. The influence of family origin on new parents' experiences extends beyond pervasive norms or family "culture." The character of her early childhood relationships may predict a new mother's quality of parenting and ease of assuming that role; the same holds true for new fathers (*see* Part Six). The sensitivity and supportiveness of a new parent's family of origin correlate with easier adjustment to parenting.[18-20]

A woman's social context shapes her emotional response to parenting: her interest in child-rearing, her attachment to the baby, her degree of self-care, and her future plans. Relationship context also plays a role in a woman's postpartum recovery in the areas of physical, social, and sexual health. As discussed earlier, women like Felicity with poor social supports and chaotic relationships are most at risk of adverse outcomes: physical pain, fatigue, diminished ability to work within and outside the home, prenatal and postpartum depression, emotional lability, and decreased sexual satisfaction.[21] Felicity herself also has a problem with her weight that makes her back pain difficult to manage and reinforces her negative self-image.

Within this social context, a new mother's worldview shifts. She suddenly has another life to protect – the world may no longer seem like such a safe place as it did a few months ago. Her view of herself, too, will shift. She may feel more dependent; she may feel frightened or deficient in knowledge. Without the frequent presence of a knowledgeable support person such as a health visitor, a new mother may find the baby's nasal congestion, milial rash, or crying overwhelming, leading her to seek help from the doctor, the health clinic, or even the emergency services, because of her fears that the baby is sick. Many providers dealing with overwhelmed new mothers will try "reassurance," yet the new mother may need exploration of the demands on her and her sense of responsibility. Conversely, some new mothers may feel more self-sufficient, more responsible for taking care of their own life obligations.

> At her postpartum visit, Samantha (*see* Part Two) was shocked to learn that she was pregnant again. She and Jack had already been having unprotected sex. Harmony, the nurse practitioner who worked with Dr. Epps, gave Samantha information about pregnancy options and encouraged her to make her own decision with follow-up in a week. Samantha, feeling overwhelmed by the idea of being pregnant again, went to talk with the nurse at the school mothers program. This nurse reminded Samantha of the healthy, responsible choices she had made in labor with the help of her support system and how those choices reflected her ability to make adult decisions. . . . Samantha ultimately decided to go to the Planned Parenthood in the city where she met with a counselor and received medication and instructions for a medical abortion.

A young mother may not have previously thought of herself as making decisions on an adult level, especially not when she finds out she is pregnant again. Nevertheless, the nurse's reminder about Samantha's new-found adult capacity and her encouragement to rely on her growing sense of self and ability for self-care enable Samantha to recognize that she *is* capable of making important decisions and is not at all ready to embark on another pregnancy.

With the addition of the new baby, the family begins to socialize with a new group of people: other parents or families with children in the same age range and similar concerns and interests. The new mother will now have more in common with other mothers and will begin to speak a common language of mothering. Baby food, diapers, teething, crying, tantrums, toilet training, and sibling rivalry are among the topics that she now finds interesting and even important. The parental couple will relate to friends in a different way – revolving around child-watching and children's play, rather than pure adult socializing. A woman's first experience of pregnancy and mothering further changes her named identity with family and friends – for the first time, she is "mom." She may feel that she is more "mom" than "wife."[22] Her identity may shift so far as to be known only in relation to her child, not even by her own name but simply as "Joey's mom." A woman who does not share the same last name with her children may hear herself called by a name that is not her own.

Pre-existing relationships may need to be reshaped to fit new patterns and needs. A career woman who leaves work after a birth or a young woman who cannot spend time with friends as before may each feel cut off from her familiar life patterns and relationships. Teens need ongoing relationships with friends, family, or other adults, such as the school nurse, for non-judgmental support, especially at moments of crisis such as a sick baby or a positive pregnancy test.[23] Samantha may feel more connected than Felicity because of her sense of community and peer support in the school-aged mothers program. Social isolation for teen mothers, on the other hand, may put a teen mother at risk for parenting difficulties.[16]

Many women seek out models – other women who have gone before, or contemporaries who are mothering in parallel – whose experiences can be observed as guides and patterns for the new mother. For Samantha, it is her cousin Alice, for Felicity her older sister. Medical providers and social workers may also play a central role in guiding and supporting a woman's adult development through the stages of pregnancy and transition to parenting.

For a maternity provider to act as a catalyst for a woman's development as a new mother requires understanding of her current state and her goals and expectations for the stages ahead. Through a series of questions focusing on relationships, a provider can learn about a woman's degree of connectedness and her expectations of parenting. For example, the often-invoked series of questions authored by Arthur Kleinman (*see* Box 3.1) to elicit a patient's belief about a particular illness can be reframed for the healthcare provider's use with an expectant mother and her partner.[24:121,25:260-1] (*See* also Part Two and the FIFE concepts for additional ways to formulate these questions.)

BOX 3.1 Health Belief Questions

1 With whom do you have your most important relationships? Who will support you in pregnancy, in labor, and as a parent?
2 How is your current relationship with your partner/father of the baby? What strengths does the relationship have?
3 How did you choose to become pregnant/parent now?
4 What do you expect that parenting will do for you and/or for your relationship with your partner? How do you think that parenting this child may change your relationship(s) with your prior child(ren), or with your parents?

5 Has the pregnancy caused you any problems in your relationships (with partner, family, etc.)?
6 What challenges do you anticipate about pregnancy/parenting? What do you fear most about pregnancy/parenting?
7 How do you think pregnancy and parenting will change you?
8 What plans do you have for yourself postpartum? (i.e. return to work, school, etc.). How do you think that parenting may change your sense of self?

(Derived from Kleinman, 1988, and Fadiman, 1997)[24,25]

The woman's responses to these questions can lead the woman-centered provider to consider different interventions. Prenatal discussion of psychosocial issues may be a means to reduce risk of postpartum stress or isolation (especially if conducted in a group setting); supportive interventions for at-risk mothers to treat depression during pregnancy or deal with relationship problems may reduce the risk of postpartum depression.[26] Parenting programs may be effective in improving outcomes for teen parents especially in the areas of improved parental knowledge and attitude, and more advanced development of maternal identity.[27,28] When parents' skills include the capacity for relationships, the ability to adapt to challenges, and the experience of support from other people in a woman's social environment, a healthy mother–baby interaction is more likely to ensue.[29] Prospective fathers who participate in antenatal interventions also have increased satisfaction with parenting and show more involvement in childcare.[30,31] Social connectedness seems to promote healthy parenting habits.

The parenting couple may share concerns with the clinician about how the relationship might change after the baby. Separately they may also worry about loneliness or boredom if one parent stays alone at home with the baby, or about whether one or the other might have difficulty coping with their new role.[32] These key topics may serve as a guide for a group prenatal class or for one-on-one discussion with a provider. The provider might schedule a worried couple for early postpartum follow-up and, if appropriate, a counseling intervention for the mother or couple. (*See* Part Six for further discussion of the impact of pregnancy and parenting on fathers.) Although systematic review has not demonstrated that universal provision of postpartum support improves maternal outcomes (mental health, physical health, or quality of life), targeted interventions such as peer support and home visitation to women at risk of depression or family problems, respectively, make a difference.[33]

Partner relations do shift with the birth of a baby. Many find that, rather than creating a stronger or "deeper" partner bond, the partner relationship may feel strained in the early transition to parenting. Particularly, the partnership may feel more platonic as the couple becomes absorbed in the many logistical aspects to caring for an infant. Family systems research has shown that, of all the relationship factors to consider, the strength of the pre-baby partner relationship is most predictive of a smooth and satisfying transition to parenting. A supportive, positive relationship between a woman and her partner (specifically, one with commitment, closeness, and an even power distribution among partners) predicts a smooth transition to parenting and low parenting stress.[19] Partnerships such as Michelle and George's are better able to anticipate the marital strain that may arise postpartum and to attend more carefully to maintaining the marital relationship.[18,34,35] When partners support each other, communicate well, solve problems and make decisions together, and strive for a balance between connectedness and ability to separate, their parenting is more likely to be effective.[29]

CHAPTER 3

Women's Gender Roles and Employment Issues in Pregnancy and Child-rearing

Tracy Kedian

The creation of a family is a profound and permanent change in a woman's life path. For the woman engaged in paid employment in the workplace, that transformation may lead to increased satisfaction as her identity shifts from worker to mother or to a combined self-image of the woman balancing work and family. Yet, at times, pregnancy and birth set an employed woman up for role strain, conflict, and overload. Many women from all walks of life struggle with the issue of work–home balance and continuously face the problem of overload. Often economic and political policies far beyond a woman's control determine how long she may spend at home after the birth, and what proportion of her waking hours she spends at work after she returns to her employed position.

> Melissa, in Martin's first few months of life, struggled with when to return to her high-powered job (*see* Part Two). After much discussion at the well-child visit with Larisa (and a normal baby exam), Melissa agreed to call her supervisor at work and see if there would be any possibility to delay her return, to do some work from home, and to return to work part-time. She felt guilty about abandoning her colleagues for so long, but also felt completely unable to consider leaving Martin

yet. . . . Melissa's supervisor was happy to hear from her but acknowledged that it would be difficult for her to be gone from the team for too much longer. They agreed that she would do some work from home for her third month postpartum, could work part-time the next two months, but then would have to return to work full-time at six months postpartum.

Rosa (*see* Part Two) was not eligible for extended parental leave, and as an undocumented immigrant, her limited insurance coverage for the pregnancy and delivery did not continue past six weeks to cover the cost of a breast pump or rental.

Kerry (*see* Part Two) had planned to stay at home for three months after Erika's birth . . . but found that she missed both the classroom and the adult companionship of her fellow teachers, and by six weeks arranged a half-day position at her old school where she could still be home in the afternoon with Erika.

Kerry, a motivated, educated woman with experience in early childhood education and a planned and wanted pregnancy, seems unlikely to develop role strain, self-doubt, or damage to self-image and respect, yet she is eager to get back to work after six weeks of full-time mothering. Melissa, a full-time engineer in a competitive field, is surprised to find out how much she wants to be a full-time mother for even longer. Rosa has little choice – she must return to work with no options. Each faces different challenges as a working woman making the transition to parenthood. National policies, at various governmental levels, will determine a woman's eligibility for maternity and parental leave and the regulations about breastfeeding. At the immediate level, the specific values and practices in her workplace will strongly affect a woman's experience of returning to work. The presence or absence of the family-friendly policies of job sharing, flex time and part-time employment reflect employers' underlying attitudes. Through the process of coming to know the woman in her context, the woman-centered provider may anticipate and assist her with the difficulties she will experience during the transition to motherhood, her return to work and the resulting changes in her view of herself.

To assist Kerry in her transition Larisa must learn about her proximal context – her immediate situation as described earlier – the foundation of how she will perceive herself as a mother. Asking women like Kerry about their motherhood expectations rooted in their family of origin experiences can enable providers to better understand each woman's challenges and to facilitate the upcoming transitions. Thus, asking "Do you want to be a mother like your mother?" enables Larisa to find out what role Kerry's own mother played in the home, whether she was at home full-time or had a career, or a combination. The responses to this question also will suggest how Kerry's mother is likely to weigh in on Kerry's own choices and what support Kerry will get for her decisions. Once familiar with this background, Larisa may anticipate that Kerry, who had a close and satisfying relationship with her own full-time mother, may have some anticipatory guilt about her plan to combine her career with motherhood. Kerry's upbringing and her own family's expectations will help her decide if she can be a good teacher while staying home part-time or if she can be a good mother while going to work.

Larisa also explores the context of Kerry's work situation. Many of Kerry's fellow teachers may already be working parents with ideas about part-time work, breastfeeding, pumping breast milk, and role combination. Kerry is therefore likely familiar with what it might be like for her to combine work and parenting in her professional culture. Surrounded with other mothers both as colleagues and as the parents of the children at her school, Kerry will have ample opportunity to talk about her choices. Research suggests that combined worker and parent roles may reinforce each other, producing a more satisfied, happier member of the workforce and community.[36] Kerry's supportive workplace is likely to foster her transition to the role of working mother. Evidence to promote such work environments comes from a 2004 study commissioned by the Women's Bureau of the US Department of Labor, *Win-Win Workplace Practices*, which showed that higher profits, improved productivity, and lower attrition can result from workplace practices that include support for "family-friendly" benefits.[37]

In contrast, Melissa and other women in competitive and often largely male professional environments, despite their relative economic security, may face more role strain as they encounter strong supervisory and peer pressures to resume "pulling their weight" in their workplace. Despite national policies for a year of parental leave in countries like Canada, competitive workplaces exert pressures on women to return to work sooner than they might prefer. For example, support from Melissa's supervisor sounds short-term at best. Research about role combination shows that women experience role conflict when their expectations clash with their perception of others' expectations.[36] Without nearby extended family or a peer group of other mothers with whom to share her concerns, Melissa is likely to feel very alone with this painful conflict. Her maternity care clinician may be her main confidante; Larisa should be attuned to ways to help Melissa find other outlets for support.

As we saw in Part Two, women like Rosa have difficulty leaving work to keep multiple prenatal appointments and must return to inflexible full-time, low-income factory jobs or potentially lose their employment altogether. They face unspoken losses in their struggle to manage in a world often hostile to them because of their race, culture, or immigration status. Such women, especially in the United States, encounter few family-friendly policies, less job security and limited recognition of the contribution of the working mother. As a non-English speaking immigrant couple, Rosa and José face a myriad of challenges. In their country they lived near both their extended families, but after immigration they have very limited support. Rosa faces a real risk of losing her job if she misses work. Immigrants, particularly undocumented immigrants, have no financial safety net. Rosa may be receiving her earnings "under the table" and have no access to sick time or job security.

Knowing that Rosa had trouble keeping some of her prenatal appointments, her provider Jonathan can inquire if her employer knew she was pregnant and ask how her employer will regard her pregnancy and time off. Understanding how little "choice" Rosa has with these issues of employment risk and financial struggle, Jonathan may find less surprising Rosa's decision to take off only one month from her job on an assembly line, a factory position that is also unlikely to provide her with time and privacy to pump breast milk. While caring for families whose experiences are so different from his own, her clinician benefits from being part of a team that includes advocates and interpreters who know and share critical facts about patients' lives. Such multidisciplinary teamwork with diverse populations is further discussed, later in Section Three of this part and also in Part Four.

Having left her first child behind in her country, Rosa may find the problem of rapidly weaning this baby and returning to work to be another loss. She may long to stay at home a bit longer but cannot because of her economic straits, immigration status, or the factory policies. Or perhaps she finds herself feeling sad at home alone with this baby, and feels that at least if she returns to work she will be able to pay some bills and send some money to her mother. To understand Rosa's feelings and expectations, Jonathan must situate her choices about returning to work within the larger context of her life.

This "distal" context is crucial. In most European countries and in Canada and New Zealand, paid parental leave available to mothers and fathers has been government policy for years. Most wealthy countries offer at least a year of parental leave. While the total extent of permissible leave and the amount paid for by government vary from country to country, the USA and Australia are the only two developed countries not to offer any paid maternity leave, and the USA and Switzerland offer the lowest total months of leave.[38] Despite the fact that women's participation in the US workforce has increased from 43% to 60% in the last 32 years,[37] pregnant and postpartum women often need insurance and disability forms completed by their medical provider to obtain more than a minimal six-week maternity leave, and may need medical support for a longer leave and for returning to work part-time. These issues depend on the specific policies of the employer as well as state and national policies. Such forces may have unstated yet very traditional or stereotyped visions of a woman's role, including a stance on who is best to care for her child.[36] Thus, governmental and societal attitudes will directly affect how a mother can combine work and childbearing, and indirectly affect the woman's sense of her own worth.

Woman-centered postpartum planning includes exploring a woman's plans for maternity leave and how these relate to her family's economic situation. In contrast to Rosa, Kerry may have short-term disability insurance or may be able to use accumulated sick-time to have salary coming in after the birth. Even so, financial constraints may be a source of stress for both of them. Melissa's concerns relate less to income and more to the pressures on her to perform as part of a team in a competitive environment. All three women face the often stressful need to make childcare arrangements. Exploration during late pregnancy visits of a woman's childcare plans can be an entry point into her concerns about returning to work. How women, couples, and families solve the issue of childcare serves as a strong indicator of the resilience of their systems and their assumptions about gender roles within those systems.

Rosa had planned that her sister-in-law, Lilia, who was living in their apartment, would watch the baby when she returned to work. However, Lilia had just found full-time work and was unavailable for this. Rosa and José decided that they would share the childcare by working opposite shifts. Rosa would be home with Eva in the daytime and work evenings; José would look after Eva in the evenings, work nights, and sleep in the daytime. Although exhausting, this arrangement enabled them to save money on childcare. José became very skilled at feeding and changing Eva and recognizing her needs. Rosa found that she was still able to nurse Eva a few times a day and when she arrived home from work. Even though her milk supply was not enough for exclusive breastfeeding, she nonetheless felt gratified that Eva still wanted her breast milk.

Ron and Kerry worked out an intricate arrangement for Erika's feeding, dressing, and transport so that Kerry could work a half day and Ron could stay involved with the baby's care despite his busy work schedule.

Melissa was exhausted from trying to "do it all" at home with more of the housework and traditional gender roles than she had expected. She felt frustrated with Kirk that he did not seem to notice this imbalance.

As couples become parents, partner roles in the home and in the relationship adjust to incorporate new lifestyle and self-care needs. Many couples, like Michelle and George as we saw earlier, find that a new division of household tasks occurs – whether tacitly or explicitly negotiated. Even in partnerships that were previously quite gender-equitable, couples often shift toward assuming traditional gender roles after the birth of a baby; the birth of a first or subsequent child may challenge their ideals and practices.[39] Many of the traditionally "female" tasks (cooking, cleaning, arranging childcare, and communicating with the children's school) are assumed as a part of motherhood. Certainly, during the postpartum period, a woman like Michelle, usually at work, may be at home more hours of the day and thus may feel she should take on more of the household tasks than a partner who is employed outside the home. But as time passes and she returns to work or other obligations, the division of labor again needs to be renegotiated. Many more fathers are now interested in being actively involved in parenting than was true in their own families of origin. (*See* Part Six.) The task of woman-centered providers is to help new parents rethink the gender roles that they have seen modeled in their families of origin, models that they may find themselves repeating or challenging as they become parents.

The issues of changing roles and return to work are intertwined. Because the majority of women with children are in the paid workforce as well,[37] many mothers will struggle with how their roles will change when they return to work and how they will manage this change. Kerry's, Melissa's and Rosa's maternity providers probably cannot have any impact on the policies at their patients' workplaces but may be able to help them be realistic (and sometimes creative) about how they each work out impending transitions and potential conflicts in roles.

Not surprisingly, factors that alleviate working mothers' role conflicts include a supportive spouse, children beyond preschool age, higher income and a lower stress job. Those that increase role conflict include the lack of a supportive spouse, decreased socialization and concerns about childcare quality.[36] Melissa, with her higher income, returns to a high-stress job and lacks social support outside her marriage. She may be a mother who requires additional counseling to face her conflicts and her marital concerns. In contrast to Felicity, the other three women – Melissa, Rosa, and Kerry – receive various kinds of support from their spouses, who face their own workplace demands yet seek ways to be involved with the new baby.

Childcare is a central preoccupation postpartum for the working mother. Often families with severe economic pressures like Rosa and José's, while perhaps outwardly embracing traditional roles, may actually engage in household management and childcare arrangements that challenge gender-typical practices.[40] While such couples swap shifts to cover childcare for financial reasons, others prefer to keep childcare within the family even if other options exist; for instance over half of employed pregnant women in one study explicitly stated that their first preference for childcare was in-home care by their spouse.[41] Increasingly, in couples with small children, some fathers are choosing to be "stay-at-home dads" – or "full-time fathers" – when the mothers are the successful breadwinners.[37]

To help decrease the risk of role strain, the woman-centered provider explores a woman's gender role ideals and expectations, the roles of each of her parents during her childhood, and her goals for her own role at work and at home after the birth. Such conversations need not be lengthy; short exchanges during prenatal visits may open the topics and pave the way for the mother to raise the issues again later as they become important. For instance, in the context of asking about childcare plans, the provider might ask, "How did your parents do childcare? What will they think about your plans?" The woman-centered provider will also be observant of the partners during prenatal care (and intrapartum care) and will inquire about their upcoming transitions as well. Quiet moments during labor are another time when the clinician might inquire about these expectations. (Partner issues will be further addressed in Part Six.)

Discussions about employment, maternity leave, returning to work, childcare, and gender role expectations may seem outside the realm of expertise of many maternity care providers. Nevertheless, the goal of being woman-centered places the woman as a whole person, not only as a reproductive being, at the center of care. Asking questions in these areas and listening hard to the answers, woman-centered providers can become familiar with the wide range of challenges for women in their arrangements of responsibilities at home and at work.

Challenging Assumptions

The next four chapters will address how healthcare systems and providers need to challenge their assumptions in order to provide woman-centered maternity care to women marginalized by society. Providers themselves may share characteristics with women on the margins (i.e. lesbian women, women with histories of abuse, women with substance abuse problems), but their histories often go unrecognized by colleagues, co-workers, and patients. Women clinicians facing these challenges experience the same stigma as their women patients, yet may hide these aspects of their lives to protect themselves and their careers. Even women providers without these shared experiences need to avoid stereotyping these vulnerable populations.

CHAPTER 1

Lesbian Motherhood: When Both Partners are Mothers

Nancy Newman

The irreversible changes of pregnancy in a woman's individual and family development are in many ways the same for lesbian and heterosexual women.* Every pregnant

---

* Women who partner with women use different words to name their orientation toward same-gendered partners. These include lesbian, gay, queer, and woman-oriented woman. Woman-centered medicine respects the terms that women use to describe themselves and their partners. For simplicity of writing style in this section, "lesbian" will denote women who partner with women.

woman faces the challenges of adjusting to changes in her body, and of reorganizing her home, work, and immediate family to welcome a new baby. Woman-centered providers will want to understand some of the additional issues facing lesbian mothers in order to offer them suitable pregnancy and childbirth care.

Lesbian motherhood is not new. Lesbian women have always become pregnant, given birth, and raised children. In the past, many lesbian mothers raised children from past relationships with men, or through adoption, often facing the risk of having children taken away if the lesbian relationship became public.[42,43] Although still at legal risk in some contexts and regions, in the early 21st century in North America, lesbian women generally find it safer and easier to get pregnant and raise children openly in the context of their committed relationships with their woman partners. Compared with 30 years ago, maternity providers today are less likely to refuse to care for an openly lesbian woman wanting to get pregnant through donor insemination. Practitioners and medical systems today show increasing awareness and acceptance of the need for respectful, affirming lesbian healthcare, although such acceptance is by no means universal.

In order to become pregnant, lesbian women need more intentional planning, often involving technology, than do fertile heterosexual couples.[44,45] Some lesbian women may choose to have sex with a male friend or casual acquaintance, or to self-inseminate with fresh sperm from a known or anonymous donor. A known donor may or may not plan to be involved in the life of a future child. Women can also choose to involve medical providers in order to access resources and technology such as sperm banks, and donor insemination (vaginal or intrauterine). Donor insemination is also referred to as "artificial insemination" in medical settings. Some lesbian women prefer to use the term "alternative insemination" or "donor insemination" because of the unnatural implications of "artificial." When providers inquire about the donor, they can ask how the family refers to the person who donated sperm, and use that terminology.

Regardless of the method, the intentional and more public process for lesbian women of trying to get pregnant can heighten the anticipation, and leave women feeling defective when their attempts are not successful quickly. In contrast, heterosexual couples often experience getting pregnant as a more informal and private process. Aware of the stresses on lesbian women and their partners who are engaged in trying to get pregnant, woman-centered providers will provide support for the couple in their process. (*See* also Part Two, Section Two, Chapter 2 on infertility.) Here is Susan, the nurse practitioner-runner we met in Part Two:

> Susan made an initial appointment for well-woman care at the woman-centered practice that had a strong orientation toward women's health. She felt comfortable at her initial visit with an older woman family physician, Judith Peters (whom Susan chose for her reputation for woman-centeredness) who inquired in an open way about Susan's sexual orientation. Susan freely told Judith that she was in a long-term committed relationship with Geri, a woman who taught at a local college. They were thinking about getting pregnant in the near future.

A few months later Susan and Geri came in for an appointment to talk more about getting pregnant. Susan decided to be the one to try to get pregnant. Through their lesbian community they learned about sperm banks and other related issues. Susan had been keeping records of her menstrual cycle and last month detected her luteinizing hormone (LH) surge using an ovulation predictor kit. Judith referred them to a colleague in the city who did donor insemination as part of her practice, and invited Susan to return for prenatal care once she became pregnant.

Susan and Geri considered using a sperm bank that would reveal the donor's identity, but eventually decided that they would use a particular anonymous donor instead because they preferred the physical characteristics of that donor. Susan and Geri thought carefully about whom to tell regarding their efforts to get pregnant and decided to tell Susan's sister and Geri's parents, who responded with the enthusiasm that Susan and Geri had anticipated.

It took eight cycles for Susan to get pregnant, longer than they were expecting, and somewhat longer than average. During that time they found resources about the emotional strain of dealing with infertility, as well as the support of lesbian mothers who had struggled with the process. Susan worried that her athletic training might have been affecting her fertility. Just before she decided not to train for the next local marathon, she became pregnant.

Pregnancy defines a woman as a sexual being, yet most often others make the assumption that she is a *heterosexual* being. As her pregnancy becomes known, either because of her physical appearance, or her disclosure, a lesbian woman will often encounter the assumption of heterosexuality by both strangers and acquaintances. Naïve questions or comments about her husband or male partner put the lesbian woman on the spot, forcing her to have to decide how open to be about her sexual identity. The decision to "come out" in such circumstances can be a complex one, influenced by how safe the woman feels in the environment, the messages she wishes to convey to her other children if present, her overall comfort in being "out," and her desire to teach about heterosexism. Similarly, when the lesbian woman registers for prenatal care, clinic forms and routine questions often assume that she has a male partner. Providers also often take for granted that a woman's first pregnancy is her debut into motherhood. As with a heterosexual woman who has adopted children, a lesbian woman may already be a mother of her partner's children, even when she herself has not been pregnant or given birth. Woman-centered care involves training staff to avoid making assumptions, as well as using intake and screening forms that do not assume a heterosexual two-parent couple. Such openness is also more respectful of *any* single woman who may not have a partner.

After finding out that they were pregnant, Susan and Geri gradually told their family and friends about the pregnancy. Susan was relieved to get support from her parents, whom she had feared might react the way they had when she first came out to them 10 years ago. In fact, after Susan told her mom, her mother wept happily about the prospects of being a grandmother and embraced Geri for the first time.

As expected, Geri's brother reacted by sending Susan a letter with quotes from the Bible to justify his disapproval.

Susan returned to Judith's practice for prenatal care, and appreciated the acceptance that she and Geri experienced from the staff, as well as Judith and the other providers. As her body revealed her pregnancy more and more, Susan also had to decide when to come out to strangers and colleagues who casually asked how her husband felt about the pregnancy. She realized that she would likely face the same kind of assumptions in the future out in public with her baby. She decided to confer with some of her lesbian mom friends to hear how they had handled such situations in front of their children.

When Susan registered by phone for an ultrasound, the hospital clerk got very flustered when Susan offered a "second mom" to list, rather than "father of baby." The phone clerk put Susan on hold and called her supervisor. When the supervisor came to the phone he apologized, saying, "The clerk didn't know what to do because the computer doesn't have that category."

As with fathers (discussed in Part Six), medical systems and providers need to integrate women's lesbian partners respectfully into the system of care. When two women are co-parenting the birth child of one of them, the non-biological mother often finds her role challenged subtly or directly. For example, the question "Who is the real mother?" suggests that one is not authentic. Likewise, adoptive mothers often hear the birth mother referred to as the "real" mother. Woman-centered providers can avoid this mistake by asking about which mother has a biological relationship with the child, when that information is relevant (i.e. genetics and breastfeeding), and by not making assumptions about what each woman's parenting roles will be in the care of the baby. Another heterosexist assumption involves ignoring the possibility of abuse in lesbian couples, a reality for women of all sexual orientations.

The ethnic and religious background of women may influence how "out" they are to themselves as well as the world around them. Research about lesbian women has focused on self-declared lesbians and has not addressed lesbian women in cultures where lesbians remain "in the closet" for reasons of safety. Providers need to be careful not to assume that the cultural standards of "out" European-American lesbian women apply to women from other countries and cultures.[46,47]

Maria Isabelle was a 30-year-old multiparous woman from Mexico City who had left her husband several years ago and immigrated to look for work. Her first two children stayed with her parents and sister in Mexico. When her provider Jonathan Rosen asked about the father of her current pregnancy, Maria Isabelle stated that her boyfriend had left her when he found out she was pregnant. She worked in housekeeping for a local hotel, and was grateful for the medical assistance she received during pregnancy. Maria Isabelle lived with "a friend" and told Jonathan that her friend would help her during labor. . . . When Maria's contractions started at 39 weeks, her friend Guadalupe brought her to the hospital to be checked. She was 5 cm dilated.

When Jonathan walked into the labor room, he greeted Maria Isabelle, and then introduced himself to Guadalupe, who was actively supporting her friend through contractions. Over the course of the next few hours, it became clear from their interactions that Guadalupe and Maria Isabelle were very close friends. Maria Isabelle invited Guadalupe to make decisions for her as the contractions became stronger. Guadalupe stayed physically close and to Jonathan's eye seemed quite affectionate at times. Jonathan learned that Guadalupe and Maria had shared an apartment since Maria had moved here four years ago and that Guadalupe was to be very involved in the child-rearing of this soon-to-be-born child.

Jonathan hypothesized that the two women were in a committed relationship that they chose to keep secret from the hospital system, and probably many others as well (family, friends, neighbors). Jonathan's own sister was partnered with a woman and raising two children, and he would have liked to show explicitly his acceptance of a same-gendered partnership to these women. He chose, however, not to address these issues directly in the context of the labor and delivery area, but rather to focus on involving Guadalupe in the birth to the extent that Maria and Guadalupe desired. Later, when he discharged Maria Isabelle and her baby, Jonathan invited Guadalupe to come to future well-child appointments.

Jonathan was somewhat aware of the different realities and cultural meanings in other countries for women who partner with women and imagined that women may not self-identify as "lesbian", even when their relationship may look like a lesbian relationship to others. (*See* full vignette in Appendix.)

A provider already sensitized to the issues of lesbian relationships and familiar with Mexican immigrants, Jonathan recognizes that he needs to discover how he can be supportive of whatever healthy relationships Maria Isabelle is creating for herself and her new baby. Rather than labeling the connection between Maria Isabelle and Guadalupe when asking about their relationship, he can match whatever language Maria Isabelle and Guadalupe use to describe themselves. Over time he can look for openings to mention lesbian parenting resources and any legal options to support a legal parent relationship between Guadalupe and the new child. If appropriate Jonathan can also ask more questions about the "boyfriend," framed in the context of the baby's or Maria Isabelle's health – for instance, "Do either of you have any concerns about the father's health or family history or any involvement by him in your lives?" In the context of their primary care relationship over time, Jonathan can learn how to name the family that will raise this new baby.

In addition to the ethnic and religious context, the legal and political environment around lesbian couples and their families strongly influences their experience of safety and well-being as they navigate the experiences of pregnancy, childbirth and child-rearing. At the present time, in a few places in the world, same-gendered couples can marry or have a civil union, and thereby be granted some or all of the legal rights of spouses and parents. Many other cultures ostracize lesbian and gay couples and their children and deny them basic human rights as well as legal supports. While a small group of countries (The Netherlands, Belgium, Spain, South Africa, Norway,

Sweden, and Canada) recognize same-sex marriage as of 2009, as well as a few states in the USA, in more conservative areas the rights of gay and lesbian parents continue to be challenged, making it clear that that families with two mothers will likely face ongoing legal struggles.[45] (See also www.familypride.org, the website for the Family Pride Coalition, which offers a summary of news, resources, etc., about political and legal current events relevant to lesbian, as well as gay, bisexual, and transgender parenting.) Woman-centered providers can encourage lesbian mothers to seek legal expertise in order to protect their families legally and financially.

CHAPTER 2

When the Context is Violence and Abuse

Cathy Kamens and Ambareen A. Bharmal

IMPACT ON THE CHILDBEARING WOMAN

> Mariluz was a 23-year-old mother of three with many life issues. Mariluz had ongoing conflicts with her own mother and had moved out as soon as she could when she was 17 with Rocky, who because of his stable job as a security guard with a good income, a car, and health insurance, seemed like an ideal partner. During Mariluz's pregnancy with Rocky's child, however, he became possessive and accused her of seeing other men when he was at work. He began calling her countless times during the day to check on her whereabouts and hassled her if her clinic visits were longer than expected. (*See* full vignette in Appendix.)

Prior and ongoing abuse of girls and women is a common experience in all cultures and all social strata. The woman-centered approach recognizes the prevalence of victimization and stays open to the discovery of such abuse in the life of a pregnant woman. The sensitive clinician understands that a history of victimization may shape a woman's experience of pregnancy and childbirth – her ability to care for herself and her body, and her ability to accept medical care and to participate in relationships with her providers. The woman-centered provider may be able to help the woman in securing a safe, protected, and fulfilling experience of pregnancy and childbirth, often a period of heightened physical and emotional vulnerability.

INTIMATE PARTNER VIOLENCE

Like Mariluz, many adult women experience intimate partner violence (IPV), often with their current or former partner or spouse or other family members. Perpetrators use physical, sexual, psychological, and emotional means to harm the woman. Such IPV can occur once or multiple times, over a short period of time or over many years.[48] Intimate partner violence is a global problem. International studies show a range of 11% to 54% for lifetime prevalence of domestic violence, with violence during pregnancy ranging from 1% to 32.4%.[49-52] Best estimates suggest that in the USA between 4% and 8% of women experience IPV during their pregnancy.[53] Such violence spans all age groups, ethnic groups, and socioeconomic groups, but certain factors may put women more at risk. Mariluz's situation is not unusual. Women who are abused tend to be younger, unmarried, less educated, more likely to have unstable housing, more likely to have fewer social supports and more stress, and more likely to have experienced childhood abuse.[49,52,54]

> Mariluz's childhood was harsh; her mother, Carmen, drank a lot and hit the children on many occasions. All four children had been placed in foster care several times during Mariluz's school years. Although Carmen finally stopped drinking and had a stable partner, her children's experiences lived on. Mariluz became pregnant from a single apparently consensual sexual episode when she was 14. This child, José, was only four years younger than Mariluz's youngest brother, and he was raised as another child in the family.

CHILDHOOD ABUSE

Sexual abuse occurs when an adult makes a child engage in sexual activities that she or he cannot comprehend, for which she or he is developmentally unprepared, and to which she or he cannot consent.[55] While all forms of child abuse have a significant impact on adults, childhood sexual abuse may particularly affect the childbearing woman, as the experience of being out of control of sexual aspects of her body can recapitulate her abuse and feel like another victimization. As with IPV, the prevalence of childhood sexual abuse varies greatly with the population questioned and how the term is defined (i.e. the age of the child, the extent of contact, etc.). The prevalence of a history of childhood sexual abuse among women ranges from 8% up to 25%.[56-8] Women from all economic and social classes can have histories of abuse.

> Melissa (see Parts One and Two) was the oldest daughter of three in a family where her father drank heavily and ultimately became an invalid after a car accident

where he was driving drunk. Her mother became the sole breadwinner and moved back in with her parents when Melissa was 12. Her grandfather began touching Melissa inappropriately when no one else was around, but she never felt she could tell her mother, who expressed being indebted to her parents for taking them in after the accident. Melissa stayed late at school and took after-school jobs that kept her out late throughout high school to be at home as little as possible, but the sexual abuse went on until she left home for a distant engineering school. As an adult, she had little contact with her family except for her mother. Five years ago she married Kirk, whom she met in school. After a year of infertility finally responding to clomiphene, they became pregnant. She had never discussed her history of abuse with either Kirk or her provider Larisa.

Jen was a 17-year-old who at seven months of pregnancy came from another town to live with her aunt. During prenatal visits with her new provider, Larisa, she hinted that something bad had happened causing her to move here, but even with gentle probing, she steadfastly refused to discuss whatever it was. "I don't want to talk about it." Larisa anticipated that labor would be difficult for Jen because she was skittish about pelvic exams and jumped when she was touched. (*See* full vignette in Appendix.)

Adult women vary in how they manage their past experience of childhood sexual abuse. Some deny, repress, or otherwise block out their past; others are constantly reminded. Those who experienced very severe abuse (repetitive events involving penetration or multiple perpetrators) are likely to suffer from chronic physical complaints and mental health problems. Survivors of such adverse childhood experiences are prone to depression, post-traumatic stress disorder, and suicidality, as well as re-victimization in subsequent abusive adult relationships.[57,59,60] When a survivor has not yet been able to take control in her own life and to work through an understanding of her past abuse, she is more likely to experience new difficult and painful events as victimizing. Women with a past history of sexual trauma are more likely to perceive the childbirth experience as traumatic.[61]

Jen presented to labor and delivery at 35 weeks in extreme pain, seemingly in active labor and almost ready to push. Her cervix, however, was not even 1 cm dilated. During the exam, Larisa saw that Jen was overwhelmed by pain, and was reacting to it with tears and agonized cries. After observation and reassurance by Larisa, Jen's contractions subsided. Much calmer, she agreed to go home. Larisa scheduled a follow-up visit for the next morning, where she hoped to unravel Jen's previous experiences and to discuss ways to help Jen cope with the fear of pain and labor.

Without an explicit awareness of Jen's likely experience of some kind of sexual violence, the labor and delivery team caring for her was unable to anticipate her feelings of helplessness and being out of control. Although Jen had not made any explicit connection between her abuse and the pain of having a baby, her overwhelming sense of victimization had permeated the atmosphere surrounding her presentation.

Whether or not Jen's abuse history is revealed, she will benefit from a prenatal exploration of her past experiences and her fears about delivery, with adequate documentation to help the future delivery team address these issues.

With one-fourth to one-half of women experiencing violence in their lifetime, the average practitioner caring for women will encounter a victimized woman *every day*, whether the history of abuse is revealed or not. The woman-centered clinician needs to approach every woman with the possibility that she has been abused. Furthermore, given this high prevalence, maternity providers should systematically employ strategies to put women in control, as much as possible, of the events surrounding their labor and birth experiences – even when *there is no explicit history of abuse*.

The rest of this section addresses some of the effects of violence on the childbearing woman, outlines some strategies for caring for victimized pregnant women, and explores the dynamics that characterize the patient-provider relationship when the woman has experienced abuse. Understanding the impact of prior abuse enables the woman-centered clinician to choose an appropriate focus for a woman's prenatal care so that her childbearing experience will be positive and healing. Part Four will address specific strategies in working with a previously abused woman during labor.

EFFECTS OF ABUSE

The effects of childhood and partner violence ripple through a pregnant woman's psychological, emotional, physical and sexual health. Depending on the severity and timing of the abuse, many issues – physical injuries, pregnancy complications, chronic pain, anxiety, depression, strained family relationships, and/or social isolation – may complicate her medical care. Representing the extreme of abuse and its sequelae, and getting more media attention, murder and suicide emerge as common causes of death for pregnant and postpartum women.[60,62–4] Risk factors for homicide include increasing severity or frequency of violence, choking, verbal death threats by the perpetrator, suicide threats by the victim or perpetrator, drug or alcohol abuse by the perpetrator, violence by the perpetrator outside the home, and access to a gun.[65,66] Less recognized are the short-term and long-term sequelae of less dramatic but more common physical, sexual, and emotional abuse of pregnant women.

Fetal well-being is also at stake for women experiencing active abuse during pregnancy. Women with a history of such abuse are more subject to medical complications such as hyperemesis gravidarum, pregnancy-induced hypertension, unexplained bleeding, prematurity, or post-maturity.[67] Over one-third of women who are abused by their partner report direct blows to their abdomen during pregnancy,[49,68] and abuse has been associated with an increased risk of low birth weight and neonatal death.[54,69,70]

During Mariluz's second pregnancy (her first with Rocky), Rocky became increasingly physically abusive. His jealousy turned into threats to kill anyone he caught her with. He became physically aggressive, pushing her and knocking her to the ground on one occasion when he was intoxicated. The next day he apologized and promised that it would not happen again. In addition to the stress from the changes in Rocky's behavior, this pregnancy was also difficult for Mariluz physically. She had frequent exacerbations of her asthma, severe fatigue, and debilitating back pain.

Not surprisingly, women like Mariluz with histories of physical abuse will rate their quality of life to be poor in physical health domains, social relationship domains, and psychological health domains.[71] They are more likely than woman without such abuse histories to experience symptoms of depression and post-traumatic stress disorder during pregnancy and to have more trouble with anxiety, sleep, and sadness.[71] The experiences of Mariluz, Melissa, and Jen draw attention to the dynamics of power and control, trust, self-respect, and the converse dynamics of helplessness and disempowerment, distrust and betrayal, and shame and stigmatization, which will be explored later.[72]

STRATEGIES OF CARE

The maternity care providers for Melissa and Jen are initially unaware of their abuse, though Larisa suspects that Jen has experienced some kind of violent, painful or shaming event. As noted previously, since the history of abuse is often unknown to the clinician, the woman-centered clinician must approach each pregnant woman as if violence and abuse are likely possibilities. The woman with a history of victimization may benefit from sharing her story with her clinician, either overtly through the healing process of breaking her silence, or implicitly through the discussion of her special fears and needs during her childbearing experience.

Fostering Disclosure

> Mariluz became more fearful as the pregnancy progressed and Rocky's abuse accelerated, but she thought maybe he would get better after his child was born or if he found a new job. She felt ashamed about the abuse and felt that the problem was her own fault. Her mother had warned her not to get involved with Rocky, and Mariluz was embarrassed to admit that the relationship was in trouble.

Prior or current sexual abuse is a source of shame that most women do not disclose easily. Survivors often feel vulnerable, out of control, and ashamed or embarrassed.[73] An abused woman will often deny the violence she endures or has experienced. Many women are too embarrassed or too afraid to bring up abuse with their providers, or may not disclose abuse because of lack of time, lack of continuity of care, fear of losing control of decision-making, lack of privacy, fear of having their children taken away, or being uncomfortable with a male provider.[74,75] A woman may not disclose a history of physical or sexual abuse during face-to-face interviews with nurses and physicians yet might disclose via a written questionnaire. (Computerized and self-completed questionnaires have proven to be more acceptable than direct questioning to women in both emergency rooms and primary care settings in Canada.)[76] While some women will reveal their abuse when directly questioned, others do not reveal abuse even when presenting with inflicted injuries.[49,51] Women with a history of abuse may avoid medical care and present late in their pregnancies, or not at all. Women who use alcohol and drugs during pregnancy may not confide their experience of abuse for fear of providers finding out about their substance use. Some women may not be aware of their abuse due to repressed memories.

For teenagers, the situation may be even more complicated. Pregnancy may be the result of ongoing sexual abuse within the family, indicating that the young woman is still in a dangerous situation. Within a confidential context, 51% of pregnant adolescents gave a history of childhood sexual abuse beginning at an average age of 9.7 years, and 44% an experience of rape at an average age of 13.3 years.[1] Teen pregnancy is thus a strong marker for a past history of sexual abuse and underscores the importance of ascertaining and guaranteeing the young woman's ongoing safety.

Survivors are more likely to share their histories if the sensitive provider attends to boundaries and demonstrates her or his own comfort in discussing abuse. Every provider must develop a comfortable way to ask about sexual abuse; some survivors have suggested using open-ended questions such as "Is there anything else you feel I should know?"[77] or "Is there anything hard for you about pelvic exams?" After a relationship with the provider has begun to form, with a woman thus feeling safe and supported, gentle inquiry during prenatal care may facilitate discussion of prior or current abuse. In the context of an ongoing relationship using attentive listening, the woman-centered clinician with an open mind and a non-judgmental attitude fosters an environment where a woman may be able to disclose past or ongoing abuse.

Even when she has a solid relationship with a provider, a woman still may not disclose her history of abuse. Over half of the sexual abuse survivors questioned in a gynecologic clinic did not think that it was relevant to their care, and only one-third *even wanted their providers to ask* about a history of sexual abuse.[58] However, in primary care settings, women both with and without a history of childhood abuse have expressed willingness to be screened and a belief that the physician might be helpful in addressing the problem.[61,78-80] The provider can show comfort with the topic of abuse and create a supportive and safe environment, but ultimately the woman must decide when and if she is ready to share her story.

> After Jen's presentation with "false labor," Larisa knew that she needed a better understanding of what had happened to Jen to cause such panic. She was sure that Jen had experienced some kind of frightening event that continued to trouble her. Larisa decided to be very direct: "Jen, I know that you don't want to tell me what happened to you before you moved here, but now it is starting to get in the way of your having a safe and trouble-free delivery. I don't know what happened to you, but I do know that someone did something to harm you and that those events still bother you a lot. Whatever happened, I know it was not your fault and you did not deserve it."

In response to this opener, Jen dissolved in tears. Chokingly, she related the story that the previous fall she had gone with a girlfriend to her first cousin's fraternity house, even though her mother had told her she could not go. She drank what was offered her and passed out, waking up to find a boy on top of her and others indicating that they had had sex with her too. Word got back to her high school. When she turned out to be pregnant, kids started to call her "a slut." She started skipping school but pretended to her mother that everything was normal, wearing baggy sweatshirts to hide her belly. When the pregnancy became obvious, her mother, a single mother who worked as a secretary in the grammar school office, felt very ashamed and insisted that Jen leave town for the rest of the pregnancy. Jen never told her mother about the gang rape at the fraternity house.

Rape is not uncommon. Around the world, one in five women will experience rape or attempted rape.[81] Family physicians' patients report rates of 25% and student health center patients over 28%.[82] In the 1980s, approximately 16% of US college women acknowledged a history of having been made to have sex against their will.[83] According to more recent statistics published by the National Institute for Justice and the Centers for Disease Control, 17.6% of women in the USA report sexual assault (not accounting for the serious under-reporting of rape and attempted rape). Fifty-four percent of these women experience the assault younger than age 18.[84] When a pregnancy is the result of rape, the woman is not able to escape or forget what happened, nor to enjoy the experience of bringing a wanted child into the world. Larisa will need to help Jen accept a referral for rape crisis counseling so that a therapist can help her begin to address the trauma she experienced.

In preparing for the intrapartum and postpartum period and looking for sources of support for Melissa, Larisa sketched out a brief genogram with her. The process of doing the genogram led to Melissa revealing to both Kirk and Larisa her past abuse. Larisa had not anticipated either this history or Kirk's lack of knowledge of it. Melissa's disclosure resulted in visible non-verbal empathy and support from Kirk, and they left the office holding hands. Melissa and Kirk's connection with Larisa was perceptibly warmer and more engaged and trusting after the genogram visit. Larisa began working with them at subsequent visits about the fact that sexual abuse survivors often feel difficulty trusting providers, and trusting their own bodies. She discussed how feeling out of control of an intimate event like a birth where her body would be exposed had a possibility of provoking anxiety for a survivor. Melissa and Kirk begin talking about ways that he could help her feel safe during labor.

As mentioned in Section One, Chapter 1, a genogram (*see* Sidebar: "Using Genograms") is a useful tool with any pregnant woman, but especially to elicit a family history of violence, sexual abuse, and substance abuse in a non-judgmental way that enables a woman to externalize the problem as a part of her family, not a personal source of shame. While providers use family history to look for genetic risk, many are unaware of using genograms for evaluating the social and emotional context of a patient's family of origin. Larisa uses genograms to explore her patients' family context. Sometimes the results can be surprising. Melissa's history of incest with her grandfather has been a long buried secret. Melissa is fortunate to have a clinician skilled in using this tool and a partner who could support her strengths in the process of disclosure and in her plans for childbirth.

Using Genograms

The genogram is more than a genetic pedigree of medical diseases and genetic disorders. The genogram enables the patient to describe and the provider to document the "history of the family," including family relationships, social relationships, and emotional relationships. The genogram facilitates the provider's understanding and the patient's awareness of the family in context of the patient.

For more information on using genograms, see McGoldrick and Gerson. *Genograms in Family Assessment.* New York: W.W. Norton; 1985.[85]

The woman-centered provider should be aware of his or her own reactions to the topic of abuse. Providers may be reluctant to bring up abuse with their patients, mostly citing lack of time and staffing issues.[86] Busy providers may find themselves slipping into a judgmental attitude toward women who may arrive late to prenatal care, who smoke, and who avoid or refuse exams. Clinicians may not appreciate that such avoidance often reflects a previously or currently abused woman's strategy to prevent the surfacing of memories and feelings she is not prepared to deal with.[67] The provider will have difficulty establishing a relationship if the woman detects direct or implied criticism of her behavior. Woman-centered clinicians should avoid any statements that blame the woman or question whether she provoked the violence, and instead focus on the fact that *"you do not deserve to be abused."*

Safety in the Context of Empowerment

When current abuse is disclosed or suspected, the most urgent issue in the care of the potentially abused woman is ensuring her safety and the safety of her baby. An effective woman-centered approach to safety ascertains a woman's risk, helps her appreciate her jeopardy, and supports her in her struggle for safety. The woman-centered clinician should attend to signals that the woman is unsafe and identify the potential dangers, the most obvious being risk of physical harm from the abuser.

The provider should elicit the woman's perspective about her safety since abused women are the best predictors of their own risk.[87] However, if the woman appears to be underestimating her risk, the woman-centered clinician can help the pregnant woman understand her vulnerability by calling her attention to risk factors such as increasing patterns of violence, worsening of substance abuse, and access to weapons, all of which have been associated with increased risk of homicide. Ongoing forced sex may be a problem, and as with Jen, the pregnancy itself may be a result of rape from such an encounter.[88]

Conveying worry and concern for her safety, without judging her or telling her what she should do, enables the woman-centered provider to provide support and help empower the abused woman in her decision-making. Thus, some questions for Mariluz might be: "What you have told me about Rocky's behavior makes me very worried for you and the baby. Can you tell when he is likely to become violent again? What do you do to get safe at those times when you can see it coming?" Group support and social service assistance are critical when the victimized woman is ready to accept these interventions. Developing a safety plan is an ideal way for a woman-centered provider to provide concrete and personalized support to the woman in a potentially dangerous situation. (*See* Sidebar: "Personal Safety Plans.")

Personal Safety Plans

The personal safety plan describes the steps the woman will take to protect herself and her children when the situation becomes dangerous. The woman should devise the plan, with assistance and support from an experienced professional. Local domestic violence services should be able to provide sample plans or templates for a personal safety plan.

The safety plan should include details on what the woman can do to protect herself in the following situations.

- During an explosive incident. (Where to have an argument? Routes to leave safely? Where to go in an emergency? Code word to signal to others for help?)
- In preparing to leave. (Keys? Money? Medications? Documents, such as birth certificates, legal papers, insurance cards? Where to go? Shelter phone numbers?)
- With a protective order. (Where to keep the protective order? When to call the police? Who to inform about the protective order?)
- When staying in her own residence. (Change locks? Change to an unlisted phone number? Plan for safety of the children? Instructions to neighbors/ landlord?)
- When at work and in public. (Who will you tell about the situation? Inform security? Have a friend or colleague accompany you when you are out? Change routes when you come and go?)

At the 32 week prenatal visit, Dr. Burman found Mariluz more anxious and asked her about the home situation. Mariluz gradually revealed what had been going on

> with Rocky. Dr. Burman convinced Mariluz to come in more frequently and sent her home with the plan for visits, normalizing it so that Rocky would not become suspicious. Over the next few visits, Dr. Burman helped Mariluz identify her strengths: she was very careful about her medical care and kept all her appointments, she took good care of her asthma, she was able to make strong connections with women friends and relatives, especially her sister Beatriz and her friend Evie, and she was good at predicting Rocky's reactions and anticipating when he would "lose it" or "blow up." Dr. Burman encouraged Mariluz to make a safety plan in case Rocky's violence escalated further before delivery. Together, they figured out that Beatriz and Evie would be good supports in the delivery room. Mariluz thought it would be hard for her to feel safe and to manage pain with Rocky present in the labor room, but did not feel she could keep him out. Mariluz agreed with Dr. Burman that she would try to indicate if and when, during labor, she wanted Rocky to leave and to communicate that to her labor support. Dr. Burman investigated the security protocols at the hospital and planned to inform the charge nurse on the day of delivery of the potential need to ask for Rocky to be removed.

Safety may also become an issue during childbirth. For the abusive partner, the delivery room is an unfamiliar place where he may feel out of control, threatening the safety of the laboring woman, the baby, and the staff. The woman-centered provider helps the woman identify her support systems, as well as potentially harmful situations. The provider works with the nursing staff to review security protocols. If necessary, the woman can be listed at the hospital anonymously, to deter an angry, abusive partner from interfering during her hospital stay.

> When Mariluz went into labor, Rocky was out with his drinking buddies. Mariluz called Evie and Beatriz to meet her at the hospital. When Rocky arrived, loud and inebriated, at the nursing desk in the labor area while Mariluz was in labor, the charge nurse called hospital security, and Rocky was escorted out of the hospital. Because he climbed into a car and started to drive away, the town police were alerted and arrested him for driving under the influence of alcohol. After delivery, Mariluz worked with the hospital social worker to take steps to be safe. She decided to file a restraining order against Rocky and to enter an anonymous shelter with the baby to be able to get back on her feet without having to worry about staying safe from Rocky. Dr. Burman encouraged her in her plan and again underscored her strengths. They discussed ways that she might keep follow-up visits without alerting Rocky to her whereabouts.

Childbirth can be an opportunity for a woman in an abusive relationship to re-evaluate her situation. Her hospitalization offers a brief period of separation and institutional support that may facilitate a choice for safety. She may also know that if she returns home, the abuse may worsen.[50,89,90] Alternatively, she may feel under pressure from the abusive partner to get home as quickly as possible, to resume her duties for the family but also to avoid any disclosure of her situation to professional staff. Although a woman may hope that the baby will "fix" the relationship, the woman-centered provider can prepare her for the reality that the demands of caring for a newborn often cause increased conflicts and stress in the relationship. Even when partners stop physical and sexual violence, they may continue to use psychological abuse and intimidation against their partners.[91] The risk of abuse of the new baby must also be assessed, as the co-occurrence of partner abuse and child abuse can reach 30%.[92]

The postpartum period is a critical time for the safety of the mother and child. An abuser may shower the woman with gifts and promises of good behavior. Longing for the idealized family, the new mother may reunite with him and put herself and the baby at later risk. For the woman who knowingly returns to a potentially abusive situation, the woman-centered clinician continues to work with her on identifying the woman's strengths and promoting specific strategies for safety. Often, the discussion of safety in terms of protecting her children will help her engage in a realistic conversation about her risk.[93]

THE DYNAMICS OF SEXUAL ABUSE AND MATERNITY CARE

Promoting safety and fostering disclosure are crucial strategies for the woman-centered clinician providing maternity care to women with current or past abuse. The dynamics of powerlessness, betrayal, stigmatization, and traumatized sexuality are frequently problematic for survivors of child sexual abuse.[72] (The term *traumatic sexualization* was used by Finkelhor and Browne to describe how children's sexuality is affected by sexual abuse.[72] We use *traumatized sexuality* to describe the after effects on the woman as an adult.) Pregnancy may bring these issues to the surface. Feelings of powerlessness and stigma may be particularly prominent at the onset of pregnancy: a woman may feel pregnancy is a kind of punishment and feel victimized, helpless, and unable to control her own destiny, especially, like Jen, if pregnancy was the result of rape. Survivors of childhood abuse are more likely to experience postpartum depression and other mood disorders after childbirth.[59,94] As with Melissa's guilt over her baby's cephalohematoma, survivors may also feel guilty if anything goes wrong during pregnancy or delivery. (*See* Part Two and the full vignette in the Appendix.)

Alternatively, pregnancy may help an abused woman feel safe, valued, and nurtured, and give her a sense of confidence in her body and her abilities – a confirmation of normalcy and a sense of self-respect.[67] Understanding the psychological sequelae of abuse and the dynamics that may exist between the abused woman and her providers allows the woman-centered provider to reframe the context of the pregnancy. Pregnancy can be a time when the caring attention a woman receives in pregnancy can promote her sense of self-worth and foster her ability to care for herself and her baby.

Powerlessness versus Control

The survivor's feelings of powerlessness may become problematic during her pregnancy and delivery. Control issues are central to women with a history of abuse. The

pelvic exam, to the pain and body exposure during childbirth, and during breastfeeding and postpartum recovery.

Likewise, returning to sexuality postpartum may be difficult for the abuse survivor. Events during childbirth may have brought up feelings and memories of abuse. The attempt to resume intercourse may cause pain, and fatigue and stress will also cause sex to be a low priority. Breast-sensitivity and milk let-down may make touch uncomfortable.[67,95] Breastfeeding may pose challenges for the abuse survivor. She may have negative associations with the sensations of suckling, secretions from the breasts, or the sensual pleasure of breastfeeding. Exposure of her breasts may be a problem. She may at times experience the baby as another version of the perpetrator who enjoys her body at her expense.[95] Continuous demands from the baby may cause fatigue or even anger. A previously abused woman may project the feeling that her baby is rejecting her when she is actually having a rather ordinary challenge in breastfeeding related to latch or positioning. The woman-centered clinician as well as lactation consultants and nurses involved in promoting breastfeeding need to be aware of this possibility when lactation seems to evoke unexpected feelings or reactions from the mother. On the other hand, successful breastfeeding may give a woman a feeling of confidence in her abilities and in her body and be a very healing experience. The woman-centered clinician follows the woman's lead in addressing concerns around sexuality and will support the woman in her decisions about lactation, as discussed in Part Two, recognizing and reminding her that she can be a good mother in many different ways.

CONCLUSION

Abuse survivors experience pregnancy differently, depending on their history of abuse, current safety, awareness of abuse, and their point in recovery. Women who are unsafe, due to involvement in an abusive relationship like Mariluz, or due to a rape experience like Jen, may feel shame, guilt and embarrassment at the history of abuse. Survivors of childhood sexual abuse, like Melissa, may compartmentalize and minimize their abuse and may use coping mechanisms such as defensiveness or dissociation to get through pregnancy and delivery. Women well into recovery may be aware of personal triggers for abuse and ways to avoid them. All these women have the potential to grow and heal through the experience of pregnancy and childbirth, with a collaborative provider attentive to their needs.

Satisfaction with childbirth can be healing to the victim of abuse, but no recipe exists to ensure a positive experience. Satisfaction is not related to the length of labor, the complications, or the type of delivery, but comes from feeling in control and well cared for.[96] Dissatisfaction is a result of feeling out of control and receiving disrespectful treatment from her providers.[61,67] The sense of accomplishment from delivering and caring for a baby can be empowering experiences for survivors of abuse who often feel incompetent. The intimacy of the clinical relationship during the many prenatal visits makes pregnancy an ideal time to address complicated social and emotional problems. By putting the woman's pregnancy in context and attending to her spoken and unspoken needs, the woman-centered provider is able to establish trust, find common ground, and provide the best medical care for a successful birth. This positive relationship may help the woman provide a safe home for herself and her baby, feel empowered by the childbirth experience, and begin to heal the psychological wounds left by violence.

CHAPTER 3

The Pregnant Woman and Problematic Substance Use

Alice Ordean and Deana Midmer

Delia was a 25-year-old G4P3 who had been on methadone since the birth of her last child. She had been skipping school and acting out and became pregnant for the first time at age 16. Her mother and stepfather threw her out of their home then. Beginning with this teenage boyfriend who had initiated her into heroin use, Delia subsequently had several other partners who were also involved in buying and using drugs. She lived with her partners or on the street, shoplifting or prostituting herself in order to pay for her habit. (*See* full vignette in Appendix).

Woman-centered care for a pregnant woman with problematic substance use refers to a treatment process that views women as principals and allows them choice and autonomy in decision-making.[97] In a woman-centered model of care, caregivers play the role of facilitator for the woman's pregnancy and birth experience, viewing birth as a process rather than an obstetrical event. Woman-centered providers emphasize and value the social context of birth, encouraging women to define their family as whomever they choose rather than along traditional bloodlines. This stance is of particular importance for pregnant women with substance abuse, many of whom are estranged from their families of origin. A woman-centered treatment process for the pregnant woman with substance use requires the development of a suitable environment where such women can comfortably engage in care.

PSYCHOSOCIAL ANTECEDENTS TO PROBLEMATIC SUBSTANCE USE IN PREGNANCY

As in most cases of women's initiation into substance use, Delia's boyfriend introduced her to heroin. Teenagers may begin to use alcohol and drugs in social settings as a way to gain acceptance by peers or to cope with school pressures. Such experimentation may also be an aspect of making a transition or separation from their family of origin.[98] When school or family relationships become problematic or when underlying family or social problems have gone unrecognized, some teens shift from minor use of alcohol and softer drugs, such as marijuana, to heavier use of cocaine or heroin.[99] Women may also begin to use substances as a way to cope with traumatic life events, such as sudden physical illness, sexual abuse, job loss or family move or other disruption. Women may use substances due to partner pressure or due to exposure in family environments where there is a multigenerational transmission of problematic drug use, with acceptance and expectation of substance use by other family members.[100] Thus, genetic, interpersonal and psychological factors may all be responsible for the initiation and maintenance of drug use among women. It is beyond the scope of this book to discuss the clinical aspects of problematic substance use in pregnancy; clinicians can find a model for the clinical management of problematic substance use in pregnancy at the PRIMA (Pregnancy-Related Issues in the Management of Addictions) Project website, www.addictionpregnancy.ca.[101]

As with a history of family violence, the genogram is a good tool to use to highlight the underlying family context. As discussed previously, a genogram is not simply a biomedical pedigree such as genetics counselors use, but rather a diagrammatic representation of family members, health and family problems, and closeness of family relationships over generations.[102] Clinicians can use this visual framework to address unresolved family problems by interpreting areas of dysfunction and then providing opportunities for therapeutic interventions. Dysfunctional partner relationships, lack of good role models for mothering, and career or job pressures all influence a woman's need for relief through substances. The previous witnessing of violence, the experience of partner violence, and/or the experience of early childhood sexual abuse – all potential contributors to substance use[103] – are relevant to the care of all pregnant women.

Another tool for providers to use in discussing and evaluating substance use with pregnant women is the comprehensive ALPHA Form (Antenatal Psychosocial Health Assessment), available at http://dfcm19.med.utoronto.ca/research/alpha. This form enables the woman-centered provider to identify more psychosocial risk factors associated with poor postpartum outcomes from woman abuse, child abuse, postpartum depression and couple dysfunction.[104]

> In her first pregnancy, Delia went to the hospital in labor with Angela, her steadfast teen friend, who was also dealing with a substance use disorder. The hospital staff refused to allow Angela to support Delia during labor because she was not family. When Delia complained of ongoing severe pain even after a shot of Demerol, one

nurse suggested she was drug-seeking and would not contact the on-call physician for further orders. The delivery was uneventful except that the baby girl was admitted to the neonatal intensive care unit (NICU) for initial monitoring due to the substance use. During labor Delia tested positive for marijuana, cocaine, and heroin, mandating the involvement of social services. Delia did not have a chance to hold her daughter, whom she named Angelica. Once the baby was stabilized in the NICU, child protection services took Angelica into custody. The hospital staff did little to ease Delia's sense of loss. No one inquired about Delia's safety on her discharge from the hospital.

BARRIERS TO TREATMENT AND MEDICAL CARE

Delia was soon back on the streets staying with friends or living in derelict buildings and within 10 months was pregnant again. She made attempts to change her life and even attended an outpatient rehabilitation center, but found that men dominated the meetings. She felt too intimidated to speak up. She could not stay clean. During this second pregnancy, Delia spent four months in the regional detention center for shoplifting. While in prison, she received methadone treatment, but was also able to "score" cocaine and marijuana through friends. This pregnancy ended with the birth of her second child, another girl, named Janine Ivette, also taken into custody because of Delia's chaotic lifestyle and ongoing addiction to heroin. She had no ongoing contact with the two girls and received no information about their well-being or whereabouts.

Pregnant women with problematic substance use find the healthcare system very difficult to navigate.[103] These women struggle with feelings of fear, guilt, and shame due to misusing substances during pregnancy. As a result, they often may not present for antenatal care until delivery. Pregnant women who do access prenatal care may not attend all appointments or may delay seeking medical care until late in the third trimester.[105] The negative attitudes of health providers lead to women sensing rejection and lack of compassion during birth, with staff attributing stereotypical motivations to the need for higher doses of analgesia.[106] Providers may feel pessimistic or hopeless when caring for long-term substance users. These feelings can engender cynical attitudes, reinforce stereotypes, and manifest in condescending behaviors. Such prejudicial treatment during Delia's first birth may have created or strengthened her feelings that the healthcare system is punitive.

Pregnant women also face the stigma of alcohol and drug use in the postpartum period. The abrupt removal of her infant by child protective services does not even allow Delia the opportunity to make a connection with her child: to hold her, cradle her, observe how she resembled her parents, say hello and say goodbye. After this traumatizing experience with the healthcare system, it is little wonder that Delia is soon back on the street.

SUBSTANCE ABUSE TREATMENT: PROBLEMS FOR PREGNANT WOMEN

Entering treatment for problematic substance use can be difficult for some women for multiple reasons.[105] Delia encounters common barriers experienced by women in drug treatment programs. Personal barriers such as her own attitudes and feelings may keep her from full engagement in the recovery process. She may feel shame at her ongoing drug use and guilt at losing her baby. Low self-esteem and few life successes act to disempower women, directly affecting their sense of self-efficacy and motivation. Overwhelmed by the constant stress of inadequate housing, disconnection from her family, lack of financial resources, and personal safety issues, Delia copes by using substances to blunt her personal pain.

The lack of adequate resources and childcare can also prevent women from entering treatment programs.[107,108] With no fixed address or safe place to stay, Delia's homelessness mandates a need for a residential treatment program. In addition, her lack of financial stability to pay for transportation costs make attendance at an outpatient program more challenging. For other women, lack of adequate childcare is a significant factor in deciding whether to attend an inpatient or outpatient program. Often the only childcare option is her partner, who may be substance-using, violent, mentally unstable, and/or otherwise unable to provide adequate childcare.

Additionally, the lack of specific programming for pregnant women is a fundamental barrier.[109] Some programs are male-dominated with no perspective on the different needs of men and women. Women, socialized to be compliant, non-complaining and obedient, often find it difficult to find their voice at mixed meetings. Men at meetings may also treat women abusively, making disparaging remarks or objectifying them. Since many women first become substance users because of their partners, women in mixed meetings may revert to their previous style of placating and acquiescing behaviors. Their sense of self may never develop if they continue to perceive themselves through a male lens and perspective. Even if there are some women-specific programs, accessibility (financial or geographic) as well as waiting lists may be the biggest barriers to women getting adequate treatment.

WOMAN-CENTERED TREATMENT PROGRAMS

Woman-centered programs provide services that recognize the needs of women and reduce potential barriers.[110,111] Women with problematic substance use require a comprehensive range of services, including healthcare (primary care, obstetrical care, birth control and sexually transmitted disease [STD] counseling), nutritional support, and assistance with psychosocial issues such as safe housing and addictions counseling (e.g. group discussions or one-on-one counseling).

The initial encounter with a woman at such a program is critical and determines engagement into care. Establishing rapport is the primary goal with empathy, respect, and genuine concern acting as guiding principles in a non-judgmental atmosphere. Providers in a woman-centered program view pregnancy as an opportunity for life changes and attention to substance-use issues. They reframe the use of substances as a symptom of a disturbed life rather than an irresponsible and immoral personal choice. This approach allows the woman to look at the context of her life: her family of origin and childhood experiences, her failed or successful life experiences, her partner relationships, and her sense of self-worth. Because of the duality of their vulnerability (as pregnant and as women), pregnant women are more likely to gain quick admission to detoxification centers, residential treatment programs, and methadone services[112] by getting priority on waiting lists. With treatment more accessible to women at this time, pregnancy becomes an optimal time to make change in their lives. Positive encounters with providers in the course of prenatal care may encourage pregnant women to maintain contact with the healthcare system to ensure improved healthcare for them and their families in the future.

> After her second pregnancy, motivated by support from Angela and other non-using friends, Delia went through a 28-day inpatient rehabilitation program and successfully initiated methadone maintenance therapy. Delia made a strong connection with the social worker in the program and revealed to her the details of her past history of victimization during childhood as well as during adolescence.
>
> Delia's first stepfather repeatedly fondled Delia from age 8 to 12, culminating in a rape at the time of her first period. Delia never revealed the abuse because her stepfather told Delia he would kill her mother if she disclosed. Delia believed him because he kept a loaded gun by the bedside. After the rape, Delia used an excuse of proximity to school to go live with her grandmother. Shortly after the sexual assault her stepfather was arrested and jailed for killing a pedestrian while driving intoxicated. During his incarceration, Delia confided the abuse to her mother, who wanted Delia to come home, but also hoped that her husband would return once released from prison. Delia chose to stay with her grandmother, and ultimately her mother broke off the relationship with her stepfather and soon started a relationship with a very strict but non-abusive new partner.
>
> Delia returned home at 14, but was already dating and having sex with boys in her school. Her first boyfriend, Junior, who was 17, was the father of her first child. He initiated Delia into marijuana use, and later into cocaine and eventually heroin. Delia used these two substances alternatively to calm her down and give her pep. She enjoyed Junior's attention and compliments and for once in her life felt special. Junior was so important in her life that Delia got a tattoo of his name on her neck. Her mother and new stepfather were furious when they saw the tattoo and began limiting her freedom. Delia retaliated by staying out all night. She began associating with heavy drug users and started using heroin on an intermittent basis. Within a month of her first use, she was not only hooked but pregnant. Junior was angry about the pregnancy, and began assaulting her and withholding drugs. When Delia told her parents about the pregnancy, they threw her out, saying that if she wanted help, she should get it from Junior. Because of shame and fear of what they would do to her, she did not tell them about the drug use or the physical abuse. With the help of her friend Angela, she made an appointment for prenatal care at the local hospital, and put on a "good girl" face for most of her

appointments. Although they asked her about physical abuse and drug use at the first visit, she denied these, and no one asked her again after the intake. Delia was only able to break off with Junior by attaching herself to an older boyfriend who used and pushed drugs. He sometimes used Delia to move drugs or forced her to have sex with others as part of drug deals.

THE RECOVERY PROCESS

Getting and staying "clean" is a life transition. The values of woman-centered care guide the recovery process: the woman is the principal, caregivers and counselors are facilitators, and recovery is a process not an event.

> Delia's revelation to the social worker of her childhood sexual abuse facilitated a deeper connection than she had previously ever made with a clinician, and she was able to voice her anger, without relapsing. She found a part-time job as a cashier at a grocery store and entered into a stable relationship with a new partner, Paco, a welder. Paco, also a former drug user, had been on methadone for the last two years. They met at Narcotics Anonymous meetings and tried to support each other in staying clean. During Delia's third pregnancy and delivery, Paco, who was very involved as a new father, supported her emotionally and financially. His presence at prenatal appointments and during labor impressed the staff who perceived Delia differently, and provided more compassionate care. Under close surveillance by the child protective services agency, she and Paco were allowed to take home her third baby, Jeromey. They both smoked cigarettes, but tried to do so outside their apartment as part of the plan to make their home safe for Jeromey. Delia's mother and stepfather became supportive grandparents, babysitting when Delia was at work. Staying drug-free was a requirement for her keeping custody of Jeromey. She had a long-term open case with the child protective agency, with biweekly caseworker visits causing her to feel very anxious. She continued to obtain methadone from the local drug treatment program, and was stable for almost one year, thus allowing her to "carry" methadone home so she only needed to attend the pharmacy three times a week. This arrangement made Delia feel very happy.

After entering a methadone treatment program, Delia is on the path to recovery yet needs to be self-vigilant for the rest of her life. Going to Narcotics Anonymous for support provides Delia with an anchor, and a safe place to express her feelings. Her positive pregnancy and labor and delivery experiences help her to soften her feelings towards the healthcare system, although she remains guarded in that environment.

ROLE OF SOCIAL SERVICES

Many women with problematic substance use in pregnancy view social services with great suspicion. The negative connotations can also extend to public health or community health nurses and other government services. Stories of horrific child removals by aggressive caseworkers do not lead substance-using women to feel trusting toward social service agencies. However, social service providers can, in fact, often be a major support for women, especially those in need of housing, financial assistance and counseling. Women who contact social services themselves (rather than being reported by others) often feel more positive and experience more control through their proactive consultation. However, for women who have had negative past experiences with social service programs, anxiety is often present. Delia has biweekly monitoring and worries constantly that some day Jeromey will also be taken away. On the other hand, her consistent good record with her methadone treatment center allows her the privilege of taking methadone home, increasing her sense of self-worth and sense of control in her life.

> A year later Delia found out that she was pregnant with her fourth child. Delia had seen multiple providers at the health center over the years and did not have a good connection with anyone except for one of the nurses, Maureen, whom she called for a variety of needs – when she needed to make an appointment, get a letter for housing, or when she or Jeromey had an acute illness. At visits, Jeromey appeared clean and well-fed and much attached to his mother. When Delia discovered she was pregnant again, Maureen was the first person she told. Once Delia had chosen to continue the pregnancy, Maureen arranged for Delia to have her prenatal intake visit at the health center with the obstetrical nurse practitioner, Harmony, who was very welcoming. Delia denied current drug use at her intake prenatal visit and agreed to a routine urine toxicology screen at that appointment. The urine drug screen was positive for marijuana. After her positive urine screen, Harmony and Maureen discussed Delia's multiple needs and wondered whether she would be better served by the Perinatal Team specializing in problematic substance use in pregnancy at the hospital across town. Delia was averse to leaving the safety of the clinic and the support from Maureen and went to the Perinatal Team with reluctance.

IS THE BEST PROGRAM THE BEST-SUITED?

At this point, Delia reluctantly accepts the referral to the specialized perinatal team. Her past experiences with the healthcare system contribute to her high degree of suspicion and distrust toward providers and community service personnel. She has reached a comfort level with Maureen and the others at the clinic, making the change to a new unit anxiety-provoking and somewhat frightening. A specialized perinatal program for women with problematic substance use would be ideal for Delia, yet, if she perceives that the staff are judging her or treating her disrespectfully, she might not remain at the hospital for medical care.

> As Delia arrived at the new clinic, the office staff greeted her warmly. They asked her to complete a short questionnaire in the waiting room. The first visit included

a general introduction to the services available and an opportunity to meet some of the providers. The staff asked questions in a sensitive manner, and Delia was relieved that she had not been "interrogated." A second appointment was scheduled for the following week. At this visit the intake nurse completed a comprehensive assessment and brought up her positive urine screen for marijuana. Delia admitted to smoking a few joints with Paco and, after being counseled about the benefits of reducing or abstaining from drug use, she decided to stop using altogether. She returned for a visit two weeks later and admitted that she had slipped and shared a joint with Paco on one occasion. The nurse treated her admission respectfully and praised her for cutting down on her drug use. Delia left with increased resolve to stop her use completely.

The care provided by the Perinatal Team exemplifies an ideal approach to pregnant substance-using women. The team gives Delia an opportunity to discuss both abstinence and harm reduction, with assurance that she would be supported in her choice. With support from the team, Delia becomes much more open to quitting altogether. The team regards her slip as part of her recovery process, with discussion about triggers and circumstances that lead to her smoking again. Delia identifies stressors in her life that incline her to use marijuana to "mellow out" and strategizes on how to manage these situations in a different way. This woman-centered approach permits Delia to become engaged with the team and allows for autonomy in her prenatal care.

INTEGRATED MODEL OF CARE FOR WOMEN WITH PROBLEMATIC SUBSTANCE USE

The Perinatal Team employs a comprehensive and integrated model of care. The obstetrical team consists of multiple providers with a variety of backgrounds including family physicians, obstetricians, nurse practitioners, midwives, nurses and clerical staff, who share a philosophy of compassionate and non-judgmental care. In addition to the obstetrical care, the team makes a wide range of complementary services available. Social workers provide help in securing safe and long-term housing, access to food banks and food stamps, and act as a liaison, on the woman's behalf, with other government or public health agencies. The social worker in conjunction with the physician approaches the pregnant woman about mandatory reporting to child protective services. Using a caring and concerned manner, this discussion includes the current legislation and general duty to report by healthcare providers. The program encourages pregnant women to self-report as a way of improving custody outcomes. Psychiatric and psychological counseling services are available to deal with any mental health or life crisis. An addiction counselor is available to provide information and support around substance use. Nutritional counseling provides one-on-one consultation around infant/child feeding and advice on eating healthy on a limited budget. The staff offer information on childbirth education with sensitivity to the pregnant woman with problematic substance use, and make available special sessions on the need for perinatal analgesia and anesthesia. Lactation consultants discuss the appropriateness of breastfeeding with respect to any substances the woman may be using. These core services are an integral part of a perinatal program specializing in providing care to women with problematic substance use in pregnancy.

A central tenet of this philosophy of care is the belief in a continuum of drug use, from complete abstinence at one end to harm reduction at the other. Every member of the team counsels the woman to make choices that will work in her life situation and supports her in her recovery process to achieve her own goal. Harm reduction focuses beyond the drug use to decreasing harm in other areas of their lives. The team views "falling off the wagon" or slips in recovery as learning opportunities to be normalized as part of the transition process. The openness and acceptance of the providers encourages the pregnant woman to disclose continued substance use rather than to hide it because of fear of reprisals. Respecting choices and offering support represent basic strategies in a woman-centered model of care.

ARE THERE MANY WOMEN LIKE DELIA?

The extent of illicit substance use by pregnant women is difficult to estimate. Like Delia during her first pregnancy, many women may not reveal their use because of the social stigma attached to disclosure. Providers may not screen routinely for substance use during pregnancy, particularly when women seeking care do not fit the stereotype of a drug user and lack discernable evidence (e.g. needle marks, smell of alcohol). Moreover, clinicians may have few skills in identifying and managing problematic substance use when they find it. Nevertheless, problematic substance use in pregnancy is a serious and growing phenomenon. Recent reports in the USA on alcohol, tobacco and other drug (ATOD) use in childbearing women find that in 2002 and 2003, 4.3% of pregnant women aged 15 to 44 used illicit drugs during the past month, 4.1% reported binge alcohol use and 18% reported smoking cigarettes. In this population, women aged 15 to 25 were more likely to use drugs than woman aged 26 to 44, and, of all ages, whites were more likely to have smoked cigarettes than blacks or Hispanics.[113] Canadian data are similar. Two Canadian national surveys found that 17–25% of Canadian women reported drinking at some point during the pregnancy.[114,115] Approximately, 5% drank until becoming aware of the pregnancy, and another 7–9% continued to drink throughout the entire pregnancy. Most women consumed 1–2 drinks and <3% reported five or more drinks per occasion. Twenty-five percent of Canadian women of childbearing age smoke, and while 20–40% of women will quit during pregnancy, 60% of these will relapse within six months postpartum.[114-16] These numbers raise concern about a growing trend of problematic substance use in pregnancy and associated negative maternal and child outcomes.

IMPACT OF PROBLEMATIC SUBSTANCE USE IN PREGNANCY ON MOTHER/FETUS/INFANT

Delia does not know whether her first two infants suffered any sequelae from her substance use. Most likely they, as with most newborns of opiate users, underwent narcotic withdrawal. Opiate use can also cause spontaneous abortion, premature labor, intrauterine growth retardation, and fetal death.[117] Cocaine use is associated with intrauterine growth restriction, premature rupture of membranes, and placental abruption resulting in prematurity and stillbirth.[118] Neurodevelopmental effects such as expressive language and verbal comprehension delay and behavior problems in childhood may also result from cocaine use during pregnancy.[119] Cigarette smoking is associated with various adverse effects, including low birth weight, spontaneous abortion, placental abruption, placenta previa, prematurity, sudden infant death syndrome,[120,121] and possible behavioral problems.[122] Cannabis has a negligible effect on birth weight;[123,124] however, adverse outcomes include premature delivery in heavy users and long-term effects such as neurodevelopmental disorders.[125] Best studied are the effects of alcohol on the fetus. Alcohol is a known teratogen, with serious and permanent effects on fetal growth and development termed fetal alcohol spectrum disorder (FASD).[126] Fetal alcohol syndrome (FAS) is characterized by growth retardation, characteristic facial anomalies and neurodevelopmental delays. Alcohol-related birth defects (ARBD) include a wide range of congenital cardiac, renal, skeletal and ocular malformations and dysplasias. Alcohol-related neurodevelopmental disorder (ARND) may present with neurodevelopmental delay, and behavioral and cognitive problems.[126]

ARE OTHER WOMEN LIKE DELIA?

Like Delia, most women report traumatic life events such as physical or sexual violence, or other chaotic family life events, preceding the start of substance use.[127] Women often use substances to cope with memories of abuse and symptoms of past trauma. Consistently, a male friend or a male partner who is a daily user initiates the woman into drug use.[128] Typically, compared with non-users, these women tend to be younger, more isolated with fewer friends or relatives to provide emotional support and have lower educational and income levels. Many women rely on social assistance or on partners or criminal activity for financial income.[129,130] Psychiatric and social consequences include depression, suicidal ideation and completion, phobias and panic disorders, eating disorders and psychosocial problems.[131,132] Children of substance-using parents are also in jeopardy: many of the 28 million children of alcoholics in the USA are at risk for abuse or neglect as a result of their parents' untreated alcohol dependence.[133]

WOMAN-CENTERED CARE

Some women are not as easy to work with as Delia. Some women come from life situations where substance use is a cultural norm and cessation is untenable. Other women can be difficult and argumentative, arriving for visits intoxicated or "high." The key point in these situations is the presence of the woman seeking care despite her many challenges. The woman-centered provider with such women acknowledges how difficult it is for them to access care: "Your life is very complicated right now. I'm so glad that you made it in to the visit today." Every visit provides an opportunity to work with the woman towards changing her life. She may not be ready in this pregnancy, but building her trust and comfort with providers may have a strong impact on her choices in the postpartum period and during subsequent pregnancies.

Caring for women with problematic substance use in pregnancy (PSUP) can be challenging and frustrating, yet also rewarding. In standard medical training, physicians learn to take charge and make decisions about treatment and care, often unilaterally. Working from a woman-centered model requires that providers collaborate with women, allowing them the lead in making decisions about any life changes relating to problematic substance use in pregnancy. Relinquishing control is a challenge for some providers, and accepting a woman's decisions can be frustrating if those decisions do not conform to the provider's perspective. Yet the rewards are gratifying. Helping a woman successfully tackle her substance use has far-reaching benefits to the woman, her fetus/infant and other children and family members. By building a woman's self-esteem and sense of self-efficacy, woman-centered providers can help her to change her view of herself and to engage in life with a greater sense of direction. Success builds success, and facilitating and strengthening a woman's positive sense-of-self will encourage her to be more optimistic and affirmative both in her short-term and long-term mothering experience.

CHAPTER 4

Pregnant Women in Prison

Anita Kostecki

Providing woman-centered maternity care for socially high-risk populations such as incarcerated and substance-abusing women poses special challenges for providers. The model of woman-centered care, focusing on understanding women in the contexts of their lives and finding common ground to create a strong collaboration, is essential to effective work in this area. Unfortunately, most systems providing maternity care for disenfranchised women do not approach pregnant inmates and addicts with relationships in mind, and individual providers are often distanced from rather than connected with these patients. Practitioners who do attempt to offer care to these patients, in settings without adequate supports from other disciplines such as social work, psychiatry, and perinatology, often find themselves overwhelmed by the complexity of the women's psychosocial and obstetrical problems.

> Chantel was a 21-year-old African-American young woman arrested on a parole violation when police raided a house where she was present during a drug deal. They took her initially to a local jail facility where her urine tested positive for pregnancy, as well as opiates and cocaine. Because of the positive pregnancy test, the jail staff transferred her to the emergency room for evaluation of possible withdrawal symptoms. Later they sent her to the regional correctional facility where on-site medical staff could continue observation for drug withdrawal, initiate methadone maintenance therapy and begin prenatal care.
>
> When interviewed by a nurse on admission to the prison infirmary, Chantel gave a history of significant substance abuse dating back to her early teenage years. She had begun to smoke both cigarettes and marijuana at age 13, and then progressed to using cocaine within a few years. Although she did not disclose more of her life history initially, Chantel herself felt that her earliest drug use began in response to her feelings of loss and depression after her mother died of a sudden cardiac event when Chantel was 12. Since her father was uninvolved with the family, Chantel was separated from her two younger brothers and went to live with an aunt who was the single mother of her two older cousins. Her aunt tried hard to raise all three girls "right" but worked two jobs and was not around the house much; the older cousins were already experimenting with drugs and made them available to Chantel at that time. Chantel's aunt had a boyfriend who was an unemployed alcoholic who made frequent attempts to fondle Chantel when he was intoxicated. He would threaten that if she told her aunt about this, he would personally see to it that she was thrown out of the house and put in foster care. (*See* full vignette in Appendix.)

Chantel's history is typical of most women in prison who have a myriad of psychosocial problems. Many come to prison from unstable housing situations, either living doubled up with others or in shelters prior to their incarceration. A majority of woman prisoners have histories of significant physical, sexual, and emotional abuse in their families of origin and/or in their teen and adult relationships. Addictions to cocaine, alcohol and heroin are common. Among women using substances, a history of past sexual abuse is almost universal.[134]

> One of Chantel's older cousins introduced her to Jason, 18, who initially seemed genuinely interested in Chantel and treated her with kindness and respect. Anxious to get away from her aunt's house whenever possible, Chantel spent more and more time with Jason and began to have sex with him. Within three months she was pregnant. When Jason found out about the pregnancy, he stopped calling or coming to see her. Certain that Jason would return once she had the baby, Chantel decided to continue the pregnancy. She gave birth to a healthy term baby boy, with one of her cousins and her aunt present as labor support. Because of her age of

14, and the fact that she tested positive for marijuana at delivery, child protective services became involved with the baby's disposition in the hospital. After interviewing her aunt, who said that she would not be able to closely supervise Chantel's parenting, the child protection worker placed the infant in temporary foster care and told Chantel that she could have the infant back if she either entered a residential teen parenting program or entered foster care herself with the baby. Uncertain of what these options meant, Chantel initially refused to do either. After leaving the hospital without her son, Chantel quickly sank into a profound postpartum depression, but received no formal evaluation or treatment.

Like Chantel, many women who are pregnant and in prison have a substantial burden of untreated mental illness including depression, suicidality, anxiety, PTSD, bipolar illness, and prolonged grief reactions, as well as personality and conduct disorders.[135-8] Over 70% of pregnant inmates have depressive symptoms above the level needed for a diagnosis of clinical depression.[134] Not surprisingly, these same women report low levels of social support prior to incarceration, with 80% stating that they were not in a relationship with a stable partner and 50% stating that they had lost an important relationship in the year preceding their incarceration.

Chantel continued to smoke marijuana and began experimenting with cocaine on the advice of one of her cousin's friends who told her it would help her stop crying and sleeping so much. She did not follow through on the suggested treatment plan to help her to gain custody of her son, and her parental rights were terminated within a year. During this time, Chantel's cocaine use escalated even further, evolving into a major crack addiction. She began to trade sex for drugs in order to support her crack habit, and was thrown out of her aunt's house after she stole money from her. She quickly became pregnant again, this time without knowing who the baby's father was. At 25 weeks of gestation she went to the hospital for abdominal pain. She underwent an emergency cesarean section delivery for placental abruption of another boy who died at two days of age of complications of prematurity. Chantel had no clear recollection of the events surrounding the birth of this second son, but does remember that the hospital staff treated her with disdain and disapproval. She received the clear message from them that because of her crack use, she had killed her baby. The staff did not encourage her to see or hold the baby and by their actions implied that she did not deserve any of the care and support that would usually be offered to a mother who experienced the loss of a baby. Chantel never found out what happened to his remains. After her discharge from the hospital, Chantel intentionally overdosed on the narcotic given to her for postoperative pain leading to admission on the psychiatric floor. When the psychiatric team thought she was stable, they sent her to a publically funded residential program for "troubled" teens.

Prior to incarceration, many inmates have received little treatment for their psychiatric conditions because of the lack of easily accessible, culturally sensitive, community-based mental health services. Additionally, indigent pregnant and parenting women may have competing needs to maintain adequate food, shelter, and routine obstetrical care and thus may not make mental health services a priority. As with Chantel, addiction may further complicate these choices.

> Feeling overwhelmed by the enormity of her losses over the preceding years, Chantel was unable to engage in either substance abuse or mental health treatment offered at the residential teen program. She ran away, and spent the next several years using drugs and prostituting, acquiring a serious heroin habit in addition to her ongoing cocaine addiction. She had two pregnancy terminations during those years, feeling that she would be unable to bear the loss of another baby. The police arrested her for prostitution at age 20 and eventually paroled her to a substance abuse treatment program where she received methadone briefly before returning to the streets. Since remaining in the program and drug-free for six months was a condition of her parole, her second arrest became inevitable.

Working to understand the previous life experiences of a pregnant incarcerated woman such as Chantel is central to connecting with her in a manner that lays the foundation for a collaborative, woman-centered approach to her care. However, providers often find it difficult to relate to chaotic stories like Chantel's. In order to find common ground, the woman-centered clinician elicits the woman's hopes and fears for *this* pregnancy. Understanding the context in which a woman conceived, whether she was using drugs or not, who the father of the baby is, what supports a woman feels she has for another baby, and how a woman feels physically may all provide insight to the woman's perspective about her current pregnancy. Focused attention on Chantel's past pregnancy experiences and outcomes enables her clinician to identify her many past losses. Whether an inmate was able to retain custody of her children prior to coming to jail also plays a large role in how she feels about herself and her ability to parent another child. Once someone like Chantel has had some time free of drug cravings, either because of methadone maintenance therapy or staying "clean" without using, she may begin to acknowledge the connections between her problematic drug use and her history of past abuse and loss. Chantel becomes increasingly aware that her substance use has been a form of self-medication to blunt the hurt and pain she has suffered. These realizations often occur only in the safety of a caring relationship, where her provider shows genuine interest and lack of fear in listening to all aspects of a woman's life story.

> Chantel was able to disclose her personal history to a supportive obstetrical nurse practitioner, Amy, in the correctional facility where she stayed for the rest of her pregnancy. Initially, she was unable even to decide whether she wanted to continue the pregnancy. She felt overwhelmed by her past life issues, complicated by apprehension, shame and guilt over being in prison again. Amy was able to listen to Chantel's fears of being unable to stay drug-free during the pregnancy and of

losing another baby. Chantel worried the child protective services agency would inevitably take this baby away, too, and that even if she gained custody of the baby, her depression would be too profound for her to be able to parent. Chantel knew that under stress, and given the opportunity, she would often choose to use drugs in an attempt to buffer her feelings of sadness and isolation from her missing family and children. Amy helped Chantel clarify her feelings about the pregnancy. Despite all her concerns, Chantel was finally able to say that she really wanted to keep the pregnancy, deliver her baby, and keep her baby and parent her child when she was released.

Finding common ground with incarcerated pregnant women like Chantel is challenging within the stressful prison environment where the priorities of correctional officials often take precedence over those of healthcare providers. Many women remain appropriately suspicious of any employee of the correctional facility; they have difficulty trusting that the health providers in such an institution are able and willing to provide a high standard of prenatal, intrapartum and postpartum care. Through her close involvement with Chantel's prenatal care, Amy demonstrates a commitment to a good outcome for both Chantel and her baby, within a reassuring and empowering relationship.

Once Chantel had decided to continue her pregnancy, Amy did a full obstetrical evaluation, in conjunction with the supervising physicians. She treated Chantel's newly diagnosed chlamydia infection and arranged a colposcopy for her abnormal Papanicolaou (Pap) smear. Chantel found out that she had hepatitis C infection, a new diagnosis for her, but she was relieved that her HIV test was negative. After adjustment of her methadone dose, her withdrawal symptoms resolved. Concern about her significant mental health and substance abuse histories led her obstetrical providers to refer Chantel to the mental health team on site who assigned her a therapist and planned a psychiatric evaluation. Chantel began to work with the social worker who looked for a residential substance abuse treatment program where Chantel could go after her release, hopefully with her baby as well.

Chantel's chlamydia, hepatitis C,[139] and abnormal Pap smear[140] are typical of the communicable diseases, especially sexually transmitted diseases,[141,142] and other subacute medical issues affecting many pregnant inmates in the USA and other countries. Many such women learn of their pregnancies only when tested on admission to a correctional facility. Those aware of their pregnancy prior to incarceration often have had limited or no prenatal care in the community, using emergency rooms for treatment of pregnancy and other conditions. Although most of these women are young and "healthy" without chronic debilitating diseases other than addiction, limited prior primary care and lack of continuity can negatively affect their health status. Frequently, their past acute medical problems have occurred in association with active drug use, limiting their ability to recall details of their specific medical care diagnoses or procedures. Woman-centered care in this context means prioritizing which details of a woman's medical history are most important and then seeking to compile prior records if possible. Amy has to be clear that Chantel may not remember all that has happened to her, and with this understanding manage her (Amy's) own sense of uncertainty, while taking on the challenge of obtaining pertinent past records or repeating evaluations for the most critical issues.

As with Delia in Chapter 3, in addition to a thorough obstetrical evaluation, comprehensive prenatal care for incarcerated women like Chantel involves a multidisciplinary team of social workers and mental health clinicians working closely with medical providers. For Chantel and Amy, this teamwork includes early completion of a mental health evaluation so that Chantel has enough time to establish a relationship with a therapist to follow her throughout her incarceration. Such evaluations can highlight the potential need for medication management by a psychiatrist. A woman who enters the correctional system already taking psychotropic medication needs prompt assessment to determine which, if any, of these medications are most appropriate to continue, particularly if she had been taking them without knowing that she was pregnant. Additionally, some inmates need urgent psychiatric evaluation for suicidality, a common problem for women inmates in general, pregnant or not.

> Chantel tried to engage with the team members working on her behalf, but admitted to feeling irritable and impatient with her life at the correctional facility. She got in trouble for arguing with some of the other inmates and correctional officers; such behavior threatened to prevent her release from prison to another less restrictive setting.

Recognizing the daily challenges of incarceration helps Chantel's provider to find common ground in her struggles of the moment. The highly structured nature of a correctional facility and the multiple environmental restrictions can create tension and fatigue. Chantel, with the expected discomforts of pregnancy, such as nausea, difficulty sleeping, or back pain, cannot easily get access to simple self-treatment measures such as healthy light snacks, extra pillows, or heating pads – all seldom available to women in jail. Amy can empathize with her normal pregnancy symptoms, inform Chantel about her rights to comfort measures, and advocate on her behalf. Amy can clarify unavailable options so that Chantel can try to adjust unrealistic expectations and exist within the rules of the institution.

> Chantel's mental health therapist, Rhonda, and Amy continued to work closely with Chantel around her lashing out at other inmates and officers. They empathized with her about how hard it was to be pregnant and incarcerated, and worked with her to get some items to increase her comfort at night and help her sleep. As it was unclear whether Chantel would be able to go to a residential substance abuse treatment program prior to delivery, Amy reviewed what would happen if Chantel delivered her baby while incarcerated. The prison social worker discussed the importance of self-control and conforming to the rules of the correctional facility so

that potential treatment programs would view her favorably. Chantel still expressed much predictable frustration with her situation, but with ongoing encouragement was able to avoid disciplinary action during her imprisonment.

Because so many incarcerated women carry the trauma of past victimizations, many feel persecuted by their controlled environment in jail and then act out in response. Some women struggle with poor coping skills due to personality disorders and/or childhood environmental deprivation. In spite of the limitations of the prison system, when the woman-centered clinician views the woman's actions in the context of her past and present life, responding to her difficult behavior becomes easier. Some of her lashing out may represent efforts to stand up for herself, feel strong, and get attention from others. Amy and Rhonda can respond to these needs by paying attention without being asked, recognizing Chantel's strengths and redirecting her energy toward self-care to the extent possible.

Encouraging an inmate to make use of existing resources for substance abuse and mental health treatment while incarcerated is one example of promoting self-care. A pregnant woman might write about her experience as a way to express her feelings as she copes with pregnancy and incarceration. (Having women write their own narratives has been a key strategy in developing participatory research for women in prison.)[143,144] Education and support groups for pregnant women in prison are available in a few settings.[145] The woman-centered provider also offers practical advice and access to opportunities for self-improvement such as adult literacy programs, parenting classes, and job training during incarceration, all of which reduce the likelihood of returning to jail. The provision of resources such as books and pamphlets on infant care and women's health issues beyond pregnancy can also empower incarcerated mothers by showing respect for their capacity to care for themselves and their children.

> Chantel had difficulty joining into group sessions on addiction, as she felt self-conscious about her drug use in pregnancy and current methadone maintenance. When some other inmates criticized her for being on methadone, she felt accused of making her baby into an "addict." Rhonda, her mental health therapist, encouraged her to continue attending these sessions, reminding her that abstaining from illicit drugs and protecting her fetus from opiate withdrawal by taking methadone were brave actions that should make her proud. Chantel was still shy about defending herself in the group setting, but did begin to write in a journal about her struggle to stay sane in prison, which she was able to share during individual counseling sessions. A portion of the journal was written as a letter to her unborn child, expressing Chantel's fervent hopes for her baby's health and strong desire to stay with her baby after delivery.

Regardless of how hard an incarcerated woman is struggling with the chaos of her own life, she almost always maintains genuine concern for her fetus and hope for her future baby's well-being. The vast majority of pregnant women in jail, despite struggles with addiction, anger at imprisonment, homesickness, and physical discomforts, express a sincere desire to have a healthy pregnancy and deliver a normal child. Many have fears about how their own substance use or other risk behaviors in the pregnancy may have affected their fetuses; the woman-centered clinician needs to explore and honestly respond to these fears. Working together with mental health and social workers, the clinician can help the woman envision herself as an empowered and capable woman who could be an effective parent, if that is her goal. Almost all pregnant inmates worry that past behaviors or current incarceration will lead to loss of custody rights.

> Chantel went to court in the third trimester of her pregnancy where the judge sentenced her to one year in prison. He left open the possibility of transfer to a supervised residential substance abuse treatment program. He did not offer parole as an option, due to her prior parole violation. If she left an assigned treatment program, she would be re-incarcerated immediately for the duration of her sentence. The social worker continued to look for open programs, but many hesitated because of Chantel's history of leaving a previous residential program. One program that did accept Chantel did not have a bed immediately available and did not know if one would open up prior to her delivery. Chantel did not have any family members or friends who were willing to provide temporary custody for the baby. She began to panic over the possibility that she would have to place her infant in foster care after delivery.

When a woman cannot transition to a residential substance abuse treatment program for mothers and their children directly from jail, the woman-centered clinician works together with her to help determine the best placement for her baby after delivery – with family, friends or in some cases foster care. Amy and Rhonda can forge stronger connections with Chantel by being willing to discuss her very real grieving process about this lost custody of her baby. Like Chantel, women feel profound sadness for the loss of family support during pregnancy and labor, for the loss of self-determination and freedom of movement both during the prenatal and intrapartum periods, and for the potential loss of a baby upon returning to a correctional facility after delivery. Working with Chantel's grief around these issues is an integral part of her prenatal care.

> Despite attending weekly psychotherapy visits, Chantel's depression began to worsen to the point that she was not sleeping or eating regularly, and she struggled to participate in the required group sessions on her unit. Amy called a multidisciplinary meeting of the mental health and social work staff working with Chantel. The team recommended antidepressant medication. Although she had previously declined medication because of fears of its effects on the baby, Chantel now accepted this option. Her psychotherapist also worked more intensively with Chantel about what it would mean to have to give up another infant, at least temporarily. After three weeks on medication, Chantel's mood stabilized. Although she

still worried about the disposition of her baby after delivery, she managed to focus on an interim plan.

In addition to restrictions experienced by pregnant inmates during prenatal care, these women face the security regulations of the correctional system as they go through the process of labor and delivery in the hospital. Rules can include the need for one or more correctional officers (male or female) to remain with a laboring woman at all times, limitations on visitors, restrictions on telephone use, and physical restraints during labor. (As of 2006, shackles during a woman's labor were forbidden in only two states in the USA, California and Illinois.)[146] In the prenatal period, a woman-centered provider can prepare the woman for what to expect at the hospital and identify any areas where the laboring inmate might still make her own choices including options around monitoring, pain management, and use of the hospital staff for support in labor. Incorporating an inmate's wishes about the timing of inductions and scheduled cesarean sections is another way to allow a woman to have some self-determination in planning for delivery. Anticipatory discussion of coping strategies to promote a sense of control at the hospital can be helpful, particularly for a woman with limited supports and a history of difficult labors and frightening outcomes.

> Chantel's caregivers discussed with her the choice of a trial of labor or an elective repeat cesarean section, and she opted to try to have a normal delivery. She went into spontaneous labor at 39 weeks of gestation, and had an uncomplicated vaginal birth after cesarean of a normal healthy baby girl. She was not restrained in labor, but could not have any family or friends present, and was discharged back to prison 48 hours after delivery.

Perinatal outcomes do not appear to be worse for incarcerated women despite their many risk factors at entry. Because inmates generally receive adequate shelter and nutrition, and have decreased access to substances of abuse, imprisonment may temporarily *reduce* some of their social and medical risk factors. Women in prison are also more likely to receive regular prenatal care than their not-incarcerated counterparts. Several studies have shown no difference in low birth weight and other perinatal outcome measures between incarcerated women and women in the community.[147] Women incarcerated earlier in pregnancy may have better perinatal outcomes that women incarcerated late in pregnancy,[148] and incarcerated pregnant women are less likely to have low birth weight infants than women in a community methadone maintenance program.[149] These reassuring statistics suggest that incarceration is not an independent risk factor for poor perinatal outcome and may even offer a protective effect. However, such statistics should not be used as a recommendation for incarceration of women with problematic substance use who are already at risk for being ostracized by society and by their families.

> After several weeks in the hospital for neonatal opiate withdrawal, Chantel's baby daughter, Iris, went to foster care while Chantel remained incarcerated. Within

three months, Chantel was able to transition to an available bed at a residential treatment program. The child protection services agency placed Iris in Chantel's physical custody there, still under the agency's legal supervision, but in her mother's care for as long as Chantel met the requirements of her substance abuse treatment plan. The program was comprehensive in its approach, recognizing that training for other life skills was essential in reducing the rate of repeat offences, so Chantel was also able to enroll in a high school completion class and begin to attend a series of lectures on parenting.

ARE THERE MANY WOMEN LIKE CHANTEL?

Chantel's story is typical of thousands of women, both in the USA and other countries. Although women represent only 10% of the total incarcerated population in the USA and 6.1% in the UK, the number of women inmates is increasing at a faster rate in both countries – in the USA, by 4.8% per year for women compared to 2.7% per year for men.[150-2] Among youth as well, a growing number of teen women are entering the US juvenile justice system, with women representing 26% of all juveniles arrested in 2002.[153] Between 6% and 10% of all incarcerated women in the USA are pregnant; 25% of women may have been pregnant within one year of entering a correctional facility.[154] The actual numbers are uncertain as women move rapidly in and out of prison without large concentrations at any one location. Despite this increasing pregnant prison population, social indifference toward incarcerated persons in general means that few resources are directed at better understanding pregnant women in prison.

Minority women are over-represented in prison; one-third of incarcerated women in Canada are aboriginal, and in the USA, over two-thirds are minority.[155] Women are usually incarcerated for drug-related crimes rather than violent ones, though violent crimes may be increasing, especially among younger women. Poverty and addiction are the underlying motives for most women's criminal acts, with 65% of mothers in state prisons in the USA reporting drug use in the month before their arrests. Many commit their offenses to get drugs or money for drugs. Twice as many incarcerated mothers as fathers report mental illness and homelessness in the year prior to incarceration.[156] Many women are repeat offenders who have spent time in the juvenile justice system.[134]

Like Chantel, pregnant inmates usually have other children as well. About 60% of inmates, both men and women, are already parents. When the mother is imprisoned, their children often live with relatives and friends rather than with their fathers. When fathers are incarcerated, their children are cared for by their mothers in 90% of the time, whereas when mothers are incarcerated, only 28% of the children are in the fathers' care.[157] Many children of imprisoned women enter foster care; others are permanently adopted out of their biological families.

The addicted, the mentally ill, and the homeless are not social priorities in most societies. Yet simply addressing these fundamental social problems can decrease the rate of incarceration of pregnant women. To break the cycle of multigenerational abuse and recurrent incarceration for pregnant and parenting women, the correctional system must go beyond providing prenatal care focused only on medical issues. A committed team of multidisciplinary providers willing to engage inmates in woman-centered care is essential to improvement of life outcomes for these women. If pregnant inmates receive care that allows them to navigate successfully the physical, psychiatric, social, and behavioral aspects of their pregnancies, they will be more likely to finish their sentences as empowered women potentially better able to parent.

Helping women remain in the community after release from jail, whether in a residential program or with outpatient supports at home, is a top priority for preventing further destruction of women's self-esteem and capacity for recovery. Reunification with children, maintenance of primary custody, and prevention of further incarceration are often goals of pregnant women in prison. Women-centered teams working within the prison setting will need more support and investigation of program outcomes to best support these goals.

Kathleen A. Culhane-Pera and Debra Rothenberg

CHAPTER 1

Importance of Culture in Woman-Centered Care

While the biology of reproduction is universal, every woman experiences events in her reproductive life cycle within the particularities of her culture. Women give meaning to life-cycle events, interpret bodily sensations, and understand health, disease, and natural processes in culturally specific ways.[158] Across cultures, the wide-ranging cultural practices around fertility and childbirth are intimately linked with the position of women in society; a woman's roles and status are affected by whether or not – and in what manner – she bears children.

As more migration occurs around the globe, bringing people of diverse cultural backgrounds together, providers of woman-centered care will need to familiarize themselves with this rich diversity, to inquire about women's cultural understandings of sex, sexuality, gender roles, fertility, pregnancy, and birth and to understand women's and families' expectations for prenatal, intrapartum and postpartum care. Systems of care, as well, will need to address barriers to quality prenatal care linked to racial, ethnic, and language differences often included under the rubric "cultural."

Woman-centered practitioners use their general understanding of culture to form hypotheses about relevant issues for particular pregnant women. They do not assume that any given woman from a specific ethnic group will believe or behave in specific ways. Rather, these providers learn the general cultural beliefs and behaviors and then ask specific women and their families about their beliefs and desires. To make assumptions based on cultural generalizations will result in errors of misunderstanding and perhaps poor medical care.

The stories progressing through the book illustrate the variety of ways in which culture, class, and power influence women's reproductive lives. These stories draw heavily on the range of cultures typical in North America – white, African-American, Native American, and Hispanic, all of which are within themselves quite varied – as well as the cultures of immigrant women, both those born in their native countries, and those born in North America but strongly rooted in their native cultures. Issues are likely to be similar for women immigrating to other parts of the world from these cultures. The countries and regions of origin included here are Albania, Brazil, El Salvador, Guatemala, Laos, Mexico, Somalia, South India, Vietnam, and West Africa, reflecting the authors' experiences, but could include many other cultures.

Culture – or the "distinctive spiritual, material, intellectual and emotional features of society or a social group"[159] – shapes the way in which women everywhere experience sexuality, pregnancy, labor, and the meaning of motherhood. Each woman's ethnicity adds to the "webs of meaning" that she weaves around these life events.[160] That each woman is not explicitly aware of the influence of her culture on her perceptions is part of the power of socialization, a process by which individuals assume that their symbolic structures and patterns of behavior are "normal" and "the right way" to be in the world.[161]

Likewise, the power of socialization into the culture of medicine creates providers who "see" their way of doing birth or providing prenatal care as the best or only way of doing so. To adequately understand the pregnancy experience from the woman's perspective, to appreciate the context of the whole person, and to find common ground requires a nuanced understanding of both the provider's own biomedically influenced cultural stance as well as the woman's cultural perspective.[162] As a biological reductionist science, medicine is often "blind" to the influences of culture, economics, and politics on health outcomes. The stories of the women in this book, however, illustrate the powerful role these factors play in woman-centered care.

For all women, but particularly for immigrant women moving from developing to more developed nations, the culture of medicine in their adopted homes can be a challenge to understand and to navigate, especially around the sensitive issues of pre-pregnancy, prenatal, childbirth, and postpartum care. Perinatal complications for immigrants from Latin America, Africa, and Asia to Westernized countries vary with the country of origin, the destination country, the time since immigration, and socioeconomic variables.[163-9] In the USA, the status of non-immigrant women who belong to ethnic/racial minorities – not always viewed in terms of "culture" – clearly affects their access to prenatal care and pregnancy outcomes. For example, African-

American and Hispanic-American women are less likely than Caucasians to receive enough early, routine, and preventive healthcare services,[170] and African-American women are four times more likely to die of pregnancy-related causes than European-American women.[171]

IMPORTANCE OF CULTURE IN PREGNANCY AND BIRTH

Pregnancy and birth reflect and reinforce larger cultural beliefs, practices, and values. In the late 1970s, Brigitte Jordan' seminal book, *Birth in Four Cultures*, compared childbirth cross-culturally and contributed to the growing "consumer birthing" movement in the USA that questioned the universal necessity of American medical systems' technological approaches to birth.[172] Her work highlights two concepts critical to understanding the importance of culture in woman-centered maternity care. First, the biomedical approach to pregnancy and birth is as culturally based as other birthing systems around the world. Second, any given culture is dynamic and ever-changing, especially when it comes in contact with other cultures.

The amazing range of cultural beliefs and practices around the world should lead providers to be curious and inquisitive when working with women from multicultural backgrounds. Woman-centered providers ask each woman and her family about their beliefs and desires and do not assume that any given woman and her family will believe, value, and behave in specific ways. Such providers are ready to understand that cultural beliefs and practices can be congruent, inconsistent, or contradictory with cultural expectations in the new dominant and biomedical cultures.

BIOMEDICAL HEGEMONY AND BIRTH AROUND THE WORLD

Around the world, human beliefs, values, and behaviors vary enormously with regard to pre-pregnancy, gestational, intrapartum, and post-partum states.[173,174] These cultural practices have roots in indigenous peoples' traditional cultures, including their beliefs and values about the place of people in nature, the natural roles of men and women, the importance of reproduction, and the process of understanding and influencing bodily processes. From the earliest of times, birth attendants were women. The transformation to the dominant technocratic model of birthing, in which technology and not women's bodily senses influence the course of birth, is an example of a hegemonic process, described by Gramsci, by which a way of life becomes dominant, infused throughout a society and widely accepted as the norm.[175] The loss of historical memory about the roots of the word obstetrician (from *obstetrix*, the Latin word for midwife) illustrates the power of this process. Complex social, cultural, and political processes combined to move birth in Western biomedical cultures from a woman-dominated arena into the male-dominated domain of obstetrics, an allopathic medical profession in which few women participated until the 1990s.[176]

Now developing countries must address the ways that technology is a double-edged sword. Certainly, tetanus toxoid, trained birth attendants, access to emergency obstetrical care, and other approaches have vastly improved maternal and infant outcomes. Nevertheless, how each culture incorporates new technologies influences whether birth empowers or disempowers the woman at the center of it. In some settings, hierarchical control over birthing replicated colonial relations between white colonizers in the role of nurses and doctors, and native people in the role of birthing women.[177] Private hospitals serving more privileged women in some countries, such as Mexico and Brazil, manifest cesarean rates among the highest in the world, exceeding even the extent of obstetrical intervention in the US or Western Europe.[178] Thus, women's control over birth and ownership of their birthing experiences is challenged by the introduction of technology around the world. In many cultures, technology stands in opposition to woman-centeredness. This process is most evident in the developed world where society's core value of technology is reflected in its medical system's approach to birth. In these societies, non-evidenced based technology now dominates births for women in almost all settings, even those who are powerful and privileged in terms of language, literacy, education, insurance, and socioeconomic class.[179]

CHAPTER 2

Cultural Issues in Birth Practices

This section describes specific cases of woman-centered care and then explores general concepts that apply to women and families from different cultures. While brief descriptions of diverse cultural practices are appropriate to portray the range of pregnancy-related experiences, ultimately providers must learn about the populations whom they serve and try to place the traditional practices within the context of the original healing system. Providers may interpret many of the practices and proscriptions as superstitious or mythical, but understanding the culture's contextual beliefs about life, death, gender, fertility, pregnancy, and birth will reveal the system's internal justification and rationality. Woman-centered providers understand the importance of inquiring about specific cultural beliefs and expectations that *all* women bring to prenatal care encounters.

PRE-PREGNANCY

Concepts of fertility and conception, like concepts of gender, vary in societies around the world. Examining cross-cultural comparisons reminds us that these categories are not "natural," "God-given," or "universal," but are socially constructed – that is, made and defined by each culture. In many parts of the world, women believe that the most fertile time is immediately before and after menstruation, because at that time "the uterus is open."[180] Indeed, belief in the scientific concept of egg fertilization by sperm during one sexual intercourse encounter is not universal. Some societies stress the importance of repeated intercourse in the development and creation of an infant. Others describe the necessity of the soul entering the fetus. Ideas about fertilization can, in fact, parallel the social structure; patriarchal and patrilineal societies stress the male role in fertilization, while matriarchal and matrilineal societies emphasize the female role in creation. Symbols of fertilization can cast light on a culture's concepts of gender characteristics. Western biomedical imagery, for example, describes the egg and sperm in passive and militaristic terms, respectively; the "small but mighty" sperm is "strong" and "on a mission in quest of the ovum."[181]

The Albanian couple Sylvie and Viktor (*see* Section One, Chapter 1) had come to Dr. Burman for their first pregnancy a year before the birth described earlier. They arrived for an urgent visit where Dr. Burman found Sylvie crying. "I have lost my baby," she murmured as tears rolled down her cheeks. Viktor explained that she had missed her period for two months and then two days previously, she had a lot of cramping and bleeding, and "lost the baby."

Knowing that miscarriages could be significant loss events, equivalent to the death of a child, Dr. Burman wondered how their cultural background might affect their interpretation of the pregnancy and their experience of its loss. Might Sylvie or Viktor blame themselves for the loss? Might they fear they could not get pregnant again? Dr. Burman knew that Sylvie felt disrespected by her in-laws and wondered how the miscarriage might affect her status in the family. After consoling Sylvie for a few minutes, Dr. Burman said, "Losing a pregnancy is very, very sad. And hard, too, in different ways. Can you tell me what is the hardest part of losing the baby for you?"

Sylvie dried her eyes and replied, "The hardest part? I am a failure . . . I cannot even have a baby for my husband." She began to cry again. Viktor put his arm around Sylvie and murmured to her in Albanian.

After a few moments, Dr. Burman provided some factual information about miscarriages, and then said, "Sylvie, I don't think you are a failure. You came to a new country and learned English and got a job. You have lived very far away from your family with only Viktor's support. You got pregnant and then handled a miscarriage at home when many women would not have been able to do that. You are a very strong and competent woman. You will get through this and then a baby will come." Sylvie offered a small smile back.

A year later, Sylvie delivered a baby girl, Elisabeth, by cesarean section. A few months later, she took Elisabeth back to Albania, where she experienced the emotional glow and social status of successful motherhood.

In most cultures, change in social status during pregnancy or after birth is a common human experience, such that in some societies, infertile individuals may never completely make the social status transition from childhood to adulthood. For Sylvie, miscarriage means not only loss but also failure. For Sylvie and Viktor as a couple, having children is an important marker of being adults in their family, and having a miscarriage threatens that transition and potentially impedes Sylvie's acceptance by her in-laws.

People's emotional attachments to a pregnancy and the fetus are common around the world, although not universal. Some cultures resist emotional attachment until the infant has been born and has lived for several days. This pattern may be a response to high infant mortality rates, but also is consistent with religious and social beliefs about life and death. Also, not all cultures acknowledge a pregnancy in the first trimester, such as Sylvie does. Women may attribute amenorrhea to menstrual irregularity until four or five months have passed, when they feel the baby move, or notice the uterine enlargement. In some societies, women do not announce their pregnant state until it is physically noticeable by others, while in other societies, women and their families celebrate a pregnancy at the first late menses, confirmed with a positive urine pregnancy test (as we saw with Kerry and Ron in Part Two).

In many Asian, Arab, and African societies, particularly agrarian societies, the number of children a woman bears is a measure of her worth. Indeed, bearing sons is of utmost importance in patrilineal and patrilocal societies, such as China. (China's law to limit parents to one child has resulted in more sons and fewer daughters, as girl fetuses may be aborted or girl infants abandoned.)[182] Conversely, bearing daughters is generally more important in matrilineal and matriarchal societies.

Mai Yer was an 18-year-old high school student known to Dr. Miller as a quiet, intelligent and respectful daughter in a Hmong family. She sought Dr. Miller's help for infertility. He learned that she had irregular periods every one to two months, had never used contraception, and had been sexually active with the same boyfriend for two years. He asked, "Do you want to have a baby now before you graduate from high school?"

Mai Yer replied, "Not really. It would be hard to juggle school and a baby."

Dr. Miller responded, "Hmmm, so can you tell me about why you don't want to wait until high school is over?"

"I am afraid I can't get pregnant," Mai Yer admitted. "And if I can't, then my boyfriend won't want to marry me, or his family won't allow him to marry me. So, I just want to know that I can get pregnant."

Dr. Miller considered his cross-cultural ethical dilemma in the context of being a woman-centered physician. Should he impose his cultural and ethical values of valuing school over pregnancy and refuse to prescribe medicines? Or should he defer to her experience as a recent refugee balancing both traditional cultural norms of the importance of fertility for a Hmong woman with new personal options to succeed academically? Or should he help her explore how traditional cultural values might be influencing her self-worth so strongly that they could be limiting her bright academic future?

Dr. Miller suggested an alternative. "If you can postpone getting pregnant for one year, I will help you get pregnant after you finish high school."

Mai Yer shook her head. "No, I need to know now if I can get pregnant," she asserted again.

So he suggested another alternative approach, to approach her fear directly, "I can do a pelvic exam and draw some blood today. Then I can explain how you can monitor your body for three months. When you return to see me in three months, I will use this information to help you understand your fertility."

She thought for a minute, and then said, "If this helps me know I can get pregnant without being pregnant, then I would be glad to try it. But if not, then I want to use your fertility medicine."

Dr. Miller smiled at her tenacity and felt that they had found common ground. (*See* full vignette in Appendix.)

While bearing children is important for men and women around the globe, the social significance of fertility and infertility varies from society to society. Some societies interpret a woman's inability to bear children as a lack of social and familial worth. Infertile women may be divorced, forced to live alone, abused, not invited to auspicious ceremonies, or pressured to commit suicide in some cultures, while in others, they may divorce their husbands and remarry, or stay married, but ultimately live an active productive life without children. The stigma of infertility can affect men also, with an infertile man being an undesirable husband in some cultures. In this example, Mai Yer feels the social pressure within her culture to be a fertile woman in order to please her future husband and his family and to feel that she is a worthwhile woman, even though becoming pregnant could interfere with her academic goals in the new culture.

Six months later, Mai Yer returned. She asked the nurse for a pregnancy test, which was positive. When Dr. Miller told her the news, he also asked, "How do you feel about being pregnant?"

She smiled back at him, "I couldn't be happier. This is what I have always wanted."

Dr. Miller responded, "And tell me, what happened?"

Mai Yer explained how her family was so concerned about her that they did a shaman ceremony for her. Since then she had not had a period. Dr. Miller asked about her school plans.

"My boyfriend and I will get married, and my mother-in-law will help with my baby until I finish high school and when I go to college next year," Mai Yer explained without hesitation. "I have already received a scholarship to college, and my husband's parents don't want me to lose it. They really know that going to college will help me and my family."

Dr. Miller made a mental note of the strength of this family's adaptation to this new country with their valuing of both fertility and education.

Control over fertility, either enhancing or limiting it, is important in every society. In many cultures, women take herbal medicines to induce fertility, create a boy or a girl fetus, delay pregnancy, or cause permanent infertility. Other fertility practices include massage, proscriptive dietary patterns, prohibitive activity patterns, and pharmaceutical preparations. For some women, having regular menses is important to health. They will prefer a contraceptive method that preserves regular menses (like a non-hormonal intrauterine device, or cyclical oral contraceptives) over methods that abolish menses or make them very irregular. For some women, if their period is late, they may take a medication to cause their menses to appear. Women may label these medicines as "fertility enhancers" rather than "abortifacients" because they believe that they cannot get pregnant without having their menses.[183]

The onset of sexual activity plays varying roles in different cultures. Whereas for Mai Yer, sexual activity was a step toward defining herself as a fertile woman, teens from other cultures hide the fact of their sexual "debut." Among Black and Latina teenage girls in Bronx, New York, most did not reveal their sexual activity to either their mothers or clinicians, but instead sought reproductive healthcare only when concerned about sexually transmitted diseases or pregnancy, an average of 13 months after onset of sexual activity.[184,185] Cultures that place a high value on chastity until marriage may mandate early marriage among young adults to prevent premarital sex. Different kinds of cultural backgrounds can lead to the same outcome: limited or no pregnancy prevention and limited or no preparation for sexual activity.

Roberta Runningbear (*see* Part One) was a 32-year-old Ojibwa woman with a complicated obstetric history who was unexpectedly pregnant. She worried aloud with her doctor about her past history of preterm birth. After a pause of silence, Dr. Miller asked her what options she was considering.

She slowly replied, thinking about each and every word, "I would have to consider having an abortion. It's never anything I thought I would do, but life brings challenges and one's options change. I know my husband would support me; he too is afraid of having another premature baby. But my mother would be upset. She is a strong Catholic and raised us as good Catholics . . . although now I go to a sweat lodge more than church. My mother would accept all of God's children as gifts, but I don't know that I can. But I don't know that I could disappoint her, either; she's helped me so much with my sick babies. And I don't know that my parents' parents or my parents' grandparents would agree with my being selfish, and considering my own needs over the baby's needs. I was always raised that we should think about how our actions influence the future, and our descendants, seven generations from now." She was quiet for a long time, then continued, "I just don't know what I would do."

Dr. Miller reassured her that they would share this journey together, whatever she decided, and suggested she come back next week, alone or with her husband, whichever she preferred, to share her thoughts and feelings. She smiled a little and agreed to return.

Culture is a critical aspect of how women address the issue of undesired pregnancy, yet women from the same culture make very different decisions in facing this event. In countries where abortions are legal, women have a range of supportive services to help them make a decision, but women may still be unable to access the services because of social constraints, such as disapproving family members or inadequate finances. Women with controlling partners or family members may face serious safety issues if their abortion is discovered; such women may choose medication abortion administered in the doctors' offices because the visits can be attributed to miscarriages.[186] In countries where abortions are illegal, a complex subculture with an underground network may enable women with means to locate abortion services.

In predominantly Catholic countries in Latin America, many women refuse any method of abortion even when a pregnancy would create havoc in their lives. But other women in these same countries, where medications are available without a prescription, buy an "abortion pill" (misoprostol alone),[187] even though use without mifepristone lowers the efficacy. The meaning of abortion may be different for married and unmarried women in some societies. For instance, unmarried women in Tunisia – where abortion is legal – face stigma and humiliation at public hospitals and choose private clinics if they can afford them.[188] In some African cultures, an abortion would be an acceptable choice for a single woman if the man were unwilling to marry her, but if she were married, the decision would fall to her husband.

Finally, women may come from a culture that publicly opposes abortion, yet under extenuating circumstances, such as concerns about the normality of the fetus, women may be able to choose an abortion. Although such a decision may not appear as a "cultural" issue, careful exploration reflects the conflict between beliefs, legalities, and realities all at play in the life and family of the woman as well as in the "culture" from which she comes. Because of a wide variety of practices and beliefs about abortion around the world, ranging from countries where abortion is routine to those where it is illegal, clandestine, dangerous, or punishable by religious authorities, the woman-centered clinician will need to ask the pregnant woman about her beliefs, the practices in her country and her culture, and the stories that she might have heard from friends and family.

Farhiyo was a 25-year-old Muslim Somali woman who fled her war-torn homeland at the age of 15. She spent the following six years in Pakistan before immigrating with her uncle and four younger brothers. Since her mother died in childbirth and her father was killed in the war, Farhiyo functioned as the surrogate parent for her brothers, keeping house and cooking meals for them and making sure the youngest had what he needed for school. When she first met Dr. Adelle Epps, a family doctor who was known among the African immigrant community, Farhiyo was working as a certified nursing assistant and going to school to become a registered nurse. (*See* full vignette in Appendix.)

Woman-centered clinicians build trusting relationships that allow them to delve deeper into patients' perspectives over time. Dr. Epps recognizes Farhiyo as a unique "key informant." As someone who straddles two cultures and is in the process of learning more about healthcare in her new country, she could teach Dr. Epps about her culture of origin. Over the years of their relationship, as Farhiyo wrestles with her identity as a Somali woman, she shares more and more with her provider, seeing her as a source of non-judgmental support for these struggles.

During Farhiyo's first pelvic examination, Dr. Epps noted the evidence of prior genital mutilation – a small stump where her clitoris should have been and a small vaginal introitus indicating that the inner labia had been sewn together. Building on the trust already in the relationship, Dr. Epps asked Farhiyo if she could tell her more about her experience of genital mutilation. Farhiyo said she had been about eight years old at the time, and had few memories of the event. When Dr. Epps asked about current symptoms, Farhiyo said that she did not now feel pain and that she did have sexual sensations in the area. Still, she was certain that she would not want any future daughter to go through this procedure, but she worried about the consequences. Would a daughter be able to find a suitable Somali husband if she was not properly cleansed and "made" into a true Somali woman?

Woman-centered clinicians who read about this cultural practice learn that female genital mutilation (FGM) consists of a variety of surgical excisions, from circumcision (clipping the clitoral hood) to infibulation (removing the clitoris and labia minora and stitching the labia majora closed, leaving a small hole for urine and menses to drain).[189] (The use of the term "female genital mutilation" rather than "female genital cutting" has been controversial. We chose "mutilation" as preferred by Inter-African Committee on Traditional Practices.)[190] Muslims and non-Muslims alike perform FGM mainly in countries in Sub-Saharan Africa including Djibouti, Egypt, Ethiopia, Sudan, Sierra Leone, and Somalia. These practices predate Islam, having begun in Egypt over 4000 years ago during the Pharonic times. The practice is not mentioned in the Qur'an and is not sanctioned by Muslim scholars.[191] In Somalia, about 98% of women are circumcised,[192] and an uncircumcised woman traditionally has few marital prospects. Efforts to change these practices take into account the social and economic context in which they have been performed.[193] Some people believe the surgery is necessary to "cleanse" a girl child, to clarify her sex by removing "remnants" of male sexual organs, and to control her sexuality.[191]

Women from these regions and cultures are key actors in the process of challenging the practice.[190] Surgical correction appears to improve health and sexual function: Somali women (living in Boston, Massachusetts) who chose to undergo surgical "deinfibulation" for pain or difficulties with urination, menstruation, or intercourse, were uniformly pleased with the result, as were their partners.[194] If and when Farhiyo becomes pregnant, her woman-centered provider needs to understand more about specific techniques for vaginal deliveries and subsequent repair of the perineum.

> Over time, Farhiyo began to address her own sexuality. She asked Dr. Epps for articles on FGM and wrote a paper on it for a class in nursing school. Despite knowing that her family would disapprove, she became sexually active with a non-Muslim man. Dr. Epps viewed her as a remarkably reflective young woman and was not surprised when Farhiyo told her that she wished she "had the bravery" to confront her family and culture. When Dr. Epps asked her if she would like more support to work through these conflicts, Farhiyo readily agreed. Dr. Epps referred her to a supportive therapist and continued to see her regularly.

The extreme act of FGM is just one method of controlling sexuality. Other cultures control women's sexuality through other means, such as acceptable clothing, proscribed behaviors, and social mores about marriage. The woman-centered clinician understands the cultural basis and delicate nature of these proscriptions and offers opportunities for women to reflect on them in a safe, supportive, and therapeutic relationship.

PREGNANCY

> Martha was a 39-year-old West African woman who entered prenatal care for this pregnancy at five months of gestational age. She had a history of two prior normal vaginal deliveries, 10 and 8 years ago in her country; one child was alive, but the second baby had died of an infection shortly after birth. The father of this baby – who was not the father of her prior children – was still in her country, and she was living with cousins. Recently arrived, she did not have legal immigration status but found out that she could obtain prenatal care through a local program. Martha spoke some English, but her provider, Dr. Epps, found her accent difficult to understand. Dr. Epps brought up the topic of screening for HIV by saying that in this country doctors recommended that all pregnant women get screened for HIV because the spread of the infection to infants can be prevented if mothers receive treatment during pregnancy and delivery. Martha nodded but started to cry. Dr. Epps was not sure what this meant. She asked Martha what was the matter, but received no answer. Realizing that the visit was going to be much longer and more complicated than the allotted time, Dr. Epps left the room to get help to arrange her later patients. When she re-entered the room, she found Martha standing with her coat on, preparing to leave. She asked Martha to sit back down and again tried to open the topic of necessary blood tests, but she felt Martha did not fully understand or could not process the information. She asked Martha if she would like an interpreter in her native language, and Martha nodded.
>   Dr. Epps called the telephone interpreter service and within a few minutes had

a bilingual native speaker of Martha's language on the phone. She explained her recommendation for HIV testing, and then Martha talked at great length with the interpreter; she became very animated and appeared upset. By speakerphone, the interpreter explained that Martha understood that Dr. Epps thought that she had HIV and that her prior baby died of HIV and now they wanted to treat her for HIV. Dr. Epps was initially stunned at the confusion and then apologized for having confused Martha. She patiently explained via the interpreter that HIV testing is a routine practice in this country and that she had no reason to think that Martha's baby had died from HIV. She went on to say that every woman who has sex is at risk for HIV, so Martha had risk like everyone else and should be tested. She did not mention that HIV is more prevalent in Africa as she felt that going in this direction would just make matters worse. Martha settled down as the three-way conversation proceeded and agreed to the HIV testing and to scheduling an ultrasound to see about the size and dates of the baby. Dr. Epps thought to ask Martha if she would like to bring her cousin with her at the next visit to interpret, and Martha responded that she did not want her cousin to know about the HIV testing. They agreed that Dr. Epps would use the telephone interpreter again at the next visit. (*See* full vignette in Appendix.)

Although Martha comes from a country where English is the national language, her first language is actually Hausa. When English is a second language for a patient, use of an interpreter can help mitigate potential misunderstandings, especially when discussing a topic as fraught with fear and myth as HIV. Additionally, women's attitudes and beliefs about HIV and AIDS may be markedly different from healthcare providers' views, who may consider discussing and testing for HIV as routine. AIDS carries significant amounts of social stigma, so that merely mentioning HIV is frightening, and discussing HIV in privacy (even from family members) is necessary.

Culture strongly affects how women react to prenatal testing, as we have seen with the reactions of three women whose stories appear in Part Two. Not everyone embraces biomedical antenatal care practices. For instance, Rosa, the 22-year-old pregnant woman from Guatemala, tries to follow all the providers' prenatal recommendations, but does not really understand much about the tests that Dr. Jonathan Rosen orders. Jackie, the 36-year-old African-American woman who sees Dr. Judith Peters, does not want an amniocentesis for religious reasons, as she would not consider an abortion. But then recall Melissa, the 38-year-old Caucasian software engineer cared for by Dr. Larisa Foster, who wants every possible test to gain the most certainty about her pregnancy.

Women may refuse standard protocols because they reject the medicalization of pregnancy or physicians' biomedical control, or because they interpret the biomedical risks differently from providers.[195,196] Women use their personal knowledge based on cultural beliefs, expectations, and interpretations of their own sensations to interpret the relevance of biomedical information to their pregnancy, rather than just following biomedical recommendations.[197] Unfortunately, some women like Rosa and Martha may not fully understand the language or meaning of proposed interventions, and therefore may refuse or submit to those tests for reasons that remain opaque to the healthcare team. The chasm of language, education, and culture separating pregnant new immigrants from the highly technical obstetrical culture requires the intense involvement of interpreters and cultural brokers on the team to bridge the gaps in any meaningful way.

When offering antenatal care, woman-centered practitioners ask women about their desires and expectations, and explain the biomedical options, seeking to find acceptable common ground. For example, women fearful of drawing several tubes of blood from arm veins may accept fingerstick tests for small amounts of blood. Women who resist the idea of pelvic exams while pregnant may be willing to defer the exam until after delivery. Women fearful of amniocentesis may agree to the procedure if their family members are present.[198] A woman who would not terminate a pregnancy with a genetic anomaly may still be willing to have an amniocentesis to prepare herself for a child with special needs.

All societies have ideas about optimal behaviors during pregnancy to ensure a healthy mother and baby. Many prohibitions are aimed at avoiding harm to the infant, protecting a mother's life, or preserving fertility. In some societies, proscriptive behaviors apply to fathers as well as mothers, and sometimes even to other family members. These proscriptions often address diet, activities, and emotions, usually consistent with larger cultural ideas about causations of health and disease. Religious beliefs and practices and the concepts of ideal roles, responsibilities, and psychological attributes derived from the kinship and gender systems strongly influence understandings of health and illness in pregnancy.

Jackie, the African-American woman from Part Two, develops gestational diabetes, and has to adjust her usual diet to accommodate the medical recommendations of a diet lower in refined sugars and carbohydrates. As we will see in Part Four, motivated by her concern for her baby as well as her own health (given that she had seen devastation from diabetes in her family members), she rises to the task, strictly following the diet and even preparing separate meals for herself and her family. Jackie is able to change her diet, a cultural set of behaviors particularly difficult to change. Diet is another area where cultural patterns may conflict with the recommendations of modern obstetrical care. Reducing the intake of carbohydrates is challenging for many women whose usual diets are high in carbohydrates. Where protein is expensive, and fresh fruits and vegetables less available, expanding the carbohydrate portion size is a typical nutritional strategy in many resource-poor settings. Whether rice in Asia; tortillas, rice and beans in Mexico; cassava, millet, or corn in Africa; or wheat, potatoes and corn in Europe and North America, carbohydrates contribute the majority of calories in the daily diet. Given the centrality of specific foods in people's appreciation of their own culture, dietary restrictions involving the staples and comfort foods of a culture – often the carbohydrates – can be particularly difficult for many women.

Pregnant women's expectations for medical attention, including biomedical prenatal care, vary around the world. In some developing countries, traditional birth attendants (TBAs) or midwives take care of pregnant women, advising them on how to eat, how to behave, and possibly how to manage their emotions and sexual relations in order to have a healthy baby. Generally, lay midwives' and TBAs' recommendations are consistent with local cultural concepts. However, as lay midwives and TBAs are increasingly officially trained in biomedical concepts, conflict and disagreement are more likely to emerge.[199]

Globalization has fostered the medicalization of prenatal care around the world. The use of obstetrical ultrasound has changed prenatal care and women's expectations of it.[200] In some European countries, several ultrasounds are required components of prenatal care, and may even occur at each visit. Elsewhere families might pay for ultrasound videotapes that document the development of their yet unborn child. Ultrasound examinations during pregnancy have become so "normal" that one North American woman used it as a metaphor. On learning that she won a lottery for a house she had not seen, she commented, "It's like having a baby without an ultrasound."[201]

In yet other countries, ultrasound has enabled parents to select male fetuses and abort female fetuses, resulting in a skewed gender ratio. The cultural conditions for women in India and China make the delivery of girls problematic, especially after the birth of one prior girl; technology here plays a complicated role. On the one hand, access to ultrasound means a woman can abort a female fetus who would become an economic burden and whose birth may jeopardize the mother's own health and safety in the family; on the other hand, becoming complicit with the preference for boys perpetuates her own diminished status and that of other girls and women.[202] Decades later, the resulting skewed gender ratio impairs young men's opportunities for marriage and the ability of their families to perpetuate their lineage.

INTRAPARTUM

> When Mai Yer planned her delivery, she hoped that her extended Hmong family would be present during her labor and birth. Anticipating that the nursing staff would object to more than two support people, she and Dr. Miller developed a birth plan to allow her family to attend.

> When Rosa from Guatemala went into labor, her husband José accompanied her to the hospital, and sat in back of the room. Dr. Rosen asked him how he was feeling, and José replied that he was upset seeing his wife in pain. "A lot of dads feel that way," Dr. Rosen commented, offering to show José some ways to help relieve his wife's pain. But José declined to hold Rosa's hand or hold her legs while she pushed. When the birth became imminent, José left the room.

Birth customs differ around the world. Birth positions vary, from squatting to kneeling, sitting, standing, rocking in hammocks, and lying on the back. The place of delivery varies, from houses to woods and fields to hospitals and clinics to birthing in water. Likewise, birth attendants vary. In some societies, women deliver alone, or only with their mothers, or with many family members present. In many societ-ies, only women are allowed to attend delivering women, and men are forbidden to participate, while in others husbands are passive observers or active participants in supporting their wives. However, even if the cultural norm is for family members to be present, some individuals may face personal emotional challenges in witnessing pain, blood, or exposure of a woman's genitals.

The role of birth assistants varies across the globe. Some traditional birth atten-dants or lay midwives perform internal examinations to assess labor progress; conduct external manipulations to help the fetus find optimal position for birth; give medi-cations to ease pain or facilitate delivery; massage the woman's abdomen, back or perineum; place binders on the upper abdomen to assist in expulsion; chant to the infant to entice its exit; or perform spiritual rituals to assist the birth. Their actions make sense within their respective healing systems' concepts of the normal and opti-mal birthing process.

Similarly, the actions of biomedically trained birth attendants – including pro-fessional midwives, family physicians, and obstetricians – are consistent with the values of biomedicine, despite notable differences between the disciplines' general approaches.[199] Generally, those cultural values include controlling nature, reducing risk, using technology to see and know, and setting up institutional guidelines to address safety and reduce medico-legal risks.[172,203,204]

> Rosa cried out in severe pain and thrashed about in bed during her strong con-tractions. Sofia Khan, her nurse, having previously discussed the possibility with Dr. Rosen, offered Rosa pain medication, but she declined, stating she wanted to deliver the baby naturally, as she had done in Guatemala. As the labor intensified, Ms Khan thought that Rosa's anxiety might be slowing her progress and again offered her pain medication, using Lupe as the interpreter. Rosa replied, with Lupe translating, that she did not know what to do. Ms. Khan wondered what factors were important in her decision, and so asked her, "What are you thinking?"
>
> Lupe translated Rosa's response: "I am afraid something is wrong. Why can't this baby come as easily as my other babies?"
>
> Ms. Khan explained through Lupe that Rosa's labor was very strong, but that it was proceeding normally.
>
> Rosa wondered, "If I take the medication, will you then have to cut the baby out?" Lupe interpreted this question for the nurse.
>
> Ms. Khan responded that medication would let her relax some but would not increase the need for a cesarean section, that Dr. Rosen would consider surgery only if the baby had difficulties and could not be born vaginally. Reassured by Lupe translating these words, Rosa accepted the medication, relaxed between contrac-tions, and proceeded quickly and smoothly to a normal delivery.

Cultural norms about the ideal expressions of pain or joy during birth are variable. In some cultures, women feel ashamed to scream or cry out in pain during labor, while in others, woman's verbal expressions of pain carry no stigma and may even be valued as a signal of a strong woman. Within the general cultural norms, individual women have their own experiences and expectations, such that some women accept their pain more easily than others. Thus, people's reactions to modern anesthetic methods vary, from women rejecting the medications and wanting to experience birth in a natural way, to women accepting medication that alleviates pain or anesthesia that ablates it almost entirely.

> Sofia Khan, Rosa's nurse, came from a Pakistani family where women do not cry out in childbirth. She herself had had three unmedicated deliveries. She admired Rosa's desire for a natural childbirth, but also thought her thrashing and wailing were unproductive. She also knew that other nurses on the floor would think that the patient was making too much noise and should get an epidural. She was glad when Rosa calmed down and had better "control."

A woman-centered clinician is aware of the power that cultural context can have on women's decisions, and helps birthing women make decisions between existing options, whether those actions are identical to traditional options, congruent with newly emerging cultural themes, or consistent with biomedical practices. Birth attendants, as well, have their own opinions and values about the appropriate way for women to act in labor, based on what they themselves have done, as well as what is condoned in the particular setting.

> Mariana from Brazil (*see* Part Two) had had an uncomplicated pregnancy until 38 weeks' gestational age when her blood pressure reached 140/90 and she had protein in her urine. Dr. Miller suggested hospital admission to evaluate her pre-eclampsia and make a delivery plan. Her husband and his mother (for whom this was the first grandchild) anxiously accompanied her and confronted Dr. Miller about her care. They talked in Portuguese, expecting Mariana to translate for them. Dr. Miller obtained a telephone interpreter, and heard the family's concerns. They particularly demanded to know why Mariana was not being offered an immediate cesarean section. Dr. Miller carefully explained the options for care, including a cervical ripening agent, oxytocin, and fetal monitoring. As they continued to be alarmed, and demand a cesarean section, Dr. Miller asked them, "What happens in Brazil?"
>
> Mariana's mother-in-law replied, "In Brazil, a cesarean is the safest, most modern, and best delivery method for people who can afford it. Anyone who can pay for it gets a cesarean."
>
> Mariana then interjected, "She is worried that you won't give me a cesarean because we can't afford to pay for the cesarean here. They think you are trying to save insurance money." She smiled, a bit embarrassed, and continued, "And I think they are worried about me and the baby. Whenever there is any problem in Brazil, they do a cesarean."
>
> Then understanding their perspective, Dr. Miller explained, "In this country, vaginal deliveries are usually the safest birthing method for a woman with pre-

eclampsia. But if something changes and I think you need a cesarean, I will recommend one. What kind of insurance you have won't make any difference."

Families' experiences of medical care in their countries of origin influence their expectations of the medical care system, including responses to monitoring, rupturing membranes, pain medications, and cesarean sections. In some countries, women may prefer cesarean operations – particularly families from higher socioeconomic groups who can afford the operations, and lower socioeconomic class families from the same countries who interpret operative deliveries as indicators of better care or as status symbols. For example, in Athens, Greece, 52.5% of native-born Greek women undergo cesareans in the public hospital setting, while in the private hospital, 65.2% of women with private insurance deliver by cesarean section.[205]

If problems arise during birth, family members around the world turn to many options. They may seek help from religious leaders and seek relief from spiritual causes. Or they may address underlying social conflicts between the birthing women and her husband or her in-laws. They may seek assistance from medical healers, and receive herbal medicines or massage. Also, they may consider biomedical interventions (whether amniotomy, oxytocin augmentation, internal monitoring, or cesarean section) when available. Who makes the decisions about intrapartum interventions is variable, from the individual women in labor, to family members, to their birth attendants. Concerns about biomedical interventions may include worries about the immediate and long-term adverse effects of the interventions on the mother, infant, and family.

> Mariana asked Dr. Miller to wait until her mother arrived the next day from Brazil, to have her assistance if the family had to decide between medical options. Dr. Miller agreed to wait because her pre-eclampsia had stabilized, so he felt comfortable delaying the plan for cervical ripening. Once her own mother had arrived, Mariana agreed to go ahead with induction, and after a night of prostaglandin gel and a day of oxytocin, she delivered a healthy daughter without further complications.

POSTPARTUM

> The postpartum nurse had difficulty administering routine postpartum practices to Mai Yer, the 18-year-old Hmong woman, because her mother and grandmother objected to vigorous uterine massage, a cold drink to quench her thirst, and an ice pack on her swollen perineum. To the postpartum nurse these were important practices to prevent postpartum hemorrhage and to provide relief. To Mai Yer's mother and grandmother, these practices endangered her short-term postpartum recovery and long-term health and fertility. Mai Yer did not know whose advice to follow or which practices were best. She found herself caught between two cultures while actively learning about both.
>
> Dr. Miller, with the assistance of a hospital interpreter, asked the family about

their concerns. Mai Yer's mother explained that blood must flow out of the uterus for the uterus to recover and be fertile in the future. However, cold water, food and air could congeal the blood in the uterus and prevent its flow, which would impair recovery. And vigorous massage could directly harm the uterus. The doctor asked what practices they wanted for their daughter, and the mother said they needed hot water, hot food, warm air, gentle massage and an abdominal binder.

Dr. Miller replied, "Thank you for explaining that to me. We can easily accommodate your needs. And then, if the uterus hemorrhages, what should we do?"

The mother said not to worry, it would not. Recognizing that Mai Yer was at low risk for hemorrhage and had not had any concerning signs or symptoms yet, Dr. Miller decided not to push that point, but rather asked Mai Yer's mother to help monitor the blood flow, particularly when Mai Yer first got up to the bathroom after delivery.

As Dr. Miller and interpreter left the room, the grandmother said to her daughter, "I don't know why the doctors and nurses don't know this. How can they be so educated and yet be so ignorant?"

Similar to the prenatal period, the postpartum period is replete with cultural prohibitions and proscriptions in order to restore and ensure health and avoid morbidity and death. Immediate postpartum concerns often focus on the blood flow, with some birth attendants performing uterine massage, others wrapping an abdominal binder above the uterus, and others applying poultices with medicines or hot cloth in order to aid uterine involution and/or prevent prolapsed uterus. Remaining indoors is common, both to protect the woman and her infant from external dangers (such as germs, wind, light, cold temperature, people, evil demons or spirits), as well as to protect society from the liminal dangerous state or polluting nature of postpartum women. The length of a woman's confinement and limitation of activities is variable, ranging from eight days to three months. Proscriptions about avoiding sexual intercourse are also common, varying from as soon as the blood stops flowing to seven days to five years or from when the child can walk to when the child is weaned from breast milk. Some societies consider menstrual blood dirty, rendering women impure and potentially harmful to others, particularly men. These cultures require initial segregation of women after delivery. Attitudes toward birth and birth products may reflect the status of women in a society. Many South Asian cultures regard the woman's blood, the placenta, and even the baby at first, as contaminated. The birth attendants who touch these things are of low status and earn only a few coins for their parts in the birth process.[177]

People have placed placentas in rivers, buried them in cattle yards or where the child is born, eaten them, or discarded them as biological waste. Some people will keep the dried amniotic sac in a cloth bag to protect the infant from evil, or they keep the dried umbilical cord stump for medicine later in life. North American hospitals have a variety of formal policies about the disposal of placentas with parents in some locations required to obtain a permit from their city or town for permission to bury "human waste."

Rosa partially weaned her daughter Eva in the first four to six weeks in order to be able to return to work without pumping; she breastfed only when she was home.

Jackie continued to breastfeed with bottle supplementation at home for many months after her delivery, which helped her lose weight and thus lowered her blood pressure.

Mai Yer chose to bottle-feed because her mother-in-law would be the primary daytime caregiver while she attended school.

Siobhan (*see* Part Two) tried to breastfeed her first child for a few days but stopped when she became frustrated with the challenges of breastfeeding with inverted nipples. She had thought she could adjust to breastfeeding in front of others, but when she had to add the nipple shield (and then the additional tubing), it became too much for her.

Women's decisions to breastfeed or bottle-feed are influenced by both cultural patterns and social factors, such as availability of space and time to pump at school or work, reactions by family members, acceptability of breastfeeding in public, and cost of formula.[206,207] Many culturally based postpartum prohibitions and recommendations are aimed at ensuring adequate breast milk supply. In some societies such as Japan, women may massage their breasts or pay professionals to perform breast massage. In others, women may avoid specific foods and specific actions that could impair breast milk production.

Many cultures discourage breastfeeding for the first several days of life in order to avoid giving colostrum and instead give pre-lacteal nourishment, such as rice water and honey, water, chamomile tea, or the breast milk of wet nurses. Health practitioners from Western cultures may interpret these practices as "anti-mother" or may not understand them because of their strong biomedical view of the importance of the nutrients and antibodies in colostrum. In contrast, women from a culture where withholding colostrum is the norm understand that to be good mothers means watching carefully until the watery "harmful" colostrum passes, so they can safely nurture their babies with "good" breast milk. Women-centered practitioners use careful cross-cultural communication to understand these mothers' concerns and behaviors in the first postpartum days when Western standards recommend a very different set of breastfeeding practices. Another common cultural conflict around breastfeeding emerges in the immediate postpartum period when many immigrant women believe in doing "both" breast and bottle – feeding and therefore give formula in bottles in the first few days because they "have no milk." Women-centered lactation consultants keep this in mind as they try to encourage exclusive breastfeeding to stimulate milk production.

While people from many cultures in the world have no qualms about breastfeeding in public, those from Euro-Anglo cultures perceive breasts as sexual objects and discourage public nursing. In these cultures, advertisements encourage mothers to buy things like a "L'ovedbaby 4-in-1 Nursing Shawl" to allow "busy moms" to "privately nurse in public . . . and in style" (http://lovedbaby.com/). In addition, multinational infant formula corporations supported the "anti-breastfeeding" attitudes, actively promoting formula feeding as the healthy choice. In 1991, UNICEF launched the Baby-Friendly Hospital Initiative to encourage the promotion of breast-feeding at all maternity centers (www.unicef.org/programme/breastfeeding/baby.htm#10 and *see* Part Five). Such initiatives need to take into consideration the varying cultural contributions to breastfeeding practices within their communities. One such special circumstance is the situation of HIV-positive women in Africa. In some countries, such as Uganda, *not* to breastfeed is taboo, so that HIV-positive women who are advised not to breastfeed to minimize risk of transmission of the virus to the newborn are identifiable and thus doubly stigmatized.

CULTURE CHANGE/ACCULTURATION

Culture is dynamic, influenced by internal conflicts and contact with other cultures. Acculturation is the loss of traditional cultural characteristics and the acquisition of the locally dominant values and practices. Immigrants tend to move along a spectrum of acculturation over time and over generations. In Part Four we will meet Alicia, a 16-year-old who had emigrated from Mexico when she was nine years old, and lives with her extended family during her pregnancy. She has a transformative experience as she progresses through prenatal care, labor, and delivery and the well-child group visits with her daughter. (*See* Appendix for full vignette.)

As a Mexican-born American, Alicia is an example of what has become known as "the paradox of Latina health," i.e. that women born in Mexico who have immigrated to the United States have better birth outcomes than women of Mexican descent born in the USA.[208] This finding has been replicated with many different Latino immigrant groups: foreign-born mothers have less risk of delivering low-birth weight babies than more acculturated women who have become more integrated into life in the USA.[209-13] Changes in diet, use of drugs, alcohol, and tobacco, and undesired pregnancy explain some of these trends, but acculturation probably plays a significant role as well.[214] However, *undocumented* Latina mothers have more low-birth weight babies than documented immigrants;[215] undocumented women may endure stresses associated with dangerous border crossings and constant vigilance about being apprehended by the authorities. They may also obtain inferior medical care, initiating care later, with poorer nutrition and less access to services that are more easily available to other citizens. Thus cultural background is not the only salient factor in immigrant birth outcome.

Around the world, immigrant women tend to fare worse in their obstetrical outcomes than native-born women in the country of arrival. For instance, immigrants to Germany,[216] Norway,[163] and the United Kingdom[217] have more complications and worse birth outcomes than native-born women. In Canada, university-educated immigrant women paradoxically do worse than those with less education.[218] Even within the same country, migrants face obstacles in obtaining prenatal care (e.g. from country to city in China),[219] and depending on the season and food availability, have worse perinatal outcomes (e.g. nomads in Kenya).[220] Thus while we may acknowledge, respect, and support cultural practices that buttress healthy pregnancies, we must also recognize the very powerful social, political, and economic factors working against good obstetrical outcomes for many women outside the dominant culture in their country or their region.

Providing Culturally Responsive Care in Woman-Centered Care for Patients and Families from All Cultural Backgrounds

All clinical encounters are opportunities for culture clashes. Women and their families who have expectations about pregnancy care and childbirth that differ from mainstream biomedicine pose special challenges. Culture clashes take place within the specific context of the social, economic and historical realities affecting both the women and medicine as well. To address these cultural and social issues and provide quality healthcare, woman-centered clinicians seek specific knowledge and skills. They look for sources of general cultural knowledge about the communities with whom they work; nurture attitudes of interest and respect; ask women and families about their cultural needs; find common ground to generate options for care; and are proficient in cross-cultural communication.[221]

Cross-cultural communication, both non-verbal and verbal, is a complex activity. The meanings attached to gestures, greetings, touches, looks, or pauses reveal huge differences in non-verbal communication across cultures. For clinicians to show respect and create a trusting therapeutic relationship, they need to know what non-verbal behaviors come across as respectful to people from different cultural groups. Perhaps nodding one's head rather than shaking hands, or speaking to the husband first rather than the pregnant woman, or looking away from a woman's eyes rather than looking directly into her eyes will communicate respect. In addition, woman-centered providers need good skills in working with interpreters for patients and families with limited English (*see* Sidebar: "Fundamentals of Working with an Interpreter"). Finally, woman-centered care includes working with bilingual-bicultural healthcare workers, community health workers, and cultural advocates as cultural brokers – people who can teach both provider and patients about the other's culture and who can help both sides improve their mutual understanding, for the benefit of the pregnant woman's health.

Fundamentals of Working with an Interpreter*

Do:

- Use professional interpreters whenever possible.
- If possible, ahead of time, situate the interpreter in the clinical situation and the relationship.
- Explain your expectations of the interpreter's role.
- Encourage comprehensive interpretation.
- Ask for the interpreter's cultural understandings if desired.
- Introduce everyone.
- Arrange everyone so that the clinician, the pregnant woman and the interpreter can all see each other. When possible, enable everyone to be seated.
- Look at the woman, not the interpreter.
- Learn and use greetings in the woman's language.
- Address the woman herself using the second person, e.g., "And how are *you* feeling?"
- Keep sentences short, breaking material into small segments and allowing time for interpretation between concepts and questions.
- Avoid medical jargon and technical language.
- Rephrase and repeat information if the woman's response suggests she does not comprehend what you are saying. Ask the woman to restate her understanding of the question in her own words if you are not sure.
- Even if the woman seems to understand some English, ask if she would like to have an interpreter.
- Use professional telephone interpretation when an in-person interpreter is unavailable.
- If you have to use a non-professional interpreter, ask for word-for-word interpretation.

Don't:

- Don't talk loudly. People who do not speak your language are not hard of hearing.
- Don't use the third person with the interpreter (e.g. what does she want?) – talk as if you were speaking directly to the pregnant woman.
- Don't try to get by with broken phrases in the woman's language. If you are not a fluent speaker of her language, get an interpreter.

- Avoid family interpreters unless absolutely necessary. Never use child interpreters or men who are family members or non-interpreter staff (custodial, dietary, etc.) as interpreters for any issues having to do with reproduction, sexual behaviors, or interpersonal violence.
- Don't settle for incomplete interpretation. If the woman gives a long utterance that the interpreter rephrases in a word or two, ask politely for full interpretation.
- Don't say things on the side in your language to the interpreter that you do not want to have interpreted (e.g. editorial comments on the situation).

*See website of International Medical Interpreters Association for current standards for professional interpreters.[222]

Discovering women's salient cultural beliefs and finding common ground requires that woman-centered providers elicit and respond to women's and families' specific cultural beliefs, values, and desired practices about pregnancy and birthing. Woman-centered providers also need to understand how women and families from various cultures are likely to react to a range of biomedical practices. Examples of areas to explore include those outlined in Box 3.2.

BOX 3.2 Exploring Cultural Beliefs, Values, and Practices

1 What ethnic, cultural, social, and religious group/s do you and your family identify with? What is your and your family's migration history?

2 How do people in your culture approach childbearing and rearing, prenatal care, intrapartum practices, and postpartum care? And how do your ideas and ideals agree with or differ from your cultural groups' ideas and ideals? How do your family members support you and your pregnancy?

3 What have you heard about how hospitals and clinics provide care for pregnant women? What expectations do you have for partnering with clinicians, clinics, and hospitals in your pregnancy and birth? How do your ideas and ideals agree with or conflict with biomedicine's ideas and ideals? How can we support your desires during pregnancy and delivery?

4 What are your ideals about decision-making for pregnancy and birth? Would you make decisions alone, or with others? If with others, with whom would you want me to talk about potential decisions?

5 What is your financial situation? Do you have health insurance? How do you and your family support yourselves? What is your immigration status? (Consider whether documented immigrants, refugees, visa holders, or permanent residents.) Does your legal status interfere with your ability to work, receive insurance, and benefit from social programs?

Asking these questions in lay language will help woman-centered clinicians achieve equitable outcomes for all women. The financial and legal questions in particular may demand special sensitivity. Women will only be able to answer these questions honestly when the provider has already established a trusting relationship – premature inquiry may result in delays or withdrawal from care if women worry that their immigration or financial status may affect their care. Undocumented immigrants are also understandably fearful of being reported to immigration authorities and may not understand why else a provider might want to know about their legal status. When woman-centered providers work with women in the context of their cultural history, identity, and family, they will most likely be able to connect with and support the women and their families. By recognizing needs derived from cultural and socio-economic factors that require focused and specific responses, professionals can help women and families understand and achieve their desired healthcare goals.

REFERENCES

1 Boyer D, Fine D. Sexual abuse as a factor in adolescent pregnancy and child maltreatment. *Fam Plann Perspect.* 1992; **24**: 4–11.

2 Menacker F, Martin J, MacDorman M, *et al.* Births to 10–14 year-old mothers, 1990–2002: trends and health outcomes. *Natl Vital Stat Rep.* 2004; **53**(7): 1–18.

3 Ventura S, Bachrach C. Nonmarital childbearing in the United States, 1940–99. *Natl Vital Stat Rep.* 2000; **48**(16): 1–40.

4 Levenson PM, Smith PB, Morrow JR, Jr. A comparison of physician–patient views of teen prenatal information needs. *J Adolesc Health Care.* 1986; 7: 6–11.

5 Coussons-Read ME, Okun ML, Schmitt MP, *et al.* Prenatal stress alters cytokine levels in a manner that may endanger human pregnancy. *Psychosom Med.* 2005; **67**: 625–31.

6 Dominguez TP, Schetter CD, Mancuso R, *et al.* Stress in African American pregnancies: testing the roles of various stress concepts in prediction of birth outcomes. *Ann Behav Med.* 2005; **29**: 12–21.

7 Jesse DE, Seaver W, Wallace DC. Maternal psychosocial risks predict preterm birth in a group of women from Appalachia. *Midwifery.* 2003; **19**: 191–202.

8 Barnet B, Duggan AK, Devoe M. Reduced low birth weight for teenagers receiving prenatal care at a school-based health center: effect of access and comprehensive care. *J Adolesc Health.* 2003; **33**: 349–58.

9 Beck M. *Expecting Adam: a true story of birth, rebirth and everyday magic.* New York: Berkley Books; 1999.

10 Dunn CL, Pirie PL, Hellerstedt WL. The advice-giving role of female friends and relatives during pregnancy. *Health Educ Res.* 2003; **18**: 352–62.

11 Engle PL, Scrimshaw SC, Zambrana RE, *et al.* Prenatal and postnatal anxiety in Mexican women giving birth in Los Angeles. *Health Psychol.* 1990; **9**: 285–99.

12 Dennis C-L. Psychosocial and psychological interventions for prevention of postnatal depression: systematic review. *BMJ.* 2005; **331**: 15.

13 Simkin P. Just another day in a woman's life? Women's long-term perceptions of their first birth experience. Part I. *Birth.* 1991; **18**: 203–10.

14 Simkin P. Just another day in a woman's life? Part II: nature and consistency of women's long-term memories of their first birth experiences. *Birth.* 1992; **19**: 64–81.

15 Malterud K, Hollnagel H. Talking with women about personal health resources in general practice: key questions about salutogenesis. *Scand J Prim Health Care*. 1998; **16**: 66–71.

16 Percy MS, McIntyre L. Using touchpoints to promote parental self-competence in low-income, minority, pregnant, and parenting teen mothers. *J Pediatr Nurs*. 2001; **16**: 180–6.

17 Knauth DG. Predictors of parental sense of competence for the couple during the transition to parenthood. *Res Nurs Health*. 2000; **23**: 496–509.

18 Cox MJ, Owen MT, Lewis JM, *et al.* Intergenerational influences on the parent–infant relationship in the transition to parenthood. *J of Fam Iss*. 1985; **6**: 543–64.

19 Matthey S, Barnett B, Ungerer J, *et al.* Paternal and maternal depressed mood during the transition to parenthood. *J Affect Disord*. 2000; **60**: 75–85.

20 Florsheim P, Sumida E, McCann C, *et al.* The transition to parenthood among young African American and Latino couples: relational predictors of risk for parental dysfunction. *J Fam Psych*. 2003; **17**: 65–79.

21 Kline CR, Martin DP, Deyo RA. Health consequences of pregnancy and childbirth as perceived by women and clinicians. *Obstet Gynecol*. 1998; **92**: 842–8.

22 Cowan CP, Cowan PA, Heming G, *et al.* Transitions to parenthood: his, hers, and theirs. *J of Fam Iss*. 1985; **6**: 451–81.

23 Richardson RA, Barbour NE, Bubenzer DL. Peer relationships as a source of support for adolescent mothers. *Journal of Adolescent Research*. 1995; **10**: 278–90.

24 Kleinman A. *The Illness Narratives*. New York: Basic Books; 1988.

25 Fadiman A. *The Spirit Catches You and You Fall Down*. New York: Noonday Press; 1997.

26 Morse C, Buist A, Durkin S. First-time parenthood: Influences on pre- and postnatal adjustment in fathers and mothers. *J Psychosom Obstet Gynaecol*. 2000; **21**: 109–20.

27 Coren E, Barlow J. Individual and group-based parenting programmes for improving psychosocial outcomes for teenage parents and their children. *Cochrane Database of Syst Rev*. 2009; **3**.

28 Bryan AA. Enhancing parent–child interaction with a prenatal couple intervention. *MCN: Am J Matern Child Nurs*. 2000; **25**: 139–44.

29 Oates DS, Heinicke CM. Prebirth prediction of the quality of the mother–infant interaction: the first year of life. *J of Fam Iss*. 1985; **6**: 523–42.

30 Hudson DB, Campbell-Grossman C, Fleck MO, *et al.* Effects of the New Fathers Network on first-time fathers' parenting self-efficacy and parenting satisfaction during the transition to parenthood. *Issues Compr Pediatr Nurs*. 2003; **26**: 217–29.

31 Doherty WJ, Erickson MF, LaRossa R. An intervention to increase father involvement and skills with infants during the transition to parenthood. *J Fam Psychol*. 2006; **20**: 438–47.

32 Matthey S, Morgan M, Healey L, *et al.* Postpartum issues for expectant mothers and fathers. *J Obstet Gynecol Neonatal Nurs*. 2002; **31**: 428–35.

33 Shaw E, Levitt C, Wong S, *et al.* Systematic review of the literature on postpartum care: effectiveness of postpartum support to improve maternal parenting, mental health, quality of life, and physical health. *Birth*. 2006; **33**: 210–20.

34 Cox MJ, Owen MT, Lewis JM, *et al.* Marriage, adult adjustment, and early parenting. *Child Dev*. 1989; **60**: 1015–24.

35 Curran M, Hazen N, Jacobvitz D, *et al.* How representations of the parental marriage predict marital emotional attunement during the transition to parenthood. *J Fam Psychol*. 2006; **20**: 477–84.

36 Shrier DK. Psychosocial aspects of women's lives: work, family, and life cycle issues. *Psychiatr Clin North Am*. 2003; **26**: 741–57.

37 Reed PS, Clark SM. *Win-Win Workplace Practices: the improved organizational results and improved quality of life: a report to U.S. Department of Labor, Women's Bureau*. Vienna, VA: Choose 2 Lead Women's Foundation; 2004.

38 Ray R, Gornick JC, Schmitt J. *Parental Leave Policies in 21 Countries: assessing generosity and gender equality*. Washington, D.C.: Center for Economic and Policy Research; 2008.

39 Franco JL, Sabattini L, Crosby FJ. Anticipating work and family: exploring the associations among gender-related ideologies, values, and behaviors in Latino and white families in the United States. *J Soc Issues*. 2004; **60**: 755–66.

40 Hochschild A. *The Second Shift*. New York: Avon Books; 1989.

41 Riley LA, Glass JL. You can't always get what you want – infant care preferences and use among employed mothers. *J Marriage Fam*. 2002; **64**: 2–15.

42 Laird J. Lesbian and gay families. In: Walsh F, ed. *Normal Family Processes*. 2nd ed. New York: Guilford Press; 1993. pp. 282–328.

43 Dean L, Meyer I, Robinson K. Lesbian, gay, bisexual, and transgender health: Findings and concerns. *J Gay Lesbian Med Assoc*. 2000; **4**: 101–39.

44 Martin A. *The Lesbian and Gay Parenting Handbook: creating and raising our families*. New York: Harper Collins; 1993.

45 Perrin E. *Sexual Orientation in Child and Adolescent Health Care*. New York: Kluwer Academic/Plenum; 2002.

46 Harper GW, Jernewall N, Zea MC. Giving voice to emerging science and theory for lesbian, gay, and bisexual people of color. *Cultur Divers Ethnic Minor Psychol*. 2004; **10**: 187–99.

47 Greene B. Ethnic-minority lesbians and gay men: mental health and treatment issues. *J Consult Clin Psychol*. 1994; **62**: 243–51.

48 National Center for Injury Prevention and Control. *Costs of Intimate Partner Violence Against Women in the United States*. Atlanta, GA: Centers for Disease Control and Prevention; 2003.

49 Valladares E, Pena R, Persson LA, *et al*. Violence against pregnant women: prevalence and characteristics. A population-based study in Nicaragua. *BJOG*. 2005; **112**: 1243–8.

50 Bowen E, Heron J, Waylen A, *et al*. Domestic violence risk during and after pregnancy: findings from a British longitudinal study. *BJOG*. 2005; **112**: 1083–9.

51 Bradley F, Smith M, Long J, *et al*. Reported frequency of domestic violence: cross sectional survey of women attending general practice. *BMJ*. 2002; **324**: 271.

52 Saltzman LE, Johnson CH, Gilbert BC, *et al*. Physical abuse around the time of pregnancy: an examination of prevalence and risk factors in 16 states. *Matern Child Health J*. 2003; 7: 31–43.

53 Gazmararian JA, Lazorick S, Spitz AM, *et al*. Prevalence of violence against pregnant women. *JAMA*. 1996; **275**: 1915–20.

54 Lipsky S, Holt VL, Easterling TR, *et al*. Impact of police-reported intimate partner violence during pregnancy on birth outcomes. *Obstet Gynecol*. 2003; **102**: 557–64.

55 Kellogg N, American Academy of Pediatrics Committee on Child Abuse and Neglect. The evaluation of sexual abuse in children. *Pediatrics*. 2005; **116**: 506–12.

56 Stenson K, Heimer G, Lundh C, *et al*. Lifetime prevalence of sexual abuse in a Swedish pregnant population. *Acta Obstet Gynecol Scand*. 2003; **82**: 529–36.

57 Dube SR, Anda RF, Felitti VJ, *et al*. Childhood abuse, household dysfunction, and the

risk of attempted suicide throughout the life span: findings from the Adverse Childhood Experiences Study. *JAMA*. 2001; **286**: 3089–96.

58 Peschers UM, Du Mont J, Jundt K, *et al*. Prevalence of sexual abuse among women seeking gynecologic care in Germany. *Obstet Gynecol*. 2003; **101**: 103–8.

59 Johnson DM, Pike JL, Chard KM. Factors predicting PTSD, depression, and dissociative severity in female treatment-seeking childhood sexual abuse survivors. *Child Abuse Negl*. 2001; **25**: 179–98.

60 Mezey G, Bacchus L, Bewley S, *et al*. Domestic violence, lifetime trauma and psychological health of childbearing women. *BJOG*. 2005; **112**: 197–204.

61 Soet JE, Brack GA, DiIorio C. Prevalence and predictors of women's experience of psychological trauma during childbirth. *Birth*. 2003; **30**: 36–46.

62 Granja AC, Zacarias E, Bergstrom S. Violent deaths: the hidden face of maternal mortality. *BJOG*. 2002; **109**: 5–8.

63 Espinoza H, Camacho AV. Maternal death due to domestic violence: an unrecognized critical component of maternal mortality. *Rev Panam Salud Publica*. 2005; **17**: 123–9.

64 Horon IL, Cheng D. Enhanced surveillance for pregnancy-associated mortality – Maryland, 1993–98. *JAMA*. 2001; **285**: 1455–9.

65 McFarlane J, Soeken K, Campbell J, *et al*. Severity of abuse to pregnant women and associated gun access of the perpetrator. *Public Health Nurs*. 1998; **15**: 201–6.

66 McFarlane J, Parker B, Soeken K. Abuse during pregnancy: frequency, severity, perpetrator, and risk factors of homicide. *Public Health Nurs*. 1995; **12**: 284–9.

67 Simkin P, Klaus MH. *When Survivors Give Birth: understanding and healing the effects of early sexual abuse on childbearing women*. 1st ed. Seattle, WA Classic Day Publishing; 2004.

68 Bacchus L, Mezey G, Bewley S. Domestic violence: prevalence in pregnant women and associations with physical and psychological health. *Eur J Obstet Gynecol Reprod Biol*. 2004; **113**: 6–11.

69 Murphy CC, Schei B, Myhr TL, *et al*. Abuse: a risk factor for low birth weight? A systematic review and meta-analysis. *CMAJ*. 2001; **164**: 1567–72.

70 Yost NP, Bloom SL, McIntire DD, *et al*. A prospective observational study of domestic violence during pregnancy. *Obstet Gynecol*. 2005; **106**: 61–5.

71 Leung TW, Leung WC, Ng EHY, *et al*. Quality of life of victims of intimate partner violence. *Int J Gynaecol Obstet*. 2005; **90**: 258–62.

72 Finkelhor D, Browne A. The traumatic impact of child sexual abuse: a conceptualization. *Am J Orthopsychiatry*. 1985; **55**: 530–41.

73 Goldstein KM, Martin SL. Intimate partner physical assault before and during pregnancy: how does it relate to women's psychological vulnerability? *Violence Vict*. 2004; **19**: 387–98.

74 Bacchus L, Mezey G, Bewley S, *et al*. Women's perceptions and experiences of routine enquiry for domestic violence in a maternity service. *BJOG*. 2002; **109**: 9–16.

75 Bacchus L, Mezey G, Bewley S. Experiences of seeking help from health professionals in a sample of women who experienced domestic violence. *Health Soc Care Community*. 2003; **11**: 10–18.

76 MacMillan HL, Wathen CN, Jamieson E, *et al*. Approaches to screening for intimate partner violence in health care settings: a randomized trial. *JAMA*. 2006; **296**: 530–6.

77 Schachter CL, Radomsky NA, Stalker CA, *et al*. Women survivors of child sexual abuse. How can health professionals promote healing? *Can Fam Physician*. 2004; **50**: 405–12.

78 Palmer SE, Brown RA, Rae-Grant NI, *et al*. Survivors of childhood abuse: their reported experiences with professional help. *Soc Work*. 2001; **46**: 136–45.

79 Walker EA, Gelfand A, Katon WJ, *et al*. Adult health status of women with histories of childhood abuse and neglect. *Am J Med*. 1999; **107**: 332–9.

80 Friedman LS, Samet JH, Roberts MS, *et al*. Inquiry about victimization experiences. A survey of patient preferences and physician practices. *Arch Intern Med*. 1992; **152**: 1186–90.

81 World Health Organization. Gender and women's health. 2009 [cited July 25, 2009]. Available from: www.who.int/mental_health/prevention/genderwomen/en/

82 Walch AG, Broadhead WE. Prevalence of lifetime sexual victimization among female patients. *J Fam Pract*. 1992; **35**: 511–16.

83 Koss MP, Gidycz CA, Wisniewski N. The scope of rape: incidence and prevalence of sexual aggression and victimization in a national sample of higher education students. *J Consult Clin Psychol*. 1987; **55**: 162–70.

84 Tjaden P, Thoennes N. *Prevalence, Incidence and Consequences of Violence Against Women: findings from the National Violence Against Women Survey*. Washington, D.C.: National Institute of Justice, Office of Justice Programs, US Department of Justice; 1998.

85 McGoldrick M, Gerson R. *Genograms in Family Assessment*. New York: W.W. Norton; 1985.

86 Mezey G, Bacchus L, Haworth A, *et al*. Midwives' perceptions and experiences of routine enquiry for domestic violence. *BJOG*. 2003; **110**: 744–52.

87 Weisz A, Tolman RM, Saunders D. Assessing risk of severe domestic violence. *J Interpers Violence*. 2000; **15**: 75–90.

88 McFarlane J, Malecha A, Watson K, *et al*. Intimate partner sexual assault against women: frequency, health consequences, and treatment outcomes. *Obstet Gynecol*. 2005; **105**: 99–108.

89 Gielen AC, O'Campo PJ, Faden RR, *et al*. Interpersonal conflict and physical violence during the childbearing year. *Soc Sci Med*. 1994; **39**: 781–7.

90 Richardson J, Coid J, Petruckevitch A, *et al*. Identifying domestic violence: cross-sectional study in primary care. *BMJ*. 2002; **324**: 274.

91 Adams D. Guidelines for doctors on identifying and helping their patients who batter. *J Am Med Wom Assoc*. 1996; **51**: 123–6.

92 Appel AE, Holden GW. The co-occurrence of spouse and physical child abuse: a review and appraisal. *J Fam Psychol*. 1998; **12**: 578–99.

93 Campbell JC. Helping women understand their risk in situations of intimate partner violence. *J Interpers Violence*. 2004; **19**: 1464–77.

94 Buist A, Janson H. Childhood sexual abuse, parenting and postpartum depression: a 3-year follow-up study. *Child Abuse Negl*. 2001; **25**: 909–21.

95 Coles J. Breastfeeding and touch after childhood sexual assault. 2006 [cited April 21, 2009]. Available from: http://eprints.infodiv.unimelb.edu.au/archive/00003007/

96 Hodnett ED. Pain and women's satisfaction with the experience of childbirth: a systematic review. *Am J Obstet Gynecol*. 2002; **186**: S160–72.

97 Midmer DK. Does family-centered maternity care empower women? The development of the woman-centered childbirth model. *Fam Med*. 1992; **24**: 216–21.

98 Carter B, McGoldrick M. *The Changing Family Life Cycle: a framework for family therapy*. Boston: Allyn and Beacon; 1989.

99 Adlaf E, Paglia A. *Drug Use Among Ontario Students 1977–2003*. Toronto: Centre for Addiction and Mental Health; 2003.

100 Stein M, Cyr M. Women and substance abuse. *Med Clin North Am.* 1997; **81**: 979–98.

101 Ordean A, Midmer D, Graves L, *et al. A Reference for Care Providers.* 3rd ed. Toronto, Canada: Department of Family & Community Medicine, University of Toronto; 2008.

102 Poon V. Genogram: a diagnostic tool for family practice. *J Can Diagnosis.* 2003: 135–47.

103 Currie J. *Best Practices Treatment and Rehabilitation for Women with Substance Use Problems.* Ottawa: Health Canada; 2001.

104 Carroll JC, Reid AJ, Biringer A, *et al.* Effectiveness of the antenatal psychosocial health assessment (ALPHA) form in detecting psychosocial concerns: a randomized controlled trial. *CMAJ.* 2005; **173**: 253–9.

105 Klein D, Zahnd E. Perspectives of pregnant substance-using women: findings from the California perinatal needs assessment. *J Psychoactive Drugs.* 1997; **29**: 55–66.

106 Carter CS. Perinatal care for women who are addicted: implications for empowerment. *Health Soc Work.* 2002; **27**: 166–74.

107 Haller DL, Miles DR, Dawson KS. Factors influencing treatment enrollment by pregnant substance abusers. *Am J Drug Alcohol Abuse.* 2003; **29**: 117–31.

108 Kelly PJ, Blacksin B, Mason E. Factors affecting substance abuse treatment completion for women. *Issues Ment Health Nurs.* 2001; **22**: 287–304.

109 Howell E, Chasnoff I. Perinatal substance abuse treatment: findings from focus groups with clients and providers. *J Subst Abuse Treat.* 1999; **17**: 139–48.

110 Creamer S, McMurtrie C. Special needs of pregnant and parenting women in recovery: a move toward a more woman-centered approach. *Womens Health Issues.* 1998; **8**: 239–45.

111 Tiedje L, Starn J. Intervention model for substance-using women. *Image J Nurs Schol.* 1996; **28**: 113–18.

112 Daley M, Argeriou M, McCarty D. Substance abuse treatment for pregnant women: a window of opportunity? *Addict Behav.* 1998; **23**: 239–49.

113 Office of Applied Studies. *Results from the 2002 National Survey on Drug Use and Health: national findings.* DHHS Publication No, SMA 03–3836, NSDUH Series H-22. Rockville: Substance Abuse and Mental Health Services Administration; 2003.

114 Anonymous. *National Population Health Survey, 1994–1995.* Ottawa: Statistics Canada; 1995.

115 Anonymous. *National Longitudinal Survey of Children and Youth, 1994–95.* Ottawa: Statistics Canada; 1995.

116 Floyd RL, Decoufle P, Hungerford DW. Alcohol use prior to pregnancy recognition. *Am J Prev Med.* 1999; **17**: 101–7.

117 Finnegan LP. Effects of maternal opiate abuse on the newborn. *Fed Proc.* 1985; **44**: 2314–17.

118 Addis A, Moretti ME, Ahmed Syed F, *et al.* Fetal effects of cocaine: an updated meta-analysis. *Reprod Toxicol.* 2001; **15**: 341–69.

119 Nulman I, Rovet J, Greenbaum R, *et al.* Neurodevelopment of adopted children exposed in utero to cocaine: the Toronto adoption study. *Clin Invest Med.* 2001; **24**: 129–37.

120 Dybing E, Sanner T. Passive smoking, sudden infant death syndrome (SIDS) and childhood infections. *Hum Exp Toxicol.* 1999; **18**: 202–5.

121 Selby P, Dragonetti R. *Pregnets: smoking cessation in pregnancy.* Centre for Addiction and Mental Health; 2002.

122 Ernst M, Moolchan ET, Robinson ML. Behavioral and neural consequences of prenatal exposure to nicotine. *J Am Acad Child Adolesc Psychiatry*. 2001; **40**: 630–41.

123 Fergusson DM, Horwood LJ, Northstone K, *et al.* Maternal use of cannabis and pregnancy outcome. *BJOG*. 2002; **109**: 21–7.

124 English DR, Hulse GK, Milne E, *et al.* Maternal cannabis use and birth weight: a meta-analysis. *Addiction*. 1997; **92**: 1553–60.

125 Fried PA, Smith AM. A literature review of the consequences of prenatal marihuana exposure. An emerging theme of a deficiency in aspects of executive function. *Neurotoxicol Teratol*. 2001; **23**: 1–11.

126 Chudley AE, Conry J, Cook JL, *et al.* Fetal alcohol spectrum disorder: Canadian guidelines for diagnosis. *CMAJ*. 2005; **172**: S1–21.

127 Adrian M, Lundy C, Eliany M, editors. *Women's Use of Alcohol, Tobacco and other Drugs in Canada*. Addiction Research Foundation; 1996.

128 Hser YI, Anglin MD, McGlothlin W. Sex differences in addict careers. 1. Initiation of use. *Am J Drug Alcohol Abuse*. 1987; **13**: 33–57.

129 Tuten M, Jones HE. A partner's drug-using status impacts women's drug treatment outcome. *Drug Alcohol Depend*. 2003; **70**: 327–30.

130 Kissin WB, Svikis DS, Morgan GD, *et al.* Characterizing pregnant drug-dependent women in treatment and their children. *J Subst Abuse Treat*. 2001; **21**: 27–34.

131 Martin SL, Kilgallen B, Dee DL, *et al.* Women in a prenatal care/substance abuse treatment program: links between domestic violence and mental health. *Matern Child Health J*. 1998; **2**: 85–94.

132 Ross H, Shirley M. Lifetime problem drinking and psychiatric co-morbidity among Ontario women. *Addiction*. 1997; **92**: 183–96.

133 Young NK. Effects of alcohol and other drugs on children. *J Psychoactive Drugs*. 1997; **29**: 23–42.

134 Fogel CI, Belyea M. Psychological risk factors in pregnant inmates. A challenge for nursing. *MCN: Am J Matern Child Nurs*. 2001; **26**: 10–16.

135 Lewis C. Treating incarcerated women: gender matters. *Psychiatr Clin North Am*. 2006; **29**: 773–89.

136 Browne A, Miller B, Maguin E. Prevalence and severity of lifetime physical and sexual victimization among incarcerated women. *Int J Law Psychiatry*. 1999; **22**: 301–22.

137 Jordan BK, Schlenger WE, Fairbank JA, *et al.* Prevalence of psychiatric disorders among incarcerated women. II. Convicted felons entering prison. *Arch Gen Psychiatry*. 1996; **53**: 513–19.

138 Teplin LA, Abram KM, McClelland GM. Prevalence of psychiatric disorders among incarcerated women. I. Pretrial jail detainees. *Arch Gen Psychiatry*. 1996; **53**: 505–12.

139 Correctional Association of New York. Healthcare in New York prisons, 2004–7. 2009 [cited May 5, 2009]. Available from: www.correctionalassociation.org/publications/download/pvp/issue_reports/Healthcare_Report_2004-07.pdf

140 Clarke JG, Phipps M, Rose J, *et al.* Follow-up of abnormal pap smears among incarcerated women. *J Correct Health Care*. 2007; **13**: 22–6.

141 Bonney LE, Clarke JG, Simmons EM, *et al.* Racial/ethnic sexual health disparities among incarcerated women. *J Natl Med Assoc*. 2008; **100**: 553–8.

142 Centers for Disease Control and Prevention. High prevalence of chlamydial and gonococcal infection in women entering jails and juvenile detention centers – Chicago, Birmingham, and San Francisco, 1998. *MMWR Morb Mortal Wkly Rep*. 1999; **48**: 793–6.

143 Fine M, Torre ME, Boudin K, *et al.* Participatory action research from within and beyond prison bars. In: Fine M, editor. *Working Method: research and social justice.* New York: Routledge; 2004. pp. 95ff.

144 Martin RE, Chan R, Torikka L, *et al.* Healing fostered by research. *Can Fam Physician.* 2008; **54**: 244–5.

145 Ferszt GG, Erickson-Owens DA. Development of an educational/support group for pregnant women in prison. *J of Forensic Nurs.* 2008; **4**: 55–60.

146 Liptak A. Prisons often shackle pregnant inmates in labor. *New York Times.* 2006 March 2.

147 Martin SL, Kim H, Kupper LL, *et al.* Is incarceration during pregnancy associated with infant birthweight? *Am J Public Health.* 1997; **87**: 1526–31.

148 Cordero L, Hines S, Shibley KA, *et al.* Perinatal outcome for women in prison. *J Perinatol.* 1992; **12**: 205–9.

149 Kyei-Aboagye K, Vragovic O, Chong D. Birth outcome in incarcerated high-risk pregnant women. *Ob/Gyn Survey.* 2000; **55**: 682–4.

150 Sabol WJ, Couture H, Harrison PM. *Prisoners in 2006. Bureau of Justice Statistics Bulletin.* December, 2007. U.S. Department of Justice, Office of Justice Programs.

151 Ash B. ed. *Working with women prisoners.* 4th ed. Women's Estate Policy Unit. HM Prison Service 2003. [cited October 13, 2009]. Available from: www.hmprisonservice.gov.uk/

152 Black D, Payne H, Lansdown R, *et al.* Babies behind bars revisited. *Arch Dis Child.* 2004; **89**: 896–8.

153 Snyder HN. Juvenile arrests 2002 *Juvenile Justice Bulletin.* September 2004 [cited October 13, 2009]. Available from: www.ncjrs.gov/pdffiles1/ojjdp/204608.pdf

154 Hoskins IA. A guest editorial: women's health care in correctional facilities: a lost colony. *Obstet Gynecol Surv.* 2004; **59**: 234–6.

155 Correctional Service Canada. Ten-year status report on women's corrections, 1996–2006. 2006 [cited November 30, 2008]. Available from: www.csc-scc.gc.ca/text/prgrm/fsw/wos24/tenyearstatusreport_e.pdf

156 Mumola CJ. Incarcerated parents and their children. Bureau of Justice Statistics: Special Report 2000: NCJ 182335. [cited October 13, 2009]. Available from: www.ojp.usdoj.gov/bjs/pub/pdf/iptc.pdf

157 Chicago Legal Advocacy for Incarcerated Mothers. Women in Prison Fact Sheet. 2007 [cited December 29, 2007]. Available from: www.claim-il.org/about.html

158 Garro L. Cognitive medical anthropology. In: Ember CR, Ember E, editors. *Encyclopedia of Medical Anthropology: health and illness in the world's cultures. Human Relations Area Files.* New York: Kluwer Academic/Plenum Publishers; 2004. pp. 12–23.

159 United Nations Educational and Scientific and Cultural Organization (UNESCO). *Universal Declaration on Cultural Diversity.* 2002 [cited November 4, 2006]. Available from: www.unesco.org/education/imld_2002/unversal_decla.shtml

160 Geertz C. *The Interpretation of Cultures.* New York: Basic Books; 1973.

161 Bourdieu P. *Outline of a Theory of Practice.* Cambridge, UK: Cambridge University Press; 1977.

162 Kleinman A, Eisenberg L, Good B. Culture, illness and care: clinical lessons from anthropologic and cross-cultural research. *Ann Intern Med.* 1978; **88**: 251–8.

163 Ahlberg N, Vangen S. [Pregnancy and birth in multicultural Norway]. *Tidsskr Nor Laegeforen.* 2005; **125**: 586–8.

164 Rizzo N, Ciardelli V, Gandolfi Colleoni G, *et al.* Delivery and immigration: the experience of an Italian hospital. *Eur J Obstet Gynecol Reprod Biol.* 2004; **116**: 170–2.

165 Wolff H, Stalder H, Epiney M, *et al.* Health care and illegality: a survey of undocumented pregnant immigrants in Geneva. *Soc Sci Med.* 2005; **60**: 2149–54.

166 Westerway SC, Keogh J, Heard R, *et al.* Incidence of fetal macrosomia and birth complications in Chinese immigrant women. *Aust N Z J Obstet Gynecol.* 2003; **43**: 46–9.

167 Sullivan JR, Shepherd SJ. Obstetric outcomes and infant birthweights for Vietnamese-born and Australian-born women in southwestern Sydney. *Aust N Z J Public Health.* 1997; **21**: 159–62.

168 Treacy A, Byrne P, Collins C, *et al.* Pregnancy outcome in immigrant women in the Rotunda Hospital. *Ir Med J.* 2006; **99**: 22–3.

169 Robertson E, Malmstrom M, Johansson SE. Do foreign-born women in Sweden have an increased risk of non-normal childbirth? *Acta Obstet Gynecol Scand.* 2005; **84**: 825–32.

170 Anachebe NF, Sutton MY. Racial disparities in reproductive health outcomes. *Am J Obstet Gynecol.* 2003; **188**: S37–42.

171 Smedley B, Stith A, Nelson A, editors. *Unequal Treatment: confronting racial and ethnic disparities in health care.* Washington, D.C.: Institute of Medicine of the National Academies: National Academies Press; 2003.

172 Jordan B. *Birth in Four Cultures: a cross-cultural investigation of childbirth in Yucatan, Holland, Sweden, and the United States.* 4th ed. Prospect Heights: Waveland Press; 1993.

173 Ember CR, Ember E, editors. *Encyclopedia of Medical Anthropology: health and illness in the world's cultures. Volume II: Cultures. Human Relations Area Files.* New York: Kluwer Academic/Plenum Publishers; 2004.

174 Shah MA, editor. *Transcultural Aspects of Perinatal Health Care: a resource guide.* Washington, D.C.: National Perinatal Association: American Academy of Pediatrics; 2004.

175 Hoare Q, Nowell-Smith G, editors. *Selections from the Prison Notebooks of Antonio Gramsci.* London: Lawrence & Wishart International Publishers; 1971.

176 Dawley K. Origins of nurse-midwifery in the United States and its expansion in the 1940s. *J Midwifery Womens Health.* 2003; **48**: 86–95.

177 Ram K, Jolly M, editors. *Maternities and Modernities: colonial and postcolonial experiences in Asia and the Pacific.* Cambridge, U.K.: Cambridge University Press; 1998.

178 Belizan JM, Althabe F, Barros FC, *et al.* Rates and implications of caesarean sections in Latin America: ecological study. *BMJ.* 1999; **319**: 1397–1400.

179 Davis-Floyd R. The technocratic, humanistic, and holistic paradigms of childbirth. *Int J Gynaecol Obstet.* 2001; **75**(Suppl. 1): S5–23.

180 Jordan B. Technology and the social distribution of knowledge: issues for primary health care in developing countries. In: Coreil J, Mull JD, editors. *Anthropology and Primary Health Care.* Boulder: Westview Press; 1990. pp. 98–120.

181 Martin E. *The Woman in the Body: a cultural analysis of reproduction.* Boston: Beacon Press; 1991.

182 Hesketh T, Lu L, Xing ZW. The effect of China's one-child family policy after 25 years. *N Engl J Med.* 2005; **353**: 1171–6.

183 Browner C. The management of early pregnancy: Colombian folk concepts of fertility control. *Soc Sci Med Med Anthropol.* 1980; **14B**: 25–32.

184 McKee MD, O'Sullivan LF, Weber CM. Perspectives on confidential care for adolescent girls. *Ann Fam Med.* 2006; **4**: 519–26.

185 McKee MD, Fletcher J, Schechter CB. Predictors of timely initiation of gynecologic care among urban adolescent girls. *J Adolesc Health.* 2006; **39**: 183–91.

186 Prine L. In sickness and health: choosing. *Fam Syst Health.* 2002; **20**: 431–7.

187 Miller S, Lehman T, Campbell M, *et al.* Misoprostol and declining abortion-related morbidity in Santo Domingo, Dominican Republic: a temporal association. *BJOG.* 2005; **112**: 1291–6.

188 Foster A. Young women's sexuality in Tunisia: the health consequences of misinformation among university students. In: Bowen DL, Early EA, editors. *Everyday Life in the Muslim Middle East.* 2nd ed. Bloomington, IN: Indiana University Press; 2002. pp. 98–110.

189 Toubia N. Female circumcision as a public health issue. *N Engl J Med.* 1994; **331**: 712–16.

190 Inter-African Committee on Traditional Practices. Report of the 6th Regional Conference/ General Assembly, Bamako Mali, April 4–7, 2005. 2008 [cited February 9, 2008]. Available from: www.iac-ciaf.com/Reports/6th%20General%20Assembly%20Report%20 2005.pdf

191 World Health Organization. Female genital mutilation: Fact Sheet No. 241. 2008 [cited January 9, 2009]. Available from: www.who.int/mediacentre/factsheets/fs241/en/index. html

192 UNICEF/UNFPA. What is female genital mutilation? What actions are being taken to prevent it? 2000 [cited January 19, 2009]. Available from: www.un.org/geninfo/faq/ factsheets/FS3.HTM

193 Kelly E, Hillard PJ. Female genital mutilation. *Curr Opin Obstet Gynecol.* 2005; **17**: 490–4.

194 Nour NM, Michels KB, Bryant AE. Defibulation to treat female genital cutting: effect on symptoms and sexual function. *Obstet Gynecol.* 2006; **108**: 55–60.

195 Markens S, Browner CH, Press N. 'Because of the risks': how US pregnant women account for refusing prenatal screening. *Soc Sci Med.* 1999; **49**: 359–69.

196 Rapp R. Refusing prenatal diagnosis: the meanings of bioscience in a multicultural world. *Sci Technol Human Values.* 1998; **23**: 45–70.

197 Browner CH, Press N. The production of authoritative knowledge in American prenatal care. *Med Anthropol Q.* 1996; **10**: 141–56.

198 Browner CH, Preloran HM. Male partners' role in Latinas' amniocentesis decisions. *J Genet Couns.* 1999; **8**: 85–108.

199 Davis-Floyd R. Mutual accommodation or biomedical hegemony? Anthropological perspectives on global issues in midwifery. *Midwifery Today Int Midwife.* 2000: 12–16.

200 Oaks L. Reproductive frontiers: ethnographic explorations of the meanings of reproductive technologies. *Rev Anthropol.* 2002; **31**: 323–38.

201 Kane M. Hard work pays off. *Worcester Telegram and Gazette.* 2006 July 26; Sect. 1.

202 Candib LM. Incest and other harms to daughters across cultures: maternal complicity and patriarchal power. *Womens Stud Int Forum.* 1999; **22**: 185–201.

203 Davis-Floyd RE. The technocratic body: American childbirth as cultural expression. *Soc Sci Med.* 1994; **38**: 1125–40.

204 Davis-Floyd R, CF. S. *Childbirth and Authoritative Knowledge: cross-cultural perspectives.* Berkeley CA: University of California Press; 1997.

205 Mossialos E, Allin S, Karras K, *et al.* An investigation of caesarean sections in three Greek hospitals: the impact of financial incentives and convenience. *Eur J Public Health.* 2005; **15**: 288–95.

206 Millard AV. The place of the clock in pediatric advice: rationales, cultural themes, and impediments to breastfeeding. *Soc Sci Med.* 1990; **31**: 211–21.

207 Van Esterik P. Contemporary trends in infant feeding research. *Annu Rev Anthropol.* 2002; **31**: 257–78.

208 Guendelman S, Thornton D, Gould J, *et al.* Mexican women in California: differentials in maternal morbidity between foreign and US-born populations. *Paediatr Perinat Epidemiol.* 2006; **20**: 471–81.

209 Callister LC, Birkhead A. Acculturation and perinatal outcomes in Mexican immigrant childbearing women: an integrative review. *J Perinat Neonatal Nurs.* 2002; **16**: 22–38.

210 Cobas JA, Balcazar H, Benin MB, *et al.* Acculturation and low-birthweight infants among Latino women: a reanalysis of HANES data with structural equation models. *Am J Public Health.* 1996; **86**: 394–6.

211 Page RL. Positive pregnancy outcomes in Mexican immigrants: what can we learn? *J Obstet Gynecol Neonatal Nurs.* 2004; **33**: 783–90.

212 Rosenberg TJ, Raggio TP, Chiasson MA. A further examination of the "Epidemiologic paradox": birth outcomes among Latinas. *J Natl Med Assoc.* 2005; **97**: 550–6.

213 Scribner R, Dwyer JH. Acculturation and low birthweight among Latinos in the Hispanic HANES. *Am J Public Health.* 1989; **79**: 1263–7.

214 Madan A, Palaniappan L, Urizar G, *et al.* Sociocultural factors that affect pregnancy outcomes in two dissimilar immigrant groups in the United States. *J Pediatr.* 2006; **148**: 341–6.

215 Kelaher M, Jessop DJ. Differences in low-birthweight among documented and undocumented foreign-born and US-born Latinas. *Soc Sci Med.* 2002; **55**: 2171–5.

216 David M, Pachaly J, Vetter K. Perinatal outcome in Berlin (Germany) among immigrants from Turkey. *Arch Gynecol Obstet.* 2006; **274**: 271–8.

217 Kothari A, Mahadevan N, Girling J. Tuberculosis and pregnancy – results of a study in a high prevalence area in London. *Eur J Obstet Gynecol Reprod Biol.* 2006; **126**: 48–55.

218 Auger N, Luo ZC, Platt RW, *et al.* Do mother's education and foreign born status interact to influence birth outcomes? Clarifying the epidemiological paradox and the healthy migrant effect. *J Epidemiol Community Health.* 2008; **62**: 402–9.

219 Shaokang Z, Zhenwei S, Blas E. Economic transition and maternal health care for internal migrants in Shanghai, China. *Health Policy Plan.* 2002; **17**: S47–55.

220 Pike IL. Pregnancy outcome for nomadic Turkana pastoralists of Kenya. *Am J Phys Anthropol.* 2000; **113**: 31–45.

221 Culhane-Pera KA, Vawter DE, Xiong P, *et al.*, editors. *Healing by Heart: clinical and ethical case stories of Hmong families and Western providers.* Nashville TN: Vanderbilt University Press; 2003.

222 International Medical Interpreters Association. Medical interpreting standards of practice. 2007 [cited May 19, 2009]. Available from: www.hablamosjuntos.org/resources/pdf/IMIA_Standards_Of_Practice.pdf

PART FOUR

Finding Common Ground in the Care of Pregnant, Laboring, and Postpartum Women

CHAPTER 1

Birth Plans

Elizabeth Naumburg and Cathleen Morrow

Pregnancy is an essentially normal process, and birth is an opportunity for a woman to appreciate her own strength, authority, and knowledge in arriving at the ultimate goal of a healthy mother and baby. Maternity care that shares these goals must be centered in the woman within the context of her family.

The woman-centered clinician seeks common ground with pregnant women through interpreting and integrating the often conflicting, widely divergent worlds of professional medicine and lay experience. The challenging process of finding common ground involves mutuality between clinician and woman, a democratic process of information sharing that leads to informed decision-making for the woman. The pregnant woman and her clinician work together toward defining the clinical issues, clarifying the goals and priorities of a collaborative treatment plan, and figuring out mutually agreeable roles for both clinician and woman.

The process of the FIFE method is an "essential precursor" to finding common ground because this method allows the clinician to explore the woman's experience explicitly and thoroughly.[1:84] The clinician simultaneously lays out the medical issues, blends these with the woman's lifeworld perspective,[2] and together with her identifies any divergent issues that can then be further discussed. The clinician's role is to present alternatives, with informed discussion of pros and cons and uncertainties, and to ascertain how well the woman understands the decisions, how she wants to be involved in her care plan, how realistic her goals are, and what her coping capacity

265

is. The hard work of effectively accomplishing these tasks transpires throughout pregnancy, with each prenatal visit making further progress.

In this part we use the model of a **birth plan** as a metaphorical and concrete manifestation of finding common ground. Historically, in the USA and the UK a "birth plan" was a written document expressing the pregnant woman and her partner's wishes about her labor and delivery. Popularized in the era when physician-centered obstetrical care employed much unproven intervention, the birth plan became a way for women to attempt to regain control of the birth process. As such, physicians often perceived birth plans as a threat to medical control and held a negative view of them.[3-5] However, studies from Australia show that birth plans can enhance communication between women and the hospital staff.[6]

Expanding this model of a birth plan to encompass the entire prenatal process and into the postpartum period is the essence of finding common ground. Indeed, the birth plan should be considered a pregnancy, birth, and parenting plan. The development of a birth plan with each woman becomes a tool for educating, empowering, and encouraging her and her family through the birth process. The collaborative process of creating a mutually agreed-upon birth plan promotes communication and decision-making that emphasize the woman's capacity to make healthy choices for herself and her family.

The woman-centered provider understands that a "birth plan" is a dynamic, evolving process, starting at the beginning of pregnancy, or even earlier as part of a woman's lifelong reproductive plan. The birth plan unfolds as preconception care merges into maternity care and beyond. Shifting emphasis throughout these many months, a birth plan viewed broadly focuses on optimum health for infant, mother, birthing couple, and family. In the best of circumstances, a birth plan can lay the groundwork for a continued relationship for the provision of lifelong healthcare to a woman and her extended family.[3]

CHAPTER 2

Prenatal Care

Elizabeth Naumburg and Cathleen Morrow

Prenatal care is a unique phenomenon of care in modern medicine. In the developed world, prenatal care consists of a prescribed set of visits over a relatively short course of time, increasing in frequency and culminating in one of life's most intense experiences. Prenatal care offers support to an essentially well woman, yet also addresses predictable and significant biomedical issues at set times during the course of the pregnancy. The visits themselves are often short, but the frequency usually allows for the range of issues that need to be addressed, in small increments, over the course of the pregnancy. The intentional use of this structure over the course of ongoing prenatal care allows the woman-centered provider to explore longitudinally a woman's goals for the pregnancy, including discussion of numerous topics that range from the purely biomedical to the woman's feelings, ideas, functions, and expectations.

Finding common ground starts with the first prenatal care visit. Traditionally, numerous provider goals such as medical history-taking and completion of forms drive this visit. Given that this visit is often a woman's first contact with this part of the healthcare system, however, the woman-centered approach also necessitates using this first visit to clarify the meaning this pregnancy holds for the woman and her family. Doing so also clearly establishes the provider's interest in understanding this woman's unique perspective.

Box 4.1 describes five steps in this crucial first visit, most of which involve seeking the woman's perspective during the process of eliciting her medical history. As described in Part Two, the woman-centered provider explores dimensions of the woman's experience such as current life stage and plans, experiences with prior pregnancies or close friends' or family members' pregnancies, the status of the relationship with the father of the baby, and myriad other crucial issues that can all play a role in shaping the meaning of this particular pregnancy experience.

BOX 4.1 The Five Steps of Evidence-based Midwifery (adapted from Page, 2000)[7]

1 Find out what is important; use open-ended questions such as, "Tell me how you feel about being pregnant."
2 Use information from the clinical examination, asking about lifestyle, nutritional status, personal and family medical history, giving evidence-based feedback on any areas of risk.
3 Describe evidence to inform decisions the woman may wish to make.
4 Talk it through with the woman and her family.
5 Reflect on outcomes, feelings and consequences.

Many providers use pre-printed forms specific to prenatal care for documenting history, physical, laboratory results, and other baseline information at this first visit. While such documentation helps with communication, risk assessment, and reminders for providers about specific protocols or guidelines, the woman-centered provider remembers to maintain a personalized tone and approach so that the woman feels in control and is not overwhelmed by the administrative needs of the forms.[7] For instance, at the point of beginning to complete the forms, the provider can state, "Part of what we need to do in this first visit is talk about and write down a lot of information about your medical and family history. This may feel tedious or repetitive. Let me know or stop me if I'm missing something important or you get confused with the order of the questions." These medically oriented forms rarely include a place for the woman's perspective beyond sometimes including a place to document items such as plans for analgesia during labor, breastfeeding, and circumcision. The woman-centered provider should see this form as a useful but limited tool, recognizing that for every stage of pregnancy there is a list of appropriate items to solicit the women's ideas and feelings, assess for problems, and plan for the future labor and postpartum period.

Mariluz's mother was raising her first child, born when Mariluz was 14 (*see* Part Three). Mariluz's doctor, Dr. Burman, had been her doctor since she was born (in fact, she was still the doctor for Mariluz's immediate and extended family). Dr. Burman cared for Mariluz in all her previous pregnancies and births and knew about her prior abusive relationship . . . After almost a year of homelessness, Mariluz finally found a place of her own and lived on her own with Rocky Junior for a year before she met Louie and had a baby with him, Louie Junior. Now pregnant for the fourth time, Mariluz had several medical issues besides her current pregnancy: poorly controlled asthma requiring frequent urgent visits, intermittent depression, ongoing heartburn, and chronic low-back pain. She needed letters to keep her electricity and phone connected as she had fallen far behind in her bills. Louie was supportive and helpful, but Mariluz vowed that this would be her last child, even if it were another boy.

The on-call doctor reassured Melissa and Kirk (*see* Parts One through Three) that they could make a first prenatal appointment with Larisa sometime in the next few weeks. They felt as if they could not wait that long but needed some time to adjust both their work schedules to fit in the prenatal appointments.

When we compare the perspectives of each of these women at the beginning of their pregnancies, we see that their providers must have flexible approaches and open attitudes towards the widely differing issues that these women bring. Mariluz, with her fourth pregnancy at a relatively young age, simply endures, feeling little of the promise or excitement that can typify some women's pregnancies. Her provider remains optimistic that this pregnancy will engage Mariluz in better self-care. Melissa embarks on the pregnancy with a radically different mindset; she experiences the delight of something long dreamed and worked for combined with the expectations of a 38-year-old accustomed to having a high level of authority and control in her life. Larisa must work with her to enjoy the process of exploring the mystery of the experience as it unfolds, assisting her in acquiring a very different set of expectations.

Mariluz's provider, Dr. Burman, with the history of an extensive and at times difficult relationship with this pregnant woman, has to balance the usefulness of the rich knowledge base about her with the burden of cynicism toward her ability to engage in prenatal care. Without exploring potential expanded life experiences and new social supports, Dr. Burman may miss an important opportunity to step back from the situation and work with Mariluz to clearly define a set of realistic goals for this final pregnancy. With multigravid women whose informational needs about pregnancy and childbirth are different from those of women having their first baby, the provider can devote more of the prenatal care time to other issues. For example, Mariluz's physician works to engage her in care for her asthma, low-back pain, heartburn, and depression in addition to her pregnancy. Dr. Burman can share with Mariluz the challenges from the provider's perspective (transportation, childcare, keeping regular appointments, taking medication regularly, and other self-care activities) while really trying to understand what might be Mariluz's primary concerns (keeping her partner engaged, having enough money to pay the bills, living with physical and psychic pain). Dr. Burman can expand the care system by referring Mariluz to counseling in order to work on her personal and family issues.

Disease-oriented goals such as establishing the best possible dating of the pregnancy and identifying any risks to the pregnancy – medical, genetic or social – often dominate the early prenatal visits. The provider must skillfully balance these goals with beginning to learn about the woman's perspective and experience thus far. Even if this pregnancy is a new "diagnosis" for an established patient, each pregnancy raises new issues to be explored. Obtaining the database that assesses the biomedical concerns, examining the woman, and ordering routine lab work are opportunities to establish a style of communication with the woman that demonstrate the provider's desire to share information and in return hear her ideas and reactions. The woman-centered provider educates the woman about basic self-care during pregnancy in the context of what the woman already practices in this area and what medical science recommends, while seeking the best balance for this individual and family. Initial visits are often longer, and may need to be more frequent than the traditional four-week span, in order to fully address the most significant issues.

Beginning with the first trimester, women have significant choices to make about prenatal care. Decisions abound, such as: where to seek care, who will attend prenatal visits, what screening tests to have, who will provide labor support, and eventually what kind of childcare to arrange. The woman quickly needs to become a decision-maker at a time where her mind may not feel as clear as before. She may feel that she is swimming in a sea of self-doubt around all the decisions; she may fear that she will be unable to meet either her own or the provider's expectations.

A woman-centered clinician needs to be adept at identifying a woman's unique strengths and abilities for such decision-making as well as the supports in the woman's own environment. Rather than having a laundry list of questions to ask or information to give about every possible issue of early pregnancy, the woman-centered clinician can target a few individualized questions based on his or her knowledge of the woman's basic context. As the history-taking, screening, and measuring occur in these early visits, the clinician begins to know the woman as a unique person.

CHAPTER 3

The Routine of Prenatal Visits

Elizabeth Naumburg and Cathleen Morrow

From the first prenatal visit, one of the woman-centered provider's responsibilities in defining the birth plan is to share plans for the typical structure of prenatal care. The provider informs the woman that visits typically occur with a specified frequency that changes and increases as the pregnancy progresses. Having learned something about the woman's pregnancy experience so far, the woman-centered provider then elicits the woman's ideas about this plan: Does this frequency make sense to the woman in question? Might she actually require more or less frequent visits? Will the woman have trouble complying with the routine? Are transportation or work or family commitments likely to be a barrier? From the beginning, in establishing these issues as part of the overarching birth plan, the woman-centered provider sets the framework that this kind of information is relevant and may save misunderstandings in the future.

The other task in defining the birth plan beginning with the initial prenatal visits is for the provider to share his or her thoughts about what is best and what is acceptable based on medical knowledge, community standards, and what the provider feels comfortable with. Larisa, for instance, chooses to write down some of her philosophy to give to women with other written prenatal materials at an early visit.

> I am a family physician. I see pregnancy and childbirth as a normal body process that most often needs no medical intervention. I see my role as supporting you in caring for yourself and empowering you through this process. Together we will be aware of and look for potential problems that can arise. Usually, I share the prenatal care of women with a nurse practitioner. If there are no unforeseen problems and I am not out of town or on vacation, I will be present for your birth. I share care with a group of family physicians who have a very similar practice philosophy. If there are medical issues that arise, I may need to consult with an obstetrician, as I do not do cesarean sections or manage complex problems without help. I attend births at the local community hospital. I would be happy to continue to care for you after your delivery and also become your new child's doctor if you have not already selected one. I look forward to working with you to help you accomplish a safe and satisfying birth experience.

This statement may provide the first opportunity to clarify whether there is basic compatibility between the provider and the woman. The pregnant woman may not be familiar with the different providers available to attend births; she may not know about hospital or birth center affiliations; she may want a home birth or a more technically oriented model.

> Kerry (*see* Part Two) came for her prenatal visit at 12 weeks, finally feeling better after her hospitalization. Larisa acknowledged first, "I'm so glad to see you are well enough now to be seeing me in the office," then said, "I have a few things I'd like to discuss today but, first, do you have any questions for me?" Kerry wondered how her weight was and whether she really still needed to try to take the prenatal vitamins that made her nausea worse. Larisa reviewed her weight gain and her normal hemoglobin results, and asked Kerry to lie back on the exam table to listen for the heartbeat while saying, "Your weight has stabilized so I am hopeful that you are past the worst of the nausea and vomiting now. You are not anemic, which is great, but let's talk more about your nutrition needs now so that we can decide together if you need to take the vitamins still." Kerry described what she had been able to eat over the last week, and Larisa showed her an easy-to-read pamphlet that summarized the expected needs for iron, protein, and other nutrients at this point in pregnancy. She mentioned that some women tolerate a chewable vitamin without iron better, and suggested that Kerry try this until she was tolerating a more regular diet.

After the first one or two often longer prenatal visits, the monthly ritual of the visits themselves can be a source of comfort and predictability. A typical sequence to find common ground at each of these routine visits includes first inquiring about and exploring the woman's current state, addressing any questions or concerns that the woman may have, reviewing labs that have been obtained in the interim, introducing topics for discussion based on the trimester, examining the woman's abdomen, listening for fetal heart tones, clarifying medical recommendations appropriate to the trimester, coming to agreement about roles and plans for the woman or provider to carry out, and planning for the next visit.

The woman-centered provider can further express his or her desire for partnership by encouraging the woman to come with a written list of questions or concerns that have come up since the last visit. Inviting the presence of the father of the baby or any significant support person, especially if the woman wishes to have that person present at delivery, can shift the experience to a more personal and less medical one. Engaging children in the process by having them help to listen to fetal heart tones and hearing their excitement about the new baby can further integrate the family into care. However, with some women and couples (like Melissa and Kirk), forging a partnership in the presence of uncertainty is difficult.

> Each visit was longer than average, as Melissa and Kirk found the waits and unpredictable part of pregnancy very problematic and always had long lists of questions and concerns. Larisa felt frustrated with their need for certainty and schedules, and tried to explain that this was just the beginning of unpredictability in their lives, but they did not hear that.

The challenge of finding common ground during Melissa's prenatal care includes clarifying the problem, goals, and roles (*see* Table 4.1). Their provider needs to see clearly that pregnancy is unlike any experience that Melissa and Kirk have ever encountered before and that they will need a new and different set of skills to negotiate this life phase. With this understanding, Larisa can redefine the work that needs to be done with the couple. Being explicit, repeatedly, about the inherent limits of knowledge and control in this life process and on into parenthood, the provider can emphasize the benefits of adapting to this experience by embracing an attitude of limited expectations. For example, Larisa comments, "There are a lot more uncertainties about prenatal care than people often realize. What do you think will help you cope with this?" Interventions include being explicit about what time the provider will have for them in a given visit ("Today we have 15 minutes; what would you like to focus on?") and the possibility of scheduling more frequent visits ("If this does not feel like enough time, we can follow up sooner."). Larisa can try to describe possible responses to particular situations and thus explore in a hypothetical way Melissa and Kirk's decision-making processes. Deliberately assigning Melissa and Kirk to seek further information through reading or the Internet promotes the self-learning that they already embrace and may in fact be therapeutic.[8,9] They may benefit most from prenatal classes or other resources that not only contain cognitive content but that also work on experiencing life as process rather than focusing on mastery. Prenatal yoga and other strategies for meditation and relaxation may be especially helpful.

Finally, sharing Melissa's care with another provider or a team that includes nurses or childbirth educators may help the primary provider cope.

TABLE 4.1 Clarifying Problems, Goals and Roles around Prenatal Care

Issue	Melissa	Dr. Larisa Foster
Problems	Long waits; unpredictability of experience; heightened anxiety about tests and symptoms; lack of control.	Long visits, repeated explanations.
Goals	Shorter waits, more predictability, reassurance, coping strategies, preparation for parenting.	Shorter visits that still satisfy, resources to teach coping strategies.
Roles	Information-gatherer, finding alternate resources, student/learner.	Linkages to alternate resources, linking to consultants if needed.

> At the 10-week visit, Melissa and Kirk, having researched the issues extensively, were ready to talk about having first-trimester screening. Larisa referred them to the local perinatal center for this testing, and a week later Melissa and Kirk were back in Larisa's office to discuss the abnormal results. They were panicking about the possibility of Down syndrome; Melissa was tearful while Kirk was trying to keep a stiff upper lip.

Addressing the loss of control during pregnancy with a woman with a high need for control means helping her from the beginning to develop a flexible stance, learning what she can control and what she cannot, and what the options might be at any moment. Women and their partners may explore many strategies to gain more control over what is happening; for Melissa and Kirk this exploration includes an insistence on first-trimester genetic screening. They are unprepared for the abnormal results. Without demeaning their anxieties, Larisa reminds Melissa and Kirk, "These kinds of test results can be very scary for parents. While we talk through what they may or may not mean, let's remember that pregnancy is just the beginning of the many uncertainties involved in bearing and raising children." Thus, Larisa responds to Melissa's request about early-trimester screening first by acknowledging openly both her self-directed learning and her likely anxiety after her carefully planned pregnancy. Larisa can also recognize Melissa's self-doubt and her obvious close partnership with Kirk in decision-making. Further suggestions for her provider about the specific issues of genetic screening will be discussed further in Part Five, Prevention and Health Promotion.

Learning when to let be, to let things unfold, to go with the flow, and when to make decisions and push for options are part of the woman's task of incorporating pregnancy into her expectations. Building on this understanding from the first stage of pregnancy helps women prepare for later changes as well.

Group prenatal visits are a strategy of care that strengthens women through connections with other pregnant women, shared experiences, and collective knowledge, thus promoting many of the concepts of finding common ground. A woman who has attended group visits can identify how she wants her care to be conducted; she can ask for what she wants. Thus, group prenatal care actualizes the core principles of finding common ground, shared decision-making, and empowerment. Providers accustomed to traditional individual prenatal visits may resist what they see as relinquishing some of the powerful connections of continuity with individual women, but given the satisfaction ratings of women who have gone through group care, a truly woman-centered provider remains open to this model's potential benefits. Part Five discusses this model of care in full detail.

CHAPTER 4

Due Dates and the Illusion of Control

Elizabeth Naumburg and Cathleen Morrow

Detailed planning for labor, delivery and the postpartum period can create an illusion of control that contrasts with the inherent unpredictability of how events actually unfold. Helping women appreciate that pregnancy and birth are both very defined in general but highly variable and unpredictable on an individual basis is a key element in finding common ground.

> Siobhan (*see* Parts Two and Three) never returned for her postpartum visit after her first child was born. She had irregular bleeding in the first few months. She and her partner Danny continued to use condoms for contraception as they had done for many years. Their son, Danny Jr., had enough health issues in the first months of life to need hospitalization a couple of times. In addition, Danny's mother became very ill and was in a coma for several weeks. Siobhan had been overweight before getting pregnant. After delivering she lost some weight, but soon began to gain again. She was too busy with family responsibilities to think much about this. When Danny Jr. turned nine months old, Siobhan realized that she could no longer attribute her abdominal sensations to gas – she was pregnant again and had been feeling fetal movement for some time. She had been responsible as a teenager, avoiding pregnancy, alcohol, and drugs, but in these past months, she had been spending so much energy on caring for her baby and mother-in-law. She was embarrassed to be pregnant again and did not want to return to her prior physicians.

It took another month before she worked herself up to call a new doctor to establish care. She first called an office recommended by a friend, but was told that they would not accept her as a patient because she had waited so long. This added to the guilt she was already feeling. She called the community health center and was relieved to speak with an understanding staff member who scheduled an appointment with a physician the next week. The day after her first prenatal appointment, her ultrasound indicated that she was further along in pregnancy than she or her doctor had thought – she had already completed 34 weeks of pregnancy. Danny accompanied Siobhan to the visit after the ultrasound. . . . The new doctor, Dr. Miller, explained to them that with dating this far into pregnancy, the due date could be off by a few weeks either way, so they would wait for her to go into labor naturally. She began weekly visits.

At the 37-week visit, they questioned Dr. Miller carefully about the anticipated due date, since they were going to have to arrange for Danny's out-of-town brother to help care for Danny's sick mother and for Danny Jr. when Siobhan went into labor.

The concept of the due date is a good example of this challenging issue. A due date is an estimate based on an idealized model of menstrual cycle, conception, and duration of gestation. When and how the due date is determined affects its accuracy. Even for women with precisely known conception dates, such as Melissa, the exact date of delivery remains uncertain. In an otherwise normal pregnancy, delivery any time two weeks before or two weeks after that estimated date is normal. Providers cannot accurately predict when a given woman will go into labor. Nonetheless, a due date has power for both the woman and the provider. For the woman the due date becomes a focus for her life for the next many months, or as in Siobhan's case, for the next few weeks. How she relates to the reliability of that date is emblematic of how she will relate to the entire unpredictable process of giving birth and beyond into parenting. For the provider the due date is a key point of time in the care of a pregnant woman that determines the timing of every other medical decision. Yet both individuals must keep in mind that it is an estimate.

CHAPTER 5

Addressing Common Symptoms in Pregnancy

Sara G. Shields

Providers need to inquire about common symptoms throughout pregnancy and while taking them seriously, normalize the typical changes – in the early stages, growing and tender breasts, increased frequency of urination, and fatigue; later in pregnancy, back discomfort, leg swelling, and heartburn. The clinician learns how this woman relates to her body by assessing the woman's reactions to these ordinary changes, which may range from ignoring or minimizing them, to anxiety about their meaning, to frustration with the initial experience of losing control over one's body. The woman-centered provider listens to these responses, acknowledges the particular impact on the individual woman's life, and supports her coping strategies while suggesting others.

> Susan (*see* Parts Two and Three) early in her pregnancy felt well enough to keep up her exercise regimen, but by about seven weeks started having more morning nausea. She kept a sports drink and crackers next to her bed to have before she got up, but most days still ended up vomiting after any more breakfast. She tried ginger tea and acupressure bands in hopes of feeling better.

Nausea can be one of the most debilitating complications of early pregnancy and can be potentially serious if persistent vomiting is also present. Willingness on the part of the woman to adapt her life to the needs of her body will be an ongoing part of the pregnancy experience. The provider can support a woman in finding workable solutions for increased rest, a more planned diet, and other interventions as needed. Part of this support includes specifically inquiring about fears about the meaning of nausea and vomiting to the well-being of the developing fetus or about the woman's ability to cope with the demands of pregnancy. Preference for and acceptance of complementary treatments such as acupressure bands and herbal teas versus interest in pharmacological solutions such as pyridoxine plus doxylamine will be areas for discussion and reveal the attitudes of the woman and her partner towards medical issues.

> Once past the first-trimester nausea, Susan felt much stronger and more comfortable, but then in her early third trimester started noticing that she felt short of breath more quickly. Judith asked both about potential danger signs such as chest pain or leg swelling, and also framed the evaluation within knowledge of Susan's experience. Judith knew that Susan was an athlete for whom physical endurance was especially important and who was not expecting to feel physically challenged by the changes of pregnancy. Susan worried that her breathing symptoms meant that her physical stamina would take longer to return after pregnancy. Knowing this, Judith was able to address her frustrations and fears directly: "You sound frustrated by not being able to do as much as you would like to or are used to, because you get short of breath. Are you worried that this means something more serious or more permanent than this current stage of pregnancy?"
>
> Judith also further described the problem by sharing more information about how she thought through possible diagnoses. "Certainly when women have trouble breathing during pregnancy, I think about both common issues such as the ways that pregnancy hormones change your breathing patterns or how the growth of your uterus makes it harder to take a deep breath. I also think about serious illnesses such as pneumonia, asthma, a heart problem, or a blood clot. At this point, based on what you are telling me about other related symptoms, my sense is that your breathing symptoms are related to the normal changes of pregnancy."

Part of seeking common ground requires avoidance of medical jargon and encouragement of the woman to ask questions when she does not understand technical language or the way that the clinician has defined the problem. Judith can ask questions such as "What have you done so far that has helped?" or "Was there anything else about this symptom that you had been worrying about?" Once Susan and Judith have defined the problem, the next stage of finding common ground is defining goals. For example, Judith can say, "Let's think about how we can work together to help you with these symptoms." Susan may want either reassurance that nothing is wrong, or guidance about what to pay attention to as more concerning symptoms, or she may want to know what else she can do during pregnancy to stay fit.

> Toward the end of this pregnancy Mariluz began having severe pain in her back on walking and found it difficult to manage her small children at home. She seemed demanding in a passive kind of way, sitting without apparent inclination to end the visit until something was decided. Using a cane and taking pain medications had not really relieved the situation. She could not bear to think she had four more weeks to go. "I can't sit, I can't stand, I can't clean my house, I can't do my kids. It just hurts ALL THE TIME," she blurted in tears.
>
> "Oh, Mariluz, you are hurting so much!" responded Dr. Burman, hearing finally

how much Mariluz's back pain was restricting her life. At this point, Dr. Burman offered the option of inducing the birth when the pregnancy reached 38 weeks, discussing the minimal risks of lung problems for the baby and the likely success of induction. Mariluz finally felt attended to and was able to go through the next 10 days of the pregnancy without any extra visits.

The experienced practitioner listens to the woman's experience, discusses the medical alternatives, and empowers the woman to make informed decisions about her care alternatives.

Addressing Specific Medical Issues: Ultrasounds, Gestational Diabetes, Smoking, Nutrition

Sara G. Shields

As prenatal care unfolds there are specific medical issues that will need discussion, some of them quite early on in pregnancy. Some common issues include use, timing, and frequency of ultrasounds; testing for and care of women with gestational diabetes; smoking cessation, and nutrition issues.

A few months after her miscarriage, Pat's home pregnancy test was positive (*see* Part Two). She and Mike were both delighted and terrified. They decided not to tell anyone right away, but called their primary provider, Dr. Miller, begging for an ultrasound as soon as possible to be able to see if the baby was okay.

Mariana was a 30-year-old Brazilian immigrant (*see* Parts Two and Three). She was the youngest child of four and the only daughter. She had been married for two years to Roberto and finally became pregnant. Her mother-in-law was able to visit from Brazil during her pregnancy and accompanied her to several of her prenatal visits. She had no medical risks and was having a medically uncomplicated pregnancy, but was quite anxious about the body changes, particularly around weight gain and stretch marks. Both she and her mother-in-law asked at every early visit about when she could have an ultrasound to know the baby's sex.

Ultrasounds, even two of them if dating is uncertain, have become a standard part of modern medical care internationally, even though the evidence for their positive contribution to perinatal outcomes is lacking.[10-12] Women often request an ultrasound only to determine the sex of their baby, with commercial enterprises available to provide that service in some communities. Early on in prenatal care, Mariana's provider needs to address the indications for ultrasound and practical issues such as cost and insurance coverage, acknowledging the possibility of the request for gender determination and the options in her community for obtaining an ultrasound that is not medically indicated. "A lot of parents ask about getting an ultrasound to know if the baby is a boy or a girl. Your particular insurance will not pay for an ultrasound just for that reason. There is a company in the next town that will do such an ultrasound for a fee. The other option is to wait, because sometimes a different reason for doing an ultrasound comes up that will make us get one later on in your pregnancy anyway." Keeping this discussion open-ended helps establish important rapport about the issue and counters frequent requests for repeat ultrasounds.

> Felicity, whom we met in Parts One through Three, was having what she thought was a routine ultrasound. Seeing the technician's solemn face, Felicity felt her heart sink, and asked worriedly, "What's wrong?" but the sonographer replied only, "I need to talk to the doctor who can then talk with you." Rafael, not having been with Felicity for their daughter's ultrasound, was puzzled, thinking this was the routine, but Felicity said, "This didn't happen before," and gripped his hand nervously while they waited. Finally, the ultrasound doctor arrived and told them that the fetus appeared to have a "space in the heart," which was sometimes a marker for Down syndrome. She mentioned the term, "echogenic cardiac focus."

As noted in Part Two, woman-centered care with ultrasound in pregnancy also means remaining cautious about the possibility of incidental and ultimately insignificant "abnormal" findings.[13,14] At the time of referring Felicity for what seems like a "routine" ultrasound, her provider Harmony can remind her of the imperfect nature of ultrasound screening. "Ultrasound feels like fun for many women and families because they get to see the baby, but we have learned that sometimes we see things that may look unusual to us but that do not have any long-term clinical meaning. If this happens to you, with the ultrasound person saying something is not normal, you may feel scared and worried and have a hard time concentrating on anything else right then. I'll try to be available to talk with you as soon as I can about any such findings so we can make a plan." Having had this conversation ahead of time, Harmony can then respond more fully to Felicity's needs when an unexpected finding does occur. Similarly, the reassuring power of a normal ultrasound cannot be overlooked, particularly for a woman like Pat who has experienced some common yet worrisome early pregnancy symptoms such as spotting.

Jackie's first three children were born 8, 10 and 12 years ago (*see* Parts Two and Three). She became pregnant unexpectedly from a brief reconciliation with her children's father, but they were not in a relationship any longer. She was a foster mother for three other children and was very active in her church. She also worked part-time as a nurses' aide. Her mother had diabetes and her father had hypertension and had had a stroke at 55 years old. Jackie was very overweight (body mass index [BMI] of 40) and had a lot of back pain even when she was not pregnant. So far she had not had diabetes or hypertension diagnosed herself, but she had severe fatty food intolerance but had been avoiding getting a gallbladder ultrasound, as she was afraid of surgery. Although she took her children to her family doctor, Judith Peters, for regularly scheduled appointments, she avoided care for herself. Jackie entered care at four months of pregnancy.

At 28 weeks, Jackie had a one-hour glucola challenge of 160 mg/dl (8.9 mmol/l) but postponed the glucose tolerance test (GTT) for two weeks, which, when she finally was able to come in fasting, showed all four values to be abnormal, giving her the diagnosis of gestational diabetes (GDM). Judith talked with her about the implications both for her and for the baby. Jackie took diabetes very seriously because of her mother's history and committed herself to following a strict diet, something she had never done before, even though this meant preparing separate meals for herself from those for her children, which was difficult to do given her work schedule. She picked up her prescription for a glucometer, and saw the diabetes nurse educator and the dietician at the hospital. At first her blood sugars remained high, and Judith worried aloud that she might need to start insulin and be transferred to a specialist. Hearing that, Jackie tried harder to deal with portion sizes and snacks, and within the next week proudly showed Judith her more normal blood sugar numbers. She admitted with frustration that the strictness of the diet was really difficult. Given her continued intermittent abdominal pain, Jackie wanted to stop checking her blood sugar so many times a day because now even her fingers were hurting.

Finding common ground for the care of medical issues during pregnancy again involves clear communication around the problem, the goals that both the woman and her provider have, and the roles that each takes in the treatment plan. For Jackie, woman-centered care also addresses the stigma that obese women face in medical care in general and pregnancy care in particular (*see* Part One). Judith needs to frame the care plan for her diabetes within the context of her other symptoms (abdominal pain) and concerns (work and family demands). Ultimately, the tenets of woman-centered care – assessing Jackie's experience within her context, as addressed in Part Two, and incorporating principles of lifelong health promotion, discussed further in Part Five – are key to devising a mutually agreeable prenatal program for Jackie and Judith (*see* Table 4.2).

TABLE 4.2 Clarifying Problems, Goals, and Roles around Medical Issues

Issues	Jackie	Dr. Judith Peters
Problem	Diet is hard; fingersticks hurt; other symptoms bother her more than diabetes symptoms; not used to caring for herself first; defensive about pre-existing obesity.	Concerns about risks of GDM given pre-pregnancy obesity; concerns about Jackie's ability to prioritize her own care and keep weekly appointments.
Goals	Avoid diabetes complications for baby and herself; avoid consultant care; address relief for other symptoms; fit diabetes monitoring into work and diet needs into family life.	Assess diabetes control; use consultation according to guidelines; engage Jackie in care plan with more frequent visits; use time wisely; avoid macrosomia.
Roles	Engage family in helping her with diet – kids can play with educational DVD (*see* Part Five); ask employer for shorter more frequent breaks to eat smaller but more frequent amounts; keep appointments.	Nutrition counseling and referral if needed; alternate educational strategies that fit Jackie's busy life (e.g. DVD for GDM, or phone/email review of blood sugars); rethink GDM monitoring needs for lifestyle; stay abreast of current medical literature and evidence-based care for GDM.

Another common area of challenge for pregnant women and providers in finding common ground relates to changing health behavior around smoking and nutrition. As with all attempts to collaborate in care, the woman-centered clinician needs to ascertain how the woman wants to be involved in her care plan, how realistic the woman's goals are, and what her coping capacity is. During this process of engaging the woman with informed decision-making, the clinician's role is to present the pros, cons, and uncertainties of each alternative, and to ascertain how well the woman understands her choices. As with Dr. Miller and Tonya below, if the woman does not seem to understand or want to engage with the issue, the provider remains flexible in just how to ask questions, and tries different approaches that openly acknowledge underlying feelings.

> Dr. Miller recognized how distrustful Tonya felt toward providers when they brought up the smoking issue in previous pregnancies (*see* Part One). He decided to take on the issue of trust directly. "Look, I know it must be hard to have to switch to a new provider, and I know doctors nag a lot about cigarettes, so it's no surprise to me that you might find it hard to trust me. I will try hard to earn your trust and to be here for you. What kinds of things are important to you in your prenatal care?"
>
> This was the first time anyone had ever asked Tonya this question, and she was astounded. "What do I care about? Me? Well, for one thing, I hate waiting. I want to get in, get checked, and get out. No sitting around waiting for hours. That's what's important for me."
>
> Dr. Miller said he would make that his first priority and, after the visit, made a notation for Tonya to have the first prenatal slot each month so that she would have the least likelihood of waiting. She came promptly for all her visits and by seven months was measurably more open toward him.
>
> "I've been thinking about what you said – about the smoking."

"Yes?"

"Well, my other kids are nagging me and my boyfriend wants me to stop, too, so I have been thinking about it."

"Would you like some help with that?"

"Yeah, do you have some ideas for me?"

Dr. Miller reviewed some of the specific behavior changes that Tonya could do to decrease her smoking, and Tonya thought a few of them might be worth trying. She said she would make some attempts before the next visit.

Other questions to ask in eliciting the woman's ideas about goals of a treatment plan include: "Can you think of ways this might be a hard plan to follow? What else can we do to make this plan easier for you? Would you like more time to think over this plan or to talk about it with others?"

Samantha the teenager (*see* Parts Two and Three) had help from the school nurse to transfer her care to Dr. Epps at the community health center. Rushing to catch the bus to get to the after-school appointments not too late, Samantha usually stopped to grab a value meal at the local fast-food place. At one visit, the school nurse saw her finishing French fries and sipping the soda and asked about her meal habits. Samantha admitted that she usually skipped breakfast although had been trying to at least drink some juice on the way to school; she had a hard time remembering to take her prenatal vitamins. The nurse called Dr. Epps to discuss Samantha's weight gain (only 10 pounds by 30 weeks) and nutrition habits. At the next visit, Dr. Epps, while reviewing Samantha's prenatal flow chart and measuring her fundus, asked about her favorite foods, her understanding of prenatal nutrition, and her access to food coupon programs or food stamps. Samantha had not had time to do the paperwork for those programs but was interested in them. She agreed to try to eat a piece of fruit and drink one small glass of milk each morning when she was helping Alice feed her cousins. She asked for chewable vitamins.

Teens may be particularly pleased to feel the inherent respect of a provider who seeks common ground with them rather than telling them authoritatively what to do.

CHAPTER 7

Alternative Models of Care

Elizabeth Naumburg and Cathleen Morrow

In North America, most women give birth in a hospital setting.[15] Elsewhere in the developed world, however, home birth is more common and recognized as a safe option for low-risk women.[16-18]

As we saw in Part Two, Ruth and Lewis are planning a home birth.

> All the grandparents supported their decision. Their provider, Judith, an advocate of low intervention in the hospital setting, supported their overall plan but worried about the negative experience they might undergo if Ruth needed to be transferred to the hospital in labor, or if the baby required hospitalization. Judith also worried that the hospital specialists would be critical of her for "allowing" her patients to plan a home birth. Ruth had an uncomplicated pregnancy, delivered a healthy baby at home with no complications except a second-degree perineal tear that the midwife repaired, and had an uneventful recovery. Ruth breastfed for 18 months, then she and Lewis decided to have a second pregnancy with the same plan.

This part focuses on the birth planning process for the conventional location for birth in the developed world, the hospital. Whether a traditional labor and delivery "ward," a single birthing suite within the hospital, or a larger unit existing within the walls of a hospital but designed to separate the family from the more disease-oriented work of a hospital, these locations comprise the place of delivery for the vast majority of families in the developed world. Providers, will, however, encounter families who desire to deliver their children in a different environment, such as at home, or at free-standing birth centers. Local custom, cultures, and the availability of alternative sites will significantly affect the type of requests that a provider may encounter.

Mainstream providers often have strong feelings about medical safety in alternative environments; such feelings may color their ability to provide unbiased advice and recommendations. Some providers believe, for example, that home birth is not safe and will simply state this as medical fact. A woman-centered approach recognizes that obstetrical authorities have exaggerated the purported dangers of home birth and minimized or not recognized the risks of hospital births.[19-21] Open, non-judgmental discussion with the woman and her support network to understand and clarify the reasons for her choices will often reveal the best way to address her specific needs. Sometimes a written document clarifying the provider's and woman's expectations around home or hospital birth may be helpful. (*See* Sidebar: "Home Birth Waiver.")

> Judith explained that because of hospital politics she would be unable to take care of Ruth if she were to develop complications and needed to come to the hospital in an emergency situation in labor. Ruth and Lewis clearly articulated that what they wanted from Judith was appropriate prenatal screening blood work initially and at 28 weeks, and physical exams, including a late-pregnancy exam to be sure all was normal and a Group B Streptococcus screening at 36 weeks. Both parties agreed that they could live with this care plan.

Whether the initial provider ultimately delivers full perinatal care or not, the process of helping a family to clarify their values, fears, and hopes for their pregnancy and delivery retains the potential for a future working relationship. A provider who feels strongly opposed to an alternative (e.g. home birth) should, at a minimum, acknowledge his or her bias and offer referral to colleagues or resources more open to discussion of alternatives.

The Sidebar "Home Birth Waiver" provides an example of a written "contract" about physician backup for home birth.

Sample Home Birth Waiver

We recognize that some women, when faced with choosing a setting and provider for care during pregnancy, choose home birth with a lay or certified midwife. Unfortunately, a woman who chooses a home birth sometimes feels excluded by the medical community for making that choice. This can cause her to be reluctant to seek out medical care when it is needed and cause her to delay getting help. We want to avoid this if at all possible, and we want all women to have easy access to quality medical care in the office or hospital, if and when they request it.

We encourage a woman anticipating home birth to schedule a "get-acquainted" visit with one of our physicians early in her pregnancy. At that visit we can become acquainted, clarify expectations, and answer any questions a woman may have about our "standby" role. We will not review your medical record or perform a physical examination since it is not our intent to advise or persuade you regarding the place you choose for birth. This is your choice.

I have weighed the relative risks and benefits of hospital versus home birth for myself, and have chosen home birth. I do not hold (practice name) responsible for my prenatal care or birth at home, but do want to have ready access to office or hospital care when I request it. I have read this waiver for home birth, and have had the opportunity to have my questions answered.

Signature of woman and provider: _____

CHAPTER 1

Planning for Labor

Elizabeth Naumburg and Cathleen Morrow

As discussions of the specific plans for labor unfold in the third trimester, the provider must balance the potential problems of labor with the opportunities for de-medicalizing birth and creating a uniquely satisfying experience. Typically, childbirth classes, concentrated in late second and third trimesters, offer ongoing specific information and provoke discussion between the clinician and the woman about common practices and potential interventions. Some women want a detailed discussion of every aspect of labor: who will be there, what will they wear, how will they move or be positioned, when will monitoring be used, what will the lighting be like, what facilities are available for showers or baths and what supports for labor might be available. The woman-centered provider can best care for well-informed women who are focused on the details of birth by scheduling one longer visit to address these issues. Reviewing the woman's idealized birth plan in writing prior to this visit can facilitate moving the discussion to assessing her flexibility, establishing her most important priorities, and reiterating the themes of control and uncertainty. Particularly for a woman approaching her first delivery, the provider's role becomes helping her and her support people to appreciate how the power of the process takes over.

> At Siobhan's 39 week visit, Dr. Miller finally had time to talk some about her prior labor experience. Siobhan remembered her first labor as long and tiring, with

painful prodromal contractions for about two days and several frustrating visits to the hospital with intense discomfort but no cervical change. She had not had any specific birth plan and was never asked about that. When she finally entered active labor she felt quickly overwhelmed and asked for an epidural, which had to be placed twice and gave her only partial relief. She had found pushing particularly uncomfortable and remembered having yelled grouchily at her nurse and other people in the room. She had not met the doctor who delivered her baby, and felt no connection to him. She had not been able to hold her son immediately because of meconium. She commented to Dr. Miller, "Wow, I hope it doesn't take as long this time. I really was tired. I pushed forever."

Woman-centered care for women who have previously given birth necessitates inquiring about the woman's own prior experiences with labor, as well as those of other women close to her. When listening to the woman's story about previous births, the provider stays particularly attentive to negative past experiences and fears, even if the provider was the woman's attendant at that time. Candid exploration of such feelings can be a healthy and constructive step toward a positive outcome for the upcoming labor.

Dr. Miller responded to Siobhan, "It sounds like it was a tough first birth for you. Second births may not take as long because your body has been through this before. What do you think would help you with this labor? Other than how long it took before, is there anything else you would like to be different?"

CHAPTER 2

Anticipation and Expectation

Elizabeth Naumburg and Cathleen Morrow

Kerry and Ron began childbirth classes weekly for a month starting at 34 weeks and enjoyed meeting some of the other couples also expecting their first baby. Before the class was over, one of the women had already delivered and brought the baby to the last class. Kerry was still noticing some nausea at this point but mostly just felt big and bloated, and while holding this other newborn was all the more eager and anxious to give birth herself. She and Ron received almost daily phone calls from the rest of their family inquiring about her symptoms, but she had had no signs of labor as her due date approached. At her 40-week visit, Kerry's mother came along. She was particularly nervous about how much longer until the baby arrived. Larisa acknowledged Kerry's mother's upcoming change in status as a new grandmother and her concern for her daughter and reassured everyone that Kerry was already a bit dilated and that the baby was healthy. They discussed the plan for monitoring her over the next one to two weeks.

Samantha started to have painful regular contractions near term, but without cervical change. She called the on-call service and the office several times and came in for several labor evaluations. At each one, the provider (who was a different provider each time) told her that this was not truly labor yet and that she did not need to be admitted to the hospital yet. Samantha was frustrated to be sent home several times when her discomfort was so intense.

The anticipation of birth can be one of the more delightful, fruitful, and genuinely connected times in a woman's and her partner's life. It can also be one of the most exasperating, uncomfortable, and anxiety-provoking periods of time in the same couple's existence. The experienced practitioner anticipates this mixture of emotions and provides specific gentle guidance, covering topics such as signs of early labor, reasons for a call to the provider or the labor and delivery suite of the hospital, and reasons to proceed to the hospital or birthing center. The discussion of how and when to contact the provider about possible labor includes reviewing the woman's thoughts about her comfort in staying at home and the risks of coming to the hospital "too soon" compared with anxiety about arriving "too late."

For both women and providers at this time, the all-important question, "Is this labor?" looms large. Helping a woman appreciate that most women with their first delivery experience some degree of latent phase labor is critical anticipatory guidance. The provider can use reassuring, positive language to empathize and allay fear and anxiety. Focus on cervical dilatation alone can be a disservice if the woman becomes discouraged about lack of dilation. The woman-centered provider with every vaginal exam discusses what Simkin calls the Six Ways to Progress: cervical movement from posterior to anterior, cervical softening, cervical effacement, cervical dilation, fetal rotation, and fetal descent.[22] In early labor when dilation seems slow, focusing only on centimeters of dilation can undermine a woman's confidence. For a woman experiencing contractions that feel as intense and strong as what she has expected for active labor, the disappointment of not being further dilated may overwhelm her coping. After acknowledging and letting her express this discouragement, the provider's task here is to "help her get her head back to where her cervix is."[22:91] Finding common ground through this frustrating time includes assessing the woman's feelings and expectations, and encouraging her with distracting activities, education about the normalcy of slow early labor, adequate hydration and rest, and comfort measures.[22:89]

Samantha came into the office for a labor check with Dr. Epps the next day after a midnight labor check at the hospital. Her cervix was now 1.5 cm and 90% effaced and anterior with the vertex at 0 station. Clearly frustrated, Samantha burst out, "I thought I'd be in labor this time. How long is this going to last? What's wrong that it's taking so long? How do I know when I'm really in labor if this already hurts so much?"

Her provider responded, "You must be exhausted. Being up all night and going back and forth with no sleep! But guess what? You really are making progress. I know hearing 1.5 cm again sounds discouraging, but compared to last night, your cervix is all thinned out. Last night it was thick as a winter coat, and now it is as thin as your sweater. And, remember how we had to reach way in the back to get to it? Now it is all the way up front with the baby's head lower. So this is REAL PROGRESS. Your body is doing some great preparation that is going to make it much easier when you get to the hospital. I am really pleased with how well this is going."

"Really? I'm so wiped out. And it feels like it will never end."

"Some of that discouragement is from feeling exhausted. Who's at home today who can help you? Let's think together about things you can do to get some rest, and who can help you with that. Your baby's doing wonderfully. Everything is going in a very good direction."

Though anticipated in the prenatal period, many women are initially overwhelmed by the early hours of labor. Experiencing the intensity of contractions, getting used to the physical environment of the labor and delivery unit, settling into a rhythm with a support person, coach, or doula, and contending with new people (nurses, shift changes, residents) all can be quite overwhelming. The familiar face of a trusted provider can be a powerful calming force even if labor is just getting under way, especially if accompanied by discussion about mutual goals and plans. Reminding the woman that this is the work she has been planning for and keeping an eye on the goal of a healthy baby are key. Reassurance about normal fetal assessment, discussions of progress, and encouragement to stay active and moving in this early stage may all be indicated.

In addition, the woman-centered provider reminds a woman and her family of the typical duration of a first labor, despite what is depicted in the media, and with that encourages more realistic expectations. The very real experiences of sleeplessness, nervousness, excitement, and physical fatigue, from the bulk of late-term pregnancy and frequent nocturnal awakenings as well as insomnia, can conspire to exhaust a woman at the end of pregnancy. Planned frequent visits, sleep agents if needed, and cervical exams can all help to reassure and allay anxieties. Educating families about the inherent risk in staying at the hospital or birth center before active labor is established can be very valuable.[23-5] While some women may find it reassuring to remain in the hospital before the onset of active labor, doing so may not be in anyone's best interest.

Because of cultural or family reasons, other women may hesitate to call about symptoms, such as leaking fluid, or wait until labor is in full force and arrive at the delivery site in an advanced stage. Such late arrival may preclude use of medical interventions typical in some settings, such as treatment of known Group B Streptococcus infection, or even the provider's ability to get there in time, or the participation of other desired support people. The decision to admit for observation, admit for active labor, or discharge to home depends on knowing well the woman's circumstances including transportation, finances, support people, distance from facility, care for other children at home, and arrangements for childcare. Having ongoing discussions about the timing of transition to the birthing site will improve but not guarantee a smoother process.

CHAPTER 3

Labor for Survivors

Cathy Kamens and Ambareen A. Bharmal

Larisa encouraged Melissa and Kirk to think about ways that he could help her feel safe during labor. Larisa asked them to write down some ideas about how Melissa envisioned labor, how those around her could be helpful to her, and how she might cope if things did not go according to plan. Kirk focused again on worst-case scenarios but from the perspective of having Melissa think through how he could help her through such possibilities.

After Jen (*see* Part Three) told Larisa about the rape that resulted in her pregnancy, they talked more about how Jen could handle labor and who she wanted to support her in this. Jen admitted that every vaginal exam was excruciating for her. They discussed that she would need some further vaginal exams once labor truly started, but that Larisa or other providers would try to minimize these. Jen asked about getting an epidural earlier rather than later in labor since she imagined that not being able to feel the exams would help her immensely.

As we discussed briefly in Part Three, planning for labor is especially critical for survivors of sexual abuse or rape, like Melissa and Jen. Prenatal care for each woman should include a discussion regarding the course of labor in a way that normalizes her fear and anxiety and, in turn, empowers her to control what she can and trust her body through the process. Since control is such an important issue for women who have survived abuse, giving them as many options as possible in determining their own care can help alleviate some anxiety over losing control, while also clearly defining that in certain circumstances or emergency situations, the provider may not be able to offer choices. Permitting a previously abused woman to demand explanations for procedures or other aspects of her care plan is a way to empower her and allow her some control in labor. A realistic, written birth plan reviewed ahead of time can help clarify the survivor's needs and communicate those needs to clinicians and staff.

The clinician can also help the survivor identify positive support persons, keeping in mind that abuse may have occurred within the family of origin and dysfunctional family relationships may exist that could cause triggers or otherwise negatively affect the experience. For example, if the survivor like Mariluz feels that her mother did not protect her as a child when she was abused, then this feeling may very well recur if her mother is there to provide support, even if the mother is saying and doing what appear to be all the right things. For many survivors of sexual abuse, a doula she has chosen prior to labor can provide the best labor support and act as a mediator between the woman and the caregivers. We will see in the next chapter on induction how having a doula is of central support to Susan.

Providers recognize that some extreme reactions during labor may be due to abuse, even if the woman has not disclosed a history of abuse. Ideally, as with Melissa, the provider would be aware prior to labor of the history of abuse and would have discussed potential ways to help the woman feel in control and comfortable with her care. When a woman's reaction during labor is out of proportion to the clinical reality, as with Jen, a provider should suspect abuse and respond with compassion and tolerance to help create an environment in which the woman feels safe and protected.

Attending to the conduct of every aspect of clinical care to assist the abused woman through the difficulties of prenatal care and delivery includes being careful about the words a provider chooses when touching the woman and performing exams. Clinicians run the risk of repeating the words and tone of the perpetrator, as in "Just relax, this won't hurt," for instance. Asking permission to perform each exam can help give the woman a sense of control over her body in these highly charged moments.

Uncertainty over how labor will progress and how they will handle the pain, as well as the unfamiliar and high-tech hospital setting, may cause a loss of control that brings out every coping mechanism the abuse survivor can muster.[26:61] She may experience triggers, such as perineal pain, certain positions, or statements made by caregivers, that bring back the fear and vulnerability she felt during the abuse. She may respond to the feeling of loss of control by fighting, resisting, or crying, or she may become withdrawn and submissive. She may completely dissociate, seeming to be out of touch and not verbally responsive, a survival technique that erases any emotional response to the labor, as well as any memories of the experience.

Unconscious mechanisms may lead to dysfunctional labor or stalled progress.[26:72–9] A prolonged prodromal labor, stalled active labor, or failure to descend in second stage may be the subconscious effect of the woman's fears – fears of pain, of losing control, of exposure to strangers, or of becoming a parent. Ideally, the provider should assess what is causing the woman to hold back, validate her feelings, and reassure her. If she is feeling out of control, helping her focus on things she can control, such as her breathing, may help. For the woman who is dissociating, having a trusted person continue to talk to her and keep eye contact may help keep her in the present. Dissociation is a coping mechanism associated with more severe abuse, longer duration of abuse, and earlier age of abuse and is not related to quality of support after abuse.[27] Simkin and Klaus's book, *When Survivors Give Birth*, has a practical and detailed chart on potential challenges in labor and possible solutions.[26:79–83]

CHAPTER 4

Induction

Elizabeth Naumburg and Cathleen Morrow

The question and timing of an induction is fraught with challenges. A woman's desires may conflict with best medical practices as defined by regional variation and consultants' opinions. Hospital systems, provider schedules, and nursing requirements on busy maternity suites may determine the timing of inductions. Neither the provider nor the woman may be able to affect this process. Major shifts in developed countries in the standard approach to induction, in the absence of conclusive evidence for improved outcomes, may lead to a wide variety of practices among providers, in the face of a range of consumer preferences for and against induction. Even in the same community, practitioners may hold divergent views about the timing of induction and cesarean section on demand. In many places a woman's request for an elective cesarean section will generate a referral to an obstetrician willing to comply. Her provider will thus lose out on the important history underlying the request, along with the possibility of an empowering opportunity of labor.

In this context, woman-centered communication assists in prevention of misunderstanding and impossible expectations. By mutually defining the problem, woman and provider are "on the same page":

➤ How will I know I am in labor?
➤ What will we do if I don't go into labor by a certain time?
➤ What is that time?
➤ What interventions might be considered if I haven't gone into labor and when might they safely be instituted?

Susan was in the final two months of her uncomplicated first pregnancy and decided to ask Judith to refer her for a primary caesarean section. Her main expressed fear was incontinence, which she was worried would compromise her running. She had read the literature on pelvic-floor relaxation and incontinence and did not want to take any chances.

At the 32-week visit, hearing Susan's request for elective cesarean, Judith began asking more details about her past medical and social history. Eventually, with careful, gentle inquiry, Judith elicited that Susan had a past history of childhood sexual abuse, and was fearful of what would happen to her in labor, feeling exposed and out of control. She had tightly controlled her diet during the pregnancy in order to avoid gaining too much weight or having a big baby. She had never had major surgery and was a bit nervous about the anesthesia, but would rather run that risk than be incontinent.

Judith listened to her fears and then with her wrote down a list of possible options and outcomes (*see* Table 4.3). They discussed trying to prevent macrosomia and perineal tears and trying to start Kegel exercises early postpartum. Judith suggested that Susan start doing perineal massage regularly until delivery and encouraged her to hire a doula for labor support. They talked about how different labor and delivery positions could decrease the risk of perineal laceration. Judith offered to strip her membranes regularly after 37 weeks in hopes of preventing a post-dates labor and to consider induction by 39 to 40 weeks if Susan had not had spontaneous labor by then. Susan agreed to try a vaginal delivery under these conditions, and at 39 weeks with her cervix already 2 cm/50%, she came to the hospital for an oxytocin induction.

TABLE 4.3 Clarifying Problems, Goals, and Roles around Induction

Issue	Susan	Dr. Judith Peters
Problems	Concern about incontinence.	Concern about unnecessary surgery.
Goals	No tears, no incontinence.	Low technology.
Roles	Perineal massage, doula.	Provide information about risks and benefits; membrane stripping; avoid post-dates.

Judith, as Susan's provider, respects her fears about a large baby and pelvic floor incontinence, and recognizes the underlying fear of loss of control of her body implied in Susan's request. Thus she offers to strip Susan's membranes each week after 37 weeks and induce her at 39 weeks. Recognizing that this approach is unlikely to be harmful to mother or baby, Judith uses this intervention to strengthen her alliance with Susan. Judith's strategy contributes to Susan's ability to feel some degree of control and allays her fears enough to allow her to proceed with a vaginal delivery (*see* Table 4.3).

CHAPTER 5

Labor Support

Debra Erickson-Owens and Judith Mercer

Continuous labor support is a crucial and integral part of any comprehensive birth plan. Multiple studies demonstrate the significant benefits both intrapartum and postpartum of the presence of a trained labor support companion, also known as a doula. (*See* Box 4.2 about an exemplary Canadian program.)[28] Although many providers may consider a support person as a resource in birth plans primarily for younger women of limited English capacity, all women can appreciate the reduction in pain, fear, and isolation that derive from the presence of a trained labor support person. Doulas may also be key labor advocates for middle-class women such as Susan who want to do everything possible to secure a normal childbirth.

What do women really want for labor support? Qualitative study shows that women want to labor in a supportive birth environment that includes a person(s) who can provide continuous physical and emotional care throughout labor and birth. Women identify three qualities that they value in the provider offering labor support. MacKinnon's model labels these the *Three Beings*:

1 Being There (physical presence)
2 Being With (emotional support)
3 Being For (advocacy).[29]

BOX 4.2 **South Community Birth Program: Working with Community Doulas**

At term when a woman goes into labor, she pages the midwife or physician on-call, as well as her assigned doula. Before labor becomes active, the doula is often in attendance in a supportive role at the woman's home. She is in contact with the on-call provider, updating on the progress of labor. The doula acts as a companion only and does not perform any clinical assessments. Frequently, the provider first attends the woman in her home during labor, assessing cervical dilation, fetal heart, blood pressure, and labor progress. All of the providers carry the equipment necessary to assess maternal and fetal well-being out-of-hospital. Admission to hospital is postponed until the labor is active, which is often around four to five centimeters

---

dilated. This plan, of course, varies depending on the labor progress. Both the provider and the doula attend the woman in labor in the hospital, and both stay until the birth is completed.[28:21]

(Permission for use granted by South Community Birth Program: www.scbp.ca)

BEING THERE (PHYSICAL PRESENCE)

Late in her third trimester, Susan with Judith's help found a doula, Rachel, to assist with labor support. Susan and Geri met with Rachel and formed a strong attachment to her. Rachel came with them for the hospital induction. The nurse encouraged Susan to use the telemetry fetal monitor that allowed her to walk and move around more. Rachel offered numerous techniques to relieve Susan's back labor: positioning, heat, massage, the lunge, and the labor ball.

Susan's labor progressed steadily, but as she entered transition at 7 cm of dilation, her back labor was particularly intense and starting to overwhelm her. Judith suggested the injection of sterile water around the sacrum as an option. Judith did this while Rachel stood at Susan's head and helped her stay focused on Geri's eyes during the stinging of the injections.

After half an hour, Susan's waters broke spontaneously and she felt a strong urge to push. Judith asked permission to examine her and found that her cervix was not quite fully dilated. Rachel helped her find more comfortable positions and blow through a few more contractions until the anterior lip finally disappeared. After 40 minutes of pushing, during which time Judith used warm compresses, and Rachel helped Susan blow through the crowning stage to stretch the perineum better, Maxwell was born, with Susan having no perineal tears.

Doulas are supportive companions who are trained experts in providing appropriate and comforting physical and emotional care for women during labor, birth, and the postpartum.[22,30-2] A doula focuses on the woman, helping her feel safe and comfortable in unfamiliar surroundings by providing guidance, physical comfort measures, continuous presence and patient advocacy.[33] The doula does not interfere with or provide medical or nursing care.[34] As an important addition to a woman's labor support, a doula can also offer support to the family members who are present and can help them provide labor support, too. The addition of a doula to the care team (provider, nurse, and family) not only benefits the laboring woman but also significantly reduces obstetric interventions.[35]

After careful listening, questioning, and understanding, Susan and Judith make a plan before labor that leaves Susan feeling empowered. Judith communicates the importance of Susan having a doula and also offers choices about induction. The trust fostered in this relationship supports Susan's confidence to labor and birth. The strong bond between Susan, Geri, and Rachel also supports Susan when labor begins. Rachel remains with Susan continuously throughout labor and assists her in the particularly challenging times of transition, early urge to push, and during second stage. Through the techniques offered by Rachel and Judith (including sterile water papules),[36-8] Susan is able to labor without analgesia and anesthesia, as she desired.

BEING WITH (EMOTIONAL SUPPORT)

Samantha's labor nurse praised her ability to cope with labor and offered her the shower to help with the pain. When the teen got out of the shower, she was already 7 cm dilated and started to panic with the intensity of the contractions. Alice, remembering her own natural labors, helped Samantha with back massages and cool facecloths and softly reassured her that everything was okay. Dr. Epps arrived to relieve the on-call provider and entered the room and knelt by the bed, looked directly at Samantha and asked how she was feeling, and then reassured her that she was coping very well with labor.

Continuous support may have especially important added benefits for other young women like Samantha, who may lack a supportive family and face many social issues.[31] Samantha's provider, nurse, and family use a team approach to labor support. By being fully present to the woman and actively listening to her, each member of the team has an important role in supporting Samantha emotionally, thereby contributing to building trust for her. The nurse praises Samantha's coping abilities and offers techniques to alleviate her discomfort. Dr. Epps, conveying a gentle, warm, and caring nature, kneels to look at Samantha directly, helping her to focus on their conversation, and shows genuine interest in how Samantha thinks her labor is going. Alice and Jack provide continuous support. This case includes many examples of emotional support such as encouragement, active listening, trust building and reassurance of a normal process. "Being With" Samantha contributes to her satisfaction with her birth experience and the bonding and nurturing of her newborn.

BEING FOR (ADVOCACY)

At 37 weeks, Jackie's consultant suggested to Judith considering induction of labor since her blood pressure while stable remained elevated. Jackie needed to wait until her sister could arrive from out of state to help her with childcare, so they decided on an induction plan for a few days later. After a long and arduous induction, when the baby's heart rate became abnormal after two hours of second stage, the consultant recommended a cesarean section. Jackie wanted her mother with her during the birth. The labor nurse prepared Jackie's mother before they went into the operating room and encouraged her to praise Jackie's hard work and endurance. The mother sat by Jackie's head and whispered to her daughter how proud of her she was.

When Mariana's blood pressure slowly increased toward the end of her pregnancy, her husband and mother-in-law demanded to know why Mariana was not being offered an immediate cesarean section. Dr. Miller carefully explained with an interpreter the options for care and recommended beginning a cervical ripening agent.

Mariana panicked and asked to wait until her mother from Brazil arrived the next day. Her medical issues had stabilized enough that Dr. Miller agreed to this delay.

These two cases exemplify woman-centered advocacy. Throughout the pregnancy and labor, the partnership that Jackie and Mariana each have with their respective providers illustrates how advocacy promotes finding common ground. As problems develop, each provider offers information and advice, answers all questions honestly and openly, and supports the woman's decisions. The provider's decision to delay the labor induction a few days until Jackie has childcare or Mariana's mother arrives demonstrates understanding, caring, and respect for the woman's needs, desires, and context.

Advocacy is not always easy. Often, medical issues and the hospital environment clash with a woman's request. For instance, if Mariana's blood pressure had continued to rise, Dr. Miller would have needed to revisit the planned delay. Whenever possible, the provider should attempt to clarify and advocate for the woman's wishes with the other members of the healthcare team.

TABLE 4.4 The Three Beings of Labor Support: Quick Techniques for Labor Support[29,39,40]

Being There (Physical Presence)	Being With (Emotional Support)	Being For (Advocacy)
Reassuring touch	Clear communication	Partnering with the woman
Holding	Eye contact	Supporting her decisions
Massage	Voice modulated to decrease stress	Interpreting the woman's wishes to others
Hydrotherapy (tub or shower)	Thoughtful and careful use of words	
Pelvic rock	Warmth and caring nature	Support for the partner and family
Double hip squeeze	Companionship	
Teaching effleurage	Encouragement and reassurance	Providing information and advice (without medical jargon)
Application of heat and cold	Praise	
Assisting with ambulation	Trust building	Coaching
Helping with positioning	Role modeling for partner	Empowering
Continuous presence	Attention-focusing	Supporting the woman's innate wisdom of her body
Creating a relaxed and safe space	Reaffirming normalcy of the process	
	Active listening	
Offering nourishment	Being fully present in the moment	
Encouraging frequent urination	Acceptance with non-judgment and tolerance	

CHAPTER 6

Relational Birth Plans and Progress

Elizabeth Naumburg and Cathleen Morrow

Labor and delivery is the place where the provider's hard work and attention to woman-centeredness often bear fruit. In the late third trimester, much of the focus of the prenatal care will have shifted toward this dynamic time. In the best of circumstances, ongoing continuity of care lays the groundwork for a relationship of trust and mutuality that persists into labor. The experienced and thoughtful practitioner will have anticipated and reinforced the inherent uncertainty of the beginning, duration, and ultimate end of this momentous period in this woman and family's life. Birth plans, both concrete and relational, should by now be well in place. Yet, despite a provider's best attention to detail, unaddressed issues or new circumstances may arise to challenge both woman and provider. The relational birth plan can help most in this instance: the recognition that we, together, can solve this problem, with a relationship rooted in mutual trust and consideration.

The concepts of labor support are particularly important when labor seems slow to start or slow to progress, as with Samantha. The relationship to time is one of the hallmarks that differentiate birth in a medical setting from physiologic birth. The medical model of birth requires the woman's body to stay "on time" or be deemed pathological; the midwifery model, in contrast, sees the woman herself as *active* in time rather than pitted against the clock.[41] Providers vary widely in their philosophy and experience of what constitutes progress in labor. For some, hospital practice or personal style may include updating every two hours a standardized "partogram" or labor graph that is on the front of the labor chart, while other providers opt to follow a more fluid assessment of how labor is progressing. Women will look to providers for this assessment, as it is impossible for the individual woman, caught up in the work of labor, to have an objective view.

> The night of her 38-week prenatal visit, Pat noticed a trickle of fluid after she got up to go to the bathroom, but this time did not think much of it since the other times she had these symptoms and saw Dr. Miller, he had reassured her. When she got up a second time a few hours later, more fluid was leaking out, however, and

> ## Potential Causes of Prolonged Labor (adapted from[22:106])
>
> - Fetal factors
>   - Macrosomia
>   - Malposition (including asynclitism)
> - Fetal-pelvic factors ("cephalopelvic disproportion")
> - Uterine factors
>   - Ineffective contractions (infrequent or insufficient)
> - Iatrogenic factors
>   - Dehydration
>   - Immobility
>   - Parenteral medications
>   - Epidural anesthesia
> - Emotional factors (fear, anxiety, tension)
> - Physical factors (exhaustion)

she wakened Mike and headed into the hospital. The resident on call confirmed that her bag of waters had broken, but she was not contracting or dilated yet. Pat wanted to talk to Dr. Miller, who would be in later that morning, before starting any induction of labor, but was worried about the Group B Streptococcus infection so agreed to start an antibiotic. Once Dr. Miller arrived, they discussed the various choices for induction, and Pat and Mike decided that they wanted whatever the doctor thought would work fastest and most safely for the baby. They wanted to try as long as they could without pain medication, as well, and had also read about the risk of infection if Pat had too many vaginal exams, so they also asked for as few as possible of these. Dr. Miller agreed but also noted that he would need to make some regular assessment of how labor was progressing in order to plan the best induction method for them.

The initial prostaglandin got Pat's labor started so that she progressed to 3 cm dilated with just one dose, her own contractions coming regularly and strongly. To help her cope with the pain, she and Mike found different positions with her ambulatory monitor attached, and also brought out their own music and pillow and Pat's favorite old nightgown and slippers. After a few hours, her contractions spaced out, and Dr. Miller suggested starting oxytocin to re-invigorate her labor. Once the contractions became more regular, her cervix still did not progress initially beyond 4 cm, and the doctor recommended an intrauterine pressure monitor (IUPC). Pat and Mike were hesitant since they wondered about increased infection risks, and Pat started thinking that everything was going in the wrong direction (induction, IUPC, what next?).

Once active labor ensues, but then stalls, the provider faces the challenge of combining adequate clinical evaluation for the etiology of labor dystocia with encouragement and emotional support. Dr. Miller needs to carefully assess fetal, maternal, and iatrogenic causes of long labor (*see* Sidebar)[22:106] and work with Pat, Mike, and the rest of the team to find solutions (*see* Table 4.5).

TABLE 4.5 Clarifying Problems, Goals, and Roles in Labor

Issues	Pat	Dr. Simon Miller
Problem	Intense labor with slow progress; discouragement and self-doubt; fear for baby's health and self-health; fear of disempowering physical intensity.	Non-progressing labor of uncertain etiology.
Goals	Recognizable progress in labor with endpoint in sight; supportive coping assistance; choices in care plan; alleviation of fear.	Evaluate clinical issues to find best treatment plan; avoid increasing risk of infection; balance over-intervention with risks of delaying intervention.
Roles	Report feelings and needs; ask about alternatives; get help from support people if needed to make decisions; reassess expectations; be willing to change positions.	Stay up to date on full spectrum of treatment options for dystocia; stay attuned to signals about how woman is coping with dystocia; ask about her fears; use empowering language and recognize disempowering situations such as supine position.[22:125]

Although providers may feel obliged to adhere to strict standards about normative values for progress in labor, addressing Pat's emotional state (maternal "well-being" not just fetal well-being) is nonetheless an essential component of her care plan. This includes recognizing a woman's verbal and non-verbal cues about her coping with prolonged labor – the 3 Rs of relaxation, rhythm, and ritual.[22:137] When Pat's responses to contractions start to lose any of these aspects of good coping, Dr. Miller needs to consider "emotional dystocia" and identify Pat's possible fears with questions such as "What was going through your head with that contraction? Do you have ideas about why your labor is slowing down?" (*see* Box 4.3).[22:137–8] Once the provider has some sense of what the woman's fears are, basic supportive strategies include restating to clarify what she means, validating her fears, offering reassuring factual information, reframing her concerns, and helping her with massage, hydrotherapy, or pain medication.[22:138]

> While Pat and Mike were thinking about the doctor's suggestion, Dr. Miller was called away to evaluate another woman in labor and returned to Pat's room after the nurse reported, "She's really not coping very well right now." Dr. Miller observed that while previously Pat had been blowing and moaning rhythmically through each contraction with Mike holding her hand, she was now tightening her brow immediately with each contraction and shaking Mike's hand away. Dr. Miller, recalling the intensity of Pat and Mike's prenatal anxiety, wondered how this might impact her labor now and asked, "I'm remembering how much you worried about your baby's health during the pregnancy. What are you thinking right now about the baby and how this labor is going?"

> **BOX 4.3 Possible Childbirth Fears that May Impact Labor Progress[22:137–8]**
> - Dread of increasing pain
> - Fear of bodily damage or disfigurement ("never being the same again")
> - Fear of uterine rupture (if prior cesarean)
> - Fear of labor harming the baby (belief that cesarean is safer)
> - Fear of loss of control, modesty, or dignity ("shame")
> - Fear of invasive procedures (including vaginal exams)
> - Fear of caregivers (particularly if strangers with power and authority)
> - Fear of being unable to care for baby ("inadequate mother")
> - Fear of abandonment by baby's father or other family, or by caregiver
> - Fear of dying that is deep and persistent

> Pat and Mike voiced their concerns about infection, and Dr. Miller reassured them that Pat did not seem to have any other signs of infection. They decided to proceed with the intrauterine monitoring, and over the next several hours the oxytocin was increased until the contractions appeared to be strong and regular with the internal monitor. However, Pat's cervix stopped dilating beyond 5 cm and started to thicken, with the baby's head still not engaged and starting to have molding. Pat was getting tired, but had not yet wanted any anesthesia. Dr. Miller recommended a cesarean section, but she and Mike were reluctant to proceed with this yet, wondering if there were anything else to try still.

At such times of change in expected birth plans, the trust established through the ongoing process of finding common ground makes the difference for a woman and her provider. The provider who understands the full context of Pat and Mike's history facilitates bridging to a consultant's care. Working with a woman-centered consultant makes this easier, but even without that, Pat's relationship with Dr. Miller is still available to add credibility to what the consultant says and to allow time and information sharing to help Pat and Mike feel comfortable with their choices.

> Dr. Miller sat down with them and reminded them of their individual past histories – how difficult it was to trust doctors, and how frightening medical settings and especially complications could be. He asked if they would like to speak with the obstetrical consultant first, before any decision was made, and they agreed.

The woman-centered provider anticipates the potential for more aggressive interventions such as oxytocin, vacuum, forceps, manual placental extraction, and cesarean section. Ideally, provider and woman will have previously discussed during the prenatal period all of these possible interventions, especially those most commonly utilized. The context of this discussion remains rooted in the woman's questions and interests and includes exploring her feelings and ideas about each. Prenatally, the woman-centered provider documents these discussions either via a formal birth plan with a listing of such "advance directives" about potential emergencies or interventions, or a checklist embedded within the prenatal forms. The provider may choose to revisit these decisions periodically during prenatal care as well as at points through labor if clinically indicated.

Unlike Pat, many women with a slowly progressing labor may be overcome emotionally and physically, but view a cesarean section as the only solution early on, even when not medically indicated as Pat's has become. Hearing the despair behind such a request, the woman-centered clinician responds by exploring the underlying feelings, ideas, function, and expectations, seeking to clarify roles and goals and find common ground in the same process iterated in Table 4.5.

Both the woman with a strongly worded non-intervention-based birth plan, and the woman with a desire for effective epidural analgesia by the time she is 4 cm, may have to contend with unpredictable outcomes. Finding common ground at such transitions is easier for a woman-centered provider who has, in open and genuine fashion, communicated a respect for each of those wishes, along with a reality-based assessment of the likelihood of their success, and a clear outline of options should their desired wishes not be achievable.

CHAPTER 7

Analgesia in Labor

Elizabeth Naumburg, Cathleen Morrow, and Sara G. Shields

Tonya had slowly learned to trust Dr. Miller through working on smoking cessation, although she still had her doubts about doctors and institutions. She told him at her 38-week visit that she wanted her epidural with the first contraction. He tried to talk about other options for pain relief, but she interrupted him, saying, "C'mon Dr. Miller, you've never had a baby, I don't want any pain. I got enough to deal with in my life."

He acknowledged, "Yes, you've had a lot of painful stuff in your life. Tell me about how you dealt with pain in your other labors."

She reported that in her first labor she had been induced for pre-eclampsia and had found the pain of "that contraction medicine" unbearable from early on because she had to stay in the hospital bed; the epidural let her sleep even though she agreed that it probably made her labor somewhat longer. For her second pregnancy her water broke at 35 weeks without labor, and she had to get induced again. She recalled getting her epidural around the same time the oxytocin started. Her third labor came on quickly at 37 weeks, her waters breaking at home with strong pains coming quickly after that, so that by the time she arrived at the hospital she was "too late" to get the epidural and then had to push without it and felt, "I just barely survived that." She said, "I'm coming with the first contraction this time. I don't want to feel anything."

Attitudes toward the pain of labor and how to handle it are culturally embedded. The shift toward routine epidural use by some women is in stark contrast to the accepting endurance of pain for other women. Women who have attended prenatal classes or spent time educating themselves will undoubtedly know about epidurals and may have definite opinions. Other women will be totally unaware of options, and some will be solidly committed to a labor without the use of analgesia. As noted in Part One, providers have similarly wide-ranging interpretations of the complicated evidence about the effects of different pain relief modalities in labor. The availability of a broad spectrum of pain relief options varies widely in different settings.

Dealing with labor pain fully challenges the woman-centered provider to find common ground: first to inquire about the woman's context, ideas, and expectations; next, to discuss clearly and carefully the medical facts about risks and benefits for all options; then to facilitate the woman clarifying her goals based on her needs and her understanding of the medical choices given what is available in their setting, and finally to delineate the roles of each support person or provider in helping the woman achieve her goals. This cycle of communication can change during the course of labor – what women need or want early in labor for pain relief can be dramatically different from their desires during the intensity of late first stage or second stage of labor.

The unique qualities of labor pain – its discontinuous nature and its clear function in accomplishing work – are key aspects of finding common ground in labor. The provider can also explain how the experience of steady progress in labor might affect a woman's experience of pain, leading to a discussion of the advantages of adopting an attitude of "let's see how it goes." Starting this discussion prenatally lays the groundwork for education about complementary approaches such as self-hypnosis, acupuncture, or the use of a doula. Such groundwork transitions with the woman's changing needs throughout labor, from the early stages through the most intense moments of the first and second stages of labor.

The visual scales often used for assessing acute pain in non-pregnant hospitalized patients have become a standard part of the measurement of a woman's experience of pain in labor. Underlying the use of standardized scales are the assumptions that patients should not experience pain, and that all pain should be relieved. The application of this approach to labor pain is problematic for several reasons:[42] first, labor pain is not pathologic; second, the experience of labor pain involves physiologic, psychologic, and sociologic aspects, not just neurophysiology; third, pain is not equivalent to suffering, which includes psychological aspects such as helplessness, fear, and inadequate coping resources;[26] fourth, the intensity of labor pain does not necessarily correlate with a bad experience of labor (a woman can report it as the worst pain ever, yet feel satisfied with the birth); and, finally, while measuring pain carries the unstated implication that it must be relieved, not everyone wants labor pain relief in the form of medical interventions.

Giving a laboring woman various modalities for coping with pain may alleviate her suffering even if the physical intensity of the pain persists. Thus if a woman perceives labor and its pain as non-threatening life experiences to be mastered, she may experience great pain but not suffer.[42] While labor hurts, not feeling the birth of one's baby is a loss for women who value the birth experience. Some women also know that interventions to relieve pain carry inherent risks of further undesirable interventions. Most of the popular visual analog scales ask the woman to reference her pain from a maximal point of "pain as bad as it could possibly be," a measure that necessarily depends on an individual woman's past experience of pain and thus is not as absolute or objective as such scales purport to be. When a woman says that her pain is 10/10 when she is in prodromal labor, the utility of such scales is obviously limited.

Simkin[26] notes that focusing solely on pain scales and removing all pain pharmacologically forces clinicians into very provider-centered labor care. Eliminating all pain for a laboring woman requires clinicians to invoke a cascade of medical/pharmacologic technologies that force her to remain in bed attached to a monitor, an epidural catheter, and an intravenous line. Her body becomes the object of surveillance for a variety of complications, and she is completely dependent on the medical system and its personnel to manage and interpret what her body is doing. This dependence is the polar opposite of the values of woman-centered care in childbirth – a method in which the provider and the systems recognize a woman's own competency and emphasize her self-efficacy. Woman-centered care assesses the importance of the labor experience, the meaning of pain to the woman, and the implication for the woman of removing that pain through medical interventions. Rather than taking power away from the laboring woman, woman-centered care places the meaning of pain in perspective and highlights the life-affirming and life-changing aspects of the woman's birth experience.

For the provider who promotes natural, or "physiological," childbirth with minimal technology, woman-centered care involves focusing on giving the woman "control" of her experience as she defines it. Such control may include supporting a woman's choice to have epidural anesthesia, as in Tonya's case. For some providers, this advocacy of technology may feel particularly challenging,[43] especially if the current maternity care system as a whole offers ready access to epidurals but not to a full range of other less technological choices.[44] For some women in the midst of active labor, making a choice about an epidural is too overwhelming, so that staying woman-centered with them may ultimately include "embracing the medical technological model."[43:174] Although such technology may increase a woman's risk of further medical intervention even including cesarean, the provider's task is to fully inform her and recognize that, for some women, freedom from pain is ultimately more empowering than the risk of operative care. Even for the provider who prefers minimal technology, labor support does not end once the woman receives pain relief from the epidural – being with and advocating for her afterward remain important.

TABLE 4.6 Clarifying Problems, Goals, and Roles in Pain Relief in Labor

Issue	Woman	Provider
Problems	Pain; lengthy labor; some routine hospital procedures prevent common comfort measures.	Difficult to watch suffering; medical knowledge about side-effects of different pain medications; lengthy labor impatience.
Goals	Coping with pain; healthy fetal outcome; empowering choices.	Healthy outcomes; empowering women in childbirth; using coping scales not just pain scales.
Roles	Keep talking about feelings and needs; ask questions when not understanding; ask for help in avoiding panic.	Stay up to date on and open to options; encourage low-tech measures; involve support people; use positive language without misinforming; work to make more options available in all settings.

The birth plan thus requires the clinician to elicit the woman's experience, to establish mutual goals, and finally to clarify mutual responsibilities in the care plan.[1] There may be times when the woman wants to take more active responsibility and times when she wants to take a more passive role in the plan. Similarly, the clinician may move between more biomedical or technical roles and more egalitarian ones. The "levels of participation in decision-making" may fluctuate depending on the woman's current capabilities,[1:91] requiring the clinician to remain flexible and responsive to these dynamic variations. For example, in early labor, Melissa feels more in control of her pain, but later during a long and exhausting second stage needs her clinician to be more active and directive: "I know you are tired now. Concentrate on every push right here in your bottom. Take a deep breath and go with it."

CHAPTER 8

Emergencies

Elizabeth Naumburg, Cathleen Morrow, and Sara G. Shields

After 10 days of hospitalization at bedrest, Evelyn (*see* Part Two) awoke late one night needing to go to the bathroom and noticed both further leaking of fluid and uterine cramping. She rang for her nurse and went into the bathroom, where she felt a particularly strong cramp and an odd sensation in her vagina. As the nurse came in, they both realized suddenly that the umbilical cord was coming out of the vagina. The nurse urged, "Evelyn, you need to lie right down while I put the head of the bed way down and call the doctors. This is an emergency. Your job is to take slow deep breaths of this oxygen so your baby gets as much as possible." Evelyn felt very scared but tried to do what the nurse said as the on-call obstetrical team rushed into the room.

The chief obstetrician saw the cord and came immediately to the head of the bed to talk to Evelyn. "The umbilical cord is coming out first. It has a good pulse, which is good. You are going to need an emergency cesarean right now. Until we get you in the operating room, you need to be upside down like this and one of us needs to put a hand in to hold the baby's head off the cord to keep it from being squeezed. It all feels weird, but stay with us."

Several other nurses and doctors were readying her hospital bed for moving quickly to the operating area, so Evelyn behind the oxygen mask just nodded, wide-eyed and asked if someone could call Ed to alert him. As they pushed her bed down the hall, the chief doctor was asking Evelyn to sign the surgical consent form, saying, "I apologize in advance that we'll have to put you to sleep for this surgery. That's safest for the baby." The doctor who was holding the cord kept Evelyn posted, "Your baby has a nice strong heart rate. You're doing a great job breathing oxygen for the baby."

Once in the operating room, Evelyn felt overwhelmed by all the rush but then remembered nothing after taking some more deep breaths until she awoke in the recovery room with Ed at her side, telling her about their 1100 g son, David. The obstetrician was there to tell her, "You did such a great job working with us in all the crazy rush that the surgery happened as fast and as well as we could have hoped for. David was vigorous at first, breathing well at first on his own but then getting a bit tired as we expect for a baby his size." Evelyn, exhausted and astonished by the emergency cesarean and anxious about David's condition, held Ed's hand tightly and nodded wordlessly.

All providers of obstetric care have faced the sudden and critical moments when rapid interventions are required to save the life of a baby, a mother, or both. At such times, woman-centered care focuses on clear, confident communication rather than lengthy discussion. Nonetheless, during emergencies, the principles of woman-centered care – seeking to understand the woman's experience and then incorporating that into a collaborative plan of care – still apply.

Martha from West Africa (*see* Part Three) arrived at the hospital's birth center in active labor at 37 weeks and told the nurse that she already felt an urge to push. The nurse examined her and quickly notified the on-call provider, Dr. Jonathan Rosen, that Martha was already almost fully dilated. Jonathan arrived as the nurse was preparing for the baby, and within minutes Martha had spontaneous rupture of membranes with bloody fluid followed within a contraction by the baby's head. Jonathan barely had his gloves on in time to catch the newborn and deliver the placenta soon after. The nurse cared for the healthy baby while Jonathan turned to deal with Martha's heavy bleeding. Martha, uncomfortable when he tried to do bimanual uterine massage to slow the hemorrhage, tried to push away Jonathan's hands but was able to nod when he urged, "Martha, look at me. You are bleeding heavily. I will need to press here on your womb to help you stop bleeding. The nurse will give you medicine, too. I am sorry this may hurt, but I need to do this to keep you from bleeding too much. Tell me if I am hurting you."

In emergencies, efficient yet clear discussion is important to both good medical outcomes and the ultimate satisfaction of mother and family. Ideally, the provider during emergencies is someone who already knows the woman, so that strong trust and an established relationship allow both anticipation of potential complications and timely woman-centered response should they occur. Realistically, the luxury of such pre-existing relationship in emergencies may not be a reality, as in both Evelyn's and Martha's cases. When the emergency provider is a stranger to the woman, finding common ground is especially challenging but even more essential. Pain control is often critical at such times, to enable an exhausted, laboring woman to hear and understand the reasoning for probable interventions. At such times, taking a few minutes to invest in an open and trusting relationship with a woman and her family is powerful insurance against unnecessary delays resulting from frightened, angry, or confused women.

For the provider with an ongoing relationship, dealing with an emergency includes not only the immediate issues but the aftermath, even days to weeks after an emergency.

Beverly was a 31-year-old African-American biochemist at a research lab in a pharmaceutical company. (*See* full vignette in Appendix). Her husband, Carleton, was a successful investment broker. She had chosen Dr. Greg Diamond's private practice for her obstetrical care. Her pregnancy was uncomplicated except for a few elevated blood pressures in the last few days before she went into labor, but her tests did not suggest significant pre-eclampsia. She finally went into labor a few days after her due date after a 24-hour prodrome that allowed her mother plenty of time to arrive to support her in labor. Beverly had planned to try for an unmedicated childbirth, and her mother strongly supported her in this goal. Carleton was nervous about Beverly's health and did not want her to suffer, but felt that the choices about pain control were up to Beverly. He was also somewhat frightened by the hospital environment, but felt that all would be under control in the tertiary care hospital attached to the medical school.

Beverly's labor was difficult. After remaining at 7 cm for several hours, she had an IUPC inserted, and oxytocin begun. At this point, exhausted and discouraged, she asked Dr. Diamond and the nurse Laura for an epidural. She proceeded slowly to full dilation, but did not feel an urge to push; as the head was descending slowly, Dr. Diamond suggested that Beverly rest to allow more descent before she began pushing. After two hours, she felt the contractions more strongly and wanted to push. Carleton and the nurse worked with her in the different positions that she could move into with the dense epidural, and finally after two hours the baby's head began to crown. Dr. Diamond, not expecting any issue with the delivery without any of the usual risk factors for shoulder dystocia, noticed that this penultimate stage seemed to take longer than usual and wanted to alert the nurse to the possibility of dystocia, but also did not want to alarm Beverly or her husband as she was working so hard to finish pushing.

"C'mon, Beverly, the head is almost out, that's it!" he said as the baby's nose and mouth finally emerged but then retracted slightly, making it hard for him to assess for a nuchal cord or suction the baby's mouth. "Okay, take a breather and let's get your legs back as far as you can. Tell me when you're ready to push again."

Beverly took a sip of water and then nodded and gasped, "Okay, let's do this finally!" Dr. Diamond attempted gentle traction on the baby's head but was not able to move the anterior shoulder. As he adjusted his hands to try alternate maneuvers for the shoulders, he looked Beverly in the eye and urged her, "Okay, Beverly, let's work together. I need you to help make more room for your baby. Push again while I do this. Carleton, hold her leg even further back – think about trying to get your heels to your ears, and Laura will push down right here on your pubic area. We also need to get some others in here to help."

Beverly kept pushing with Carleton, looking on worriedly, moving her legs back and urging her on. Dr. Diamond still did not feel the shoulders budge, and he looked back directly at Beverly. "Okay, you're doing great. I need to put my hand in here now and may need to do a few other things that may be uncomfortable, but we need to get the baby out. Bear with me, and keep working with me." Another obstetrician and the perinatal team arrived to help as, finally, after repeating the Woods' maneuver, with the nurse on a stool applying suprapubic pressure, Dr. Diamond was at last able to extract the posterior arm. "Here he is. Great work!" he told Beverly as baby Jackson emerged at last, limp and not yet crying. While Dr. Diamond clamped the umbilical cord and offered the scissors to Carleton to cut it, he added quickly, "I can feel that he's got a solid heartbeat, but needs some help to breathe. Take a look while I let our newborn team take over."

The pediatric team was in the delivery room for the birth and received the baby who responded quickly to stimulation and blow-by oxygen. But when Dr. Diamond peeked in between the nursery staff to see the baby in the warmer, he recognized the brachial palsy immediately. While he felt relieved that the baby was finally out, he also noted in himself the usual complex feelings that come with a complication – guilt mixed with anxiety – the knowledge that there would need to be long discussions with this couple and the grandparents about the palsy. He said softly to the neonatal team, "Let me tell them about the arm."

Taking a deep breath, Dr. Diamond walked over to Beverly, and looked at Carleton and Beverly together, and began, "Your baby is doing fine – he's breathing well, has lots of oxygen, his heart sounds good. But there is a problem – he's not moving his arm. We see this sometimes after a hard delivery when the nerve to the arm gets stretched as we get the baby out. I'll bring him over in a minute so you can hold him. He's fine otherwise."

"What does this mean? Is he going to be paralyzed?" shot out Carleton, fearing the worst.

"To be honest, we don't know yet whether this problem with the arm will last – sometimes the nerve recovers fully and sometimes it doesn't. The injury is called a brachial nerve palsy. The whole arm is not paralyzed, but with this palsy the hand and arm can't do some movements controlled by that nerve."

"Is he going to be all right?" asked the grandmother.

"Overall, the baby is fine, but we can't say about the arm yet," Dr. Diamond repeated. "Here, let me show you." By this time the nursery staff had begun to leave, and Dr. Diamond picked up baby Jackson in some blankets and brought him over to Beverly and Carleton. He carefully pointed out the baby's good color and tone, and then showed how the baby did not move his right arm. Everyone looked frightened, and he realized that he had perhaps jumped too far ahead. "You are all tired, and Beverly must be exhausted. Let's take a little time to hold Jackson and feed him and wonder at him, and we can talk about the arm later. Let's just welcome him for now." The nurse stepped in and helped Beverly position him next to her on the bed, pointing out all his newborn features and encouraging her to look at his hair and toes and eyes. Gradually, the atmosphere in the room relaxed as the nurses completed their postpartum routine. Dr. Diamond stepped out of the room, pointedly telling the nurse that he would be back after completing his notes.

After Beverly had a chance to nurse the baby, she slept a while, and then remembered about Jackson's arm. She felt anxious about it but just wanted to have a chance to be with the baby and hold him and love him, and did not want to think about it all the time. She trusted Dr. Diamond, and did not think he was to blame. But she also knew that her mother, who could be militant about any adverse event, might start talking about whose fault it was. Beverly really did not want "to go there."

Many providers spend little to no time anticipating or discussing such life-threatening possibilities in detail during the prenatal period, yet in the course of discussing uncertainty, woman-centered providers express to women the possibility of sudden, unexpected risk arising, which will require intervention with limited explanation. Larisa offers the following anticipatory guidance at the 36-week visit:

> Though highly unlikely, there are times, during the course of a delivery when things can suddenly and unexpectedly go wrong. These might be related to your health, or the baby's. As you and I have talked about many times, labor and delivery is different for everybody, and though we have talked about options and possibilities, we both have to accept that there are possibilities that we might not anticipate. If such a thing happens to you, I might not have the time to explain well to you what is happening, and you might not have much choice — we may simply need to do, very quickly, what is best for you and the baby. You will know that it is serious, however, by the way we are talking to you, and I pledge to give you every bit of information I safely can. You will be amazed, as I always am when such a thing happens, at how strong and powerful you will be able to be, to do whatever is needed to protect yourself and your baby.

CHAPTER 9

Finding Common Ground during Postpartum Care

Martha Carlough and Sara G. Shields

Kirk reminded the nurse that Melissa had asked not to have the eye medications given right away so that she and Martin could look wide-eyed at each other after Melissa's perineal laceration was repaired.

One of Alexandra's sisters (*see* Parts Two and Three) brought out her camera just as the baby was born and followed the baby to the warmer snapping photos, while the other sister held Alexandra's hand during delivery of the placenta. Helen encouraged the maternity nurse to allow an extra family member into the delivery room so that Alexandra's mother and third sister could come celebrate the new arrival.

As Pat was wheeled into the operating room, Mike reiterated to Dr. Miller that one of the points in their birth plan was Pat's desire to have immediate skin-to-skin contact with the newborn, in hopes of promoting breastfeeding. "Is there a way to do this for her even with a cesarean section?" Mike wondered. "We read somewhere about trying to do that in the operating room. Of course, only if the baby is okay," he added. Dr. Miller nodded and agreed to ask the surgeon and the nurses about this. While Pat was being prepped on the table, he discussed this plan with the rest of the medical and nursing team and offered to assist with the infant's care however he could to make this happen.

The first hours to days after childbirth are often a time for rest, for both provider and woman, and for welcoming the new baby into the family. In the hospital delivery setting, this moment is also a time when routines and protocols often take precedence over an individual woman's desires or needs. The woman-centered provider blends these routines with the woman's wishes regarding such care as immediate skin-to-skin contact, breastfeeding on demand, no separation of infant and mother, eye prophylaxis, bathing, duration of stay, sibling visitation, etc. Women themselves may have learned about the benefits of bonding strategies like skin-to-skin contact[45-8] that may not be part of hospital routines. Ideally, with the framework of a flexible perinatal birth plan, the provider and the woman anticipate these important choices so that the process of finding common ground is well established before the postpartum period. Again a key component of such a birth plan involves anticipating unexpected outcomes that may influence some of these issues.

DISCHARGE PLANNING

"When the mother leaves the hut the first time after birth, she emerges dressed specially to meet the community. Sedately, she walks to the market, where she is greeted with songs such as were sung to the warriors returning from battle."

(Wachagga people of Uganda)

On postpartum rounds the next day, Alexandra was breastfeeding well but told the resident working with Helen that she was having a lot of pain in her lower abdomen when she tried to sit up, stand up, or move around at all. Her sister pressed the resident, "What's wrong? I never had this problem after my babies." When the resident examined Alexandra, her uterus was not tender, but she winced with midline pressure over her lower abdomen. The nurse reported that Alexandra had not been out of bed except with help and that she limped, doubled-over, to the bathroom only with assistance. The resident told Helen that he thought Alexandra's problem was due to not getting out of bed enough postpartum. Helen, knowing Alexandra and the family, doubted this conclusion. She re-evaluated Alexandra with the resident present and saw that even with both sisters helping, Alexandra's discomfort was beyond the usual. On exam, Helen found the pain to be located in the pubic symphysis, not in the abdomen and pointed out this difference to the resident. She diagnosed pubic symphysitis and arranged for a physical therapist to see her since Alexandra lived in a third-floor apartment and would need to manage stairs to be discharged. The therapist agreed with the diagnosis and arranged for daily sessions in the hospital for three more days until Alexandra could begin to tolerate stairs with the use of a special girdle and enough pain medication. Alexandra wanted to avoid too much medication while she was breastfeeding but was also frustrated with the long hospital stay and with the continued pain. Helen had to carefully document all of these findings to justify the longer stay to the administrators.

On the third postpartum day, Dr. Miller took a moment to ask Pat what she knew about her own mother's deliveries. Pat looked sad and said she did not know. Dr. Miller encouraged her to call her aunt in another state to find out if her aunt remembered about her mother's deliveries. . . . Neither Pat nor Mike felt ready for the planned discharge on the fourth day. Pat had trouble with continence, and walking around even just the hospital room hurt her incision; her milk was just coming in and her breasts hurt, especially as Madeline latched on. The nurses and doctors reassured her that everything was healing appropriately, but she and Mike were dubious. They wanted to stay another night in the hospital and see the hospital lactation consultant another time. Dr. Rosen (who remembered this couple's heightened anxiety from before) was seeing the hospital patients that day and decided to ask Dr. Miller to call in to their hospital room to discuss a discharge plan further. Dr. Miller listened to their concerns and offered to call the next day to see how everything was going, and to arrange for an experienced postpartum visiting nurse to come within the next two days to see them at home.

Postpartum care providers need to recognize that both emotional and physical support for new mothers, particularly for first-time mothers, is often woefully limited in Western culture. For fortunate new mothers, as with Alexandra, support comes from a woman's mother and older sisters or older women in the family. More at risk of lack of support are immigrant women whose mother may be very distant; women, who because of societal mobility live far away from their families of origin; or women like Pat, whose mother died long ago. (Pregnancy and delivery may trigger renewed sadness in women whose mothers have died. The woman-centered provider will address this at various times in the prenatal and postpartum period.) This lack of systemic or societal support often manifests in challenges to or disagreements about finding common ground with postpartum birth plans. The woman-centered provider's task remains collaborating with the mother and her family to match their preferences and needs with clinical judgment, expertise, and evidence, as well as marshaling resources as needed. This provider is not simply a servant doing whatever the woman requests,[1:95] but rather a partner with medical knowledge that can inform the woman's choices. Helen recognizes that Alexandra has medical needs not met by routine timing of postpartum discharge. Dr. Miller, Pat's provider, actively listening just as he did throughout prenatal and intrapartum care, engages Pat and Mike in a discussion of the underlying problems of trust and the upheaval of life with a newborn, and articulates a team approach using community resources. Dr. Miller also recognizes how bereft a new mother might feel when she can no longer ask her own mother questions about how childbearing felt for her.

In most cultures worldwide, women change significantly when they become mothers not only in their own eyes, but also in the eyes of their family and community. In many situations, women return to society with a higher status and responsibilities that expand in many new directions. Woman-centered postpartum care both immediately and into the first year after delivery continues the paradigm of seeking common solutions that empower women as they assume these new roles. The postpartum period is a critical time for supporting informed decision-making for new mothers and their families. Several aspects of this time facilitate such collaboration: the frequency of contact with healthcare providers, the high motivation for health education that may affect long-term habits and goals, and the opportunity for providers to build longitudinal relationships with parents, baby, and extended family.

Many cultures have deeply rooted traditional and complementary care practices centered in the postpartum and neonatal period. Part Three reviews some of these practices. Even in situations where cultural issues may seem less influential, the intersection of biomedical culture with family beliefs and healthcare practices should not be underestimated. Emergency visits for newborn concerns by new mothers often represent a moment where biomedical approaches and family beliefs can come into conflict. Careful inquiry into what family members are saying or recommending often uncovers contradictions that are confusing and anxiety-provoking for the new mother: e.g. "You don't have enough milk – that's why he's crying."[49]

Two critical areas of postpartum care that benefit from a common ground approach are breastfeeding and postpartum depression. The woman-centered provider dealing with these issues looks first, as always, to integrate understanding the woman's experience with information sharing about her choices during this time. As Part Two outlines, exploring the woman's unique experience by inquiring about her feelings, ideas, function, and expectations is an essential part of how the provider ascertains the woman's perspective during the postpartum period.

> On the day of discharge Dr. Miller invited questions from the grandmothers about how both Mariana and Veronica were doing and learned that neither grandmother had breastfed her children. . . . The family went home with plans for a home visit

by a nurse the next day and an office visit five days later. At that visit Mariana focused on breastfeeding while everyone else peppered Dr. Miller with lots of questions about the baby's mild facial rash, her yellow stools, and her sneezing. He acknowledged that taking care of a newborn could feel overwhelming even with experienced grandparents around, and commented on how well Mariana was able to focus on Veronica's needs in the midst of this and how involved each grandmother was in ways that supported Mariana's healthy choice of breast-feeding. They talked about the immediate concerns but also about ways for both Mariana and the rest of the family to find answers to future questions in between appointments.

Here the woman-centered provider first observes the context of Mariana's family involvement. Seeking to ultimately empower her parenting skills, Dr. Miller antici-pates the importance of the grandmothers' influence and specifically addresses their needs for information about the importance of breastfeeding. Next, he assesses the mother's coping ability and avoids being proscriptive by explicitly discussing self-directed ways to learn more about her newborn. Dr. Miller does not abdicate all responsibility for decision-making to the woman but rather remains open to offer-ing assistance in her decisions, her ability to cope, and her ability to make changes to achieve goals.

Samantha was feeding Kyle both formula and breatmilk when Shereen visited them at one week postpartum. Shereen weighed Kyle and explained that he was already very close to his birth weight and that most babies lose some weight in the first week and then gain it back. She watched Samantha breastfeed and gave her a few pointers for positioning and latching on. While doing this, she talked about Samantha's diet and encouraged her to drink enough herself. Shereen could see Alice in the kitchen listening in, and invited her to come watch Kyle nurse and hear his swallowing. They talked a bit about Alice's own breastfeeding experi-ences, which were short-lived due to her perception of a limited milk supply. On the way out, Shereen thanked Alice for all she was doing and her important role in Samantha and Kyle's lives.

Most women want to have a "label" for what is going on or a specific diagnosis as soon as possible. As happened with Samantha, women often develop their own hypoth-eses, and sometimes solutions, before seeking care. During this vulnerable time of caring for a new baby, trusted relatives and friends greatly influence self-health prac-tices, even when the new mother may have wanted to do something differently. Just as Shereen does with Samantha's family, the woman-centered practitioner acknowl-edges and respects these practices as a first step in finding common ground.

At four weeks, Samantha came to the clinic with Kyle for his first well-baby exam. Without her own car, she nonetheless maneuvered her donated car seat and dia-per bag into a local taxi and was proud of herself for arriving "put together" and on time. She still felt tired and anxious, and to calm herself reached for a cigarette outside the clinic door, then regretted this. Samantha knew Dr. Epps disapproved of her smoking and had encouraged her to quit during the whole pregnancy, but somehow she just could not. But now, when holding Kyle after smoking, Samantha thought not only about her health but also the harm her habit might have on his health. She decided to ask Dr. Epps for help with quitting smoking for good.

A second important step in finding common ground is understanding and respecting the woman's expectations for what should happen during medical visits and what should be discussed. The timing is critical, particularly with issues of behavioral change where self-motivation and readiness are crucial to any intervention. Providers need to be sensitive not only to their own sense of urgency, but also to the woman's readiness and understanding of what it might take to change.

Kyle had gained a pound (0.5 kg) since Shereen had gone out for the home visit, and was thriving. Samantha proudly talked about still breastfeeding. She also talked with Dr. Epps about lots of things – what it was like to be out of school with a baby, any symptoms or concerns about postpartum depression, plans for using condoms if she became sexually active again, and basic baby care issues. At the end of the appointment, Dr. Epps asked if she was still smoking, and Samantha sheepishly said, "Well, yes, but now I really want to quit." The doctor reminded her that it was never too late to quit, that it could take a few tries, and that there would be major health advantages for both her and Kyle. They reviewed specific interventions, like identifying smoke-free spaces at home and avoiding trigger situations. Dr. Epps asked if Samantha would come back and talk about this again in a month, and also inquired if Shereen could make another home visit to check on her. Together they set a complete quit date for one month later. Samantha was relieved to be able to talk about her smoking and have a plan, and agreed that what they had outlined sounded like a good plan.

The health provider often assumes the responsibility to define a problem, and to educate and inform about the risks involved in behaviors that affect health. One of the tenets of finding common ground, however, is for this to be a two-way conversation and for women to feel honored, respected, and included even at the level of defining the problem. Women are more often ready to accept advice and to make changes if information is targeted to what they are thinking and what they care about. During pregnancy, Samantha could not think about the possibility of quitting smoking even though she knew it was bad for her own and her baby's health. She felt she had no other coping mechanisms for this stressful time. Now, in the postpartum period, as she holds her infant son, she realizes that she needs to make a different choice. Her self-confidence in her ability to care for Kyle and to be a good mother gives her the strength and commitment to think about quitting smoking. She can also see more clearly how her smoking habit had affected her pregnancy and weight gain, and can clarify that having healthier behaviors for herself would contribute to better health over the long term for her newborn son as well.

Most cultures invent systems of support for new mothers and infants involving the family and community. Woman-centered postpartum care understands the role that these informal systems play in addressing the mother's physical recovery and the new parents' emotional and life-cycle changes, which endure well beyond the few days in the hospital. Aware of the enormity of the challenges facing the new mother, the woman-centered clinician can encourage her to maximize supportive care from a variety of sources among her friends, family, and community. Clinicians familiar with community resources can connect young women with each other in postpartum or lactation support groups, and modify standard postpartum care for better assessment of psychological recovery and contraceptive needs. Ideally, again, addressing postpartum issues should be part of the perinatal birth planning described above.

CHAPTER 10

Consultation and Perinatal Teams

Lawrence M. Leeman and Paul Koch

If medical risks develop during the course of pregnancy or labor and delivery, primary providers often need to consult with specialists. Establishing plans for such consultation proactively is another type of system-wide birth plan that incorporates the fundamentals of finding common ground. In addition to physician specialists, the involvement of other consultants, for example, nutritionists, lactation consultants, physical therapists, or social workers, may become necessary for appropriate coordinated care. Women with atypical perinatal issues, both medical and psychosocial, benefit from arrangements such as standardized clinical forms, guidelines for assessing risk, on-site consultation or coordination of travel and communication with off-site clinicians, and regular multidisciplinary meetings to discuss care plans. All of these aspects of multidisciplinary care become key to finding common ground in a comprehensive perinatal care plan.

Ramona was a 28-year-old Latina woman whose first child was born six years ago in her home country by cesarean section. (*See* full vignette in Appendix.) She had waited to get pregnant again because it had taken her a long time to recover from her first delivery, and because she had immigrated and tried to further her education, including learning English. When she came for her first prenatal visit, she told Dr. Burman that her first labor lasted for two days but that the reason for the operation was that the baby, who weighed 7 pounds (3.2 kg), had had problems with his heartbeat that made the doctors decide to do the cesarean when she had been almost ready to push. She already told Dr. Burman that she really wanted to avoid a cesarean, because of how exhausted the surgery and the new baby made her feel. Dr. Burman briefly discussed the choices and referred Ramona to her colleague, Dr. Rosen, who consulted for women who wished to have a trial of labor after cesarean. Ramona and her husband, who also spoke some English, came to the consultation appointment scheduled late in the day after work, after the interpreters had left, and met with Dr. Rosen without interpretation. Dr. Rosen discussed the risks and benefits of vaginal birth after cesarean. Ramona had brought the operative report from her country that her cousin had been able to help her obtain. She and her husband were firm that this would be their last child, and wondered if she needed to have a repeat cesarean in order to get a tubal ligation. After this consultation, Ramona came to her next appointment with Dr. Burman uncertain about what she would ultimately choose. She said her husband became nervous about the risks of uterine rupture and wanted her to have another surgery. She was not ready to give up on her body yet and dreaded the exhaustion of another post-operative course. She had cousins and friends who had described complications of repeat cesarean, making her anxious about these possibilities as well. She and Dr. Burman agreed that they would continue to discuss her choices throughout the pregnancy. By the time Ramona was eight months' pregnant, she was reconsidering what might happen if her pregnancy continued 10 days past her due date, the way she had with her first baby. She remembered the difficulty of waiting and wondering, and the long labor induction process. She and Dr. Burman talked about a plan should her pregnancy go past her due date. She decided that if she went into labor on her own she still certainly wanted a trial of labor, but if she had little chance of doing that by her due date, she would like a repeat cesarean after all.

Lisa (*see* Part Two) and her husband Randy went to the regional high-risk perinatal center to meet with the obstetrical and neonatal specialists about the gastroschisis of their fetus. These doctors discussed with them a plan for both prenatal care and immediate newborn surgery, and sent an initial consultation report to Dr. Rao. At her 28-week visit at the regional center, the perinatologist noticed that Lisa appeared anxious and tired and asked her about plans for support. When her tears welled up, he made a call to the perinatal social worker Reina who began meeting regularly with Lisa (and Randy when he could make it) after her prenatal appointments to provide emotional support.

In mid-pregnancy Judith referred Jackie to the obstetrical specialists for her multiple risk factors, but Jackie returned from this consultation saying she would not see them any more because they only talked about how fat she was and did not deal with her concerns about her back pain and her gallstones that appeared on her ultrasound. She felt that they were prejudiced against her because she was black, as she felt interrogated about substance abuse and because they immediately brought up the possibility of cesarean and sterilization without asking her if she would want more children after this pregnancy. When Jackie's blood pressure rose late in her pregnancy, Judith discussed this additional problem along with her other risk factors and recommended additional consultation with the obstetrician specialists again. Jackie, remembering her prior experience, was very opposed but finally agreed to see one specific consultant who had worked closely with Judith in other situations. The consultant agreed to co-follow Jackie with alternate visits with Judith for management of her blood pressure . . . When Jackie made no progress in second stage, Judith asked the consultant to assess her for an assisted delivery by the consultant. The consultant evaluated Jackie and thought that the baby was posterior and too high to safely attempt an assisted vaginal delivery and recommended a cesarean section instead.

Dr. Miller asked if Pat and Mike would like to speak with the obstetrical consultant first, before any decision about cesarean was made, and they agreed. Dr. Miller was pleased that the day's ob consultant was Dr. Greg Diamond, an old friend with a very patient and reassuring style. He reviewed the obstetrical case with Greg, but also reviewed the couple's personal difficulties with trust. Greg spent 20 minutes with Pat and Mike, and after some time by themselves, they agreed that they would like to move ahead with the cesarean.

Obstetrical collaboration, consultation, and referral occur commonly and throughout the perinatal period. Ramona initially plans a trial of labor after cesarean but becomes ambivalent about that decision after she and her husband have an obstetric consultation early in pregnancy; they ultimately may transfer care late in pregnancy for a planned cesarean if she goes past her due date. Lisa's unexpected fetal anomaly means that she will need high-risk multidisciplinary care that necessitates transfer of care at the time of diagnosis. Jackie has an initial obstetrical consultation midway through her pregnancy due to her obesity, fibroids and advanced maternal age; unhappy with this visit, she is reluctant to have another third-trimester consultation when she develops gestational diabetes and hypertension. Eventually, she needs further consultation during labor for an abnormal fetal heart tracing and non-progressing labor. Pat also requires an intrapartum consultation with an obstetrical consultant due to labor dystocia. The consultant reinforces her primary provider's recommendation, and performs a cesarean delivery. In all of these situations, the principles of woman-centered care apply.

Consultations can be broadly divided into inpatient and outpatient consultations and may be for obstetric or non-obstetric indications. Consultation request of an obstetrician by a family physician or nurse midwife is a special type of consultation, which may result in the transfer of care for subsequent antenatal care and childbirth, co-management, or recommendations with return of the woman's care to the primary provider.

CATEGORIES OF CONSULTATIONS

Consultations typically fall into one of the following four categories:

➤ informal consultations
➤ single consultations
➤ collaborative management with the consultant
➤ transfer of care to the consultant.

Informal Consultations

These questions usually come under the categories of diagnosis, management or prognosis in family medicine in general.[50] A provider asking a specialist colleague about a general approach to women with a specific concern is an example: "Do you wait 18 hours to start antibiotics on a woman in labor with ruptured membranes without Group B Streptococcus screening results, or do you begin them earlier if you do not think she will be delivered by 18 hours after rupture of membranes?" These consultations can be reassuring for the generalist, as they support his or her plan of care if the consultant agrees. One study demonstrated that having a well-thought out question and specific plan in place for curbside consultations may result in a definite response to the question and less chance of recommendation for formal consultation by the consultant. Depending upon the clinical scenario, the woman may not be made aware of an informal consultation.

Although they may be convenient for the referring physician, "curbside" consultations are fraught with peril for the referring and consulting physician and for the woman. Typically, the danger is construed as a medicolegal issue, but such consultations also pose a problem for woman-centered care. A woman-centered consultation should include transparency in the consultation process as part of the partnership of finding common ground. The referring physician may assume a doctor–patient relationship between the consultant and the woman when in fact none exists without the consultant interviewing and examining the woman, in addition to reviewing all diagnostic information pertaining to her care. The consultant might be tempted to give recommendations based on incomplete information, leading to misdiagnosis or treatment. The woman may not feel that either her concerns or questions were addressed or that she fully understood either the reason for an additional opinion or the recommendations that were made without her directly hearing them. If the woman is told that a consultant agreed to or suggested the treatment plan and an adverse outcome occurs, she may seek legal recourse despite lack of a direct relationship.[51] A recent analysis of a national legal malpractice case database and the medical literature found that courts have ruled that no doctor–patient relationship exists with an informal consult.[52]

Single Consultations

This type of consultation, such as Ramona's and Jackie's first consultations, entails the consultant interviewing and examining the woman once and providing recommendations to the referring provider for further diagnosis or care. The primary provider continues to assume responsibility for the woman's care and can act as a known and trusted "translator" of the consultant's advice. Examples include consultation about a trial of labor as in Ramona's case, discussion of multiple medical risk factors such as in Jackie's case, or issues such as referral for amniocentesis or targeted anatomic ultrasound for abnormal genetic testing, or genetic counseling regarding teratogenic exposures. The benefit of a one-time consultation is that the primary provider remains the main caregiver, so that the woman does not have repeated visits with the consultant. Problems may develop if the primary provider does not recognize the need for a re-referral to a consultant, leading to unnecessary delays in diagnosis if the woman's condition worsens or a new clinical concern develops. In woman-centered single consultation, both the referring provider and the consultant remain open to both the woman's request for possible additional consultation as well as the potential medical need for such follow-up.

Collaborative Management with the Consultant

In collaborative care for obstetrical risk issues, the primary provider continues to provide most of the prenatal and delivery care, but a specialist assumes care for or makes significant decisions about specific complications such as multiple gestations, diabetes mellitus, or abnormalities in fetal heart rate tracings in labor. As in Pat's case, this process may include temporary transfer of care for a specific procedure that the primary provider does not perform (e.g. external cephalic version, forceps, cesarean delivery). Most important in such collaborations are transparency and open communication: the woman must understand clearly the plans and contingency plans, and communication must be open and clear between all parties. The woman must be able to initiate communication that will be heard and respected by both the primary provider and the consultant. Conflict, both overt and hidden, among the physicians, makes transparency and open communication impossible.

Transfer of Care to the Consultant

Transfers may occur at any time during pregnancy, labor, and delivery, depending on the skills of the primary provider and the resources available in the specific location. In transfers during pregnancy, the consultant assumes responsibility for the remainder of prenatal, intrapartum, and postpartum care. In very remote areas of some countries, for instance, women may move close to the hospital at 36 weeks in order to deliver with specialty attention. Transfer of care during labor, as for Pat and Jackie, often occurs when the woman requires a procedure for which the primary provider is not trained. In both situations, the consultant needs to bear in mind that the primary provider will eventually resume care, and will need a clear understanding of any issues that will require follow-up. Some primary providers, in collaboration with the consultants, may prefer to resume postpartum care immediately after an operative delivery by a consultant; others will resume care later when the woman is ambulatory. In settings where a woman or her fetus require highly specialized services, such as with Lisa, consultation may require transfer to a tertiary care facility if necessary, such as for a 28-week preterm birth, HELLP syndrome at 30 weeks, or an infant anticipated to need pediatric surgery soon after birth. Again, detailed communication to the primary provider is critical for the woman's long-term care and for her satisfaction with the process. Providers such as Dr. Rao, who will not only remain Lisa's primary doctor but will also ultimately be Anthony's physician, need regular updates from consultants after a woman has been transferred to their care, particularly after delivery for discharge planning. In some specialty settings with many referred patients, nurses provide phone follow-up to primary care providers.

REASONS FOR CONSULTATIONS

The overriding reason for any consultation in medicine is for the health and welfare of the patient. Primary maternity care providers usually refer women to consultants for the following reasons.

1 Lack of certainty of diagnosis – for instance, ambiguous ultrasound findings, an atypical presentation of pre-eclampsia, or labor dystocia.

2 Need for a specific procedure that the primary provider is not qualified or trained to do, i.e. a cesarean or instrumental delivery, amniocentesis, external cephalic version.

3 Lack of improvement or stabilization in the woman's condition despite standard diagnostic and therapeutic interventions by her primary provider (e.g. worsening pre-eclampsia despite standard treatment).

4 Hospital or health delivery system credentialing requirements for specific complications of pregnancy or delivery or for specific procedures.

5 A disagreement in management between the woman, and possibly her family, and the primary provider; or at the woman's request for other reasons such as her family's insistence.

6 The development of a complication in pregnancy requiring specialty care in a different hospital for optimal outcome, i.e. preterm labor in a woman with a 28-week gestation fetus in a rural/community hospital without a level III nursery or neonatologists.

7 A potentially life-threatening – or health-threatening – complication, i.e. HELLP syndrome, acute fatty liver of pregnancy, or peripartum cardiomyopathy, requiring multidisciplinary intensive care.

8 Multiple medical, obstetric or surgical problems requiring a consultant's input into the overall prenatal management of the woman and possibly collaboration or transfer of care. Jackie, with her age, obesity, gestational diabetes, and newly developing hypertension, is an example of this situation. Although any of the risk factors alone may not necessarily require consultation, Jackie's multiple risks may benefit from consultation to ensure an optimal pregnancy outcome. The local standard of care and expectations of the medical community, as well as Jackie's

choice of a maternity care provider, influence this decision.

9 For the care of identified risk factors, consultation occurs not necessarily with single physicians but with specialized perinatal teams and services such as:

a Prenatal care coordination services that make home visits for a pregnant woman, initiate a comprehensive risk assessment including biopsychosocial factors, ensure follow-up office and lab visits, monitor a woman's adherence to treatment and medication regimens, and make referrals as necessary to appropriate community agencies such as nutrition programs.

b Gestational diabetes programs that provide health and diet education, glucometer teaching, and instruction in use of insulin or oral hypoglycemic medicines.

c Substance abuse treatment programs that include drug abuse counseling, social work services, psychiatric care and methadone maintenance when needed. The prerequisites of such a program are discussed further in Part Three.

TYPES OF OBSTETRICAL CONSULTANTS

In the USA, family physicians or midwives may use a variety of obstetrical consultants including obstetrician/gynecologists, perinatologists, and family physicians with fellowship training in obstetrics. The choice will depend upon local availability, the type of obstetrical issue, and the woman's preference. Traditionally, obstetrician/gynecologists have been the primary obstetrical consultants, but the increased number of maternal-fetal medicine (MFM) specialists has resulted in an increased availability in many practice settings.[53,54] The willingness of obstetricians to provide consultation to family physicians has depended upon local practice patterns and whether they have viewed family practice maternity care or midwifery as undesired competition. On the other hand, perinatologists who do not offer routine obstetrical services may not perceive family physicians or midwives as competitors and may be supportive consultants. Recently developed fellowships in family practice obstetrics and maternal and child health in the USA over the last 20 years have produced a growing supply of family physicians with training in operative and high-risk obstetrics. Such fellowship-trained physicians practice collaboratively with other family physicians, offering maternity care themselves and consultations for obstetrical complications or operative delivery.

The consultation process differs based on the structure of the maternity care system in various developed nations. In the UK, hospital-based midwives are the typical primary maternity care provider, with consultant obstetrician gynecologists limited to complicated patients. Home births are an accepted part of the national maternity care systems in the Netherlands[55,56] and the UK[57,58]; however, in the USA, home births are primarily attended by direct-entry midwives who may have minimal integration with hospital-based physicians or midwives.[20] The Canadian system supports a variety of roles for midwives and of consultative possibilities for obstetrician gynecologists who consult to both midwives and family doctors doing obstetrics.

The consultative process may be significantly different in countries outside the

USA or Europe. Health care in many developing countries is decentralized. Women may have lack of access to transportation or finances that would allow them to receive medical supervision of their prenatal care or have a medically trained birth attendant. The primary focus may be on getting adequate nutrition and potable water, rather than identifying need for care for pregnancy complications. Maternal mortality due to complications of gestational hypertensive disorders, obstetrical hemorrhage, obstructed labor, and sepsis are primary concerns. The primary goal of consultation may be to obtain technological maternity care resources (blood banking, operative facilities, intravenous antibiotics) that are not available at the home or village level where most births in the rural developing world occur.[59] In developing nations striving to assure the presence of skilled birth attendants at all deliveries, a dire shortage of trained personnel often limits access to consultation in emergencies. In these settings, the training of "obstetrical technicians" who can perform cesarean sections in rural hospitals creates the possibility for the kind of consultation that can reduce maternal morbidity and mortality.[60]

Whatever the process or healthcare system, the woman-centered provider develops a clear understanding of the obstetrical consultants available in the community and knows how the various consultants interact with patients, particularly around giving women choice in prenatal care and childbirth. As noted earlier, woman-centered care requires transparent disclosure with any pregnant woman early in prenatal care about these systems of referral. Once consultation becomes indicated, the woman-centered provider's task is to make explicit to the pregnant woman the goals of consultation and to give her choice, if possible, in the consultant and the process. If the consultant is to become the clinician for childbirth, the primary provider will need to initiate discussion about how the transfer will affect her birth plan. If she has transferred from a family physician who offers mother and baby care to an obstetrician/gynecologist, the woman and provider should determine if the family physician will be able to follow the infant. Medical complications requiring transfer of the mother may require that she deliver in a hospital with a neonatal intensive care unit or one that may be geographically distant from her home. In the latter situation the task of the woman-centered referring provider includes assistance with medical concerns such as a consultation with a neonatologist and a tour of the NICU as well as with individualized concerns such as housing, travel, and coping with employment and family needs during extended or distant hospitalizations.

PROBLEMS IN CONSULTATION AND TRANSFER

Woman-centered consultation presents a challenge when the woman is uncertain or ambivalent about the process, and when consultation triggers the potential for conflict. Ideally, the woman-centered provider, already knowing the woman's experience of this pregnancy and committed to finding common ground when problems develop, discusses the potential need for such consultation as a routine part of prenatal care, as noted above. This anticipatory discussion smoothes the transition if and when consultation becomes necessary.

Jackie felt that her obstetrical consultants conveyed a negative attitude toward her because she was an obese African-American woman. She viewed their questions about sterilization and substance abuse as evidence of racist stereotyping.

Ramona would be communicating with her obstetrical consultant through an interpreter. She wondered if he would be more eager to perform a cesarean, as he would then be paid more for the delivery.

Pat was distrustful of physicians other than her family physician due to her perception of prior physicians' failures in diagnosing her mother's and husband's past illnesses. She wondered if her family physician's recommendation for a cesarean was a good one.

A pregnant woman may have a number of different reactions when her provider suggests referral to a specialist for complications of pregnancy or labor. Her woman-centered provider carefully explores her reaction. First, she may be concerned that her pregnancy is no longer healthy and that she now has a "high-risk" pregnancy. She may have feelings of abandonment from her physician, with whom she may have placed complete trust for the care and welfare of her and her fetus. She may have financial or time concerns if the consultation requires travel to another community. She may have substance abuse issues that interfere with her ability to comply with visits to a specialist. On the other hand, she may perceive referral to a specialist as a sign of thoroughness and diligence from her provider, or may appreciate a second opinion on a point of disagreement such as management of subsequent deliveries with a history of shoulder dystocia, or fourth-degree laceration, or cesarean delivery.

Perinatal consultation presents numerous potential opportunities for conflict. A pregnant woman may decline to go to a specialist because she does not believe anything is wrong; she may have financial, transportation, or childcare barriers; she may not want to see another physician. Cultural differences or misunderstandings, including lack of interpreters, or use of family interpreters, may interfere with the consultation process. The specialist may disagree with the current or proposed care plan and recommend transfer of care or interventions contrary to the plan that the woman and her primary provider have made. The referring provider may feel compelled to refer to whoever is on call in the hospital for intrapartum complications, even though she or he prefers collaboration with another obstetrician on an elective basis due to personality or practice-style differences. Any of these conflicts are potential sources for the woman to receive either suboptimal care or undergo a negative pregnancy or birth experience.

Other sources of conflict in consultation include issues related to the woman's specific birth plan. Although at times obstetrical complications may necessitate changes in this plan, the woman may have had specific desires regarding delivery or immediate newborn care that the consultant may not honor. Examples include desire to ambulate in labor, push in alternative positions, utilize a doula, avoid episiotomy, and have immediate skin-to-skin newborn contact. The woman may feel undervalued as a woman and a person if the practice style or high volume of patients in a referral clinic lead a consultant to embrace a technical, rather than woman-centered, approach to her care.

Many unanticipated or complex events in maternity care make it appropriate for the primary maternity care provider to transfer part or all of the obstetric care to an obstetrician. Nevertheless, the primary provider may feel varying degrees of reluctance to transfer the woman for various reasons: because of the significant time and effort he or she has invested in caring for the woman, his or her disagreement over scope of practice limitations in the local healthcare system or hospital, his or her recognition that a significant financial loss will occur with transfer of care, or because of feelings of responsibility of "seeing things through" with his or her patients.

Conflict may arise from a consultant's viewpoint as well. The consultant may feel that the referring maternity care provider is practicing outside the scope of his or her expertise, or should not be providing maternity and delivery care at all without obstetrics board certification. The consultant may feel that the consult request was late in the prenatal course or late in the labor process, and that the consultant would have managed things differently much earlier. The consultant may feel that the referring provider provided insufficient information. On the other hand, the consultant may feel that certain requests for consultation are unnecessary, and that the referring maternity care provider could have handled the issue without having specialist involvement at all. If the woman is reluctant to go to the consultant, the consultant may perceive the woman as hostile or uncooperative. At times, a consultant may be hesitant to provide consultation or surgical backup, based on his or her own malpractice experience or assessment of a high probability of an unfavorable pregnancy outcome; such a stance may lead to inadequate care.

Jackie's experience with obstetric consultation is initially negative. She feels that the consultants do not address her main concerns of low-back pain and gallstones. Judith discusses with her the specific reasons for referral, including what the consultant would not address: "I am concerned about the effect of your weight, fibroid tumors on your uterus, and family history of diabetes on your pregnancy. I would like to seek the opinion of a specialist with experience in managing pregnancies with these problems so I can take the best care of you and your baby possible. The consultant will not address your low-back pain or your gallstones. After your pregnancy we can talk to a general surgeon about gallbladder surgery." However, even when providers think that they have adequately prepared women for what to expect from a consultation, miscommunication is common. The consultant may not receive the written referral in a timely way and may therefore not know what question the primary provider is asking. Consultations that take place at another facility or at a tertiary care center may provoke anxiety in the woman, who may know of other women who had complications requiring admission there or who may feel intimidated by such institutions. Large obstetrical services with many providers including trainees may make the woman feel anonymous and keep her from developing trust with the consultant or in the process. Woman-centered providers whose consultants are part of a large service may need to make special efforts to clarify communication so that the woman feels that someone has personally addressed her problems and will communicate back to her provider.

Thus, for Jackie, subsequent reconnection with the consultant and the close collaboration during her complicated labor become possible because of her relationship and trust with Judith as the primary provider, who recommends following the consultant's guidance and who remains closely involved in her prenatal, delivery and postpartum care. In Ramona's case, Dr. Burman as her primary provider has to assist her in making a complicated decision about a repeat cesarean versus trial of labor after cesarean, with serious potential complications with either choice. The consultant's role is more limited during her prenatal care, as the consultant assesses her past operative obstetric history and counsels her on the relative risks and benefits of either choice. The referring provider should anticipate the need for an interpreter to ensure that the couple's understanding of the information is accurate, and to assure that the consultant can perform an accurate assessment of the woman's unique situation. Ramona's husband is concerned about uterine rupture, but perhaps the language barrier or the challenge of interpreting complex statistics prevent him from understanding the small absolute risk of this complication. Dr. Burman plays a key role in clarifying Ramona's and her husband's concerns about the potential delivery method and complications. The woman-centered approach is dynamic and flexible, with an open dialogue over several visits, finally arriving at the wait-and-see decision about spontaneous labor. As part of this process of finding common ground, Dr. Burman clarifies that Ramona can have a sterilization procedure regardless of her choice of delivery method and that such a procedure after a vaginal birth has less operative risk than a repeat cesarean.

Pat's case requires a consultation for a second opinion regarding her physician's recommendation for cesarean delivery due to arrest of labor. Despite a strong relationship with Dr. Miller, the couple has a strong distrust of physicians from prior perceived misdiagnoses. Hearing similar advice from a second physician ameliorates this mistrust; thus Dr. Diamond did not provide a different level of care but did provide additional reassurance that the recommendation for cesarean was correct.

ADDRESSING THE PROBLEMS

Adopting the method of woman-centered maternity care, the provider can remain an effective advocate for the woman's best interest during and after transfer of care. First and foremost is clarifying the woman's understanding of the reasons for transfer of care. The referring provider should function as a reliable source of clinical information for the consultant so that the consultant can develop the most accurate assessment of the woman's overall health, pregnancy, and labor. The woman-centered primary provider has detailed insight into the past medical history, family support structure, health beliefs, and past experience of the woman with health care; communicating such information to the consultant, the primary provider gives valuable assistance in the overall care of the woman. The woman-centered consultant attempts to develop a maternity care plan that incorporates the woman's choices with regards to her prenatal care and delivery. If the consultant is to assume primary care at the time of delivery and postpartum care, he or she will need to discuss issues such as labor support, pain control, breastfeeding, and postpartum contraception. The referring provider can assist by providing this information when known.

The woman-centered provider who also does newborn care can stay clinically involved after transfer of care by providing neonatal resuscitation, if needed at birth, and assuming ongoing care for the newborn. Depending upon the clinical situation, the woman-centered provider may also offer postpartum care in the hospital setting or after discharge. During the prenatal course, the woman-centered provider who does general medical care may continue to participate in the care of a pregnant woman who has had transfer of obstetric care by seeing her in the office for treatment of non-obstetric health issues such as asthma, musculoskeletal injury, or depression. Counseling the woman that she will remain under the care of the specialist for a time-limited or event-limited period can provide reassurance that her primary provider is not abandoning her. "I haven't been trained to do cesarean sections so the obstetrician will deliver your baby by cesarean for the placenta previa, but I will be present in the operating room to attend to your baby, visit you every day in the hospital to care for your baby, and see you in the office for your postpartum care."

Although the consultant may have accepted the woman in transfer of care for an obstetrical problem, the referring provider may be able to best work with the woman to prevent future health complications. Whether or not Jackie's prenatal care ultimately remains with a specialist, Judith clearly plays the key role in reducing her future health risks, by promoting breastfeeding, diet, and exercise to decrease her risk of developing Type II diabetes mellitus. The referring provider can obtain glucose tolerance testing at six weeks and then annually, in addition to assessing her cholesterol panel and any other cardiovascular risk factors. (*See* Part Five.)

Models of successful collaboration between family physicians and obstetricians are valuable resources to sites seeking to improve their consultation process. The University of Michigan developed a model of inpatient FP–OB collaboration for the provision of inpatient maternity care with high concordance between the stated and realized goals of consultation.[61] In some settings family physicians with advanced training in obstetrics share responsibility with obstetricians for the management of routine labor patients on busy university training services.[62] The key components of a successful collaboration are as follows: well-established, clear guidelines of reasons for obstetric consultations; collegial, not competitive, professional relationships where both parties enjoy mutual respect for their each other's clinical competence; and excellent communication between the referring and consulting providers. Interspecialty hospital committees (e.g. Maternal and Child Health or Obstetrics Quality Assurance committees) that look at maternity care from a systems perspective, offer case reviews, and run periodic morbidity and mortality conferences that can also promote high-quality maternity care.

The ideal consultation occurs when both the referring primary provider and the consultant remain woman-centered. Effective, respectful communication between the primary provider and consultant results in optimal maternity care and includes all aspects of the woman-centered method: putting in context the individual woman's prior healthcare experiences, belief system, ethnic and cultural background; eliciting her definition of the issues and her expectations of the consultation process; and incorporating all of this into a mutually delineated care plan. The practice of woman-centered care in the consultation process can often result in a higher level of satisfaction and a reduction in the disempowerment that women often experience during the unforeseen development of medical complications during pregnancy.

The absence of a true evidence base in obstetrics often means that there is no single right approach to medical and obstetrical decisions. The very real varieties in birth customs based in culture, region, and individual philosophy can result in enormous uncertainty for women during pregnancy. In fact, the relationship between provider and woman may be the one constant that helps to find answers in the face of an inherently capricious process. In the best situation, skilled providers, both in primary and specialty maternity care, can together assist women and their partners in embracing the unknown and the unfolding of their new lives as parents, and as creators of the brand-new human being before them.

REFERENCES

1 Stewart M, Brown JB, Weston WW, *et al.*, eds. *Patient-centered Medicine: transforming the clinical method*. 2nd ed. Oxford: Radcliffe Medical Press; 2003.

2 Mishler EG. *The Discourse of Medicine: dialectics of medical interviews*. Norwood, NJ: Ablex; 1984.

3 Lothian J. Birth plans: The good, the bad, and the future. *J Obstet Gynecol Neonatal Nurs.* 2006; **35**: 295–303.

4 Perez PG, Capitulo KL. Birth plans: are they really necessary? Pro and con. *MCN: Am J Matern Child Nurs.* 2005; **30**: 288–9.

5 Reime B, Klein MC, Kelly A, *et al.* Do maternity care provider groups have different attitudes towards birth? *BJOG.* 2004; **111**: 1388–93.

6 Moore M, Hopper U. Do birth plans empower women? Evaluation of a hospital birth plan. *Birth.* 1995; **22**: 29–36.

7 Page LA. Putting science and sensitivity into practice. In: Page LA, editor. *The New Midwifery: science and sensitivity in practice*. Edinburgh: Churchill Livingstone; 2000. pp. 7–44.

8 Anderson L, Lewis G, Araya R, *et al.* Self-help books for depression: how can practitioners and patients make the right choice? *Br J Gen Pract.* 2005; **55**: 387–92.

9 den Boer PCAM, Wiersma D, Van den Bosch RJ. Why is self-help neglected in the treatment of emotional disorders? A meta-analysis. *Psychol Med.* 2004; **34**: 959–71.

10 Crane JP, LeFevre ML, Winborn RC, *et al.* A randomized trial of prenatal ultrasonographic screening: impact on the detection, management, and outcome of anomalous fetuses. The RADIUS study group. *Am J Obstet Gynecol.* 1994; **171**: 392–9.

11 LeFevre ML, Bain RP, Ewigman BG, *et al.* A randomized trial of prenatal ultrasonographic screening: impact on maternal management and outcome. RADIUS (Routine Antenatal Diagnostic Imaging with Ultrasound) Study Group. *Am J Obstet Gynecol.* 1993; **169**: 483–9.

12 Ewigman BG, Crane JP, Frigoletto FD, *et al.* Effect of prenatal ultrasound screening on perinatal outcome. RADIUS study group. *N Engl J Med.* 1993; **329**: 821–7.

13 Mitchell LM. Women's experiences of unexpected ultrasound findings. *J Midwifery Womens Health*. 2004; **49**: 228–34.

14 Van der Zalm JE, Byrne PJ. Seeing baby: women's experience of prenatal ultrasound examination and unexpected fetal diagnosis. *J Perinatol*. 2006; **26**: 403–8.

15 American College of Nurse Midwives. Home birth in the context of current challenges facing the US maternity care system. 2008 [cited January 10, 2009]. Available from: www. acnm.org/siteFiles/policy/Home_birth_in_context.pdf

16 BirthChoiceUK. Basic maternity statistics. 2008 [cited January 10, 2009]. Available from: www.birthchoiceuk.com/Frame.htm

17 Amelink-Verburg MP, Verloove-Vanhorick SP, Hakkenberg RMA, *et al*. Evaluation of 280 000 cases in Dutch midwifery practices: a descriptive study. *BJOG*. 2008; **115**: 570–8.

18 Janssen PA, Lee SK, Ryan EM, *et al*. Outcomes of planned home births versus planned hospital births after regulation of midwifery in British Columbia. *CMAJ*. 2002; **166**: 315–23.

19 Fullerton JT, Navarro AM, Young SH. Outcomes of planned home birth: an integrative review. *J Midwifery Womens Health*. 2007; **52**: 323–33.

20 Johnson KC, Daviss BA. Outcomes of planned home births with certified professional midwives: large prospective study in North America. *BMJ*. 2005; **330**: 1416.

21 Vedam S. Home birth versus hospital birth: questioning the quality of the evidence on safety. *Birth*. 2003; **30**: 57–63.

22 Simkin P. *The Labor Progress Handbook: early interventions to prevent and treat dystocia*. 2nd ed. New York: Blackwell; 2005.

23 Austin DA, Calderon L. Triaging patients in the latent phase of labor. *J Nurse Midwifery*. 1999; **44**: 585–91.

24 Greulich B, Tarrant B. The latent phase of labor: diagnosis and management. *J Midwifery Womens Health*. 2007; **52**: 190–8.

25 McNiven PS, Williams JI, Hodnett E, *et al*. An early labor assessment program: a randomized, controlled trial. *Birth*. 1998; **25**: 5–10.

26 Simkin P, Klaus MH. *When Survivors Give Birth: understanding and healing the effects of early sexual abuse on childbearing women*. 1st ed. Seattle, WA Classic Day Publishing; 2004.

27 Johnson DM, Pike JL, Chard KM. Factors predicting PTSD, depression, and dissociative severity in female treatment-seeking childhood sexual abuse survivors. *Child Abuse Negl*. 2001; **25**: 179–98.

28 South Community Birth Program. *The South Community Birth Program Final Report: 2003–6*. Vancouver, BC; 2006.

29 MacKinnon K, McIntyre M, Quance M. The meaning of the nurse's presence during childbirth. *J Obstet Gynecol Neonatal Nurs*. 2005; **34**: 28–36.

30 Hunter LP. Being with woman: a guiding concept for the care of laboring women. *J Obstet Gynecol Neonatal Nurs*. 2002; **31**: 650–7.

31 Rosen P. Supporting women in labor: analysis of different types of caregivers. *J Midwifery Womens Health*. 2004; **49**: 24–31.

32 Walsh L. *Midwifery: community-based care during the childbearing year*. Philadelphia: W.B. Saunders; 2001.

33 Pascali-Bonaro D, Kroeger M. Continuous female companionship during childbirth: a crucial resource in times of stress or calm. *J Midwifery Womens Health*. 2004; **49**: 19–27.

34 Hotelling BA. Is your perinatal practice mother-friendly? A strategy for improving maternity care. *Birth.* 2004; **31**: 143–7.

35 Scott KD, Berkowitz G, Klaus M. A comparison of intermittent and continuous support during labor: a meta-analysis. *Am J Obstet Gynecol.* 1999; **180**: 1054–9.

36 Anderson FWJ, Johnson CT. Complementary and alternative medicine in obstetrics. *Int J Gynaecol Obstet.* 2005; **91**: 116–24.

37 Huntley AL, Coon JT, Ernst E. Complementary and alternative medicine for labor pain: a systematic review. *Am J Obstet Gynecol.* 2004; **191**: 36–44.

38 Labrecque M, Nouwen A, Bergeron M, *et al.* A randomized controlled trial of nonpharmacologic approaches for relief of low back pain during labor. *J Fam Pract.* 1999; **48**: 259–63.

39 Higginson WS, Camacho CK. *The Art and Science of Labor Support.* March of Dimes Nursing Module; 2003.

40 Simkin P. Supportive care during labor: a guide for busy nurses. *J Obstet, Gynecol Neonatal Nurs.* 2002; **31**: 721–32.

41 Simonds W. Watching the clock: keeping time during pregnancy, birth, and postpartum experiences. *Soc Sci Med.* 2002; **55**: 559–70.

42 Lowe NK. The nature of labor pain. *Am J Obstet Gynecol.* 2002; **186**: S16–24.

43 Surtees R. Midwifery partnership with women in Aotearoa/New Zealand: a poststructuralist feminist perspective on the use of epidurals in 'normal' birth. In: Stewart M, Hunt SC, editors. *Pregnancy, Birth and Maternity Care: feminist perspective.* 1st ed. Edinburgh: Books for Midwives; 2004. pp. 169–83.

44 Declercq E, Sakala C, Corry M, *et al. Listening to Mothers II: Report of the Second National U.S. Survey of Women's Childbearing Experiences.* New York: Childbirth Connection; 2006 October.

45 Carfoot S, Williamson P, Dickson R. A randomised controlled trial in the north of England examining the effects of skin-to-skin care on breast feeding. *Midwifery.* 2005; **21**: 71–9.

46 Carfoot S, Williamson PR, Dickson R. A systematic review of randomised controlled trials evaluating the effect of mother/baby skin-to-skin care on successful breast feeding. *Midwifery.* 2003; **19**: 148–55.

47 Moore ER, Anderson GC. Randomized controlled trial of very early mother–infant skin-to-skin contact and breastfeeding status. *J Midwifery Womens Health.* 2007; **52**: 116–25.

48 Smith J, Plaat F, Fisk NM. The natural caesarean: a woman-centred technique. *BJOG.* 2008; **115**: 1037–42; discussion 42.

49 Candib LM. The family approach at each moment. *Fam Med.* 1985; **17**: 201–8.

50 Bergus GR, Randall CS, Sinift SD, *et al.* Does the structure of clinical questions affect the outcome of curbside consultations with specialty colleagues? *Arch Fam Med.* 2000; **9**: 541–7.

51 Cetrulo CL, Cetrulo LG. The legal liability of the medical consultant in pregnancy. *Med Clin North Am.* 1989; **73**: 557–65.

52 Olick RS, Bergus GR. Malpractice liability for informal consultations. *Fam Med.* 2003; **35**: 476–81.

53 Coustan DR, Schwartz RM, Gagnon DE, *et al.* The distribution, practice, and attitudes of maternal–fetal medicine specialists. *Am J Obstet Gynecol.* 2001; **185**: 1218–25.

54 Sisson MC, Witcher PM, Stubsten C. The role of the maternal–fetal medicine specialist in high-risk obstetric care. *Crit Care Nurs Clin North Am.* 2004; **16**: 187–91.

55 Wiegers TA, Keirse MJ, van der Zee J, *et al.* Outcome of planned home and planned hospital births in low risk pregnancies: prospective study in midwifery practices in the Netherlands. *BMJ.* 1996; **313**: 1309–13.

56 Anthony S, Buitendijk SE, Offerhaus PM, *et al.* Maternal factors and the probability of a planned home birth. *BJOG.* 2005; **112**: 748–53.

57 Kitzinger S. Letter from Europe: home birth reborn. *Birth.* 2008; **35**: 77–8.

58 Royal College of Obstetricians and Gynaecologists/Royal College of Midwives. Joint statement #2: Home births. 2007 [cited May 18, 2008]. Available from: www.rcog.org. uk/resources/Public/pdf/home_births_rcog_rcm0607.pdf

59 Campbell OM, Graham WJ. Strategies for reducing maternal mortality: getting on with what works. *Lancet.* 2006; **368**: 1284–99.

60 Rosenfield A, Min CJ, Freedman LP. Making motherhood safe in developing countries. *New Eng J Med.* 2007; **356**: 1395–7.

61 Berman DR, Johnson TR, Apgar BS, *et al.* Model of family medicine and obstetrics-gynecology collaboration in obstetric care at the University of Michigan. *Obstet Gynecol.* 2000; **96**: 308–13.

62 Pecci C. A collaborative model for maternity care. 2007 [cited January 5, 2009]. Available from: www.fmdrl.org/index.cfm?event=c.AccessResource&rid=1183

PART FIVE

Prevention and Health Promotion

Most healthy women have healthy pregnancies. Although women in every culture seek medical care during pregnancy, they do so to ensure the best outcomes for themselves and their babies, not because pregnancy represents a disease state.

During standard prenatal care, the routine of frequent medical visits to a clinician makes pregnancy an ideal time to focus on health promotion and disease prevention. Many of the traditional behaviors that clinicians ask of pregnant women are good for general health promotion: e.g. balanced nutrition, avoidance of tobacco and alcohol, adequate rest and exercise. Woman-centered perinatal care includes the recognition that health requires an integrated understanding of the whole person and that health promotion and disease prevention require the collaborative effort of patient and clinician seeking common ground. Prenatal care also usually includes an emphasis on prevention of problems through risk assessment and risk reduction or avoidance. Successful woman-centered care must blend attention to the pregnant woman *and* to the baby and not become fetus-centered care, ignoring the woman in the process.

To pursue a woman-centered model of health promotion during the period before, during, and after pregnancy, clinicians assess these components of the woman's world:

1 eliciting the woman's experience of health and illness, particularly around her sense of responsibility for and control over her own health
2 identifying the woman's potential for health especially with regard to personal goals and values
3 screening for current disease and potential for disease
4 understanding the longitudinal value of the patient–clinician relationship and how each shapes the other's world
5 assessing both the woman's context and the clinician's office context. (Adapted from Stewart, 2003)[1]

We will discuss these components by first addressing pre-conception care, contraception and options counseling; then by reframing obstetric risk assessment and discussing genetic screening. We will offer innovative strategies in prenatal care and education that link to the concept of lifelong empowerment. We will then examine maternity care systems as they affect our ability to deliver woman-centered care and, finally, we will put all the steps of finding common ground together to address lifelong health promotion that can begin as part of pregnancy care.

CHAPTER 1

Pre-conception Care

Sara G. Shields

Earlier in their relationship Siobhan and Danny (*see* Parts Two through Four) used condoms the majority of the time, and had needed emergency contraception only a few times. They chose to use condoms with Plan B as a backup method after Siobhan's medical provider had talked with her about making choices that worked for her. Siobhan felt that the counselor at the family planning clinic was non-judgmental when she said, "It's hard to use condoms all the time; maybe you should have a backup method just in case." Siobhan told Danny that the counselor had even used the metaphor that "people buy car insurance without planning to drive into a tree," and so everyone should have post-coital contraception at home "just in case we need it." Danny felt that was a good plan, and appreciated that no one was blaming him for their occasional contraceptive lapses. After five years together, they decided they felt ready to start a family. Although she did not have regular healthcare to get a pre-conception visit, Siobhan found some information on the internet about getting pregnant and started taking multivitamins.

Woman-centered pre-conception care incorporates the concepts of health promotion and preventive health within the framework of understanding the woman's context and experience. The main barrier to having more opportunities for even the simple step of pre-conception folic acid supplementation is the frequency of unplanned pregnancies around the world. Thus any woman-centered pre-conception strategy should begin with excellent contraceptive care, so that getting pregnant is a deliberate act that a woman chooses and prepares for. Reframing pre-pregnancy care this way avoids treating all women as potentially about to be pregnant, a state that limits their activities on multiple levels. Rather than viewing all women as potential reproducers, woman-centered providers work with young women in anticipation of sexual initiation to understand their choices in contraception and the importance of planning their pregnancies. For women who have method failures or other unintended pregnancies, woman-centered options counseling and access to abortion services are also part of pre-conception care.

Many other pre-conception risks involve characteristics such as tobacco use or obesity that remain refractory to provider-based interventions. Woman-centered care to address these issues means avoiding subtle messages of blaming the woman. The provider considers the broader issues of poverty, racism, and violence that constrict women's capacity to plan pregnancy, choose healthy lifestyles, and effect change such as weight loss, tobacco cessation, or sobriety. Less commonly, for instance for women with chronic illness such as epilepsy or Type I diabetes, specific medical interventions before conception might truly make a difference in their obstetric outcomes. Woman-centered pre-conception care for these women not only follows the recommended guidelines for such interventions but also emphasizes careful contraception counseling. Unfortunately, many of the specialist providers who address the specific management of these diseases do not feel comfortable with addressing sexuality or contraception, but referrals back to the woman's primary provider for pre-conception care may not be priorities for the woman or the specialist. As a result, even for women with chronic diseases, unplanned pregnancies are still an issue.[2-4]

CHAPTER 2

Contraception Counseling

Marji Gold

An emphasis on self-efficacy and empowerment is also important in terms of health promotion around fertility planning. Woman-centered providers address options for choosing a method, having a backup strategy, considering the partner's plan and the woman's own life plan, and understanding the available resources.

> Six months after Joshua's birth, Jackie (*see* Parts Two, Three, and Four) came in for a visit to check her blood pressure. Her provider Judith, remembering that Jackie had never decided on a birth control method after Joshua's birth, asked now about that. Jackie replied that at this point in her life she did not want to have any more children, but she did not want to have more surgery either, and she was not sure if she would want to have children in the future. She did not want a method that might interfere with sexual spontaneity, nor one with hormones. After discussing her options, Jackie decided on an intrauterine device (IUD). Judith asked her to come back the following week to have it placed.

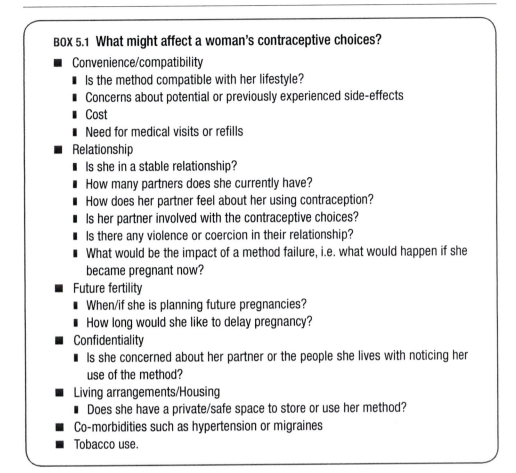

BOX 5.1 **What might affect a woman's contraceptive choices?**

- Convenience/compatibility
  - Is the method compatible with her lifestyle?
  - Concerns about potential or previously experienced side-effects
  - Cost
  - Need for medical visits or refills
- Relationship
  - Is she in a stable relationship?
  - How many partners does she currently have?
  - How does her partner feel about her using contraception?
  - Is her partner involved with the contraceptive choices?
  - Is there any violence or coercion in their relationship?
  - What would be the impact of a method failure, i.e. what would happen if she became pregnant now?
- Future fertility
  - When/if she is planning future pregnancies?
  - How long would she like to delay pregnancy?
- Confidentiality
  - Is she concerned about her partner or the people she lives with noticing her use of the method?
- Living arrangements/Housing
  - Does she have a private/safe space to store or use her method?
- Co-morbidities such as hypertension or migraines
- Tobacco use.

Contraception is a continuum of choices made up of a variety of effective methods of pregnancy prevention that are related to the timing of sexual intercourse. Understanding the woman's plans for future or near future childbearing affects the choice of method also. Permanent methods such as male and female sterilization, as well as long-term but reversible methods such as IUDs, do not require the woman to remember to use them. All the other methods involve some active participation by the woman herself. To frame an explanation of how different methods work, the provider can describe them to the woman in relation to three different times: pre-coital, intra-coital, and post-coital.

Kerry (*see* Parts Two, Three, and Four) began dating Ron in college and wanted foolproof contraception then. When she went to her primary care doctor, she was pleased that the doctor started the visit with a discussion of confidentiality – how she recognized that it was a small community and that she knew how important it was for Kerry to receive medical care in a place that respected and protected her private decisions. The doctor presented Kerry with several options, helping her imagine how each one would work with her lifestyle and her need to keep her sexual activity hidden from her parents and family. Kerry wanted a very effective method, since she did not believe she could have an abortion if she got pregnant accidentally. She chose to take the pill, since her doctor had explained that she would be able to get refills if she just called the office, and so the pills were easier for her than using the injection, and she did not want anything like an IUD that would stay inside her body.

Apart from sterilization, **pre-coital contraceptives** include IUDs and hormonal methods. Hormonal methods – injections or implants of long-acting hormones, birth control pills, the contraceptive patch, and the vaginal ring – all require a woman's active participation. She must remember them at times when she may not be sexually active. Their advantage is that they do not interfere with sexual activity, and some may be kept private from her sexual partner if necessary.

Intra-coital contraceptives include condoms (male and female), the diaphragm, and the cervical cap. Women choosing intra-coital methods must be willing to think about and be able to actively use their contraception immediately before and/or during sexual activity. Consistent condom use also requires the complete cooperation of the woman's partner, which she cannot always guarantee. Moreover, condoms do break and fall off. Immediate access to "emergency contraception" or EC is a logical complement to intra-coital methods.

Post-coital contraception is another way of describing emergency contraception, also commonly known as the "morning-after pill." Although an IUD can prevent unintended pregnancy if it is inserted within five days of unprotected sex, most people think of hormonal pills for post-coital contraception. The woman-centered provider helps women see that this method is a responsible choice in the continuum of pregnancy prevention. Because of systems problems (e.g. inability to pay for, fill or refill a prescription for oral contraceptives), or changes in contraceptive plans between office visits, many women require EC for unplanned or unprotected intercourse. In many countries, EC is legally available over the counter, but in the United States as of 2009 it is only available without prescription to women over 18, and then only at some pharmacies.[5] Where EC is not accessible to sexually active women under 18 using intra-coital methods, providers should offer prescriptions for EC frequently. A woman-centered approach dispels the beliefs that needing such contraception makes a woman promiscuous or irresponsible and in fact supports a woman's efforts to prevent unintended pregnancy in whatever way makes the most sense in the context of her life and her personal beliefs.

After Erika's birth, Kerry worried that with her busy schedule she might miss doses of oral contraceptives. She was glad to hear that other hormonal options were possible even while breastfeeding. She knew Ron was anxious to have another child soon. After discussing her choices, she opted for the hormone-infused vaginal ring, deciding that even though the manufacturer listed this device as "safety unknown" during lactation, the hormones in it were the same as those in standard birth control pills.

Alexandra was a teenager who did not want her parents finding out that she was going to start to have sex. She said she and her boyfriend would probably have sex at his cousin's house. She seriously considered an IUD, but ultimately decided to try the long-acting medroxyprogesterone injection.

For women dealing with issues of violence and abuse, woman-centered contraception care is especially important. Understanding issues of control for the abused woman starts even before pregnancy with pregnancy planning, contraception, and pre-conception care, keeping in mind that sexual intercourse is not consensual for many abused women and that abusive men may try to exercise complete control over a woman's fertility. Coitus-dependent contraceptive methods such as diaphragms and condoms may not be within a woman's control, and some abusers will even sabotage their partner's birth-control methods to maintain control, by throwing out her pills or damaging her diaphragm.[6] For women who are in abusive relationships, long-acting birth control methods such as progesterone injections or implants or an IUD may be the only way to prevent an unintended pregnancy and actually allow the woman control over her reproduction. Discussing abuse issues during contraceptive care is vital for effective pregnancy planning.

CHAPTER 3

Options Counseling

Sara G. Shields

Delia (*see* Part Three) knew she did not want to get pregnant, but contraception and getting an IUD placed had never seemed to be a priority during her visits, which focused instead on keeping her free of drugs and taking care of her son. When she discovered she was pregnant for the fourth time, Maureen was the first person she told. Maureen suggested Delia talk to one of the providers about her options with this pregnancy. Delia was not sure she wanted another child. However, after meeting with Dr. Adelle Epps and talking about having an abortion or having another child, Delia decided to continue with the pregnancy.

Woman-centered options counseling challenges providers to remain non-judgmental and supportive in assisting a woman like Delia through the crisis of unintended

Where Are Your Right Now?

Imagine that the line below contains all the ways you could feel about the best choice for you. Where are you today? Put an X on the point on the line.

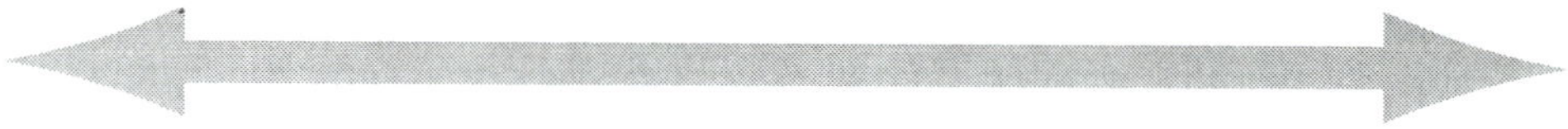

100% sure I
want to continue
my pregnancy

100% sure I
want to have
an abortion

FIGURE 5.1 Where are you right now?[7:3]

pregnancy even when her decision goes against what the provider thinks is her best interest. This particular challenge is well suited to the model of finding common ground.

Centering on the values of empowerment, dignity, informed choice, and self-determination, the woman-centered provider addresses feelings, ideas, function or context, and expectations when exploring options with a woman undecided about her pregnancy. Using a pictorial representation (*see* Figure 5.1)[7:3] of a woman's initial feelings about continuing or ending the pregnancy may be helpful to start the conversation, with further questions guided by the individual woman's responses and needs (*see* Box 5.2). The woman-centered provider pays close attention to denial and ambivalence as emotions that may be especially strong and are also particularly important for the woman to accept and work through as part of her decision-making.

BOX 5.2 Starting Points[8]

- How are you feeling about this pregnancy?
- Prior to finding out you were pregnant, what were your feelings about abortion/adoption/parenting?
- Under what circumstances do you believe abortion, adoption, parenting is okay? Not okay? Why?
- Under what circumstances would you like to become a parent?
- What are your goals for the next year? Five years? How would each alternative help or hinder the achievement of these goals?
- What part of your circumstances frightens you the most?
- What is the worst thing you think might happen?
- How would you like things to turn out for you ideally?
- It can be helpful to some women to look at what they believe and separate that from what they have been taught to believe. "You've said what your church's/boyfriend's/parent's beliefs are. Could you tell me more about what you yourself believe at this time in your life?"

Sorting Out Feelings

The idea of becoming a parent makes me feel ___ because ___.

The idea of having an abortion makes me feel ___ because___.

The idea of arranging for an adoption makes me feel ___ because___.

(Reproduced with the kind permission of Elsevier.)

The woman-centered provider's other task throughout this process is to offer accurate information about alternatives. As part of this conversation, the provider needs to understand the woman's context including, at the moment of diagnosis, whom she plans to tell first or involve in her decision and, later on, who knows about her pregnancy so far. Once she mentions specific people, the provider can review either how she thinks these people will react or how they have already reacted and how supportive they have been. If she has kept the pregnancy a secret or intends to, she may not yet have fully explored her options.[8] This knowledge about her context then leads into discussing her ideas and expectations by asking, "What have you heard from these people about your choices? What questions do you have about your choices?" These questions allow further information-sharing to center on the individual woman's needs and knowledge gaps.

In the finding common ground process, the provider and woman clarify mutual goals and roles (*see* Table 5.1). As part of this, the provider revisits how a woman feels when she considers each of her choices. One of the most challenging aspects of options counseling for providers is staying neutral and non-directive. To best do this, a woman-centered provider needs to be clear about his or her own values around the various options and to understand how these values may affect the counseling process.[8]

TABLE 5.1 Options Counseling

	Woman	Provider
Problem	Crisis of unintended pregnancy.	Difficulty in keeping personal values and biases out of the counseling process.
Goals	Make a decision and act on it.	Empower and provide support; stay disinterested while acknowledging one's own values.
Roles	Define how the pregnancy is a problem; explore options.	Listen actively, know and give accurate information; assist the woman; help her feel she is not alone; respond neutrally; stay connected through decision and afterwards, regardless of her choice.

Particularly when reacting to a woman's responses, the woman-centered provider remains vigilant about staying neutral, with phrases such as "Tell me more what is concerning you" or "It is common for women to have mixed feelings about this" or "Some other women I work with have made this decision. How would that work for you?"[8] Some questions that further foster this exploration are in Box 5.2.[8]

Regardless of what a pregnant woman chooses about continuing her pregnancy, her woman-centered provider respects her decision. If the counseling provider at the moment of decision is also the woman's primary caregiver, then he or she will support the next stage, either doing post-abortion care or continuing prenatal care or facilitating adoption if she chooses to keep the pregnancy and release the baby. Woman-centered care at this time also involves working with the pregnant woman around choices of when and if to tell her family. Such work may include referrals for assistance if the family reaction leaves her without housing or financial support. If the provider also cares for other members of the woman's family and the woman wants them to be aware of her decision, the family-oriented provider can help the family take the "long view," for instance, reminding a young woman's mother that she herself was pregnant at 16. The woman-centered provider familiar with the woman's family also explicitly guarantees the confidentiality of her decision if she chooses to have an abortion and not tell her family.

CHAPTER 4

Woman-Centered Risk Assessment

Josephine Fowler, Sara G. Shields, and Lucy M. Candib

A woman who has chosen this pregnancy or decides to keep an unplanned pregnancy enters the prenatal care system with both strengths and risks. Screening for risks, a key component of health promotion and prevention in woman-centered care, must involve careful history-taking and not just routine blood work. While many risk-scoring systems assess for biomedical pathologies in an attempt to identify women at high risk for poor perinatal outcomes, psychosocial factors such as abuse, depression, and lack of social support turn out to be better predictors of such outcomes or of the need for interventions. Thus the screening history must include such psychosocial issues, including the relational, psychological, and sexual histories, often ignored in strictly biomedical approaches.

> Sabrina was a 26-year-old Haitian woman with diabetes who entered prenatal care at nine weeks of gestation at the University Hospital obstetrical clinic. She lived with her husband, father-in-law, aunt, and younger sister. Both her parents had died in Haiti after she had migrated three years ago. Her husband worked full-

time, and Sabrina stayed home with her family who "helped take care of her." Both Sabrina and her husband reported no history of tobacco, alcohol, or drug use, and no history of physical or emotional abuse. Her husband related that Sabrina had witnessed her brother's death in Haiti. They attended church "unless she's sick." According to her husband, Sabrina spoke English and Creole, but he did all the talking during the interview. (*See* full vignette in Appendix.)

RISK ASSESSMENT

Risk assessment is defined as the evaluation of human activities – medical, psychological, social, socioeconomic, and environmental – and their impact on the perinatal outcome for mother, infant, and family. Any development during the ongoing pregnancy may affect the ultimate outcome and lead to increasing morbidity and risk of mortality; therefore, risk assessment continues throughout the pregnancy and throughout the postnatal period. A woman-centered approach to risk assessment complements the traditional obstetric list with both an assessment of psychosocial factors and with an assessment of the strengths that women and their families bring to the process of care. As will become clear, the case of Sabrina contains multiple medical and psychosocial risk factors for both mother and baby, but even the basic history enables us to make a preliminary assessment (*see* Table 5.2).

TABLE 5.2 Prenatal Risk and Strength Assessment

Initial medical risk factors	Other risk factors	Strengths
Risk of hemoglobinopathy for Sabrina's racial group.	Death of Sabrina's parents in Haiti since her immigration.	Early prenatal care.
Incomplete history (immunizations, tuberculin testing status, etc.).	Witnessing her brother's death.	Intact couple, husband involved, with some extended family and support (evidenced by church involvement).
	Lack of primary care.	Bilinguality of at least one family member and possibly Sabrina.
	Unemployment.	Husband is employed.
	Unclear why family needs to take care of her.	
	Unclear why husband does all the talking.	
	Unclear immigration status.	

The resident working at the obstetrics clinic, Dr. Mary Thibeault, was able to use an interpreter to learn more of Sabrina's medical history. In Haiti they had lived too far from a doctor to get medical care. Since immigrating, Sabrina reported, "I take some pills for my sugar." Her husband recalled that "she had some infection in the last two years that caused her to cry, yell, and scream at us," and required a brief hospitalization in the local hospital two to three times. On discharge from the hospital, she had been given medication, but they did not now recall the name. She stopped taking the medication once she started to feel better.

Dr. Thibeault suspected that Sabrina had uncontrolled diabetes, among her many other problems. The resident sought help from Dr. Greg Diamond, the clinic supervisor that day, with her worries about the complexity of Sabrina's issues. He supported her plan to get screening blood tests, and pushed her to consider Sabrina from a strength-based perspective (*see* Table 5.3).

TABLE 5.3 Ongoing Prenatal Risk and Strength Assessment

Additional medical risk factors	Additional psychosocial risk factors	Additional strengths
Presumed diabetes, unclear control.	Unknown literacy and education levels.	Prior contact with Western medical system.
Recent infections?	Probable poverty (low-income status).	Prior experience with taking medication.
Possible psychiatric illness.		Family involvement with hospitalization.
Unknown medications.		
Inconsistent medication use.		

Dr. Thibeault suggested that Sabrina have some specific prenatal testing done. The results showed the following:

Random blood glucose 256 mg/dl (14.22 mmol/liter)
HbA1c 11.0% (average blood glucose 314 mg/dl or 17.5 mmol/l)
Creatinine 1.0 mg/dl (88.4 µmol/l)
Blood type: O negative
HIV: negative
Tuberculin skin testing: negative
Hemoglobin electrophoresis: Hgb AS

Sabrina's confirmed diagnoses of uncontrolled diabetes and sickle cell trait raised her anxiety. This increased tension made her family more fearful that Sabrina's mental illness might recur either during or after the pregnancy. Nonetheless, with the assistance of the public health nurses and advocates, Sabrina kept all her appointments with Dr. Thibeault.

Sabrina had five years of primary education and could read numbers and dates and simple instructions. Her husband had a legal work permit, but Sabrina did not have legal resident status. Nevertheless, she was open in developing a relationship Dr. Thibeault, who assured her that keeping these appointments would give her the best chance to stay healthy herself and have a healthy baby. Sabrina liked the fact that Dr. Thibeault had a French name even though she did not speak French. For her part, Dr. Thibeault was pleased that Sabrina came for all her appointments, smiling and looking happy to see Dr. Thibeault. Coming to the clinic, she thought, was one of Sabrina's strengths. But the resident worried about how to follow up on Sabrina's many problems. Dr. Diamond suggested that Dr. Thibeault involve the perinatal team in the high-risk clinic, which could provide a comprehensive approach to diabetic education, nutrition counseling, and social work, and could facilitate genetics and psychiatric consultations, all assisted by the French Creole interpreter.

TABLE 5.4 Mid-pregnancy Risk and Strength Assessment

Medical risk factors	Other risk factors	Strengths
Poorly controlled diabetes in first trimester and likely prior to conception.	Undocumented immigrant.	Strong connection with primary care physician and team.
Rh negative.		Success in keeping appointments.
Hemoglobin AS (sickle trait).		Ability to read and write numbers and dates.
		Husband's legal status.

Many of the obstetrical and perinatal risks to Sabrina and her infant are obvious at her first prenatal visit, and many others emerge during the course of her care. Based on this multifactorial risk and strength assessment, Dr. Thibeault, supervised by Dr. Diamond, offers interventions personalized to Sabrina's needs, using an integrated team to address her complicated psychological context as well as standard medical practices such as blood work, genetic counseling, and ultrasound (*see* Box 5.3).

Keeping a strength-based approach will assist the team caring for Sabrina to see her multiple issues in the rich and complex context of her life experience. A strictly risk-based approach, on the other hand, consistently views pregnancy itself as a high-risk event, a catastrophe always around the corner. Prenatal care then turns into a continuous hunt for pathology while overlooking the woman's biopsychosocial strengths and capabilities. Medical slang refers to patients with many problems as "trainwrecks" – implying that the accidents have already happened and that prevention is hopeless. In contrast, Dr. Diamond encourages the resident and the team caring for Sabrina to approach her problems by close collaboration, relationship building, and taking advantage of her strengths and those of her family.

BOX 5.3 Projected Interventions for Sabrina's Risks and Strengths

- Use of French Creole interpreter
- Nutrition evaluation and education
- Diabetic teaching and assessment of self-care skills
- Further evaluation of renal function
- Obtaining old records
- Counseling regarding risks of congenital anomaly, potential genetics consult
- Blood type and hemoglobin electrophoresis for husband, Rhogam at 28 weeks if he is Rh+, genetics counseling if he has sickle trait as well

- Ongoing antenatal surveillance (explanation and permission for ultrasound, amniocentesis, fetal echocardiogram)
- Psychiatric consultation and ongoing psychiatric follow-up about potential for depression
- Social worker consultation regarding immigration issues and insurance coverage
- High-risk obstetrics consultation.

Although Sabrina's diabetes control improved, her HgbA1c remained around 8.0. At 38 weeks an ultrasound showed her baby weighed almost 8.5 pounds (3.9 kg). After talking with Dr. Diamond, Dr. Thibeault called the interpreter to help her explain the risks of a big baby at delivery, and Sabrina agreed to proceed toward delivery. After a short induction, she delivered a nine-pound (4 kg) boy named Josue who had minor hypoglycemia that resolved with feeding. The staff encouraged her to breastfeed and explained that this would help lower her blood glucose. Sabrina and her family were happy with the good outcome and appreciated all of the team's efforts. As Dr. Thibeault was going off call after the delivery, the family presented her with a painting from Haiti.

TABLE 5.5 Initial Postpartum Risk and Strength Assessment

Medical risk factors	Other risk factors	Ongoing strengths
Risk of newborn hypoglycemia after maternal diabetes.	Medical team's lack of knowledge of Haitian cultural approaches to childcare, feeding, and health care practices.	Normal delivery without complications with healthy term newborn.
	Sabrina's uncertain knowledge regarding lactation.	Nurses' encouraging early feeding as treatment for mild hypoglycemia.
		Hospital and provider with resources to assist with initial lactation efforts.
		Availability of cross-cultural interpreter services for immediate postpartum care.

The morning after delivery, the nursing staff paged the obstetrical team because Sabrina began yelling and throwing utensils at the visitors and staff and shouting at her husband. Dr. Thibeault could not calm her down either, so she called the hospital psychiatrist to evaluate Sabrina for risk of harm to herself and to her baby. Dr. Thibeault had never seen a woman with an immediate postpartum psychosis – it was more frightening to her than many obstetrical emergencies that she had seen and managed. She was greatly relieved when the on-call psychiatrist came immediately. The psychiatry consultant recommended antipsychotic and antidepressant medication, and within 24 hours Sabrina no longer appeared to be a risk to herself or the baby. The nurses also called the social worker to assess whether baby Josue would be safe at home. The social worker suggested to Dr. Thibeault that the team notify the child protective services agency to do a home evaluation. After an additional day of observation during which Sabrina's milk came in and her psychological status stabilized, Sabrina and Josue went home with her family with plans to follow up with Dr. Thibeault, the behavioral health team, and the public health team. The immediate plans included ongoing diabetes care, management of depression, parenting education, newborn education, postpartum education, and contraceptive counseling. Josue was scheduled for a visit within three days to assess breastfeeding and weight gain and maternal and family adjustment.

TABLE 5.6 Ongoing Postpartum Risk and Strength Assessment

Medical risk factors	Other risk factors	Ongoing strengths
Postpartum psychiatric illness.	Previous inconsistent medication use for psychiatric problem.	Easily managed apparently psychotic symptoms enabling mother and baby to go home together with family.
Ongoing adult diabetes risks.	Previous inconsistent self-care for diabetes.	Easy access to supportive consultants and social services.
Family planning needs.	Departure from hospital without a clear contraceptive method.	Availability of a wide variety of supportive and educational services.
Taking psychiatric medications during lactation.		Sabrina's and her family's ability to make strong linkages with clinical teams and physicians.
		Sabrina's motivation to become and stay healthy for the baby's sake.
		Ongoing strengths listed in Tables 5.2–5.4

Woman-centered risk assessment in pregnancy thus emphasizes a strength-based assessment through the process of integrating both traditional medical risks and psychosocial risks, and connecting this interactively with inquiry about the woman's self-perception of risk. This latter step is essential because women perceive risk in pregnancy differently from providers, as Stahl and Hundley note: "Health-care practitioners, on the one hand, tend to rely heavily on epidemiological assumptions in discussing risk. Women's understanding of risk, on the other hand, tends to be far more contextual, individualized and embedded in their social environment and everyday lives."[9]

Self-perception of risk is important to understand for at least two reasons: first, women with a high-risk label are more likely to have negative psychosocial state scores than women who see themselves as low-risk,[9] as Sabrina does in terms of fear and anxiety related to her medical illnesses during pregnancy. Second, self-perception may affect a woman's capacity or motivation for behavior change.[10] In a provider-centered assessment of risk, providers may focus more on medical diagnoses at the exclusion, for example, critical non-biomedical factors, and not recognize the dichotomy between a woman's own risk assessment and her provider's assessment, with subsequent struggles in both creating and achieving treatment plans.[11] A woman-centered approach understands the need to explore fully how a woman understands her own risk, and how to provide education and information in approaches that acknowledge her true worries and help her modify her health-related behaviors.

Doing woman-centered risk is more than just including the woman's self-perception, however. Multiple issues complicate even this extension of standard risk-assessment practices.

➤ Traditional obstetric risk scores do not predict poor outcomes accurately.[12]

➤ These outcomes may not be well defined either for mother or baby, and parents may perceive outcomes differently from providers (*see* Box 5.4).

➤ Otherwise healthy women may get flagged as high risk with potential adverse outcomes.

➤ Psychosocial factors such as poverty and social support may have more impact on preterm birth than medical factors.

➤ Interventions to ameliorate identified risk may not change outcomes or may be too complex to implement or measure.

BOX 5.4 Possible Poor Outcomes to Measure when Assessing Risk

For the fetus/baby:
- Congenital anomaly
- Intrauterine fetal demise
- Neonatal loss
- Prematurity (including "late preterm" infants at 35 to 37 weeks)[13]
- Low birth weight
- Failure to thrive
- Poor mother–child attachment
- Other neonatal morbidity
- Perinatal mortality
- Infant mortality.

For the mother:
- Premature delivery
- Delivery complication (this used to include cesarean delivery, but now with high cesarean rates, this form of delivery can hardly be called a complication, but rather an expected intervention)
- Maternal morbidity
- Maternal mortality
- Postpartum complications, including postpartum depression
- Short inter-pregnancy interval
- Unsuccessful breastfeeding.

Furthermore, rote use of a standardized risk checklist (as is common in obstetrical care) depersonalizes and decontextualizes the woman's experience, which may lead providers not only to overlook her individual strengths but also to blame her for behaviors that have multidimensional explanations, as in Sabrina's case.[14] Woman-centered risk assessment weaves support and reassurance into an interactive process between woman and provider, regardless of what is checked off on a form.[9] A woman-centered provider determines pregnancy risk "with" women and not "for" women."[11] The question "Is there anything about your health or your life that you think puts you at risk for this pregnancy?" can open up fruitful areas for discussion.

For other women whose problems are less obvious than Sabrina's, risk assessment can be a challenge to woman-centered care. Extensive research addresses how to identify women in early or mid pregnancy with medical risk factors for any of the later serious obstetrical complications in order to avert the problem. The glucola challenge test to detect early gestational diabetes (GDM) is one familiar prediction/prevention strategy, but there is some debate about its usefulness in changing outcomes.[15,16] Demonstration of the utility of the glucola challenge has been slow to emerge, and is confounded by many false positives that in themselves suggest some impaired glucose tolerance. Nevertheless, proving that something could be done about abnormal tests has been much more difficult. Does knowing that someone has or is at risk for gestational diabetes enable us to prevent a pregnancy or neonatal complication? Or, put another way, if dietary change can keep a woman euglycemic, will that reduce her risk?[17] And how successful are we in promoting dietary change?

At the other extreme, we know that alcohol and tobacco use in pregnancy are associated with definite complications, but even when we know the predictive nature of these risk factors for neonatal morbidity, we still lack proven strategies for halting these risks. In contrast, treatment of infection during pregnancy (HIV, syphilis, gonorrhea) definitely reduces the risk of fetal and neonatal infection. In short, there are risk factors we can identify and treat (infection), risk factors we can try to identify in advance but not necessarily have success in treating (GDM), and risk factors we can identify but not change at all.

Many immutable non-medical factors are associated with higher risks of the above biological complications (age, race, social class, race, ethnicity, education, immigration status). Prior obstetrical, gynecological, and medical problems are obvious predictors that require management but cannot be averted. Sabrina's pre-existing diabetes and psychiatric illness are among the problems that must be considered serious risks to both her and her baby's well-being. Along with problematic substance use, other psychosocial risks are difficult to establish and even more difficult to treat: intimate partner violence, low social support (social isolation), and depression are among the obvious. Low social support early in pregnancy is also, in itself, a risk factor for depression and poor quality of life in pregnancy.[18]

As Sabrina's story demonstrates, combinations of risks pose even more complex problems: the pregnant woman with pre-existing diabetes who smokes and is depressed; the non-English-speaking socially isolated grand multiparous immigrant woman who gets no prenatal care out of fear of bills and detection of her a woman's undocumented status; or the woman with pre-eclampsia whose partner abuses her physically; the minority woman with a prior stillbirth who lives in a sector without public transportation, accessible medical care, or adequate grocery stores. The interaction between such variables is complex; for instance, one study found lower birth weights among pregnant women with low support who smoked but no significant difference in birth weight between women smokers and non-smokers with high support.[18] Low support by itself was associated with a 200 g reduction of birth weight (excluding prematurity); and women with low and medium support in early pregnancy had almost twice the frequency of pregnancy complications as women with high social support.[18]

Overall, then, risk in pregnancy has three components: a review of a woman's medical and personal history to identify issues that may make a poor perinatal outcome more likely for her; a discussion of potentially unsafe behaviors or exposures to avoid during pregnancy; and a discussion of risk derived from standard screening tests that attempt to identify treatable problems and prevent adverse outcomes. The second issue is pertinent to both lay and medical people who interact with pregnant women or potentially pregnant women. The third is particularly relevant for woman-centered providers when they offer genetic testing either via blood samples, ultrasounds, or both.

Woman-centered care needs to avoid the common trap of "distortion of risk when the fetus is in the room"[19] with fetus-centered risk "trumping" all other possible risks or considerations. For example, a pregnant woman with acute abdominal pain that is likely to be appendicitis may receive inappropriate treatment if her providers focus on the small risk of radiation exposure to the fetus at the expense of avoiding the necessary diagnostic x-rays for the mother's health.[19] Employers remove any reproductive-age women from jobs with poorly understood occupational exposures. Hearing simplistic one-sided messages from the media and other lay sources about medicines in pregnancy, women with medical illnesses such as asthma, seizures, or depression often stop taking medications necessary for their own health when they learn that they are pregnant.

To avoid risk distortion, woman-centered providers need to use numerical data to seek informed decision-making within the context of an individual woman's life and values. Rather than dichotomizing risk or blindly applying a single standard of care, this approach permits women to choose from a "range of reasonable options" that compare a continuum of risks.[19]

Such issues become particularly pertinent in the discussion of risks and benefits for women considering invasive genetic testing during pregnancy, as will be discussed in the next chapter. Here again, woman-centered risk assessment considers the woman's context and values, developing a multidimensional framework that personalizes and empowers each woman in her choices in these complicated medical arenas.

CHAPTER 5

Genetic Testing

Joan M. Bedinghaus

The burgeoning technologies of genetics can present some special challenges for woman-centered maternity care. This section will discuss an approach to prenatal genetic testing using all five components of the patient-centered clinical method – understanding the woman's experience, finding common ground, considering lifelong health promotion goals, elucidating the family context beyond the biomedical pedigree, and acknowledging the patient-provider relationship that influences the care.

> Larisa referred Melissa and Kirk (*see* Parts One through Four) to the local perinatal center for first trimester genetic testing. The following week they were back in Larisa's office to discuss the abnormal results. They were panicking about the possibility of Down syndrome; Melissa was tearful while Kirk was trying to keep a stiff upper lip. Larisa planned a long visit and calmed them with a description of the statistical uncertainties of the testing. They discussed the options of chorionic villous sampling or waiting a few more weeks to have an amniocentesis as early as possible by the perinatologist who came to their town once every two weeks for consultation. They decided on the latter option to minimize risks. Larisa arranged the consultation and alerted the specialist to the couple's high anxiety level. Although Melissa had some cramping immediately after the amniocentesis, she tolerated it, but then they faced the waiting period for the final results. They both poured themselves into their work during this time to avoid having to worry too much. Finally the results returned normal.

> When Rosa came for her 16-week visit, Dr. Rosen asked if she had any questions about the quadruple screen that was explained in a Spanish patient education handout in the prenatal packet. Rosa smiled, "No, doctor." Filling out the lab order form, Dr. Rosen then asked if anyone in Rosa's family had had any babies with the specific birth defects for which the test would screen. Rosa hesitated a bit, but said no. He next asked if Rosa would want an amniocentesis if the test were

abnormal. Rosa looked blankly at him and said in Spanish, "I don't understand." Dr. Rosen decided then to find Lupe to help describe the possible next steps of the test in Spanish. Rosa, on hearing that one step was to insert a needle in her uterus, looked astonished, and began to shake her head no. Lupe, translating for Dr. Rosen, also mentioned the choice that some women make to have an abortion if the testing proved abnormal. Rosa looked a little perplexed when Dr. Rosen then asked, "Do you want this blood test today?" since she thought that any blood test the doctor was offering must have been necessary and not a choice. Lupe asked him to help clarify why Rosa got a choice about having the test, unlike the other blood work she had earlier in pregnancy, and Dr. Rosen realized that he had to explain that some women who know they do not want to abort choose not to have this particular blood test so that they do not have to worry about the possibility of incorrect results. Still a little puzzled, Rosa eventually chose to have the screen done.

EXPLORING BOTH THE DISEASE AND THE ILLNESS EXPERIENCE

Some women are aware of problems that run in their families, and may have already thought long and hard about the implications of testing and the outcome of an affected pregnancy. For others, the identification of risk may be a profound shock.

Some forms of screening for anomalies and genetic disorders have become such a routine part of prenatal care that women may undergo such testing without a considered discussion of the implication of abnormal results. Yet maternal serum screening for neural tube defects and trisomy has significant false positive (5–10%) and false-negative (10–20%) rates.[20,21] A more complex screening strategy has recently been adopted in some maternity care settings that combines ultrasound (for nuchal translucence) and serum marker testing (for free beta-HCG and pregnancy-associated plasma protein A) at 11–13 weeks with quadruple screening at 15–18 weeks.[22,23] Waiting until both first and second-trimester measurements are completed to calculate an overall risk result detects 95% of affected pregnancies with a 4% false-positive rate. The strategy of offering chorionic villus sampling to women with an abnormal first-trimester screen has a slightly higher false-positive rate (4.9%), but the pregnant woman usually prefers earlier identification of an affected pregnancy. Both of these strategies, with their multiple parts needing specific timing and the need for specially-trained ultrasonographers, can be problematic to implement and also require that women enter prenatal care early enough in the first trimester to have time to explain and arrange for the testing.

Most women and indeed many clinicians do not have a good understanding of the concepts of risk, false-positive and false-negative tests, and uncertainty in medical decision-making.[24-26] Chorionic villus sampling and amniocentesis provide a yes-or-no answer, but screening tests produce a probability. The interpretation of that probability depends in part on the ease of imagining the outcome (e.g. if the woman knows a child with a neural tube defect) as well as by the way the risk is presented.[24] The communication of the probability of having an *affected* child results in a perception of higher risk and more decisions to proceed with further testing than the converse, if the clinician presents the probability of having an *unaffected* child. The woman's estimate of her own risk prior to any counseling is the strongest predictor of her post-counseling interpretation of risk.[27] Patients and providers comprehend risk more readily when risk is expressed as natural frequencies or rates (e.g. "Five or six per thousand pregnancies of 35-year-old women are affected by a chromosomal defect.") than as percentages or risk ratios.[24,28,29] Clinicians may calculate risk objectively, but patients understand it in very individual and personal ways.[30] Referring to the customary practice of recommending amniocentesis when the risk of Down syndrome is the same as the risk of a miscarriage provoked by amniocentesis, Berkowitz expressed the woman's viewpoint beautifully:[31:1447]

> There may be inherent appeal when beneficence (detecting an anomaly) and malfeasance (causing an iatrogenic pregnancy loss) are quantitatively matched. However, the more germane question is whether a 0.5% risk of losing a normal pregnancy is the same as a 0.5% chance that the fetus has Down syndrome.
>
> These rates may be the same, but the adverse outcomes are very different. For some patients who have struggled with infertility for years the thought of losing a karyotypically normal fetus may be devastating, whereas raising a child with Down syndrome is less concerning. For others, the notion of having a developmentally disabled child may be overwhelming, whereas fears of being able to conceive another pregnancy are not as relevant. These 2 data points are not equivalent in any meaningful sense, other than being numerically identical.

Thus the woman-centered provider avoids blindly equating outcomes that may feel vastly different for each woman, such as her risk of having an infant with Down syndrome, compared with her risk of pregnancy complications from invasive testing. The usual genetic screening discussion for women over 35 needs to avoid a cookbook approach and assess more completely, for example, the feelings and values of a 35-year-old multiparous woman who in her first pregnancy in her twenties accepted the clinical recommendation for an amniocentesis after an abnormal maternal serum marker screen and then miscarried a normal fetus.

Once a doubt has been raised about the health of the pregnancy, the workup and the wait for confirmatory test results often take several agonizing weeks. If the test proves to be a false positive, the pregnant woman may resent having been "put through" the process. However, studies looking at whether women who have undergone a workup for a false-positive test are likely to refuse testing if subsequent pregnancies have yielded inconsistent results.[32,33] Even when subsequent testing reveals no abnormality, the pregnancy may afterwards be experienced as "damaged" or at risk.[34,35] Melissa and Kirk are well educated and informed, but are still panic-stricken when their prenatal screen is positive. Their apparent faith in technology helps them be comforted by reassuring results in subsequent testing.

Conversely, women may perceive a normal screening test as a guarantee of a healthy baby,[30,34] when in fact the false-negative rates are also significant (4% for integrated first and second-trimester screening). Frank [36] recounts his own experience as a family physician with a family that was initially angry at the birth of a child with Down syndrome after being reassured by normal serum marker screening.

In many healthcare systems, clinicians automatically refer women with potential genetic risks, including those who are at risk simply because of their age, directly to genetic counselors to discuss in more detail their family histories and risk issues. Such referrals can facilitate a thorough evaluation in a setting that allows more time for explanation and education than many busy clinicians may have. Trained genetic counselors practice non-directive counseling, in which they explain risks and present options but avoid pushing any particular decision on the pregnant woman or couple. Before making such automatic referrals, a woman-centered clinician should explore, at least in brief, what each woman already knows and expects about choices in care based on such counseling. [37] Such discussion may need to begin pre-conception if individual risks warrant, or at least early in the pregnancy to allow time for exploring values and choices well before the urgency of advancing gestational age demands rapid decision-making. Ideally, the clinician will know the genetic counselors' approaches and have open communication with them in order to keep the discussions as woman-centered as possible.

Women like Rosa are unlikely to be familiar with the idea of a false-positive test, as well as with the amniocentesis procedure or with an understanding of why a genetics consultation might be indicated. Conversely, the genetic counselor may neither be familiar with the cultural considerations affecting the woman's decision-making[25,38] nor have the trust and understanding that have developed in a long-term patient–clinician relationship. [39] Genetic counselors' non-directive stance may not suit the needs of ethnic minority and immigrant women. Browner analyzed the communication between genetic counselors and immigrant women from Mexico concerning amniocentesis following abnormal alpha-fetoprotein (AFP) results. In addition to misunderstanding medical jargon and having problems with translation, many of the women indicated that "the counselor's reluctance to directly recommend an intervention [was taken as] a sign that the intervention was not truly needed."[38] They also found reluctance among the counselors to challenge mistaken beliefs about spina bifida and Down syndrome if the counselors thought the beliefs were culturally determined. The interviewed women expressed feelings of not being heard by the counselor, and a tendency to trust their providers, with whom they had an ongoing relationship of trust, more than the genetic counselor. Interviews with women in California's AFP testing program also revealed complex relationships among ethnicity, acculturation, religiosity, language and attitudes toward abortion "which shape the meanings of the test decision for individual women."[40] A health worker who can explain such concepts in a woman's native language and idiom is invaluable, but clinicians must also recognize that the interpreter's style can also have an impact on the woman's decision-making. [41]

Through such multidimensional evaluation of the woman's context and values, woman-centered genetic assessment avoids assumptions about how a woman understands risk. Such steps are essential to achieve the collaboration of "finding common ground," which is necessary in moving forward toward the crucial decisions about an affected pregnancy.

FINDING COMMON GROUND

Decisions about terminating or continuing an affected pregnancy derive from deeply held beliefs about the personhood of the fetus and mother, the prevention of suffering and disability or the acceptance of it. When a woman and her clinician hold different values on these issues, this difference can strain the patient–provider relationship. Women may believe that the only reason to identify an affected fetus is to abort the pregnancy. If abortion is not an option they want to consider, they may refuse prenatal testing.

However, other potential benefits of prenatal diagnosis include the possibility of making plans for a special-needs baby. For example, knowing in advance would enable a woman to deliver a fetus with myelomeningocele identified after abnormal AFP screening, or one with Down syndrome who may need cardiac surgery, at a hospital equipped to perform the necessary surgery. When the condition is one for which no treatment exists, the family may benefit by being prepared for the outcome, emotionally and socially (e.g. plans to return to work may be modified in anticipation of a severely ill child).

In some countries and cultures, genetic testing and abortion for gender selection are common. Some physicians and ethicists see gender selection as simply another area of reproductive choice.[42] Given that gender selection is frequently selection for a male child, some see the selective abortion of female fetuses as violence against women. The practice is banned in many countries, but is widely practiced, with about 840 girls born in China for every 1000 boys[43] and birthrates in India for girls after a firstborn girl about 750 for every 1000 boys.[44] Women themselves may feel compelled to abort a female fetus because of maltreatment they might experience if they deliver girl babies, or they may be compelled to have more children than they wish in order to finally produce a male. Women-centered care requires at least a careful exploration of the woman's reasons for requesting such a choice.

INCORPORATING PREVENTION AND HEALTH PROMOTION

Rationally, the better time to assess and manage risk for genetic diseases and birth defects is before conception. Ideally, the woman and the clinician would initiate folate supplementation, control of pre-existing diabetes, and identification of genetic carrier status (when available) before a woman becomes pregnant. The insurance coverage for pre-pregnancy genetic testing is variable. A woman-centered provider will also take these issues into account when advising women and their partners, and advocate for coverage when necessary.

UNDERSTANDING THE WHOLE PERSON WITHIN THE CONTEXT OF THE FAMILY

Women may begin prenatal care already knowing about a disease that runs in the family, or the clinician may discover the risk when collecting a careful family history. Parents may feel guilty about carrying "tainted" genes, or angry at a parent or partner for carrying the gene. Women in general do not always understand what illnesses in their family history might be relevant to prenatal genetic screening. Careful gathering of pedigree information for three generations, including at least all first cousins, is necessary to pick up an inheritance pattern the woman or her partner may not have been aware of. When women or their partners come from very complex families, with half siblings and step-parents, interpretation of the potential genetic concerns is difficult for both the provider and the woman.

Although clinicians may think of prenatal genetic testing mainly in the context of chromosomal anomalies and inherited diseases, women may request genetic testing to determine paternity (which is also offered directly to consumers via the Internet.) New technologies of DNA fingerprinting to establish paternity are widely available and popular. Most Internet sites (83%) offering direct genetic services provided parentage tests, while only 13% offered health-related services.[45] In the USA, federal and some state laws require women who receive public assistance to name their children's fathers to their state's human services agency, which in turn compels fathers to pay child support. This requirement has fueled the demand for testing (and contesting) paternity. Questions about paternity are embedded in complex psychosocial webs involving disputes about custody and child support, troubled couple relationships, and legal qualification for welfare benefits. Because of the mixture of fetal and maternal DNA in the sample, errors are frequent in prenatal testing of fetal DNA done on maternal blood, further complicating the issues.[46] Whenever possible, the clinician should carefully explore the reasons a woman (or her partner) requests paternity testing, and the possible consequences of the results, before ordering the test.

ENHANCING THE DOCTOR–PATIENT RELATIONSHIP

In the example of Melissa and Kirk, Larisa adapts to their demanding style and need for control over their prenatal testing, which probably contributes to the trust that allows Melissa to later disclose her history of sexual abuse. In the example of Rosa, the difficulty of explaining risks and procedures through a translator could easily tempt a provider to present this as just another routine test. But breezing through the explanation of serum marker testing, then having to explain a positive result to a woman upset by the threat to her pregnancy, would damage the relationship badly. Given the different implications in various cultures for bearing an abnormal child, the need for exploration of these issues in the woman's native language is critical, as Dr. Rosen finally recognizes. As prenatal screening has become routine, and other kinds of genetic screening (such as newborn screening for cystic fibrosis mutations) have become increasingly more available, woman-centered providers will need, more than ever, to take time to ensure that women give truly informed consent.

CHAPTER 6

Group Visits: Empowerment

Krista Farey

Restructuring the method of prenatal care or certain office or hospital systems may help reinforce the goal of self-management and empowerment for pregnant women. For example, group prenatal visits are one way to structure care to specifically address these issues. Although group medical visits in general have been touted as a busy provider's answer to saving time and maximizing the volume of patients seen,[47] the woman-centered goal of group prenatal visits is far more effective. Ideally, group visits set up an interpersonal dynamic with a collaborative approach that empowers all the participants and de-emphasizes the traditional power hierarchy of clinician and woman. Such empowerment is particularly important in activating women and their families around behavioral and lifestyle changes such as nutrition and smoking cessation that require individual motivation and action for self-care. The leveling of hierarchy in group visits can also empower staff toward more collaborative team approaches.

Alicia became pregnant when she was a shy, overweight, stay-at-home 16-year-old, who could articulate little about her vision for her future except that she hoped to be a good mother. She had immigrated from Mexico when she was nine and lived in a small house with her parents, siblings and various extended family members. She entered prenatal care at the local community health center where the staff enrolled her in a Spanish language prenatal group; she was both the youngest and the only bilingual participant. In the group, 12 women due in the same month received care together in a series of 10 two-hour meetings. Alicia quickly learned how to check and chart her own weight, blood pressure, and urine sugar and protein, and was soon enjoying helping the other women do this. In the group discussions, she learned from the older women about being pregnant and being a parent, and did reflective self-assessment exercises that asked her to look seriously at her resources and aspirations. She began to reflect honestly about ways to realize her goal of being a good mother. She had said she could not attend school because of not having her required vaccines; soon after joining the group, she asked for and kept an appointment for the immunizations that could be safely given in pregnancy; such as tetanus, polio, influenza, or hepatitis B. She completed the first year of a high school equivalency academic program before delivering a healthy baby girl, Jennifer. She was so inspired by the pregnancy and birth experience that she decided to become a nurse, quickly finishing her high school equivalency degree and enrolling in the associate degree nurses' aide program at the local community college.

By this time her prenatal group had transformed into a well-child care group, in which Alicia continued to be a great support to the others. For instance, she visited with Maria, another young and isolated recent immigrant who was able to overcome a very profound postpartum depression with the group's and Alicia's support. Carefully observing the babies at group, Alicia was the first to notice subtle motor delays in her own daughter, facilitating an early referral to the tertiary care center and enrollment in weekly multidisciplinary therapeutic interventions. As baby Jennifer grew increasingly skilled and engaged, Alicia blossomed into a very busy, motivated and loving young mother, who consciously tended to both her daughter's and her own development. Alicia played on a soccer team, held a job in a welding shop, and had almost finished with the nursing program. Now a volunteer assistant at the clinic's prenatal care groups, Alicia was considering working at the clinic as a nurses' aide or continuing her education to become a midwife, or a doctor. (*See* full vignette in Appendix.)

Alicia is participating in a prenatal care group designed to be woman-centered. Her group visits are based on the CenteringPregnancy® model, a model of group prenatal care developed by Sharon Schindler Rising and others, with the explicit intent of conducting prenatal care in a woman-centered and empowering way.[48] Group prenatal care has been successfully implemented through both this and other models in many conventional clinic and hospital-based practices, private offices and health maintenance organizations.[48,49] This model, based on facilitated group interaction, emphasizes self-assessment, education, relaxation, self-care and community building. The philosophical roots of CenteringPregnancy® group prenatal care draw on general feminist theory and the philosophy of midwifery, as well as standard guidelines on prenatal care such as the document *Caring for Our Future: the content of prenatal care.*[50] Recommendations from this report included a greater emphasis on early and continuing assessment, health promotion, psychosocial interventions and reducing barriers to participation in prenatal care, all features that lend themselves to a more woman-centered approach.

The concept of group prenatal care is based on the premise that reorganizing prenatal care into group care might make it more successful in meeting its essential objectives and also might reduce barriers to care. Many advantages derive from group care. Groups are generally appealing and fun for women; groups provide affiliation, build community, increase motivation for learning, decrease isolation and offer a vehicle for social change.[48] Facilitated groups are a better educational method for adult learners than individual lessons, by encouraging active participation, enabling participants to learn from each other and providing more time to present and assimilate educational material.[51,52] Prenatal care in groups expands the time available for education (20 hours of contact in the 10 group model), allowing greater depth in learning conventional prenatal topics, and time for experiential learning in relaxation, exercise, and artistic expression. Group prenatal care also places women in a greater position of power, by emphasizing self-assessment, self-care, and participation in the community and by de-emphasizing professional control of care and surveillance for pathology, in what are, for most women, healthy pregnancies without major medical problems.[48,53]

Participation in a prenatal group usually begins when a woman enrolls in prenatal care and is offered the option of group care. If she is interested and able to participate she will first have one or two individual visits with a clinical care provider, where initial history, physical exam, and lab analysis will be obtained and results reviewed. Starting between 12 and 16 weeks, her periodic clinical care switches to the group setting, with additional individual visits for those who need them. Each group is comprised of up to 12 women who have due dates within one to two months of each other and share a common language. Staff includes one physician, nurse practitioner, physician assistant or midwife, and a second professional who may be a nurse, medical assistant, medical educator, or community health worker. Community volunteers may also participate. Membership of each group is generally stable for the duration of the pregnancy. Some groups choose to include partners and other support people, and older children may sometimes attend.

Each group meets for 10 sessions over a six-month period, each session lasting one and a half to two hours. In a typical schedule, the first four sessions occur every four weeks when the women are all about 16, 20, 24 and 28 weeks of gestation, and the six subsequent sessions occur every two weeks at about 30, 32, 34, 36, 38, and 40 weeks' gestation. Each session includes self-assessment, an individual physical assessment done by the clinician with each woman individually as a pullout from the group, a facilitated educational discussion of one or more topics related to that time in pregnancy, and a time for community building, such as sharing of refreshments, having a group baby shower, and exchanging phone numbers to organize reminder calls, snacks, and shared transportation. At the first group meeting, the women and any other participants agree on basic ground rules for group participation, including confidentiality, and learn the mechanics and logistics of group care.

The following scenario is an example of what happens in a typical group meeting:

It was 9:00 on Tuesday morning; Mercedes Burman, a family doctor, and Alex, a medical assistant, were setting up for group. This was to be the fourth session in the series, focusing on contraception, signs of false and true labor and relaxation. The two facilitators discussed the morning's plan, prepared the written materials, set out the supplies and arranged the chairs in a circle with a small table for food in the center. Alex put some relaxing music on the CD player. Mercedes entered recent lab results in charts and made preparations for future testing and future appointments.

The facilitators were in a group care room, decorated with posters that illustrated fetal growth, promoted breastfeeding, and advertised the local support organization for women confronting domestic violence. An exam table sat behind a screen in one corner, and a basket of toys and books to entertain small children was in another corner.

At 9:20 women began to arrive for the 9:30 group. Each one checked her weight, dipped her urine and took her blood pressure, recording the results in her chart. They chatted, helping each other, and exclaiming about the growth in each other's bellies since the last visit four weeks before. Alex waddled around trying to make his belly look 28 weeks to be "part of the group," and the women giggled at him happily. For snacks, Marta had brought a spectacular rainbow gelatin salad and others asked how she made it. Sheela had brought pungent-smelling fritters and a bowl of fresh strawberries.

The women sat down and completed a written self-assessment on contraceptive experience and plans. One by one, each woman went to the exam table behind the screen, where Mercedes briefly checked on the woman's medical issues, measured her fundal height, checked the fetal heart tones and recorded the results. She then answered specifically individual questions, while deferring other more general questions to group discussion.

At 9:40, Alex began the group session with a guided relaxation, some stretching and a check-in of how people were feeling. One woman remarked that she was feeling very short-fused and then gasped with astonished delight to learn she was far from the only one experiencing this. Another reported feeling some tightening in her abdomen at times. Alex then referred them to the handout on distinguishing true from false labor, and they discussed together their experience with this symptom, and what to do if they suspected preterm labor.

Mercedes joined the circle at 10:00 when all 12 individual exams and assessments were completed. She raised the questions that had come up during the individual exams. "Why do they say I shouldn't eat fresh cheese?" "My uncle died last week – will my sadness hurt my baby?" Mercedes asked the group what they thought. One woman knew and told the others about the kinds of food that could carry *Listeria* and what harm it could do. The women held many different opinions about the effect of grief on a fetus, but most agreed that the baby must experience something of what the mother experienced and also of how she processed that experience.

At 10:15, they broke into two groups to discuss contraception. Mercedes joined one group where they learned about tubal ligation, vasectomy and IUDs, inserting an IUD into a plastic model pelvis, and Alex was with the other group as they went over hormonal and barrier options, passing around samples of many products, and rolling condoms onto bananas. Afterwards a partner thanked Alex for the demonstration, as he had always been afraid to ask how to use condoms. Then the groups switched. When they were all back together, Tina announced that breast-feeding alone was sufficient contraception for her. Several others expressed great concern that such a plan was unrealistic, and told stories of women they knew who had become pregnant relying on breastfeeding for contraception. Tina asked more questions about IUDs.

As the group neared its 11:00 close, they discussed the next meeting, planned who would bring snacks, and distributed appointment and lab slips. Mercedes and Alex thanked all participants for their contributions, and many participants thanked staff and others. From 11:00 to 11:30, most of the women chose to stay and chat and eat, while Mercedes and Alex worked on individual issues and put supplies away. When the women left at 11:30, the staff finished the charting, billing forms and cleanup, evaluated the session, and developed a basic plan for the next one.

Restructuring care in this way, as the example illustrates, creates a woman-centered, empowering context in which the true goals of prenatal care can be better realized and outcomes improved. Evidence is accumulating to document the improvement in outcomes.[54-6] The groups cover all the core content of prenatal care, with flexibility in the order and emphasis of topics based on the needs and interests of each unique group of participants. These women are learning, assimilating what they learn, and teaching it to others. They show greater retention of educational content than women in conventional care. They are gaining skills and confidence at eating well, exercising appropriately, and managing stressors and family dynamics. They are building community support networks. They enjoy prenatal care, are eager to participate, and their responses on assessment tools of patient satisfaction show greater satisfaction than women in routine care.[48] They are learning skills that some of them will apply to healthcare professional work in the future. Participants have commented, "I learned more than I could ever tell by coming to group," and "It was nice because you knew that there were people who were really concerned, who were going through the same thing." Group care can be so appealing that some women may preferentially seek care in a center where it is available.

Multicenter outcome trials have also shown that women participating in group prenatal visits have a longer duration of pregnancy and their babies have higher birth weight than women in individual care.[53,56] A large prospective cohort study[53] involving a matched cohort of women served by public clinics showed significantly increased birth weight among preterm infants, with duration of preterm pregnancies two weeks longer in group-care women than in individual-care women. The most recent randomized study confirmed these results with a dramatic 33% reduction in preterm birth rate among inner-city African-American women receiving group care compared with women in conventional care.[56] Group prenatal care also offers benefits to staff and healthcare organizations. Staff feel empowered through group participation and multidisciplinary team building; they report increased work satisfaction and decreased sense of burn-out.[48] Productivity can be increased, as illustrated in the scenario, where 12 women were seen in three hours. Group care can also bring efficiencies of flow through registration and lab, and utilizes fewer exam rooms. These potential increases in productivity and efficiency carry a potential for improved cost-effectiveness.

Interest and support are building for restructuring prenatal care into group models. As of 2009, over 2500 healthcare professionals have trained in group prenatal care with the CenteringPregnancy model alone, and over 300 sites in the US, Canada, the UK, and Sweden were providing group prenatal care in this model, including community health centers, hospitals, private offices, and HMOs.[57] (Also, personal communication, Sharon Rising May 6, 2009). Providers have implemented group prenatal care successfully, in both English and in Spanish, with women from a wide range of socioeconomic and educational backgrounds. Many sites continue to participate in multicenter collaborative outcome studies funded by organizations interested in improving perinatal outcomes, including the March of Dimes and the National Institute of Mental Health. The Centering Healthcare Institute (CHI) (www. centeringhealthcare.org) provides professional training in group prenatal care as well as networking opportunities for those who have been trained. The CHI continues to follow implementation sites, gather data, and measure outcomes, with the goal of transforming prenatal care into a more woman-centered process with improved results for women and their families, healthcare professionals and healthcare institutions.

CHAPTER 7

Office and Institution Issues

Sara G. Shields

OFFICE STAFF

Health promotion and disease prevention also involve understanding the woman's interactions with the contexts of the office and hospital or other institutions that are part of maternity care. This process involves considering support staff, office systems, childbirth education options, and finally hospital routines and programs that both prevent errors and promote healthy outcomes and behaviors.

> Delia had been on methadone since the birth of her last child. She had lost custody of her first and second babies because of her unstable lifestyle; staying drug-free had been a requirement for her keeping her third child Jeromey who was 18 months old. She had a long-term open case with the child protection services agency. Delia had seen multiple providers at the health center over the years and did not have a good connection with anyone except for one of the nurses, Maureen, whom she called when she needed to make an appointment, get a letter for housing, or when she or her son had an acute illness. Maureen was the first person she told that she was pregnant again.

Women like Delia or others with significant psychosocial issues may connect best with an interpreter or other advocate or nurse, making such support people more central figures in a woman's prenatal care than the physician or midwife. A woman-centered provider thus must encourage a woman-centered approach by all staff who work with pregnant women and their families. This mandate may require formal office policies, hiring strategies, and/or training for staff about the principles and practice of such care, particularly in dealing with women with more complex psychosocial needs.

> Rosa was assigned to Lupe, a Mexican-born bilingual case manager who had worked for the local perinatal program for the last decade. Lupe helped Rosa and José find donations of baby clothes and a crib through a local church program. When labor began, Rosa first called Lupe who was on call for translation and labor support. Lupe notified the on-call physician and met Rosa when she came to the hospital well along in her labor. Lupe translated for the hospital staff and showed Rosa how to find comfortable positions while the nurse was checking the fetal heart beat. After the birth, Lupe stayed on, translating and helping Rosa get Eva to the breast while the nurse was finishing paperwork. During the postpartum hospital stay, Lupe came in for one session of discharge teaching and helped with making the necessary postpartum appointments. She also taught Rosa how to use a manual breast pump.

Woman-centered health promotion for immigrant women or other disempowered women involves a continuum of staffing across office and institutional sites and longitudinal staffing throughout the peripartum period. The bilingual, bicultural staff members facilitate health promotion about breastfeeding by the office provider, the intrapartum nursing staff, and the postpartum staff and provider. The case manager or advocate can help prevent breastfeeding failure by facilitating breast-pump training and access, weaving together her knowledge of local insurance coverage, cross-cultural issues, and the local work community, as well as breastfeeding basics that she has learned through her years of doing this work. She also serves as a "cultural broker," explaining the woman's reality to providers who may not grasp the difficult realities of her life.

OTHER OFFICE ISSUES

What are other ways that offices providing perinatal care can be more woman-centered in the area of health promotion and prevention? No one general answer meets the particular needs of each woman – effective woman-centered health promotion must be individualized. Patient-centered education reflects the variety of adult learning styles, offering many different venues for learning – for instance, some women might learn better by reading, others by video or personal explanation, some in group visits or others on their own, some in the context of their partner or family, others just with other pregnant women.

Rosa with her third-grade education and minimal English skills will likely learn more from individualized, language-appropriate verbal teaching with a bilingual, bicultural educator, or through videos in her native language, than from written pamphlets or questionnaires. Her deference to the authority and hierarchy of medical providers may prevent effective education done just by a physician, so that follow-up reminders or discussions with staff who are more like her peers may be less intimidating for her. Like Alicia, she may benefit most from group prenatal care with peers from her culture and in her native language.

If computerized strategies are used for health promotion, any user interface needs to be at the right literacy and language level, particularly for those women who may not have had much computer experience.

> The African-American nurse in Judith's office found a reference on the Internet to an interactive educational DVD about gestational diabetes for women of color. She asked Judith about purchasing it, and they found some extra money in their supply budget to get one copy. The nurse called Jackie to see if she could come in early for her next appointment to view the DVD; Jackie said she would need to bring her kids along, so together they all watched the DVD and used its interactive lessons.

Flexibility in office environment and design can also be woman-centered in relation to health promotion. If waiting rooms can be more child-friendly, women such as Delia can more consistently attend appointments without having to worry about childcare for older children. Child-oriented health education toys and books (such as a children's book about breastfeeding) can facilitate intra-generational health promotion. Woman-centered health promotion also includes intentionally planning a private space for nursing mothers who are waiting for provider appointments. Using newer technologies such as interactive DVDs can motivate a family like Jackie's not only about tertiary prevention in dealing with her immediate risks from GDM but also in risk reduction around general nutrition issues.

Designing educational strategies specific to prenatal waiting rooms may provide an opportunity not only for additional general education, but also specifically for prevention of prematurity.[58] Such a program may include literacy-appropriate posters, magazines, and pamphlets; short, targeted videos about recognition of preterm labor and also about general health behaviors such as smoking cessation that may reduce a woman's risk of preterm delivery; or nurse-facilitated group discussion about clinical topics with an emphasis on process not just content.[58] One challenge with a focus on preterm prevention is to help women attend to potentially concerning symptoms without overemphasizing risk and frightening women about common discomforts of pregnancy that are not indicative of preterm labor.

Another method of woman-centered health promotion and preventive care involves office "tickler" systems. Even in an office that provides primarily infant care, reminder cards on baby's charts at appropriate well-child visits can facilitate promoting both infant wellness (such as reminding the mother to get a flu vaccine if she has an infant under six months of age during flu season and has not already herself been vaccinated) and well-woman care (such as reminders for mothers to schedule their own annual check-ups around the time of an infant's one-year check-up). Furthermore, if infant care providers ask about a woman's current contraception use, they may detect her risk of short interpregnancy interval, which has been linked to an increased risk of subsequent preterm birth.[49,60] If the infant's provider is not the mother's clinician, this provider can facilitate referral for the mother to obtain needed care.

A woman-centered approach to other aspects of medical records can facilitate health promotion as well. Prenatal record templates customized to a woman-centered philosophy prompt providers to inquire regularly and systematically about each woman's preferences for her care, such as timing of appointments, choices about labor support people and intrapartum care, and decisions about postpartum and newborn care. Periodic inquiry into contraception and interpersonal violence can be built into medical records forms both during maternity care and in children's medical records. Increasingly, pediatric care providers are recognizing their need to ascertain the personal safety of the mothers of their patients.[61]

> Evelyn (*see* Parts Two and Four) was a 29-year-old G2P1 who had a young toddler at home and also worked as a night shift nurses' aide in order to supplement her spouse's income as a taxi driver. They juggled childcare and jobs, so that it was easiest for her to have early morning appointments for prenatal care on her way home from her night work while her husband Ed was at home with their daughter before leaving for his day job.

Appointment strategies that acknowledge women's home and work demands are important. In the immediate postpartum period, when rest and contagion-prevention are key health issues, medical providers need to evaluate new mothers and babies in timely ways. Either home visits should be arranged to avoid disrupting a newly formed family's schedule, or office visits should be as prompt and efficient as possible so that the new family can get back home to rest. Although large studies have not shown differences in medical outcomes comparing hospital-based postpartum visits with more expensive home visits, women prefer the latter in terms of satisfaction with care.[62,63] Another potentially woman-centered option is the continuation of prenatal group visits into the early newborn period and through the first year of well-child visits (*see* www.centeringhealthcare.org/pages/centering-model/parenting-overview.php).

Guidelines for prenatal care in office settings vary tremendously,[64,65] reflecting local variation, but they also lack standardization with potential to over-emphasize risk, miss opportunities for individualized education,[65] and lead to ineffective or costly testing or evaluation.[64] Ultimately, woman-centered health promotion and prevention in prenatal and postpartum office settings blends such guidelines with the individualized strategies discussed above.

FORMAL CHILDBIRTH EDUCATION

Many of the above-mentioned office design issues involve strategies that directly or indirectly educate women and families about healthy behaviors during maternity care and beyond. Some form of more formal childbirth education (CBE) is also a traditional part of prenatal care, and indeed in some countries is a required component of prenatal care.[66] While in the USA and European countries such as Sweden,[66] the majority of nulliparous women still participate in such formal CBE classes, this number has declined over the last few years in the USA, and most American multiparous women do not participate in these classes: 70% of first-time mothers and 15% of multiparous women in 2002 took classes, with rates of 56% and 9% respectively in those groups in 2006.[67,68] Less than one-third of women in one Canadian province[69] and less than one-quarter of Italian women[70] attended prenatal classes.

Classes in childbirth preparation originated with Lamaze classes in the 1950s in an effort to help women better prepare themselves for the pain of childbirth. Theoretically, CBE prepares women and families prenatally for healthy birth and parenting, and thus is quintessential health promotion and prevention. Early studies of CBE suggested important effects on woman-centered outcomes such as reduced maternal fears, increased self-esteem, or improved mother–infant relationship.[71] However, more recent studies that try to assess whether or not CBE "makes a difference" are mostly descriptive rather than experimental and vary dramatically in which outcomes are measured – for instance, women's satisfaction with classes, use of coping strategies or pain medication, health behaviors such as smoking, preterm birth rates, or breastfeeding rates. Such diversity combined with flawed methodology in these recent studies contributes to the lack of clear conclusions about the effectiveness or value of more contemporary CBE.[71]

Nowadays in the USA, most pregnant women who attend childbirth classes do so in a hospital-based setting rather than in independent or home-based settings.[68] Childbirth educators in hospital classes may feel pressure to teach in ways that orient women, or couples, to typical practices and policies at the specific hospital rather than fully evidence-based practices.[72,73] Talks by physicians, anesthetists, and nurses in the hospital setting may serve to prepare women for *what to expect* rather than to emphasize the woman-centered goals of empowerment and choice in the birth experience. Furthermore, attendance at childbirth classes in the USA reflects health disparities: married white women with more education and higher income are more likely to have attended classes with 75% of these initiating breastfeeding.[74] Similar socioeconomic disparities exist in studies of prenatal education attendees in Canada and Europe.[66,69,70] Why low-income women from communities of color do not attend such classes is less clear, but the usual barriers of language, transportation, need for childcare, work schedules, and feeling out of place or intimidated may be relevant. Additionally, traditional childbirth education labeled "family-centered" may focus overtly on couples and lead to single mothers feeling isolated and unwelcome. Hospitals that address these disparities with classes in other languages at flexible times and with community support may have better attendance overall including participation from usually marginalized groups.[75]

Woman-centered childbirth education avoids dogma or stereotyped labels about either natural birth or technology-laden birth.[76] Emphasizing attendance at such classes as a measure of a woman's adherence to a prenatal care plan may overrate the expected effects of "techniques" such as breathing patterns, etc., and/or blame women for not using these techniques adequately during labor. The other challenge of woman-centered CBE is to prepare women for normal, healthy birth and parenting experiences, emphasizing normalcy, while also offering some discussion of unexpected outcomes without overstating these or increasing fear or anxiety. The goal of woman-centered CBE thus is not to require strict adherence to one method or to distort fears or risks, but to offer basic information, teach decision-making strategies, and empower women and their partners in learning about their bodies, assessing their fears, and making healthy choices (*see* Box 5.7).[75]

BOX 5.7 Standards for a Family-Centered Perinatal Education[75]

- Courses offered encompass the entire childbearing year.
- In order to meet the changing needs of families during the childbearing year, educational offerings include early pregnancy, mid-pregnancy, and late pregnancy classes, as well as postpartum and parenting information.
- The long-term emotional significance of the childbearing experience is addressed in all courses.
- Classes reflect the cultural needs of the participants.
- Class size facilitates the group process, with an ideal size of 6–10 couples and a maximum of 12 couples.
- Teachers employ a variety of teaching strategies during each class to meet the needs of different types of learners.
- The Lamaze class series for first-time parents includes at least 12 hours of instruction with emphasis on skills practice (especially positioning and relaxation), comfort measures, and knowledge of alternatives.
- Classes include discussion of consumer rights and responsibilities for making informed choices based on knowledge of alternatives.
- Family input and evaluation of class content and process is actively sought and used to improve classes.
- Childbirth instructors are certified.

Woman-centered childbirth educators can provide a balanced and evidence-based perspective on the interventionist atmosphere of hospital birth – that induction and early epidurals may lead to an increased risk of cesarean; that there may be subtle effects on breastfeeding from epidurals/regional anesthesia; that women have choices about trial of labor after cesarean and should push for them; that early skin-to-skin newborn contact benefits breastfeeding mothers.[77–83]

Childbirth educators who espouse woman-centered ideas, yet work in settings or with providers where intrapartum routines may prevent a full range of choices, may feel that they walk a tightrope when focusing their teaching on natural birth for women who mostly deliver within the medicalized birth setting.[84] Nonetheless, certain strategies may help promote woman-centered goals.[85,86] For instance, the educator can offer early-pregnancy classes rather than the traditional third-trimester ones, to begin teaching woman-centered self-advocacy that may help women seek alternatives in care before they are so close to delivery that it feels too late.[86] The educator can encourage women to complete patient satisfaction surveys, which many hospitals attend to more than in the past, and to discuss any care concerns with nursing supervisors or other hospital administrators. Community programs such as women's health advisory boards can include certified educators to help promote woman-centered care throughout a community's health institutions.[85]

Of particular relevance to woman-centered caregivers, a woman's sense of satisfaction with birth, especially with regard to pain and pain relief, relates most strongly to her personal expectations, the amount of support from her caregivers, the quality of the patient–caregiver relationship, and the woman's involvement in decision-making – all key aspects of woman-centered care! As noted earlier, fewer women attend childbirth classes than in the past,[68] and childbirth preparation does not emerge as a major factor in women's assessment of their experience.[87] These findings support the development of new strategies for strengthening of clinical relationships and fostering women's choice and involvement in decisions – aspects of care emphasized in group prenatal visits and in the conscious application of woman-centered care described throughout this book.

HOSPITAL ISSUES

> One of Larisa's friends from residency joined the Indian Health Service (IHS) and provided comprehensive care at one of their hospitals. When Larisa went to visit on vacation, she found that whole extended Native American families came to the hospital for births in their family, and that a sizable group of family members were allowed into the delivery room. Larisa wondered why this more flexible policy was not available to her for the families in her practice. She decided to find out how to change the policy at her hospital.

Hospital routines and protocols are often rigid due to institutional policies and needs, but a woman-centered approach to these may facilitate health promotion. Specific examples include use of guidelines for intrapartum care, visitation rules in labor and delivery or postpartum, and policies about mother–newborn skin-to-skin contact and other practices related to breastfeeding. A woman-centered provider can work within hospital committees to address such policies.

Guidelines for intrapartum care and for common outcomes such as induction, augmentation, or unplanned cesarean contribute to health promotion through objective criteria that providers and women can understand for various childbirth issues. While, in principle, adhering rigidly to guidelines seems inherently non-woman-centered, in practice, certain guidelines can promote woman-centered care by reducing error or reducing unnecessary surgery with its potential sequelae. For instance, when certain Canadian hospitals instituted programs to review all inductions, the rate of elective inductions decreased.[88] Similarly, hospitals with intrapartum care guidelines, particularly for low-risk primigravida women, have more vaginal deliveries.[89] Multidisciplinary involvement in such programs with both nurses and physicians becoming stakeholders in the goal of reducing the rate of cesarean section may increase success rates.[90–92]

Woman-centered maternity care incorporates national programs or guidelines that promote healthy childbirth practices. For example, in the USA, the Institute for Healthcare Improvement (IHI) brings together multidisciplinary groups to address issues of healthcare quality and medical error reduction. In the 1990s one of their programs focusing on maternity care involved 28 participating organizations that committed over the course of one year to addressing systematically their cesarean section rates in trying to meet Healthy People 2000 goals.[93] Many of the conclusions of this collaborative project bear rethinking in a woman-centered framework.

Although now a decade old, this collaborative program has valuable lessons for woman-centered maternity care approaches. The current IHI work in the perinatal arena has taken a different focus, shifting to address the issue of medical error and patient safety in keeping with the Institute of Medicine's 1999 *To Err is Human* report.[94] Thus, current strategies look at perinatal morbidity and mortality and continue to emphasize nurse–physician communication issues and root-cause analysis of poor outcomes.[95] This emphasis on patient safety, while essential, approaches normal labor and delivery from a very hospital-based, risk-based philosophy, assuming that normal birth parallels other hospital-based care such as surgery or acute medical care in terms of risk issues. The application of surgically derived strategies such as "failure to rescue" to the obstetric arena ignores the fact that the perinatal care of low-risk healthy women and their babies requires different measures to look at risk issues. In the latest projects, emphasizing "induction" and "augmentation" protocols as the main strategies uses two highly technological approaches to birth.[95] Woman-centered care includes not only insisting on protocols or standards for those two clinical measures, in hopes that institutions will have lower induction or augmentation rates, but also incorporating some of the neglected recommendations of the prior IHI report that focus more on the human interactions such as labor support and avoidance of early admission in labor.[93] A recent similar national guideline from the UK in 2007 incorporates many of these concepts.[96]

National strategies can also promote perinatal wellness through woman-centered systems of care. For instance, the Mother-Friendly Childbirth Initiative expands the better-known breastfeeding-oriented Baby Friendly Hospital program of the World Health Organization to focus on provider and institutional practices that promote healthy childbirth for both woman and baby (*see* Boxes 5.8 and 5.9). An individual woman-centered provider can work with nurse managers and hospital administrators to promote these kinds of programs and to consider other hospital guidelines that affect women's health intrapartum and postpartum.

BOX 5.8 The Baby Friendly Hospital Initiative (From: www.babyfriendlyusa. org/eng/10steps.html)

Ten steps to successful breastfeeding for hospitals:
1 Maintain a written breastfeeding policy that is routinely communicated to all healthcare staff.
2 Train all healthcare staff in skills necessary to implement this policy.
3 Inform all pregnant women about the benefits and management of breastfeeding.
4 Help mothers initiate breastfeeding within one hour of birth.
5 Show mothers how to breastfeed and how to maintain lactation, even if they are separated from their infants.
6 Give infants no food or drink other than breast milk, unless medically indicated.
7 Practice "rooming in" – allow mothers and infants to remain together 24 hours a day.
8 Encourage unrestricted breastfeeding.
9 Give no pacifiers or artificial nipples to breastfeeding infants.
10 Foster the establishment of breastfeeding support groups and refer mothers to them on discharge from the hospital or clinic.

BOX 5.9 Ten steps of the Mother-Friendly Childbirth Initiative (From: www. motherfriendly.org/mfci.php#step4)

A mother-friendly hospital, birth center, or home birth service:
1 Offers all birthing mothers:
  ▪ unrestricted access to the birth companions of her choice, including fathers, partners, children, family members, and friends;
  ▪ unrestricted access to continuous emotional and physical support from a skilled woman – for example, a doula, or labor-support professional;
  ▪ access to professional midwifery care.
2 Provides accurate descriptive and statistical information to the public about its practices and procedures for birth care, including measures of interventions and outcomes.

3 Provides culturally competent care – that is, care that is sensitive and responsive to the specific beliefs, values, and customs of the mother's ethnicity and religion.

4 Provides the birthing woman with the freedom to walk, move about, and assume the positions of her choice during labor and birth (unless restriction is specifically required to correct a complication), and discourages the use of the lithotomy (flat on back with legs elevated) position.

5 Has clearly defined policies and procedures for:
- collaborating and consulting throughout the perinatal period with other maternity services, including communicating with the original caregiver when transfer from one birth site to another is necessary;
- linking the mother and baby to appropriate community resources, including prenatal and post-discharge follow-up and breastfeeding support.

6 Does not routinely employ practices and procedures that are unsupported by scientific evidence, including but not limited to the following:
- shaving;
- enemas;
- IVs (intravenous drip);
- withholding nourishment or water;
- early rupture of membranes;
- electronic fetal monitoring.

Other interventions are limited as follows:
- Has an induction rate of 10% or less;
- Has an episiotomy rate of 20% or less, with a goal of 5% or less;
- Has a total cesarean rate of 10% or less in community hospitals, and 15% or less in tertiary care (high-risk) hospitals;
- Has a VBAC (vaginal birth after cesarean) rate of 60% or more with a goal of 75% or more.

7 Educates staff in non-drug methods of pain relief, and does not promote the use of analgesic or anesthetic drugs not specifically required to correct a complication.

8 Encourages all mothers and families, including those with sick or premature newborns or infants with congenital problems, to touch, hold, breastfeed, and care for their babies to the extent compatible with their conditions.

9 Discourages non-religious circumcision of the newborn.

10 Strives to achieve the WHO-UNICEF "Ten Steps of the Baby-Friendly Hospital Initiative" to promote successful breastfeeding.

Hospital policies significantly affect the success of breastfeeding, requiring woman-centered providers to advocate at the institutional level for proven routines to achieve breastfeeding rates higher than many US hospitals reach. Such changes include not only promoting the steps of the Baby Friendly Hospital Initiative but also altering delivery room guidelines to promote initial mother–baby contact and limiting mother–baby separation as much as possible. With research suggesting the potential for short and long-term benefits of early and prolonged skin-to-skin contact,[82] hospital policies need flexibility about offering such contact in all birth situations, including in the operating room[97] with either mother or father.

> Jackie's son Joshua's initial Apgars were stable, but he ended up in the intensive care for a couple of days when he developed mild respiratory distress. Jackie's blood pressure remained high postpartum with ongoing proteinuria, such that the consultants, with Judith's agreement, recommended continuing 24 hours of magnesium sulfate therapy to prevent eclampsia, and antihypertensive medications. The long induction, this medication, and her post-operative pain all left Jackie feeling drugged, exhausted, and unable to cope with breast-pumping or visiting Joshua much in the neonatal intensive care unit. Her postpartum nurse nonetheless reminded Jackie to pump at least every four hours; each time the nurse came to record vital signs, she brought fresh pre-labeled bottles for the electric pump at Jackie's bedside. The nurse then stored the milk so that Joshua could have it when he became ready to eat. The NICU was on a different floor of the hospital, which made the trip even harder for Jackie. Finally, by the middle of the second day, her pain was better and her intravenous medications were finished, so she was able to spend a bit more time with Joshua, but she was still not able to start nursing him directly until he was over 72 hours old.

When mothers and babies like Jackie and Joshua are separated for medical reasons in the initial postpartum days, hospital routines need to foster breastfeeding and visitation in order to promote health in this time period. Incorporating pumping into the routine of vital signs or medication dosing emphasizes its importance. Individual providers can encourage hospital participation in national quality improvement programs such as the Vermont Oxford Network, a collaborative that focuses on newborn infant care (www.vtoxford.org/home.aspx); or the California Perinatal Quality Care Collaborative (www.cpqcc.org), a group that sets benchmarks for breastfeeding rates and other perinatal outcomes; or in programs like the Baby Friendly Initiative.[97,98]

> Just as the doctors were all readying to enter the operating room for Sylvie's cesarean section (*see* Part Three), Sylvie's bilingual cousin Anna arrived, and Sylvie asked the nurse if she could also be in the OR to help translate. The nurse discussed this with the consultant who agreed to have both Viktor and Anna present as long as they kept out of the anesthesiologist's way.

> While examining Alexandra's newborn daughter Jasmine, Helen talked with the various family members in the room, commenting on this new daughter's place in this family of strong women. Helen found out that all of Alexandra's sisters had breastfed at least short term, even though their mother had not. She asked

Alexandra's oldest sister to help bring Jasmine back to the new mother and talk to her about the first breastfeeding.

Flexibility around the number of family members with a woman in labor empowers healthy family dynamics that then encourage the incorporation of the new baby into the extended family system. For a woman like Sylvie exhausted and supine for her cesarean, the choice to have the two family members she wants with her for this birth is also empowering. For Alexandra's family, Helen both recognizes the dynamics and uses the energy of the newborn moments to briefly but emphatically discuss the benefits of breastfeeding.

Finally, other specific hospital routines can support or compromise health promotion during women's initial postpartum experiences in ways that woman-centered care needs to recognize. For example, adequate privacy and space in postpartum rooms allows and encourages fathers or other family support to stay through a mother's hospitalization and thus be more integrally involved with these early stages of parenting. The push to have around-the-clock rooming-in at one level exemplifies mother-friendly care,[99] yet needs to be combined with enough facilitative teaching and support that new mothers gain self-confidence in early newborn care and do not feel overwhelmed.[100] On the other hand, environmental issues in hospitals such as ambient noise or unnecessary interruptions may affect a new mother's already tenuous sleep patterns.[100,101]

CHAPTER 8

Pregnancy as an Opportunity for Lifelong Health Promotion

Pamela Adelstein

Women-centered risk assessment and risk reduction in pregnancy go beyond issues pertinent just to the fetus to incorporate long-term health goals for the new mother and family. The longitudinal aspects of perinatal care and of the patient–clinician relationship offer the possibility of ongoing work in prevention and health promotion.

Smoking cessation for a woman and her baby (and for the partner) is an ideal example of how a relational context can facilitate health promotion. Prenatal discussions of birth control and breastfeeding frame the later decisions and strategies. The hours and days of the labor, birth, and immediate postpartum period are also a time when modeling of health promotion decisions can take place – for instance, helping the new breastfeeding mother think about the potential hazards from medications, or discussing the risks and benefits of labor anesthesia.

Before encouraging a woman to focus on prevention during the pregnancy and beyond, the provider must understand how the woman approaches her health promotion and illness prevention. Consider again the case of Jackie, unexpectedly pregnant with her fourth child and dealing with several medical issues both before and during her pregnancy (*see* Parts Two through Four).

Whatever connection Judith can make during her first prenatal visit with Jackie becomes central to strengthening the foundation of their ongoing patient–provider relationship both in pregnancy and beyond. While this connection and relationship will intensify quickly during the course of short-term prenatal care, this trust will mostly bear fruit over time, in long-term health promotion and disease prevention for Jackie.

At the first visit, as a way to initiate the relationship that now involves Jackie's own care rather than her children's, Judith first acknowledges the magnitude of the experience that she and Jackie will share. "Together over the next few months we'll focus on ways to help you have a healthy pregnancy and a healthy baby." She then comments on Jackie's strengths – competencies that she will draw on as a pregnant woman, and ultimately as a mother of a newborn. "I've mostly seen you here as the busy caretaker that you are, keeping all the needed appointments with your own kids and your foster kids, and juggling all that with your nursing work. I'm impressed by how much you can give to others, especially around their health needs."

Just as with Sabrina's care, woman-centered maternity care providers have a unique opportunity to make positive contributions to the self-image of the women like Jackie by emphasizing these strengths. Because Jackie is so busy caring for others, she may not feel appreciated or receive positive reinforcement from those around her. Her provider can acknowledge these attributes. Thus over the first couple of visits, Judith shares her impression of Jackie as a matriarch, and inquires if Jackie shares this vision of herself. Judith can emphasize the strong web of support Jackie has built for herself within the community and within her church. As Judith learns more about Jackie, she can address potential topics like how pregnancy fits into her self-concept, where she finds the strength to fulfill all of her responsibilities, and what motivates her in her multiple roles.

The next step is attention to what Jackie gives to herself. Judith from the beginning emphasizes, "All that we're talking about focuses on your prenatal health. But really this is all about ways to help you in general be healthier long term, and to help your family be healthier too." She points out that while Jackie is extraordinarily busy, she needs to care for herself, and pregnancy affords this opportunity to slow down and focus inward. She reminds Jackie how important she is to so many other people, and how she herself deserves preventive care to keep herself healthy.

Questions that can elicit Jackie's methods of self-care include: When she is not caring for others, what does she think about? How does she replenish herself? In her moments alone, what dreams does she have for herself, her family, and for her unborn child? In discussing these issues, working with a trusted provider, Jackie can be her own catalyst for healthy lifestyle changes. As a sense of her own self-efficacy increases, her ability to make behavior changes strengthens: "the more capable people judge themselves to be, the higher the goals they set for themselves and the more firmly they remain committed to them."[102:635] In a meta-analysis of determinants of a healthy lifestyle, Gillis discovered that women who feel more responsible for and more in control of their own health are better able to adopt a healthy lifestyle.[103]

> After examining Jackie at the first prenatal visit, Judith was concerned about Jackie's large fundal height, her late presentation to care, and her advanced maternal age. She wanted Jackie to have the maternal serum marker screening, see the genetics counselor and get a detailed ultrasound. Jackie did not see the logic in many of these tests, as she would not consider abortion.

To build an alliance with Jackie, Judith explains that she respects Jackie's decisions. With her first connection emphasizing Jackie's strengths, Judith then begins to address her medical concerns, addressing both risk identification and risk reduction. To avoid overwhelming and alienating Jackie and to facilitate long-lasting change, the doctor addresses these risk factors incrementally, at every step assessing Jackie's self-perception of risk and preparing her for ongoing discussions about changes.

> At 28 weeks Jackie developed gestational diabetes. While upset, she was actually not surprised. She had checked her blood sugar with her mother's glucometer after a big family meal and knew that it was running high. She was worried about possibly requiring insulin.

Judith has used the foundation of ongoing prenatal care to plant the seed for the behavioral change that will be needed for Jackie to deal with this new diagnosis and its potential health impact both during pregnancy and beyond. The doctor begins by explaining the risks of gestational diabetes. While providing factual information, she stresses the need for honesty and partnership in treating Jackie's GDM.

Judith asks about barriers to change and works together with Jackie to break down these barriers and create new goals. One barrier is the feeling that dietary change is very difficult, and another is Jackie's fear of needing fingersticks and shots for the rest of her life. However, reflecting on what they have already discussed about Jackie's strengths as a matriarch, Judith appeals to Jackie's ability to accomplish many things simultaneously in the other areas of her life, and to the potential for Jackie to have some control over her illness. As further impetus for change, she reminds Jackie that she is a role model to her children and community.

> At 33 weeks Jackie had her blood sugars under control. She had met with the nutritionist and was checking her fingerstick glucose levels regularly – she had

done a great job managing her GDM. At this point a new problem arose: Jackie's blood pressure was rising. Jackie was reluctant to see a specialist as Judith recommended.

Jackie's actions in controlling her diabetes again demonstrate her underlying strengths. Judith compliments her, asks her how she feels about her achievement, and inquires about what she thinks it took for her to accomplish this. These responses can be applied to help her attain other health-related goals. The doctor points out that Jackie has seen other specialists (i.e. the nutritionist), with rewarding visits.

Judith and her obstetrical consultant followed Jackie closely in the subsequent weeks of her pregnancy and recommended induction of labor at 37 weeks when her blood pressure remained elevated. The labor was difficult, with Jackie ultimately needing a cesarean.

Judith accompanied Jackie into the delivery room to do the initial care for baby Joshua, who was at first vigorous and healthy. She encouraged Jackie to hold him right away, and to try nursing as soon as possible. Jackie was not sure she could cope with the immediate post-operative pain and still breastfeed but heard how good that could be for his health so kept trying, even when Joshua had to go to the intensive care unit with respiratory problems and she had to pump rather than nurse him directly for three days. At the time of discharge from the postpartum floor, Jackie was still hypertensive to the point that Judith recommended continuing antihypertensive medication at least until her check-up. They discussed options, with Judith careful to reassure Jackie that the medicine she chose was safe with breastfeeding.

Throughout the challenges of Jackie's complex antenatal and intrapartum course, her provider continues to emphasize her proven strengths and resilience. Knowing the long-term health benefits for both Jackie and Joshua of breastfeeding, Judith pays special attention to encouraging lactation, particularly during the difficult first few postpartum recovery days.

Jackie's blood pressure stayed up past her six-week check-up visit. At that visit she was very proud to still be breastfeeding; she was supplementing with formula to give herself a break when she was dealing with all the other kids, but she liked that she had been able to keep up with the nursing longer than with any of her other birth children. Her 10 and 12-year-old daughters, delighted with their new baby brother, accompanied their mother to this visit to help with Joshua, and Judith noted that both girls were overweight also. She suggested that Jackie have a screening test for Type II diabetes and that the whole family work with the nutritionist on weight issues. The doctor also recommended that Jackie continue to take an antihypertensive medication but that they have a plan for follow up to reconsider that decision over the next several months.

At six weeks postpartum Judith highlights two significant accomplishments – Jackie's commitment to breastfeeding, and the involvement of her daughters in the care of their new brother. While congratulating Jackie, Judith continues to encourage her to set the bar for her health even higher. Such successes, or mastery experiences, create a strong sense and belief in one's personal efficacy.[102] Thus, for Jackie, each goal she attains enables growth in her sense of self-management, empowerment, and potential to focus on prevention. Judith also capitalizes on Jackie's phase of life – her focus on her children – and on the potential a newborn baby brings to think about a whole family's long-term health. With Judith framing the discussion accordingly, still emphasizing Jackie's role as a matriarch and family role model, Jackie may be more receptive to incorporating exercise and healthy food choices into her family life.

> At six months post-partum, Jackie struggled to fit exercise into her daily routine with her new baby and her other children; the winter months were the hardest given the short days, but she tried to walk with the baby. By a year from Joshua's birth, she had returned to her pre-pregnancy weight and was able to wean off her antihypertensive medications.

Judith reinforces how far Jackie has come in a short time, how she has done a great job taking care of herself, and how these lifestyle changes are now integrated into her daily routine. She suggests that Jackie set new goals regarding her health promotion, and expresses her belief that, based on her recent successes, Jackie is fully capable of attaining them. She also checks in with Jackie about how her daughters are doing with their lifestyle modification.

This vignette illustrates how woman-centered maternity care, using the tools of understanding the pregnant woman's experience and finding common ground, can promote both prenatal and lifelong health. Jackie's story illustrates how even an apparently high-risk pregnancy for a woman with several medical issues can be a significant motivating factor for behavioral change for both herself, her family, and future generations.

CONCLUSION

The prenatal and immediate postpartum periods offer a unique opportunity for health promotion and disease prevention. Pregnant women generally understand the intimate and intricate connections between their health and their baby's health and are open to learning about wellness and self-care during this time. Rather than bombarding women with dogmatic or dire warnings about risk, woman-centered care emphasizes women's positive behavior and seeks to guide women in healthy decision-making that will empower them throughout their pregnancy, their early parenting stages, and their ongoing life choices, including around pregnancy planning issues. Woman-centered systems of care in hospital and office settings further integrate such wellness messages with flexible and responsive programs and protocols.

REFERENCES

1 Stewart M, Brown JB, Weston WW, *et al.*, editors. *Patient-centered Medicine: transforming the clinical method.* 2nd ed. Oxford: Radcliffe Medical Press; 2003.

2 Charron-Prochownik D, Sereika SM, Wang S-L, *et al.* Reproductive health and preconception counseling awareness in adolescents with diabetes: What they don't know can hurt them. *Diabetes Educ.* 2006; 32: 235–42.

3 Falsetti D, Charron-Prochownik D, Serelka S, *et al.* Condom use, pregnancy, and stds in adolescent females with and without type 1 diabetes. *Diabetes Educ.* 2003; 29: 135–43.

4 Leguizamon G, Igarzabal ML, Reece EA. Periconceptional care of women with diabetes mellitus. *Obstet Gynecol Clin North Am.* 2007; 34: 225–39.

5 Cantor J, Baum K. The limits of conscientious objection – may pharmacists refuse to fill prescriptions for emergency contraception? *N Engl J Med.* 2004; **351**: 2008–12.

6 Eyler AE, Cohen M. Case studies in partner violence. *Am Fam Physician.* 1999; **60**: 2569–76.

7 Runkle A. *In Good Conscience: a practical, emotional and spiritual guide to deciding whether to have an abortion.* 1st ed. San Francisco: Jossey-Bass Publishers; 1998.

8 Singer J. Options counseling: techniques for caring for women with unintended pregnancies. *J Midwifery Womens Health.* 2004; **49**: 235–42.

9 Stahl K, Hundley V. Risk and risk assessment in pregnancy – do we scare because we care? *Midwifery.* 2003; **19**: 298.

10 Gupton A, Heaman M, Cheung LW. Complicated and uncomplicated pregnancies: women's perception of risk. *J Obstet Gynecol Neonatal Nurs.* 2001; **30**: 192–201.

11 Heaman M, Gupton A, Gregory D. Factors influencing pregnant women's perceptions of risk. *MCN: Am J Matern Child Nurs.* 2004; **29**: 111–6.

12 Honest H, Bachmann LM, Sundaram R, *et al.* The accuracy of risk scores in predicting preterm birth: a systematic review. *J Obstet Gynaecol.* 2004; **24**: 343–59.

13 Engle WA, Tomashek KM, Wallman C, *et al.* "Late-preterm" infants: a population at risk. *Pediatrics.* 2007; **120**: 1390–8.

14 Krane J, Davies L. Mothering and child protection practice: rethinking risk assessment. *Child Fam Soc Work.* 2000; **5**(1): 35–45.

15 U.S. Preventive Services Task Force. Screening for gestational diabetes mellitus: U.S. Preventive Services Task Force recommendation statement. *Ann Intern Med.* 2008; **148**: 759–65.

16 Tuffnell DJ, West J, Walkinshaw SA. Treatments for gestational diabetes and impaired glucose tolerance in pregnancy. *Cochrane Database Syst Rev.* 2003: CD003395.

17 Tieu J, Crowther CA, Middleton P. Dietary advice in pregnancy for preventing gestational diabetes mellitus. *Cochrane Database Syst Rev.* 2008: CD006674.

18 Elsenbruch S, Benson S, Rucke M, *et al.* Social support during pregnancy: effects on maternal depressive symptoms, smoking and pregnancy outcome. *Hum Reprod.* 2007; **22**: 869–77.

19 Lyerly AD, Mitchell LM, Armstrong EM, *et al.* Risks, values, and decision making surrounding pregnancy. *Obstet Gynecol.* 2007; **109**: 979–84.

20 Malone FD, Canick JA, Ball RH, *et al.* First-trimester or second-trimester screening, or both, for Down syndrome. *N Engl J Med.* 2005; 353: 2001–11.

21 Wapner R, Thom E, Simpson JL, *et al.* First-trimester screening for trisomies 21 and 18. *N Engl J Med.* 2003; 349: 1405–13.

22 ACOG. ACOG Practice Bulletin No. 88: Invasive prenatal testing for aneuploidy. *Obstet Gynecol.* 2007; **110**: 1459–67.

23 Alfirevic Z, Sundberg K, Brigham S. Amniocentesis and chorionic villus sampling for prenatal diagnosis. *Cochrane Database Syst Rev.* 2003: CD003252.

24 Gates EA. Communicating risk in prenatal genetic testing. *J Midwifery Womens Health.* 2004; **49**: 220–7.

25 Hunt LM, Castaneda H, KB DEV. Do notions of risk inform patient choice? Lessons from a study of prenatal genetic counseling. *Med Anthropol.* 2006; **25**: 193–219.

26 Bramwell R, West H, Salmon P. Health professionals' and service users' interpretation of screening test results: experimental study. *BMJ.* 2006; **333**: 284.

27 Shiloh S, Sagi M. Effect of framing on the perception of genetic recurrence risks. *Am J Med Genet.* 1989; **33**: 130–5.

28 Paling J. Strategies to help patients understand risks. *BMJ.* 2003; **327**: 745–8.

29 Gigerenzer G, Edwards A. Simple tools for understanding risks: From innumeracy to insight. *BMJ.* 2003; **327**: 741–4.

30 Carroll JC, Brown JB, Reid AJ, *et al.* Women's experience of maternal serum screening. *Can Fam Physician.* 2000; **46**: 614–20.

31 Berkowitz RL, Roberts J, Minkoff H. Challenging the strategy of maternal age-based prenatal genetic counseling. *JAMA.* 2006; **295**: 1446–8.

32 Spencer K. Uptake of prenatal screening for chromosomal anomalies: impact of test results in a previous pregnancy. *Prenat Diagn.* 2002; **22**: 1229–32.

33 Weinans MJN, Kooij L, Muller MA, *et al.* A comparison of the impact of screen-positive results obtained from ultrasound and biochemical screening for Down syndrome in the first trimester: a pilot study. *Prenat Diagn.* 2004; **24**: 347–51.

34 Alteneder RR, Kenner C, Greene D, *et al.* The lived experience of women who undergo prenatal diagnostic testing due to elevated maternal serum alpha-fetoprotein screening. *MCN: Am J Matern Child Nurs.* 1998; **23**: 180–6.

35 Weinans MJ, Huijssoon AM, Tymstra T, *et al.* How women deal with the results of serum screening for Down syndrome in the second trimester of pregnancy. *Prenat Diagn.* 2000; **20**: 705–8.

36 Frank S. But . . . what about the tests? A failure of the negotiated model of care? *Fam Med.* 1992; **24**: 243–4.

37 Bernhardt BA, Haunstetter CM, Roter D, *et al.* How do obstetric providers discuss referrals for prenatal genetic counseling? *J Genet Couns.* 2005; **14**: 109–17.

38 Browner CH, Preloran HM, Casado MC, *et al.* Genetic counseling gone awry: miscommunication between prenatal genetic service providers and Mexican-origin clients. *Soc Sci Med.* 2003; **56**: 1933–46.

39 Browner CH, Preloran HM. Expectations, emotions, and medical decision making: a case study on the use of amniocentesis. *Transcult Psychiatry.* 2004; **41**: 427–44.

40 Press N, Browner CH. Characteristics of women who refuse an offer of prenatal diagnosis: data from the California maternal serum alpha fetoprotein blood test experience. *Am J Med Genet.* 1998; **78**: 443–5.

41 Preloran HM, Browner CH, Lieber E. Impact of interpreters' approach on Latinas' use of amniocentesis. *Health Educ Behav.* 2005; **32**: 599–612.

42 Dahl E. Sex selection: laissez faire or family balancing? *Health Care Anal.* 2005; **13**: 87–90.

43 Chan CLW, Yip PSF, Ng EHY, *et al.* Gender selection in China: its meanings and implications. *J Assist Reprod Genet.* 2002; **19**: 426–30.

44 Jha P, Kumar R, Vasa P, *et al.* Low female[corrected]-to-male [corrected] sex ratio of

children born in India: national survey of 1.1 million households.][erratum appears in Lancet. 2006 May 27; **367**(9524): 1730]. *Lancet.* 2006; **367**: 211–8.

45 Gollust S, Wilfond B, Hull S. Direct-to-consumer sales of genetic services on the Internet. *Genet Med.* 2003; **5**: 332–7.

46 Wenk R. Testing for parentage and kinship. *Curr Opin Hematol.* 2004; **11**: 357–61.

47 Bronson DL, Maxwell RA. Shared medical appointments: increasing patient access without increasing physician hours. *Cleve Clin J Med.* 2004; **71**: 369–70.

48 Rising SS, Kennedy HP, Klima CS. Redesigning prenatal care through CenteringPregnancy. *J Midwifery Womens Health.* 2004; **49**: 398–404.

49 Noffsinger E, Sawyer D, Scott J. Group medical visits: a glimpse into the future? (Enhancing your practice). *Patient Care.* 2003; **37**: 18–27.

50 United States Public Health Service. *Caring for our Future: the content of prenatal care.* Washington, D.C.: Department of Health and Human Services 1989.

51 Freire P. *Pedagogy of Hope: reliving pedagogy of the oppressed.* New York: Continuum; 1992.

52 Tennant M. *Psychology and Adult Learning.* London: Routledge; 1996.

53 Ickovics JR, Kershaw TS, Westdahl C, *et al.* Group prenatal care and preterm birth weight: results from a matched cohort study at public clinics. *Obstet Gynecol.* 2003; **102**: 1051–7.

54 Carlson NS, Lowe NK. CenteringPregnancy: A new approach in prenatal care. *MCN: Am J Matern Child Nurs.* 2006; 31: 218–23.

55 Baldwin KA. Comparison of selected outcomes of CenteringPregnancy versus traditional prenatal care. *J Midwifery Women's Health.* 2006; 51: 266–72.

56 Ickovics JR, Kershaw TS, Westdahl C, *et al.* Group prenatal care and perinatal outcomes: a randomized controlled trial. *Obstet Gynecol.* 2007; **110**: 330–9.

57 Massey Z, Rising SS, Ickovics J. CenteringPregnancy group prenatal care: promoting relationship-centered care. *J Obstet Gynecol Neonatal Nurs.* 2006; **35**: 286–94.

58 Tiedje LB. Teaching is more than telling: education about prematurity in a prenatal clinic waiting room. *MCN: Am J Matern Child Nurs.* 2004; **29**: 373–9.

59 Conde-Agudelo A, Rosas-Bermudez A, Kafury-Goeta AC. Birth spacing and risk of adverse perinatal outcomes: a meta-analysis. *JAMA.* 2006; **295**: 1809–23.

60 Smith GC, Pell JP, Dobbie R. Interpregnancy interval and risk of preterm birth and neonatal death: retrospective cohort study. *BMJ.* 2003; **327**: 313.

61 Holtrop TG, Fischer H, Gray SM, *et al.* Screening for domestic violence in a general pediatric clinic: be prepared! *Pediatrics.* 2004; **114**: 1253–7.

62 Escobar GJ, Braveman PA, Ackerson L, *et al.* A randomized comparison of home visits and hospital-based group follow-up visits after early postpartum discharge. *Pediatrics.* 2001; **108**: 719–27.

63 Shaw E, Levitt C, Wong S, *et al.* Systematic review of the literature on postpartum care: Effectiveness of postpartum support to improve maternal parenting, mental health, quality of life, and physical health. *Birth.* 2006; **33**: 210–20.

64 Bernloehr A, Smith P, Vydelingum V. Antenatal care in the European Union: a survey on guidelines in all 25 member states of the community. *Eur J Obstet Gynecol Reprod Biol.* 2005; **122**: 22–32.

65 Haertsch M, Campbell E, Sanson-Fisher R. What is recommended for healthy women during pregnancy? A comparison of seven prenatal clinical practice guideline documents. *Birth.* 1999; **26**: 24–30.

66 Fabian HM, Radestad IJ, Waldenstrom U. Characteristics of primiparous women who are not reached by parental education classes after childbirth in Sweden. *Acta Paediatr.* 2006; **95**: 1360–9.

67 Declercq E, Sakala C, Corry M, *et al. Listening to Mothers: Report of the First National U.S. Survey of Women's Childbearing Experiences.* New York: Maternity Center Association; 2002.

68 Declercq E, Sakala C, Corry M, *et al. Listening to Mothers II: Report of the Second National U.S. Survey of Women's Childbearing Experiences.* New York: Childbirth Connection; 2006.

69 Hoskins R, Donovan C, Merhi S, *et al. Examining Prenatal Services in Newfoundland.* CIET Canada; 2000. Report No.: SR-CA-nfl2-99.

70 Spinelli A, Baglio G, Donati S, *et al.* Do antenatal classes benefit the mother and her baby? *J Matern Fetal Neonatal Med.* 2003; **13**: 94–101.

71 Koehn ML. Childbirth education outcomes: an integrative review of the literature. *J Perinat Educ.* 2002; **11**: 10–9.

72 Morton CH, Hsu C. Contemporary dilemmas in American childbirth education: Findings from a comparative ethnographic study. *J Perinat Educ.* 2007; **16**: 25–37.

73 Tumblin A. How I teach evidence-based epidural information in a hospital and keep my job. *J Perinat Educ.* 2007; **16**: 68–9.

74 Lu MC, Prentice J, Yu SM, *et al.* Childbirth education classes: sociodemographic disparities in attendance and the association of attendance with breastfeeding initiation. *Matern Child Health J.* 2003; 7: 87–93.

75 Westmoreland MH, Zwelling E. Innovative perinatal education management service: developing a family-centered, hospital-based perinatal education program. *J Perinat Educ.* 2000; **9**: 28.

76 Blumfield W. Lamaze and Bradley childbirth classes. *Birth.* 1997; **24**: 132–3.

77 Baumgarder DJ, Muehl P, Fischer M, *et al.* Effect of labor epidural anesthesia on breastfeeding of healthy full-term newborns delivered vaginally. *J Am Board Fam Pract.* 2003; **16**: 7–13.

78 Halpern SH, Levine T, Wilson DB, *et al.* Effect of labor analgesia on breastfeeding success. *Birth.* 1999; **26**: 83–8.

79 Henderson JJ, Dickinson JE, Evans SF, *et al.* Impact of intrapartum epidural analgesia on breast-feeding duration. *Aust N Z J Obstet Gynaecol.* 2003; **43**: 372–7.

80 Torvaldsen S, Roberts CL, Simpson JM, *et al.* Intrapartum epidural analgesia and breastfeeding: a prospective cohort study. *Int Breastfeed J.* 2006; **1**: 24.

81 Leeman LM, Plante LA. Patient-choice vaginal delivery? *Ann Fam Med.* 2006; **4**: 265–8.

82 Moore ER, Anderson GC, Bergman N. Early skin-to-skin contact for mothers and their healthy newborn infants. *Cochrane Database Syst Rev.* 2007: CD003519.

83 Roberts RG, Deutchman M, King VJ, *et al.* Changing policies on vaginal birth after cesarean: impact on access. *Birth.* 2007; **34**: 316–22.

84 Lothian J. Concerns about the institutionalization of childbirth education. *Birth.* 1997; **24**: 133–4.

85 Bingham D. Helping hospitals change: Part 1: what childbirth educators can do. *J Perinat Educ.* 2005; **14**: 39–44.

86 Bingham D. Helping hospitals change: Part 2: childbirth education techniques to empower women. *J Perinat Educ.* 2005; **14**: 51–5.

87 Hodnett ED. Pain and women's satisfaction with the experience of childbirth: a systematic review. *Am J Obstet Gynecol.* 2002; **186**: S160–72.

88 Harris S, Buchinski B, Grzybowski S, *et al.* Induction of labour: a continuous quality improvement and peer review program to improve the quality of care. *CMAJ.* 2000; **163**: 1163–6.

89 Alfirevic Z, Edwards G, Platt MJ. The impact of delivery suite guidelines on intrapartum care in 'standard primigravida'. *Eur J Obstet Gynecol Reprod Biol.* 2004; **115**: 28–31.

90 Caesarean Section Working Group. *Attaining and Maintaining Best Practices in the use of Caesarean Sections: an analysis of four Ontario hospitals.* Ontario Women's Health Council; 2000.

91 Clark SL, Belfort MA, Byrum SL, *et al.* Improved outcomes, fewer cesarean deliveries, and reduced litigation: results of a new paradigm in patient safety. *Am J Obstet Gynecol.* 2008; **199**: 105.e1–7.

92 Chaillet N, Dube E, Dugas M, *et al.* Evidence-based strategies for implementing guidelines in obstetrics: a systematic review. *Obstet Gynecol.* 2006; **108**: 1234–45.

93 Flamm BL, Berwick DM, Kabcenell A. Reducing cesarean section rates safely: lessons from a "Breakthrough Series" Collaborative. *Birth.* 1998; **25**: 117–24.

94 Committee on Quality Health Care in America, Institute of Medicine. *To Err is Human: building a safer health system.* Washington, D.C.: National Academy Press; 1998.

95 Cherouny P, Federico F, Haraden C, *et al. Idealized Design of Perinatal Care. IHI Innovation Series white paper.* Cambridge, Massachusetts: Institute for Healthcare Improvement; 2005.

96 National Collaborating Centre for Women's and Children's Health. Intrapartum care: care of healthy women and their babies during childbirth. 2007 [cited May 13, 2008]. Available from: www.nice.org.uk/nicemedia/pdf/IntrapartumCareSeptember2007main guideline.pdf

97 Spear HJ. Policies and practices for maternal support options during childbirth and breastfeeding initiation after cesarean in Southeastern hospitals. *J Obstet Gynecol Neonatal Nurs.* 2006; 35: 634–43.

98 Grizzard TA, Bartick M, Nikolov M, *et al.* Policies and practices related to breastfeeding in Massachusetts: hospital implementation of the ten steps to successful breastfeeding. *Matern Child Health J.* 2006; **10**: 247–63.

99 Hotelling BA. Is your perinatal practice mother-friendly? A strategy for improving maternity care. *Birth.* 2004; **31**: 143–7.

100 Martell LK. Postpartum women's perceptions of the hospital environment. *J Obstet Gynecol Neonatal Nurs.* 2003; **32**: 478–85.

101 Morrison B, Ludington-Hoe S, Anderson GC. Interruptions to breastfeeding dyads on postpartum day 1 in a university hospital. *J Obstet Gynecol Neonatal Nurs.* 2006; **35**: 709–16.

102 Bandura A. Health promotion from the perspective of social cognitive theory. *Psychol Health.* 1998; **13**: 623–49.

103 Gillis AJ. Determinants of a health-promoting lifestyle: an integrative review. *J Adv Nurs.* 1993; **18**: 345–53.

PART SIX

Enhancing the Clinical Relationship in Woman-Centered Care in Pregnancy and Childbirth

CHAPTER 1

Introduction

Lucy M. Candib

The clinical relationship between the pregnant woman and her provider is so crucial to woman-centered care that we can view woman-centered work as a specific area within the domain of *relationship-centered care*. Paying attention to the feelings, ideas, function, and expectations of the pregnant woman, the clinician conducting woman-centered care will inevitably find himself or herself drawn into focusing on the relationship. At its best, prenatal care forges a strong bond between the woman and her provider through the multiple visits focused on prevention and health. Prenatal care is unique in adult health care for the frequency of personal contact in the absence of disease.

Gayle Stephens described those clinical problems and conditions that require a therapeutic relationship; included in his list are those that:

➤ are associated with marked anxiety or mood change
➤ result from life change, conflict, or stress
➤ may require risky diagnostic or therapeutic procedures
➤ arise from conditions that may be managed electively
➤ involve habits and lifestyle
➤ require moral or ethical decisions.[1]

The diagnosis of pregnancy, the provision of prenatal and postpartum care, and attendance at labor and delivery are all clinical processes that meet Stephens' criteria for health issues that require a therapeutic relationship. All of these conditions require that the clinician *know the patient's name* – meaning that the clinician must move beyond standard procedures and algorithms for diagnosis and treatment. (Stephens cites Adolph Meyer for this theme that knowing the patient's name is essential to knowing a person.[2])

Clinical relationships move through broad trajectories. The initial phase may be characterized by getting to know one another, setting the style of interaction and boundaries, clarifying roles, and establishing a database with closed-ended and factual questions. During this phase the patient may be assessing whether the clinician is the right person to meet his or her needs. In the middle phase the patient validates this choice of clinician and builds up a history of his or her caring. The patient and clinician get comfortable with one another, moving to a more empathic relationship based on shared knowledge, asking questions to clarify the meaning of specific interactions, and relating based on growing familiarity with one another. By the mature phase – or consolidation phase – of clinical relationships, clinician and patient have negotiated a variety of boundaries: of knowledge, power, and the extent of their relationship.[3] They will likely have worked through difficult episodes, misunderstandings, or clinical setbacks, and can reach levels of mutual trust, commitment, and acceptance, with potential for deeply based healing.

Maternity care compresses these phases into a shorter trajectory based on the length of pregnancy and the increasing intensity and frequency of visits. Relationships will naturally be different for a woman who knew the provider before pregnancy compared with someone who enters prenatal care and meets the provider for the first time.

> Susan (*see* Parts Two through Four) felt comfortable at her initial visit with Judith Peters . . . who inquired in an open way about Susan's sexual orientation. Susan freely told Judith, who used her first name with her patients, that she was in a long-term committed relationship with Geri, a woman who taught at a local college . . .

Prenatal care telescopes the phases of the clinical relationship as the woman and her family come to know the clinician in a concentrated way during the childbearing year. Some women, like Susan, carefully choose their clinician prior to pregnancy; others make such choices and enter into care only after they are pregnant. Other women may have little or no choice owing to limitations of geography, access, and insurance. If the standard practice at a crowded city hospital maternity clinic is for pregnant women to see a different provider at each visit, then little opportunity will emerge for the development of a patient–clinician relationship. (We will address this dynamic later under the discussion of continuity.) More typically, when the pregnant woman and the clinician meet for the first time at the initial prenatal visit, this longer and more intensive visit serves to lay the groundwork for the relationship to follow. In the first and sometimes second prenatal visit, when the provider takes a full history and conducts a physical including a pelvic exam, the woman begins to learn about the clinician. At the same time, the provider begins to know the woman and to find out about the context of this pregnancy and the strengths and fears the woman brings to the experience.

The pace of visits accelerates as the pregnancy approaches term. As the reality of impending labor looms, the woman and her family can consolidate their relationship with a consistent provider, making final arrangements and commitments to each other. Labor acts as the proving ground. The time and energy invested in building the relationship foster the depth of trust that allows the clinician to form a team in labor with the woman and her designated family. For everyone involved, the birth is the culmination of their hard work together, and the beginning of a new phase of the relationship and also family life. During the postpartum period, with its predictable stresses and fatigue, the clinician can rely on the already sturdy relationship to support the mother's competency and the participation of the partner, promoting their mutual sense of accomplishment. Whatever the birth experience, the clinician can highlight to the woman and her partner their strengths at this vulnerable time. For providers such as family doctors who offer continuing primary care, the relationship changes and expands as the focus comes to include the baby. Ideally, maternity care providers who do not continue care beyond the postpartum period learn to conduct the closure of the relationship – either during the hospitalization or at the completion of postpartum care – in a way that conveys respect and appreciation for the woman's strengths and her family's qualities.

CHAPTER 2

The Elements of the Woman-Centered Clinical Relationship

Lucy M. Candib

The critical elements of the woman-centered clinical relationship for the provider are:
➤ compassion, including empathy and caring
➤ attention to power in the relationship including the issues of trust and safety
➤ continuity and constancy
➤ healing
➤ self-awareness
➤ transference and counter-transference
➤ and during prenatal care, relationship with the woman's family as she defines it – the father of the baby or the mother's partner and other family members.

These same elements – using somewhat different language – are central to all patients, but this chapter will focus on how the clinician can best implement these aspects during woman-centered care in pregnancy and birth.

COMPASSION, EMPATHY AND CARING

The practitioner of woman-centered care does not function only at a cognitive level. Recognizing that feelings and expectations (as well as ideas and function) are key elements of the woman's experience, underscored by the newness and uncertainty of pregnancy, the provider responds with compassion, empathy, and caring. Women having their first baby enter prenatal care with unique fears and expectations based on what they know from friends, family, and the media. As we have seen in earlier chapters, the timing of the pregnancy and the woman's relational context strongly affect how she responds to being pregnant. Prior experiences (miscarriage, infertility, exposures, etc.) or new symptoms may create heightened anxiety, at times problematic for the provider who does not yet have a secure relationship with the woman or the couple.

> At her first visit, Pat (*see* Parts Two and Four) had lots of questions about treatment and about the dental x-rays she had before she knew she was pregnant. She called several times between each visit to ask about additional concerns . . .

Pat's provider faces a challenge in addressing her concerns about miscarriage, especially as she is already worried about an early prenatal exposure. Showing compassion may be especially hard when the provider thinks that nothing can be done to alleviate the anxiety; waiting is hard for all to tolerate. Women who are particularly anxious, demanding, or frightened during prenatal care may need the provider to provide an anchor of underlying stability and confidence – not that everything will be perfect but rather that the woman and her partner are not alone with their anxiety.

Maintaining a stance of empathy can be difficult when the woman's agenda is very different from the provider's. The medical provider's agenda usually incorporates surveillance and sometimes limitations in activities because of medical concerns; while the woman, too, wants to know if everything is all right, she also has questions about the meaning of various symptoms and whether any kinds of activities or restrictions are appropriate. Women and their doctors may have very divergent viewpoints on smoking tobacco or marijuana, drinking alcohol, or taking benzodiazepines during pregnancy. As we saw in Part Four, finding common ground requires skills at balancing these differing concerns. Conveying empathy for the woman's concerns is more difficult when there is a marked mismatch between the preoccupations of the provider and those of the woman or couple. In these instances, getting and keeping the relationship on track is more difficult. Young providers and providers in training may be so anxious about whether everything is normal that they heighten the woman's anxiety about the process; when sufficiently upset, women may even change providers if they feel the provider does not hear them or does not take them seriously, or is too anxious himself or herself.

Getting past these different sources of concern to show caring and connection in the relationship is the job of the provider. With a new patient, the provider can show concern through questions that attend to the woman's basic social, emotional, and economic safety. As we have seen throughout the vignettes, asking about her family and about who cares about her is a way to ground the relationship and show clear interest in her as a person. Asking some specific questions about her family of origin and her support system, sometimes while completing a genogram (as Larisa did with Melissa in Part Three), not only provides information to the clinician but also serves to show the woman a level of caring and concern that extends to her life beyond the pregnancy.

For women who already have an ongoing and compatible relationship with their provider, the first prenatal visit reconnects them and affirms the relationship they have established. The known provider can more quickly jump to the woman's thoughts and feelings about this pregnancy and help her think about how she will build it into her life, assuming that she is planning to keep the pregnancy. Even when a woman has less history with her provider, some prior connection is helpful in putting the relationship on secure footing. A provider may benefit from harking back to prior encounters with the family to establish a sense of connection. Established providers in small communities may have attended other family members' births or have been involved in other ways in the extended family's care. Providers are, of course, not perfect and do not remember everything.

> Jackie (*see* Parts Two through Five) was annoyed that Judith did not remember that she would never consider an abortion, so "Why should I have these tests [quadruple screen and ultrasound] anyway?" Judith nonetheless encouraged Jackie to see the genetic counselor and get a detailed sonogram.

Judith's obvious concern about Jackie's well-being and the normalcy of the pregnancy is able to overcome Jackie's annoyance, a feeling that in itself is perhaps a defense about not having sought care earlier in the pregnancy. Thus, when the relationship is working well, trust can grow with mutual knowledge of each other.

Women having subsequent pregnancies are more aware of what to expect from their providers but may also have preconceptions about how doctors are.

> When Dr. Miller asked Tonya (*see* Parts One and Four) about quitting smoking, Tonya responded, "All you doctors are on my case about the smoking. I smoked for all three of my pregnancies. After all the stuff I went through, it's no wonder I smoke. They tried to say my baby died of sudden infant death syndrome because I smoke. But my other two babies were fine."

Here Dr. Miller will have to work hard to establish the new relationship and find a way to show that he takes Tonya's viewpoint and feelings seriously, especially since he knows that smoking is harmful for both mother and fetus.

ATTENTION TO POWER IN THE CLINICAL RELATIONSHIP: TRUST AND SAFETY

The woman-centered relationship in maternity care inspires trust because the clinician shows a readiness to share power and a commitment to the woman's self-efficacy. The physician model of care may not promote women's agency during prenatal care and delivery, perhaps because of the reliance on the biomedical model, or perhaps because physicians are accustomed to consolidating their power and are less comfortable with a democratic relationship.[4] Midwives are more likely than obstetricians or family physicians to promote birth plans;[5] midwives and family physicians are more likely than obstetricians to believe that women's self-confidence and determination are key determinants for a successful birth.[5] Pregnant women feel a greater sense of personal control when clinicians encourage them to be fully educated about the issues and make time to discuss options and offer alternatives. Being able to make decisions about her maternity care sets the stage for a woman to continue as a decision-maker as she enters motherhood.[4]

Establishing trust is crucial to a relationship that must weather so much clinical uncertainty. Trust may not come easily when women have historical reasons why they might be suspicious of medical providers. As we saw in Part Four, Dr. Miller has to address Tonya's distrust of him directly. First he recognizes the legitimacy of her distrust:

> "Look, I know it must be hard to have to switch to a new provider, and I know doctors nag a lot about cigarettes, so it's no surprise to me that you might find it hard to trust me."

And then he makes an effort to put her in charge:

> "I will try hard to earn your trust and to be here for you. What kinds of things are important to *you* in your prenatal care?"

This approach enables Tonya to let him know that what she cares about is not having to wait:

> "I hate waiting. I want to get in, get checked, and get out. No sitting around waiting for hours. That's what's important for me."

Tonya's initial response to Dr. Miller may be based on her prior experiences of doctors, perhaps other white male authorities who tried to tell her what to do. Providers who limit how much patients have an active say in decisions are likely to generate significant levels of dissatisfaction.[6] Staying in charge may be a priority for Tonya. Dr. Miller's strategy to put Tonya first opens the *possibility* that she *might* consider trusting him down the road. Other women may not have an individual provider whom they can identify as their own:

> . . . the school nurse arranged for Samantha (*see* Parts Two through Four) to get prenatal care through a school-mothers' program and its connection to a prenatal clinic. The doctors there were busy and harried, and Samantha did not like going there or talking to them about her family or the baby's father . . .

Providers who adopt the stance of the "critical parent" may find it especially difficult to establish trust:

> Jen was a 17-year-old who knew she was pregnant but had not told her mother because she was sure she would be thrown out of the house (*see* Parts Three and Four). She missed school to go to the hospital in the city where she had scheduled a prenatal visit at the hospital she had heard was the best. There she had an intake visit with the nurse and was scheduled to come back for her first appointment with the doctor. After missing that appointment, Jen finally came in for a visit with Dr. Mary Thibeault at 19 weeks because of a bad cold. She had not gained much weight and had not been taking her prenatal vitamins as directed. She looked very tired. And, in fact, she had started smoking. Dr. Thibeault scolded Jen, and in a reprimanding tone, asked her why she had missed her appointment, why she started smoking, why she was not taking her prenatal vitamins, and why she was not taking care of herself. Jen just shrugged her shoulders and smiled in a defeated way, providing no satisfactory answer. She left the office verbally agreeing to keep her next appointment, but really feeling that it was not worth the effort of skipping school and traveling to the city.

Dr. Thibeault uses her power as a doctor to admonish the patient. By not starting from a position of empathy ("It must be hard for you to keep appointments . . . you must be really stressed to start smoking while you are pregnant . . ."), Dr. Thibeault loses the opportunity to promote trust and instead distances herself from Jen as yet another powerful person telling her what to do. In particular, as discussed in Part Three, women who have past or ongoing experiences of abuse by partners or authority figures are likely to have far more difficulty trusting medical providers. When pregnant women do not "behave" in ways that clinicians believe are optimal for maternal and infant well-being, providers may respond with lectures, criticism, and reprimands. This strategy not only does not work; it also undermines the development of trust and makes it difficult, if not impossible, to find out what is really going on in the woman's life.

Providers can err not only by being authoritarian or paternalistic. Unfortunately, the patient–provider relationship in maternity care can itself become abusive. Nurses and medical students frequently witness verbal objectification of pregnant women ("the section in Room 219"), condescending appellations ("honey," "sweetie," etc.), and misogynist language, especially around obesity. Rough and disrespectful vaginal exams during labor can feel like a violation of the woman's rights and body. At the other end of the spectrum, relationships can become abusive when a provider gets confused about the intimacy of the patient–clinician relationship and begins to touch women sexually. Such examples of abuse rarely come to light, but some providers take advantage of women's vulnerability during the puerperium to make sexual advances that confuse and harm the woman. In Canada, 3% of men obstetrician/gynecologists report having had a sexual relationship with a patient and 10% know of another obstetrician-gynecologist who has had such a relationship.[7] Women with a history of prior abuse are more likely to be vulnerable to such abuse; conversely, clinicians need to be watchful not to get enmeshed with patients in dynamics that could be construed as abusive.[8,9] All clinicians have a personal and moral responsibility to scrutinize their own behavior for the potential for abuse as well as a social responsibility to protect patients from abuse by colleagues.

Establishing trust becomes even more critical toward the end of the pregnancy.

> When Susan entered her last trimester of what was an uncomplicated pregnancy, she decided to ask Judith to refer her for a primary cesarean section. Her stated primary fear was incontinence, which she was worried would compromise her running. . . . At the 32-week visit, hearing her request for elective cesarean, Judith began asking more details about her past medical and social history. Eventually, with careful, gentle inquiry, Judith elicited that Susan had a past history of childhood sexual abuse, and was fearful of what would happen to her in labor, feeling exposed and out of control.

The maternity care providers for Susan, Pat, and Melissa do genograms as a way to understand the women's experiences and reactions. Through the elicitation of their genograms in the last trimester, both Susan and Melissa disclose a history of childhood sexual abuse. Women with serious symptoms of fear of birth who request cesarean section have a high likelihood of past abuse (over 63% among Norwegian women with these characteristics).[10] As noted above with Jen's case, women with histories of abuse may find it more difficult to trust their clinician. Providers need to find ways to build trust in very explicit ways and to establish constancy and reliability as central aspects of their practice if they are to build lasting relationships with women who have experienced abuse. As reviewed in Part Three, when up to one-third of women have an abuse history, then all pregnant women, indeed we could argue, *all patients*, need to be approached as if trust were a very critical issue.

Concerns about trust peak at the time of labor and delivery. The laboring woman is particularly vulnerable to feeling and being out of control, due to the reality of labor pain and the possibilities of highly technical interventions, potential misunderstandings, and real emergencies.

> When Pat's labor stopped progressing, Dr. Miller recommended a cesarean section, but she and Mike were reluctant to proceed with this yet, wondering if there was anything else to try still. Dr. Miller sat down with them and reminded them of their individual past histories – how difficult it was to trust doctors, and how frightening medical settings and especially complications could be. He asked if

they would like to speak with the obstetrical consultant first, before any decision was made, and they agreed.

Directly addressing anxiety and fright with Pat and Mike enables Dr. Miller to work through the decision to do a cesarean and to alleviate their persistent concerns about whether they could trust these doctors, in contrast with those in the past.

As we have seen throughout the vignettes, trust is critical to relationships; it is also about safety in relationship. Much is written about patient "safety" from an institutional point of view, with safety defined as a property of settings and systems that function to prevent medical error and thus prevent morbidity and mortality. We will focus here on the interpersonal, emotional safety that is critical to a woman-centered clinical relationship. Woman-centered care also incorporates the broader safety issues that are under providers' control to best protect women from medical risk, but still needs to address unnecessary emotional and psychological risks.

> . . . As expected, Geri's brother reacted by sending Susan a letter with quotes from the Bible to justify his disapproval (of her pregnancy and lesbian relationship). Susan returned to Judith's practice for prenatal care, and appreciated the acceptance that she and Geri experienced from the staff as well as the providers . . .

Judith and her staff provide an environment that is safe for lesbian patients and that enables Susan, in this example, to establish the relationship of trust that she ultimately needs when her fears emerge around childbirth. Providing a safe relational environment in the office, at the hospital, in the delivery room, and postpartum is the obligation of the woman-centered clinician to the woman who faces unparalleled vulnerability during the childbearing experience. Trust is not enough, however; systems need to be in place to make the settings as well as the relationship safe and sensitive to issues of bias and vulnerability. Unfortunately, change in attitudes and institutions is difficult to effect, such as hospital registration procedures (Susan's experience as discussed in Part Three) or insensitivity of colleagues to patients' concerns about racism (Jackie's experience as discussed in Part Four).

At times, as when Jen presented in false labor (*see* Part Three), it is impossible to establish an atmosphere of emotional safety, especially for a woman who may have substantial but unexplored experiences of powerlessness or abuse in her history. This work is even harder if the provider on call has no prior relationship with the woman. Attending to power issues by focusing on a woman's strengths is key in the work with previously abused women, and is central to transforming healthcare environments from being victimizing to promoting safety and health. But a focus on strength is difficult to implement if no one in the caring environment *knows* the patient ("knows her name").

> Mariluz presented to labor and delivery with irregular contractions at 37½ weeks, a few days before her scheduled induction for her severe back pain. Unfortunately, Dr. Burman was out of town. The resident on call found Mariluz to be 3 cm dilated

and −3 station, with no change after an hour of observation. The resident discussed this with the on-call attending, and they agreed to send her home. Mariluz was clearly upset and begged to stay. She tried to tell them that this was how her labors usually began and that she was going to have her baby that night, but they told her that she could return if the contractions became stronger or more frequent. Two hours later the delivery floor received a call that a woman had delivered on the ambulance ride in to the hospital. The resident rushed to the ER to find Mariluz on the stretcher with her baby wrapped in ambulance blankets and the placenta still inside her uterus with the umbilical cord hanging out. The resident approached her to deliver the placenta, but Mariluz snarled, "Don't you touch me. I told you I was in labor." The resident had to call in the attending to the hospital to deliver the placenta.

At her postpartum check-up, Mariluz appeared depressed. When Dr. Burman asked her about her childbirth experience, she collapsed into tears. She kept reliving the experience of being sent home and then being delivered by strangers in the ambulance, focusing on how the hospital staff ignored her when she said she was in labor.

In this example, hospital policy about labor checks and perhaps the inexperience of a trainee result in a plan that does not recognize the woman's knowledge of her body or respect her substantial strengths. Instead of the anticipated planned induction and delivery with support from a familiar clinician, Mariluz experiences an unsupported crisis delivery in an ambulance – underscoring her feeling of being out of control and powerless. She asserts herself in the only way possible: refusing to let the resident deliver the placenta. Her anger about this experience reverberates with her history of abuse.

The strong focus on the woman in woman-centered care requires that the clinician have a good understanding of self and broad tolerance for uncertainty. The clinician will need to be able to interpret for the woman that the uncomfortable is not necessarily the serious; that the serious is not necessarily apparent; and that the process and the outcome are not completely predictable or controllable. The more that certainty is essential to the woman, the more frightening will be the uncertainty of the process to her; the more that uncertainty is difficult for the practitioner, the more unable the practitioner will be to reassure the woman and her family. The clinician who can comfortably communicate the inherent uncertainties in medicine to the woman is more likely to be able to build a real partnership with joint decision-making.[11] As seen in Parts Two, Three, and Four, Larisa's work with Melissa and Kirk – from their earliest visits seeking the causes and treatment of infertility to their need for certainty about genetic testing, to Melissa's growing awareness of how her need for control may relate to her history of abuse – shows a clinical maturity and emotional sensitivity that serves this couple well. For a woman to develop sturdy trust in the clinician, she must see trustworthy handling of the inevitable uncertainties in prenatal care and evidence of the clinician's commitment to shared power in their work together. As the woman gains confidence in the constancy, the respect toward her, and the skill of the provider, she will grow in trust that the provider will act in her and her child's best interest at each step.

CONSTANCY, CONTINUITY AND COMMUNICATION

Constancy means that the clinician maintains a reliable and predictable clinical approach and caring manner that the woman can depend on – not that the clinician is always available and always the same. With time, the woman comes to know that she will be able to get attention from the provider for important issues. Like Winnicott's description of the "good enough" mother,[12] the "good enough" clinician maintains a consistency of practice that removes some of the uncertainty from each clinical encounter and fosters the woman's own mothering capacity. "Mothers who have it in them to provide good enough care can be enabled to do better by being cared for themselves in a way that acknowledges the essential nature of their task."[12:591] Constancy also includes the fact that the clinician has his or her own life, takes time for himself or herself and family, and takes vacation and other time periods away from work. We will address this further in Part Seven.

Continuity in maternity care is the practice of maintaining that constancy of relationship across time and sometimes across locations. Continuity across systems is also important; around the world, continuity in integrated systems of care delivery for mothers and infants has the potential to reduce maternal and infant mortality.[13] Within general medical care, continuity has multiple meanings depending on the domain under scrutiny. In primary care, the meaning usually focuses on:

> the relationship between a single practitioner and a patient that extends beyond specific episodes of illness or disease. Continuity implies a sense of affiliation between patients and their practitioners (my doctor or my patient), often expressed in terms of an implicit contract of loyalty by the patient and clinical responsibility by the provider.[14:1219]

Continuity is a value in all human relations.[15] When subjected to critical review, continuity of care is associated with improved patient satisfaction,[16] although continuity alone does not improve satisfaction unless the patient has trust in the clinician.[17]

Three kinds of continuity are distinguishable: informational, management, and relational.[14] All three of these areas are key in maternity care. *Informational continuity* requires that the woman's clinical data be available from one visit to the next (i.e. the medical record and laboratory data) and between one setting and the next (i.e. between office and hospital and back to the office again). For informational continuity of paper records, women have expressed a preference for the low-technology strategy in which they carry their own medical records from one site to another.[18] However, in high resource settings, electronic medical records (EMRs) are likely to become universal. Computerized prenatal records have significantly improved the continuity of prenatal records between the office and the labor floor (from 16% unavailable to 2% unavailable in one inner city setting),[19] but the impact of the clinician's electronic data entry on the woman-centeredness of the prenatal visit remains uninvestigated. In settings where EMRs maintain the information, woman-centered strategies are essential to keep the provider's focus on the woman and not the computer. In contrast, *management continuity*, with its clinical focus, requires consistency in the plan of care, both in prenatal care, when primary caregivers and consultants need to agree on plans, and especially during labor, when a constantly changing plan is disconcerting and worrisome to women and their supporters.

Relational continuity offers "an ongoing therapeutic relationship between a patient and one or more providers."[14:1220] Relational continuity is usually the meaning understood by patients and clinicians when using the term *continuity of care*. What constitutes relational continuity in maternity care varies greatly around the world and even within given institutions. In many parts of the world, one team delivers prenatal care and another team attends labor and delivery. After delivery, the new mother usually returns to the original ambulatory team for postpartum care – effecting continuity of ambulatory care. However, in sectors of the English-speaking world, some prenatal care providers attend births *and* do postpartum care – some general practitioners in England, some family doctors and obstetricians in the USA and Canada, and some midwifery and obstetrical services in Canada and Australia. These providers have opportunities for relational continuity across settings.

> Another year passed, and Delia learned that she was pregnant with her fourth child. She had seen multiple providers at the health center over the years and did not have a good connection with anyone except for one of the nurses, Maureen. Delia was not even sure who her primary provider was.

While measures of continuity vary from study to study, nevertheless, in every maternity setting where it has been measured, women consistently appreciate continuity in *prenatal* care and rank it as one of the measures of satisfaction.[20-4] Lack of continuity with prenatal providers has been associated with women's dissatisfaction.[25] What women value about continuity of prenatal care is a provider who gets to know them and can remember them from one visit to the next. The personal relationship with the provider, a real connection, is more central to a pregnant woman's satisfaction than seeing the same person at every prenatal visit.[26,27] Here the clinical relationship looks like a "sustained partnership,"[28] not characterized only by number of visits, but rather by the whole person focus and the clinician's knowledge of the woman ("knowing her name"). Thus a clinician who can connect quickly and deeply with a woman may offer more of the benefits of continuity to a pregnant woman than a breezy clinician who may see the woman more times but with less depth.

> When Delia discovered she was pregnant again, Maureen was the first person she told. Maureen arranged for Delia first to meet with Dr. Epps to discuss options, and then to have her prenatal intake visit at the health center with the obstetrical nurse practitioner, Harmony. Harmony's unassuming and welcoming attitude helped Delia feel more connected to the prenatal program.

Little is known about whether continuity of provider from prenatal care through labor (the attendance of the primary prenatal provider at the birth) affects the rate of intervention during labor itself. The presence of a doula throughout the labor affects the rate of intervention and cesarean.[29] What would be the effect if the clinician attending a woman's labor were a known and trusted person?

Instead, much of continuity literature in maternity care compares midwifery teams with midwifery/physician models or compares midwives with physicians, and may therefore reflect more satisfaction with the overall midwifery model, including elements of the gender of the provider. For instance, some studies suggest that continuity of the intrapartum midwife team with the prenatal midwife team is associated with some increased satisfaction compared to a doctor-led model without continuity, but continuity prenatally is most important.[30,31] Continuity of team midwifery care (compared to midwives and physicians) across prenatal, labor/delivery, and postpartum care led to fewer admissions during pregnancy, more prenatal education, fewer drugs in labor, fewer episiotomies, and less need for infant resuscitation. Women were also more pleased with such continuity of team midwifery care, but it is unclear whether that satisfaction related primarily to the continuity or to the team midwifery model.[32]

Within midwifery care, one Australian study found that among women who were randomized to either continuity of midwifery care across all three domains or to standard midwifery care, those who had a familiar midwife during labor had a significantly higher feeling of control and a more positive birth experience compared with women who labored with an unfamiliar midwife.[33] On the other hand, another structured review of continuity found no evidence that women attended in labor by a familiar midwife were more satisfied than those with an unfamiliar midwife. Women wanted consistent care from caregivers whom they trusted, but most did not value continuity of caregiver for its own sake.[34] Those women who had such continuity valued it, but those who did not have it did not value it, a finding consistent with the fact that women in childbirth tend to prefer what they know, making it difficult to evaluate their preferences.[35] In the UK, women especially value continuity of midwifery care between prenatal and postpartum care, possibly more than continuity with the delivering midwife.[36] For midwives themselves, continuity improved their job satisfaction and sense of autonomy without necessarily creating a meaningful partnership.[37]

While pregnant women value continuity, many also recognize that having the same provider for labor, delivery, and postpartum care may be unrealistic.[38]

> Amanda was a 28-year-old G3P2 office manager who connected strongly with her primary midwife, Helen, who worked part-time doing prenatal and postpartum work including home visits, but relied on the coverage system on the nights she was not on call to be able to have time at home with her family. Amanda was a bit disappointed that Helen could not guarantee being with her in labor, but liked that Helen was a mother herself. Amanda tried hard to have all her prenatal appointments with Helen, even if it meant that Amanda had to change her own work

schedule to be available on the days Helen was in the office. At her 39-week visit, Amanda was having some cramping and requested a cervical exam; her cervix was 2 cm dilated and partly effaced. Helen predicted that Amanda might go into labor before her next visit, and they joked about how the baby could share a birthday with Helen's daughter in two days. Amanda went into labor the next evening and gave birth to baby Kate on the predicted day; they went home from the hospital the following day, and Helen visited them later that week at home where they shared birthday stories. (*See* full vignette in Appendix.)

Studies of physician continuity in maternity care have received less attention. One study of low-income pregnant women randomized to a continuity setting versus a standard clinic setting found that continuity itself was not associated with improved outcomes, but rather that earlier prenatal care at the continuity site combined with increased visits led to better outcomes. These increased visits correlated with better maternal weight gain and improved Apgar scores, higher infant weight gain, and less neonatal morbidity.[39] Thus the impact of physician continuity of maternity care remains uncertain and would be challenging to measure in today's maternity care settings.

Jackie avoided medical care for herself although she felt well connected through her children's appointments with her family doctor, Dr. Judith Peters. At these well-child visits, Judith tried to remind Jackie about getting her own health care as well.

Midwifery studies confine the meaning of continuity to the circumscribed period of pregnancy, birth, and postpartum care[36] and do not transcend the childbearing period. For family physicians who have long-term relationships with women and their families, continuity can have multiple additional aspects: through the woman's life span, including prior pregnancies and this one; during this pregnancy in prenatal and postpartum care, not including birth; prior to pregnancy as well as during prenatal, birth, and postpartum care; and all of the above linked to seeing the mother during her children's well-child visits. Very long-term providers may also have the joy of caring for women, their infants and growing children, and then across generations when those children become parents themselves.

Unfortunately, studies of physician continuity in maternity care have not systematically examined the relationship of maternity care with long-term continuity preceding or after pregnancy-related care. One limited study of low-income mothers showed that continuity of provider from maternity to well-child care enhanced completion of immunizations at seven months.[40] In many settings, however, the shorter obstetrical stays and the splitting of care between different specialties (i.e. obstetrics and pediatrics) often result in failure of tracking and neglect of continuity of caregiver for the family's medical needs. Coordinated attention from known caregivers in a familiar, convenient setting can be central for continuation of breastfeeding, persistence in contraceptive method, and establishment of ongoing well-child care, especially for disadvantaged populations like adolescents.[41]

Mariluz had a lifetime relationship with Dr. Burman who was aware of her child-hood and marital abuse. Dr. Burman had known Mariluz and her family for over 25 years. While this meant that many aspects of the history were familiar to Dr. Burman at any time, it also meant that if Mariluz arrived for a visit for herself with two children in tow, she usually hoped they would be seen for their illnesses rather than sent to urgent care. . . . Most of the time, Dr. Burman could accommodate Mariluz's needs for continuity of care, but at times, superimposed on Mariluz's own medical problems and intermittent depression, the expectation felt burdensome to the doctor. Usually, however, they were able to balance these demands based on their long history together. . . . Mariluz kept every appointment for her children, and their immunizations were always up to date.

Although Mariluz can barely read, she can be clear about her needs verbally and non-verbally, and proves herself to be an effective agent for herself and her children with Dr. Burman even when it is not convenient for the doctor. Dr. Burman's choice to work with Mariluz under these circumstances supports the finding that greater continuity over time and visits tends to invoke a greater sense of responsibility in the provider.[42] Dr. Burman recognizes Mariluz's strengths and finds ways to adapt to Mariluz's often indirect style of communication.

Little is known about the impact in maternity care of such long-term continuity as Mariluz enjoys with Dr. Burman. An unpublished study by Ron McCord, cited by Stewart,[43] showed that having attended the delivery of a woman's child but *not* the provision of care during pregnancy was associated with positive rating of the current relationship between doctor and patient. On the other hand, in the Netherlands where midwives attend most deliveries, Dutch families still expect their general practitioners (GPs) to make contact at the time of a birth in the family, not specifically to examine the newborn, but as part of the GP's overall task – to see how the family was coping and to welcome the baby. Such a contact would show the GP's commitment to the woman's family.[44] Thus, satisfaction with long-term continuity of care is no doubt influenced by cultural and regional expectations as well as past experiences with a given provider or group of providers.

Despite extensive writings about continuity within midwifery and obstetrical care, many questions remain unanswered about the role of continuity of primary care clinicians in maternity care:

➤ How important is it to the pregnant woman that a known provider attend the birth?

➤ How important is it to the providers that they attend their own patients' deliveries?

➤ Does continuity of provider (from prenatal care, or from preceding primary care) affect the birth process?

➤ What happens in the clinical relationship if the doctor offering prenatal care attends the birth compared to when he or she does not attend the birth but continues as the woman's or family's doctor?

The absence of research about the role of maternity care within longitudinal relationships in family medicine is striking, considering the importance that continuity itself plays in the definition of family medicine. Extrapolation from the literature focused on maternity care, however, would suggest that women's preference for continuity in care, however defined in their setting – prenatal/postpartum without delivery care, or prenatal/labor/delivery/postpartum – should make continuity a goal of woman-centered perinatal care. (At the same time, providers must attend to the disruptive impact in their own lives and families of offering continuity in delivery care, as discussed in Part Seven).

Communication is part of the clinical relationship, but it is not the relationship itself. Woman-centered clinicians need skills in talking about hard things: an abnormal test; the risks of a procedure; miscarriage; a birth that did not go well. In areas outside of obstetrics, doctors lack skills in talking with patients about major medical decisions involving life-threatening illness and tend to focus on technical issues; they avoid the very areas patients care about most: their values, wishes, fears, and functional status.[45] Yet in prenatal and delivery care these may be the most important areas. The ability to connect at the values level is critical. Openness to questions, empathy, active listening, and giving feedback and explanations are among the communication skills that pregnant women around the world value in their care providers.[38,46] For low-income African-American women, clarity, continuity of care, trust, and a close relationship with the provider are the factors that determine whether communication is effective.[47] Women from various literacy levels in this vulnerable population appreciate clarity in communication from their providers, especially in making medical information understandable – "breaking it down."[47]

Communication is not just about verbal skills – it includes presence, non-verbal behaviors, expression of feelings, and attentiveness to the woman's unspoken feelings, as well as the words that are exchanged. Women from various cultures and with a range of educational backgrounds may expect and respond to different styles of communication. We can learn from those instances when communication does not work – vulnerable populations appear to be especially at risk, often because of differing underlying assumptions. For instance, pregnant adolescents differ from maternity care providers in what they view as motivations and barriers to prenatal care, with teenagers seeing the problems as part of the system (finances, transportation, and waiting times) while their providers tend to view the problems as intrinsic to the adolescents (depression, fear of procedures, and issues at home).[48] Such a chasm in understandings is likely to lead to poor communication. Low-income African-American women seeking prenatal care at an urban hospital identified trouble with transportation, poor coordination, being slotted into a routine, and power trips by the provider as impeding family-centered care – in this instance meaning coordinated care of mother and infant.[49] In contrast to routine or anonymous care, these pregnant women wanted personal attention. In high-risk situations such as a premature baby or a neonatal loss, being assisted with extra resources or special support for lactation helped make women feel special. For this group of vulnerable women, care that made them feel *extraordinary* was key.[49]

In other settings as well, women want to feel known as a person and have "a special relationship" with their midwife who has time for them or is "there" for them. Similarly, women visited by their general practitioner at home postpartum feel special.[38] The skilled woman-centered clinician will convey to each woman that she is special, using communication in words and gestures, allowing for questions and answers, thus building a relationship sturdy enough to withstand unpredictable events. With the woman's permission, the inclusion of partner and family in these communications can strengthen the bond with the provider.

Increasingly, physicians are recognizing that poor communication provokes a significant portion of litigation; this finding is particularly applicable to obstetrics, a specialty at risk in the USA and increasingly elsewhere for high-stakes litigation and expensive malpractice insurance.[50] Concerns about malpractice have led some obstetrical providers to avoid communicating with patients after a bad outcome. However, in the wake of the Institute of Medicine's report *To Err is Human*,[51] many organizations now recommend that providers let patients know how sorry they are about an untoward outcome without implying guilt or fault. The sooner that providers start talking to patients after a bad event, listening and supporting, and sharing the loss, the less likely that patients will see the doctors as cold, uncaring, distant figures whose conduct warrants a legal suit.[50] In the event of medical error, full disclosure, including apology, reduces the frequency of litigation and reduces the size of monetary awards from juries.[52]

HEALING AND CONNECTEDNESS

Optimally, pregnancy and delivery are healthy, happy moments in a woman's life cycle, but unpredictable or unwanted events sometimes require that the woman go through a process of healing to recover from the reproductive events. Healing in woman-centered relationships has the characteristics of connectedness and commitment. The goal of healing is to restore a sense of coherence, wholeness, and connectedness after disruption in life caused by serious illness.[53:94] In early pregnancy, the woman faces the task of incorporating the changes brought by pregnancy or the decision about termination into this moment in her adult development. Both induced abortion and miscarriage require that the woman go through a process of loss and reassessment of her priorities. Clinicians caring for women like Sylvie (*see* Part Three) and Pat (*see* Part Two), who both went through miscarriages prior to their successful pregnancies, need to incorporate an understanding of these changes in their clinical work and to be able to reflect on how such losses might affect later pregnancies.

The provider in an established relationship with the woman is ideally situated to help her interpret and integrate these events into her sense of herself as an adult woman in her own life trajectory, relationship, and family. Knowing Pat's history of her mother's death when Pat was a teenager, her pregnancy termination immediately thereafter, and the miscarriage of her unplanned pregnancy, Dr. Rosen is prepared to help Pat address the high levels of anxiety she is likely to face with her next pregnancy.

Likewise clinicians must work with women to incorporate experiences of operative delivery into their self-understanding:

> Sylvie (*see* Parts Three and Five) underwent an uncomplicated primary cesarean section when her labor did not progress. The next day with Viktor present in Sylvie's room, Dr. Burman underscored Sylvie's strength and resilience in labor and commented to Viktor, "What a strong and powerful wife you chose!"

Following delivery, the childbearing woman usually faces the task of integrating a healthy new baby into her and her family's life. Dr. Burman finds a way to define her difficult labor and delivery experience as evidence of Sylvie's strength and stamina. Sometimes, however, a woman must address her damaged self-esteem if the birth did not go well, if her body has changed or been changed in ways that feel deforming or betraying, or if a baby is not perfect. If a woman suffers the loss of her idealized birth experience or the loss of the idealized baby, then reintegration is an important role for the clinician to facilitate. Healing in this context involves helping her to restore her lost sense of connectedness to herself as woman, partner, and mother – as a competent, lovable, beautiful human being. While prenatal care and birth do not necessarily involve "serious illness," unanticipated surgery, loss, or sickness of either mother or child does require a healing relationship. Just as disease can disrupt a person's sense of coherence, a pregnancy or birth gone awry, or interpreted that way, also requires a healing relationship. The wise clinician knows that not just the healer but also the partner, the family and at times the wider community is involved in recovery. The healing relationship must extend into the woman's support system. Thus, fostering connectedness means involving the partner in prenatal care and birth, or when there is no stable partner, strengthening the woman's connections with her family of origin or other support system.

> Nancy Nguyen, a 22-year-old G2P1 Vietnamese-born woman who spoke English, came in for a regular prenatal visit at 32 weeks having felt decreased fetal movement for a few days. Dr. Burman was unable to hear the fetal heart tones and walked her over to the ultrasound suite, where an ultrasound revealed no visible heartbeat. Dr. Burman quietly said, "The baby has no heartbeat," and let the words sink in. She called the Vietnamese perinatal advocate who quickly joined them and began talking to Nancy in Vietnamese and helped her to call her husband and family. A few days later, Nancy came to the hospital for induction; Dr. Burman assisted Nancy in the otherwise uncomplicated delivery eight hours later of her stillborn baby girl. Nancy and her husband Tam chose not to see or hold the baby after the birth. The nurses took a photo of the baby for Nancy to look at when she was ready.
>
> The morning after the delivery, Dr. Burman found Nancy subdued and tearful; Tam was present along with their two-year-old toddler, Amy. Nancy said that she was not yet ready to look at the picture and that she wanted to wait until Amy was

not present. Dr. Burman talked to Nancy and Tam about how husbands and wives may grieve differently and show their grief differently. She noted that often spouses do not talk with each other about how sad they feel because they do not want to upset the other, with one result being real loneliness in their loss. Dr. Burman emphasized how normal it is to cry and to feel empty and sad, and that these feelings might linger for a few months, and might be different for each of them. (*See* full vignette in Appendix.)

Dr. Burman hopes to promote healing by enabling the couple to support each other through the process of grief. She is familiar with how grief often plays out differently according to gender. As we will see, by being explicit about gender, she enables Tam to take a major role in addressing the loss, matching Nancy's major role in physically suffering the painful induction and delivery.

The woman-centered provider for childbearing women and their families must be prepared to connect with the process of loss and grieving, whether this be about miscarriage, fetal demise, an imperfect baby, or the loss of an affirming experience. *Any* untoward event or experience that does not somehow match the woman's expectations or hopes may require the woman to go through some amount of postpartum processing and healing, even if baby is "fine." As with Mariluz, or with Pat in the example below, providers need to be able to reset their own measure of loss for each woman – and not dismiss a miscarriage, for instance, after attending another woman's stillbirth – and not disconnect from a difficult delivery experience because, "after all, she got a healthy baby."

Knowing about Pat's experience of loss of her mother as a teenager, and her anxieties about medical care, Dr. Miller was sorry to have to conclude that she needed a cesarean. He had really wanted for her to have the delivery she had dreamed of and felt sad to have to transfer her care, although he had total confidence in Greg, the consultant. Even though he had maximized Pat and Mike's control over the decision-making, he still knew she would be disappointed and might feel that she herself had somehow been inadequate to the challenge.

Leaving the hospital that night, after staying to greet and examine nine-pound (4 kg) baby Madeline, he found himself relieved to know that such a big baby would not have fit through Pat's pelvis even if he had pushed her to labor for more hours. He thought hard about how best to address her likely disappointment and decided to focus on this couple's strengths when he saw them the next morning after the cesarean.

The next day, after reviewing how the night had gone and admiring baby Madeline, he reflected out loud to Pat and Mike, "You know, I have to hand it to you all. You made a really good decision on having the cesarean when you did. If you had labored another six or eight hours, you would have had very little left to give her today. What's more, you two showed fabulous teamwork as a couple all day yesterday, and amazing flexibility in coming to the decision around the cesarean.

Teamwork and flexibility – those are what it takes to be great parents, and you two really have it. Madeline is a lucky little girl!" Dr. Miller hoped this would be a successful approach to what might be a tough postpartum recovery.

SELF-AWARENESS

Attending a birth and helping to make it an affirming event for a woman is a peak experience in the work of a clinician. Offering continuous woman-centered care during the childbearing year, at delivery, and beyond is one of the richest sources of satisfaction for clinicians who provide maternity care. Intuitively, many providers believe that the mutual trust and confidence between the known woman-centered clinician and the woman can decrease the anxiety during labor and facilitate shorter labors with less intervention; however, research findings so far document primarily the effectiveness of continuity by nurses, doulas, and lay women companions in reducing intervention.[54-7] The choice to try to attend "continuity" deliveries makes the relationship between clinician and pregnant woman more tightly bonded and sometimes more "special" than non-obstetrical patients. These positive benefits keep clinicians involved in delivery care for many years.

A high degree of self-awareness is essential for the long-term successful conduct of such work due to multiple potential tensions around relationships in the clinician's world. The long hours and unpredictable nature of maternity care may require the clinician to be unavailable to his or her own family for extended periods. Labors can go on for many hours, and inductions often take place over several days. Deliveries often occur at night, with the clinician frequently needing to have office hours the following day. Doctors may be called for a delivery with urgency, only to find a woman in desultory labor. The commitment to attend the labors of one's own patients can cause an internal conflict for the provider between home and office responsibilities and allegiance to the pregnant women. Practitioners need to be able to recognize when personal and family needs, fatigue, and value judgments may cloud their clinical judgment. The clinician cannot provide connected and insightful care when feeling conflicted about not being at home for a sick child, or when facing criticism from a spouse about unavailability, or when drained by excess clinical work in the office or at the hospital. The decision to rely on covering colleagues in order to participate in a family event, and risk missing a delivery and jeopardizing the relationship with the woman built up over months of care, can also create guilt in the clinician. Conversely, when commitment to patients consistently intrudes in family life, marital and parenting relationships are likely to suffer. These complex feelings require not only self-awareness but also the capacity for open communication with colleagues and family to be able to make the best choices for all involved. (*See* Part Seven for further discussion on these choices.) When such insight and communication are lacking, the experience of chronic fatigue, isolation from family, and at times an inhospitable hospital environment may undermine the clinician's potential to provide longitudinal woman-centered care.

Clinicians must also think about their own values and experiences as they set about caring for women making different choices. A provider who herself had an epidural for her own labor may find it difficult to identify with the woman who is committed to the challenge of an unmedicated childbirth. Conversely, the provider who is a staunch believer in natural childbirth must set aside his or her own viewpoint when caring for a woman like Tonya who plans on choosing epidural anesthesia for an uncomplicated labor.

> Tonya told Dr. Miller at the beginning of the third trimester that she wanted her epidural with the first contraction. He tried to talk about other options for pain relief, but she interrupted him, saying, "C'mon, Dr. Miller, you've never had a baby, I don't want any pain. I got enough to deal with in my life. . . . I'm coming with the first contraction this time. I don't want to feel anything."
>
> Dr. Miller knew that Tonya was likely to have a short labor and with support could easily have another delivery without an epidural. However, he recognized how strongly Tonya felt about getting an epidural for this birth. Part of really listening to her, and hearing her, was accepting this choice even though it was not the one he would recommend. He realized that Tonya's ability to control this issue, like having control over waiting at the office, gave meaning to what "woman-centered" meant for her care. Contrary to his usual practice, he smiled and suggested to her, "You'd better come in right away this time so we can get that epidural started as soon as we are sure it's labor."

The woman-centered provider can become emotionally invested in helping the woman and her family to achieve their goals during labor and delivery. Nevertheless, the clinician needs to develop ways to discuss with the woman and her partner the unpredictability of labor, the possibility of unexpected events, and the need for unanticipated interventions without being negative or "stacking the deck" by implying that this woman in particular is at heightened risk. Some may argue that such "just in case" discussions play into the over-medicalization of modern maternity care, but in fact, this kind of anticipatory guidance is not cooptation but rather essential care since labor *is* unpredictable.

> Ruth (*see* Parts Two and Four) breastfed her first child for 18 months, then she and Lewis decided to conceive again, with the same plan for midwifery care and home birth. Ruth's periods were somewhat irregular while she was breastfeeding, so that when she began to have tender breasts and morning nausea and confirmed her pregnancy with a home test, she thought she might already be a few months' pregnant. When she returned to Judith for the same prenatal monitoring that she had with her first pregnancy, Judith suggested an ultrasound to confirm her dates. As with her first pregnancy, Ruth and Lewis were reluctant to do this and declined. When they returned to Judith at 28 weeks, Ruth's fundal height was lagging significantly, and she reported that her midwife had been noticing the same finding, along with less weight gain than expected. Ruth's explanation was that this pregnancy was somewhat more difficult for her, with a busy toddler

and juggling work schedules. She and Lewis agreed to get the ultrasound, which showed a smaller fetus than expected for her presumed dates. The ultrasound report recommended follow-up ultrasounds and consideration of antenatal monitoring for possible intrauterine growth retardation. Ruth and Lewis came back to Judith with the report to discuss the findings. They continued to be very reluctant about doing a lot of monitoring, thinking that this would be just a slippery slope to interventions and hospital birth that they so much did not want, and yet they were worried that maybe something really was going on with the baby.

At times, the clinician experiences tension between the wishes of the woman and the dictates of usual practice in that setting. In settings increasingly characterized by technological strategies of monitoring, standardized guidelines for care may call for interventions that transgress the woman's expressed desires. The woman-centered provider may find himself or herself in the position of "guarding" the woman against unwanted and intrusive medical intervention, trying to advocate for her against the "system." Uncritical adoption of standard procedures without individualizing them to the woman's preferences and clinical condition (especially with regard to elective choices such as intravenous infusions, fetal monitoring, induction, and augmentation) may lead to a cascade of interventions that may not in fact be in her best clinical interest. The choice to enter the sequence of technical interventions may cause emotional distress in the woman or couple, including feeling betrayed by the clinician (with erosion of the relationship), feeling robbed of a normal experience, and feeling that unnecessary intervention may also have caused irreversible adverse consequences.

Judith knew how strongly Ruth and Lewis felt about the possibility of technical intervention, and proposed a compromise: Ruth would cut her work hours in half and increase her caloric intake. Judith would see Ruth weekly, in addition to her midwifery visits. Judith believed that if the baby turned out to be growth-restricted over the next few visits, Ruth and Lewis would recognize the slower fundal growth and at that point would agree to further evaluation. They agreed to Judith's plan, which they felt took their concerns into account but still paid attention to the concerns raised on the ultrasound. Fortunately, Ruth's fundal height continued to grow during her weekly assessments.

Working on safety *and* working on the relationship at the same time become essential. Clinicians will need to balance their allegiance to the woman and her goals with the requirements of providing safe care in technical settings that she might not find supportive or that she might actively reject. At the same time, if the clinician loses objectivity in recognizing complications, his or her attempt to avoid clinical interventions may adversely affect the course of labor, the maternal–fetal outcome, and the patient–clinician relationship. Thus, relationship-centered clinicians need to be able to interpret and monitor their own issues around the relationship; especially when complications dictate the need for consultation and/or transfer. Connected clinicians need personal strategies to handle these feelings of reluctance and make timely and appropriate decisions for their maternity patients' clinical needs.

Generalist clinicians are likely to feel satisfied when they can practice in a way that values their relationship with the patient.[58] With challenging patients, holistically oriented (as opposed to biomedical) practitioners may be more comfortable responding to patients' emotional distress.[59] Self-awareness is crucial when trying to discern the feelings and expectations of women or couples that feel demanding to the clinician: Melissa's and Kirk's need for certainty, Pat's and Mike's level of anxiety, Mariluz's dependence and feeling of betrayal.

> Dr. Miller was pleased that the day's obstetric consultant, Greg Diamond, was an old friend with a very patient and reassuring style. He reviewed Pat's obstetrical case with Greg, but also reviewed the couple's personal difficulties with trust. Greg spent 20 minutes with Pat and Mike, and after some time by themselves, they agreed that they would like to move ahead with the cesarean.

Most clinicians will not have the advantage of a prior friendship with their obstetrical consultant. Nevertheless, collegial relationships with excellent communication are critical to high-quality maternity care (*see* Part Four). The deliberate development of mutually respectful relationships between maternity care providers and their obstetrical consultants is crucial to smooth, transparent, and appropriate delivery of care for the mother and baby.

COUNTER-TRANSFERENCE AND TRANSFERENCE, INCLUDING THE ROLE OF THE GENDER OF THE PROVIDER

Counter-transference in the largest sense is a term referring to all the thoughts and feelings generated in a clinician as part of his or her work with a patient. Maternity care has the potential to stimulate many opportunities for experiencing and revealing reactions that fall under the rubric of counter-transference. For instance, at times providers may choose to disclose their own experiences to patients in an effort to build connection, model strategies, or gain credibility.[60] Women providers may be particularly likely to share their maternity and mothering experiences with their women patients.[61] Nevertheless, providers need to be circumspect about what they share – how does what they disclose fit into a given woman's prenatal care? How might it help her? The provider needs to be aware of his or her own blind spots and triggers in order to make sure that the content and direction of any self-disclosure serve the needs of the pregnant woman and her family, not the clinician's needs.[62,63]

> Hearing Susan's request for a primary cesarean section, Judith thought back to her own obstetrical experience many years ago, which left her with significant stress incontinence; a persistent but minor annoyance in her busy and physically active life. Judith considered sharing this fact with Susan, who herself was a nurse practitioner, but then thought the better of it; Susan had enough on her mind. "What

good would it do Susan to hear from me that incontinence is something you can live with? She would probably get even more fixated on a cesarean!"

Instead, at the 32-week visit, Judith learned about Susan's past history of child-hood sexual abuse and her fear of labor.

Transference is a term emerging from the language of psychoanalysis to describe how a patient transfers the intense feelings from early childhood relationships with a parent onto the authority figure of the physician. Transference occurs in small ways in all kinds of clinical relationships, not just psychotherapeutic ones. Sometimes maternity care relationships can evoke strong transference reactions in pregnant women. For instance, relationships with teenagers often involve transference when the authority figure of the clinician becomes another parental figure. Or, as with Mariluz, Dr. Burman has been able to provide some of the constancy and continuity in Mariluz's life that her own mother had been unable to give. Nevertheless, for the birth of Mariluz's fourth child, when Mariluz went into labor before the planned induction, Dr. Burman was unable to be present, recapitulating Mariluz's experience of a maternal figure who did not come through for her.

Dr. Burman decided that a clear, deliberate and focused apology would be appropriate. She took Mariluz's hands and looking directly at her stated, "I am so sorry I wasn't able to be there for you. I really wish I could have been. You must feel so disappointed and angry. Let's try to work really hard on these feelings and see if we can help you feel better."

Dr. Burman has to recognize her own sense of guilt for being unavailable, while putting in perspective her long-term relationship with Mariluz and her extended family. She also needs to be able to use herself in relation to Mariluz to promote healing. Knowing that Mariluz's relationship with her mother is still mired in conflict, she chooses to make an apology about not "coming through" for Mariluz. She hopes that such an apology can provide a healing moment to help Mariluz move through her long-term disappointments with her mother. Woman-centered providers in long-term relationships with patients need to acknowledge their own and the woman's potential sense of loss and disappointment when they cannot be available for a delivery.

The gender of the clinician can often stimulate feelings of transference. For instance, all of us are a little prone to see older men doctors as father figures and older women doctors as maternal figures. Most of the time such attributions are not problematic, but women with problems stemming from their families of origin may have gender-related problems with authority figures. Those women who have experienced poor mothering or an abusive mother may relate better to a caring male provider; women who have experienced physical or sexual abuse from male figures may refuse to deal with male providers and may consider all male figures as abusive. Thus both men and women providers can generate explosive transference issues in vulnerable women. Explorations during pregnancy of women's history of abuse will be helpful in clarifying the importance of the clinician's gender to that particular woman. When women's responses to ordinary clinical interactions seem out of proportion to the situation – inappropriately needy or distant and aloof – transference is frequently at work. Clinicians are rarely aware of these patient-held expectations and thus may not know when they are walking through an emotional minefield, full of buried hurts and losses.

Women clinicians appear to have the advantage over men clinicians in providing maternity care because of their shared experience of womanhood. Women providers who have had children have the possibility of sharing that experience with pregnant and laboring women and may gain credibility or camaraderie through the process.[60] Even women providers who have not had children seem to have an advantage despite not having gone through the birth process. In the psychosocial area, women providers are also more likely to know about conflicts in patients' close relationships.[64] Communication and touch are two areas where gendered practice may favor the woman provider. The characteristics of woman-to-woman communication in clinical settings typically include heightened sharing and partnership building and frequent mutual interruption,[65] although gendered communication in obstetrics and gynecology may differ.[66] Because of reduced patient fears about sexual abuse or exploitation by women providers, women clinicians are more free to touch patients and offer tactile human supports during labor – such as rubbing the laboring woman's backs, legs, or thighs – without arousing concerns about inappropriate touch. Men clinicians have to develop skills to facilitate the other support people (family members, doulas, nursing staff) to provide this tactile support.

Women's expectations of stereotypical gendered behavior may also favor women providers. Women may have more positive expectations of a woman provider and feel less nervous, embarrassed, or intimidated by the pelvic exam, making the whole interaction easier for a woman provider. Conversely, women's anxieties about being seen and examined by a man may make the pelvic exam more challenging for a man to perform and interpret. Many women would prefer not to be examined by men, and many cultures prohibit any man besides a husband from seeing a woman disrobed, preventing men from offering obstetrical care in those cultures. Insecure or jealous male partners of pregnant women may be less threatened by a woman provider. (However, if a woman provider identifies that a pregnant woman is at risk from her partner, and the partner becomes aware that she knows, he may attempt to force the woman to change providers.)

On the other hand, male providers have the unique opportunity to connect with the woman's male partner or the father of the baby in ways that can strengthen the heterosexual family unit when it is not abusive. David Stoller, a family doctor in the USA, describes showing a husband how to massage his wife during labor – involving a disconnected and remote father in the birthing process through modeling caring as a manly behavior.[67] Men clinicians' ability to teach other men how to become better partners and better fathers is an area meriting extensive exploration.[68]

Persistent stereotypes about gender may hinder both men and women providers. Women patients may have exaggerated expectation of a woman provider to be warm, motherly, or accommodating in ways that a woman provider may never be able to achieve during the brief clinical interactions of prenatal care. A controlling male partner may not respect a woman clinician and may undermine her management as well as the strength of his partner. Women clinicians may be perceived as "soft," emotional, or indecisive when they are waiting out a difficult situation. Conversely, men may be perceived as cold, distant, or uncaring if they are less expansive or less communicative than women when in fact they are actually shy, or formal, or cautious. Male providers being appropriately careful around issues of touch and privacy may be misperceived as aloof; conversely, they may be viewed with exaggerated power or strength that is likely to be disappointing if all does not go well. Perhaps as a result of these potential misperceptions, men clinicians committed to maternity care actually spend more time than women clinicians do at the first prenatal visit, perhaps showing extra commitment to making the relationship work.[66]

While the gender of the provider can be problematic, at the same time, each gender brings unique strengths to clinical work. In our attempt to achieve gender equity in medicine, we have often ignored what we can learn about gender strengths and what the genders can teach each other in medicine. Both men and women providers can become experts in sharing clinical power and in generating trust that can sustain the uncertainties of pregnancy and delivery. Both men and women have the opportunity to connect with the woman and her partner and promote a rapport that derives from their differently gendered experiences of adulthood. Women clinicians have much to teach men about how to improve communication for improved patient satisfaction. Honest expressions of empathy and caring do not need to be restricted to one gender. Thoughtful reflection on their own experiences as men and women and awareness of the family and culture of the woman and her partner can enable clinicians of both genders to forge strong connections with the birthing woman and her chosen family.

Clinicians bring other specific attributes beyond gender to the clinical relationship. Some of these characteristics are inherent; others can be adapted to the circumstances. Some patients will connect well to a given provider because of such attributes; others will feel less confident as a result of them. Young maternity care providers who themselves are in the childbearing phase of family life often care for pregnant women and families whose issues are remarkably parallel to their own experience. This shared life-cycle experience can result in tight bonds between young providers and young families; for instance, residents in training often connect most strongly with the families of their "continuity deliveries." Comfortable self-disclosure may result: pregnant and parenting women family doctors often share their own experiences with their patients.[60] Some women will find young clinicians less intimidating. On the other hand, older clinicians may seem more confident or more trustworthy because of greater experience. Older providers, both men and women, can join with the parents of the woman and her partner and promote a rapport that derives from a longer view of the life cycle. Grandparents are likely to feel reassured by a more senior clinician. More experienced physicians may be better able to handle emotional distress, common during pregnancy and postpartum periods, and older clinicians are more likely to know about personal conflicts in patients' lives.[64] Age and experience, however, are not always an advantage. In some areas of medicine, clinicians out of training for the longest time may be less likely to follow evidence-based guidelines for screening or treatment than younger practitioners.[69] Whether this finding is true for maternity care providers and how it affects the relationship is not clear.

THE RELATIONSHIP WITH THE PARTNER AND FAMILY IN WOMAN-CENTERED CARE

Lucy M. Candib, Nancy Newman, and Joseph Stenger

Patient-centered care incorporates the involvement of family and friends.[70] Woman-centered care therefore must understand the role of the partner – the father of the baby or another parental figure in the family unit. These relationships may be taken for granted or ignored. Men have often been excluded from and continue to feel uncomfortable in maternity care settings. Some fathers do, in fact, pose a risk to the mother and baby, and astute clinicians will be watchful for the signs of a controlling relationship that might make a woman vulnerable to violence. Nevertheless, for most non-abusive families, the integration of the other parent or other supportive adults into the clinical work is central to building a safe environment for the pregnant woman and for the new baby. The conscious and thoughtful involvement of the woman's partner in caring activities during her pregnancy sets the stage for him or her to take on a nurturing parental role. Successful incorporation of the father (or the mother's current partner) and the extended family into a woman's maternity care encourages the formation of a network of loving adults waiting to receive the new baby.

Because the woman herself may have a more established relationship with the clinician than her partner, when complications occur, the clinician must find a way to integrate the partner into an open discussion of the problems that have occurred.

> Beverly's son was born with a brachial palsy after a difficult shoulder dystocia (*see* Part Four). During the subsequent 48 hours, Dr. Diamond reviewed over and over in his mind how the labor had gone and what had happened during the delivery. He knew that the family was wondering about whether he should have done a cesarean section. Even though he felt anxious about bringing it up, he decided to address it directly when he came to see Beverly for discharge on the second postpartum day. Carleton was there helping prepare for going home.
>
> After his usual postpartum care discussion and exam, Dr. Diamond added, "I would like to talk to you now about what happened with the delivery. I think now is a good time if you are okay with that, since you are both here." Beverly and Carleton nodded their assent.
>
> Dr. Diamond proceeded to pull up a chair and began, "I am really sorry about Jackson's arm. I am guessing that you both may be wondering whether we should have done a cesarean section to get Jackson out . . ." He paused, and Carleton admitted that he had been thinking about that.

Dr. Diamond continued, "Let me share with you my thinking about this. We do cesareans usually when the baby shows sign of distress, or when the baby won't come out. In Beverly's situation, although the labor was progressing slowly, we had no advance warning that there would be a problem with the birth – the baby was not especially big, and Beverly has normal bone size."

He paused again, and Beverly, holding Jackson in her arms, nodded again. Dr. Diamond went on, "Could we have done a cesarean? Sure, but what would I have been telling you then? That maybe the baby wouldn't fit? That there's a chance of a complication? All that would have been true, but I couldn't know it for sure. This is one of the big uncertainties. Sometimes we can't know until the birth itself. We did what we thought best at the time."

He waited, watching their faces, and then went on, "Think about it for a while. I know it's hard that your baby isn't perfectly normal. I know that you or your family may want to blame someone. I take full responsibility for allowing you to have a vaginal delivery, and this injury is a complication of that delivery. I still hope it will completely resolve, but there is no way to know in advance. You will be the first to know. In the meantime, most parents want the babies to be seen by a pediatric neurologist, but to be honest, there is nothing to be done right now to change how it will come out . . . I am so sorry about this complication – I know it must be very hard for you."

Three months later Jackson was still not moving his right arm. While Beverly's mother still thought that the doctor should have performed a cesarean and prevented the nerve injury to his arm, Beverly and Carleton were more ambivalent and felt that although they did not understand the risks in advance of an injury from a vaginal delivery, they were disinclined to begin a lawsuit against Dr. Diamond or the hospital. They had heard about some surgery to move a muscle in the arm to enable the baby to move the hand and arm more normally, and they wanted to look into it when Jackson was a bit older. Beverly was fond of telling Carleton, who loved tennis, that Jackson could still be a champion left-handed tennis player.

In this instance, Beverly and Carleton benefit from Dr. Diamond's clear explanation of the events and his open acceptance of responsibility for having chosen to do a vaginal birth with the resulting injury. They are not mired in accusation and blame although Beverly's mother, one step removed, might still have tried to push the issue. Nevertheless, Dr. Diamond is less likely to be subject to litigation from this family because of his thoughtful relational approach that integrates the father into the process.[71]

As we saw earlier with Mariana in Parts Two and Four, the baby's grandparents, especially the grandmothers, can play a pivotal role in a woman's postpartum and breastfeeding experience. Familiar with extended families, the clinician recognizes family patterns of interaction and actively engages with the family members present.

On the day of discharge Dr. Miller arrived to see Mariana when both her mother and her mother-in-law were in her room. With the interpreter's assistance, he asked the grandmothers how they thought Mariana and baby Veronica were doing and learned that neither grandmother had breastfed her children. He reviewed lactation and invited their questions.

Partnering with the wide array of women and their families in woman-centered care requires that providers be knowledgeable about the typical beliefs among the women they care for, as well as aware of their own personal and professional cultural beliefs and values. Using "the family approach at each moment,"[72] Dr. Miller is able to connect with the grandmothers (who might have been positioning themselves to oppose breastfeeding), to elicit their questions and concerns and to secure their support.

Woman-centered care in the context of a woman's family means working with her family as she defines it – the father of the baby or the mother's partner and other family members. "The woman is free to designate whom she chooses to be part of her birth experience without limiting herself to the strict confines of the traditional family."[73:230] The astute clinician will pay attention to the various people whom the mother brings with her during prenatal care visits, making introductions and inquiring about their concerns and expectations for the mother and baby. This process of building connections to members of the support system will pay off during labor and delivery and later on during the first stressful weeks at home.

As fully described in Part Three, in working with lesbian parents, the clinician develops a relationship with the pregnant woman's woman partner that recognizes the centrality of her role.

> When Jonathan walked into the labor room he greeted Maria Isabelle (*see* Part Three), and then introduced himself to Guadalupe, who was actively supporting Maria during contractions. . . . Guadalupe stayed physically close and to Jonathan's eye seemed quite affectionate at times. . . . Jonathan focused on involving Guadalupe in the birth to the extent that Maria and Guadalupe desired ("no" to cutting the cord, "yes" to holding the baby soon after birth). And as he discharged Maria Isabelle and her baby, Jonathan invited Guadalupe to come to future well-child appointments.

Jonathan is particularly sensitized to the issue of lesbian mothers because of his knowledge of his own sister's family. Yet he restrains himself from making any open statement about Maria and Guadalupe's relationship, allowing them to reveal themselves at their own pace. His words, actions, and non-verbal communication all demonstrate his acceptance of Guadalupe's central role in Maria Isabelle's life. (*Author's note: Nancy Newman provided this example and discussion.*)

The clinician will best appreciate the specifics of the couple's relationship by first-hand observation in the office. Latent relationship conflicts between the partners will often surface during the stress of labor and around the birth. Identifying such tensions prenatally will be helpful to defuse such strains and can potentially ease labor for the woman and therefore for the clinician.

Felicity's ultrasound was abnormal (*see* Parts One through Four). Rafael was much less overtly worried than Felicity about the minor abnormality, focusing instead on Harmony's reassurances and wanting to get on with things during the pregnancy. He came to most but not all the later prenatal visits, when his work schedule allowed, and commented more than once during these visits when Felicity was anxious about hearing the baby's heartbeat, "Man, Felicity, you need to chill out or the baby's gonna feel your nerves inside." Harmony did not pay much attention to this comment the first time Rafael said it, but at the next visit when Rafael said, "All this stress is making you get fat, Felicity," Harmony noticed that Felicity flinched at this and decided to acknowledge the remark. "Sometimes tensions build up during pregnancy, and no one wants to talk directly about what's going on. You two seem a little tense with each other."

Some clinicians routinely elicit the inevitable tensions in the couple's relationship as a routine part of prenatal care. One midwife devotes a visit in the third trimester to what she calls "clearing the cobwebs."[74] She asks each member of the couple what each hopes and fears that the other will do during labor. Making explicit how they hope to support each other and how their expectations mesh or conflict allows an open discussion of these aspects of their relationship. Anger and fear within the couple can adversely affect the progress of labor. Facilitating a conversation about their views and expectations can allay the problem of such conflicts arising during the stress of labor. If group prenatal visits include the partners, the facilitating provider can attend to the subtleties of how the couple relates in front of the group, and can also incorporate these sorts of relationship discussions within a group format.

CHAPTER 3

Relationships with Fathers

Lucy M. Candib and Joseph Stenger

INVOLVEMENT OF FATHERS IN PRENATAL CARE AND BIRTH

Some readers may wonder why we would talk about fathers in a book on woman-centered care. The answer is complex. When a pregnant woman wants to have the father of the baby involved during a pregnancy, and when he, too, seeks that involvement, the woman-centered clinician has a responsibility to support that goal. "Making the father feel involved" can be a key element of a woman's sense of satisfaction with prenatal care.[23] But facilitating a father's involvement is not simple; helping him become comfortable in a medical setting can be a challenge. Clinicians often recognize that women tend to be the arbiters of how and when to seek healthcare for their families and usually initiate interactions with clinicians.[75] Men who may be avoidant about their own medical care may feel even more acutely uncomfortable in a medical office, especially if the focus is on a sexual or gynecological matter. Some of the discomfort may stem from feeling incompetent and disempowered. Men may reflect this discomfort either in bravado, saying that a doctor's office is a woman's place, or by adopting a passive role toward the medical system.

Danny accompanied Siobhan (*see* Parts Two through Five) to the visit with Dr. Miller after the ultrasound. Danny felt awkward to be in an office full of pregnant women and wished he could become invisible. At the same time he was worried that Siobhan had begun prenatal care so late. He was afraid that there might be a problem with the baby since she had not been taking prenatal vitamins or eating the way she would have if she had known that she was pregnant.

When Dr. Miller came into the exam room, he immediately approached Danny and shook his hand. "Danny, isn't it?" he asked. Danny was impressed that the doctor knew his name. After reviewing with both of them the normal ultrasound results, which showed Siobhan to be approximately 34 weeks pregnant, Dr. Miller turned to Danny and asked him how he was doing with the pregnancy.

> Danny surprised himself by confiding how worried he was about the baby and about Siobhan. The doctor said, "I am really glad you came today and let me know that. Even though it is late in pregnancy, everything looks fine. I know you have a lot going on now with your mother being sick and all, but I want you to know that you're always welcome at visits here."

Getting fathers to appointments often requires the active facilitation of the clinician. Their involvement requires the provider to do more than passively acknowledge a father's presence if he happens to be present for a prenatal visit. Explicitly inviting fathers to come in, gentle insistence on their participation as an expected and helpful part of prenatal care, and providing accommodation for their availability for appointments – all are ways to encourage the involvement of fathers in the clinical relationship. When the partner does come in for prenatal appointments, the clinician can further his participation by genuine welcome (including learning and remembering his name). The provider can apply the patient-centered method to inquire into the father's own feelings, ideas, function, and expectations about the pregnancy and the upcoming labor. Appealing to his caring feelings toward the pregnant woman and his aspirations for the child-to-be may help the clinician to overcome the father's reluctance to be directly involved. Asking questions that invoke his expertise with this particular pregnancy can evoke a sense of competence in what is often for him an uncharted situation. The clinician's eye contact with the father, and questions directly to him as well as to the woman about the progress of the pregnancy, can serve as powerful ways to normalize his participation in prenatal care. Avoiding condescension while not assuming too much about his level of knowledge and experience requires a delicate balance. Closing the visit with a statement of how helpful the partner was and how welcome he will be at future visits goes a long way toward enabling him to return the next time.

> Danny and Siobhan decided that they really liked this new doctor, and Danny made an extra effort to attend the next prenatal visit. Again Dr. Miller called Danny by name and asked him how his mother was doing. Danny was touched by his interest.
>
> "Tell me about how the first delivery was for you," Dr. Miller asked Danny directly.
>
> Danny answered, "Well, it was pretty fast because the baby had pooped in the water, and they had to rush him over to a bunch of doctors, but I did get to cut off the extra cord from his belly button."
>
> "Well, let's hope the water's nice and clear this time so that you can both hold the new baby right away and you can cut the cord again," Dr. Miller responded.

The presence of the partner during prenatal care, medical procedures, and tests can enhance his empathy for the woman's physical and emotional stresses. Such witnessing by the partner will at times move him from a perception that the symptoms and discomforts of pregnancy are "no big deal" to a perception of the woman's bravery and strength. Respect for her experience can translate into his greater involvement and support for her in overcoming the hurdles of pregnancy (especially if medical problems arise) and in coping with the demands of caring for and nursing the newborn. Fostering the father's involvement is likely to be positive for both the mother-to-be and for the clinician when labor ensues. The promotion of a sense of competence and teamwork among the couple and caregiver helps to allay anxiety once the pain and hard work of labor arrives and can be a crucial element when couples face a loss.

> When Dr. Burman visited Nancy and Tam on the day of discharge after their still-birth, she asked how they were doing with the sadness and saying goodbye to the baby. Nancy reported solemnly, but with an edge of pride, that Tam had held the baby. She had still not even looked at the picture. Tam said that he had wanted to see and hold the baby. It was clear that he did this for both of them, and that Nancy felt together with him in this process. The doctor commented how Tam's action showed how he could be strong for Nancy, just as she was strong in sustaining the delivery. Dr. Burman recognized that Tam's choice to claim the difficult and painful role of seeing and holding their dead baby, which Nancy did not feel she could do, was a way in which he strengthened their relationship and their recovery.

Involvement of fathers in prenatal care, labor, and early postnatal care includes both exploring their thoughts, feelings, and experiences and also actively engaging them through direct physical involvement. In prenatal care and labor, hands-on involvement can be a practical way for a father to engage in the process. Some ways to incorporate his physical involvement during prenatal care include showing him the size and growth of the uterus; showing him how to find the fetal parts and locate the fetal heart tones; drawing the fetus on the mother's abdomen; and having him feel the fetal head through the abdominal wall. During labor the provider can show him how and where to massage, provide cloths so he can cool or wipe his partner's brow, and show how he can support her in various positions during the second stage. At the delivery he can help ease the baby out, cut the cord, and hold the baby during any procedures that the mother needs. Often physically placing the father in a close and supportive position ("Joe, why don't you stand over here and try this . . .") and showing him how and where to support the mother is enough to engage a man who is feeling marginal or sidelined back into the active process of labor support. Even when the maternity care provider has not previously met the woman's partner, the clinician can apply these physical strategies to strengthen his involvement.

Often in hospital settings, fathers feel intimidated by the medical activities after the birth and are reluctant to step in close to the baby.

> Beverly went into labor after a 24-hour prodrome. . . . She had planned to try for an unmedicated childbirth. Carleton was nervous about Beverly's health and did not want her to suffer, but felt that the choices about pain control were up to Beverly. He was also somewhat frightened by the hospital environment, but felt

that all would be under control in the tertiary care hospital attached to the medical school.

José accompanied Rosa (*see* Parts Two, Three, and Five) to a couple of her prenatal visits when he could fit them into his two-job work schedule. He nodded nervously when Dr. Rosen asked if José would be coming into the labor room. . . . Yet when Rosa proceeded to full dilation and quickly delivered a 5 pound 11 ounce girl, Eva, José stepped out of the room just before vigorous Eva was born, unable to tolerate staying to watch the birth.

During prenatal care, providers often pay little attention to the partner's transition to fatherhood. For instance, Rosa's provider has not asked José about his expectations for his role in the birth itself, and does not anticipate that he would be so nervous that he would leave the delivery room.

After delivering the placenta and assuring Rosa that she had no need for stitches, Dr. Rosen stepped out of the room to invite José back in. The nurses were busy cleaning up Rosa. Dr. Rosen brought José over to the warmer and scooped the baby up in a blanket and put her in José's arms. She looked right up into his face. José melted into a huge smile. Even the nurse commented, "Look how happy she is in her daddy's arms."

Putting the baby in a father's arms or drawing him close to the warmer and encouraging him to touch the baby and showing him how the baby responds to his voice are physical strategies to involve a father like José. Praise for his efforts, his competence, and his active presence builds confidence for the future.

A further clinical goal in the inclusion of the father in prenatal care and delivery is to enhance within the couple the sense of shared experience, of collaborative decision-making, and of teamwork.

Kirk reminded the nurse that Melissa had asked not to have the eye medications given right away so that she and Martin could look wide-eyed at each other after Melissa's perineal laceration was repaired.

The partner himself needs support and information throughout pregnancy, labor, and the newborn period, including ongoing discussion about sexuality throughout the childbearing year. The provider can invite the father into decisions about contraception when such a discussion would be culturally appropriate.

On the morning of Siobhan's discharge from the hospital, Danny came in with the car seat. At just that moment Dr. Miller came in to do her postpartum check. He greeted Danny with a big smile, and said, "Well, perfect timing. Now that I have you both here, let's talk about the important thing – sex!" Siobhan and Danny both laughed.

"So what were you two planning to do this time?" the doctor asked, still smiling.

"I guess condoms didn't work so well, this last time around," said Danny.

"I was thinking about an IUD," offered Siobhan. "I'm afraid of gaining weight with the shot."

"Can't you feel that thing if it's in there?" asked Danny. "I mean, couldn't *I* feel that thing?" he added sheepishly.

"Good question," responded Dr. Miller, proceeding to explain about IUDs and their strings. After a brief discussion, the couple agreed that Siobhan would use progesterone-only oral contraceptives until she could have an IUD insertion at her postpartum exam.

For those couples who have completed their childbearing, providers can raise the possibility with fathers of vasectomy as a preferable option for permanent sterilization.

WHEN PARTNERS CAUSE HARM

In any discussions of partners, clinicians must recognize that women frequently experience violence at the hands of their partners (*see* Part Three). The postpartum period is a common point for abuse to begin, often for the first time in the relationship.[76,77] Although abuse overall is likely to decrease between 3 and 24 months postpartum, *severe* abuse is in fact more likely to escalate.[77] Not all abuse is physical: threatening and controlling behaviors and emotional abuse can be damaging, as well. Such abuse can occur in any ethnic group and any social class. Maternity care providers need to be skilled in asking all women about abuse.

Melissa was exhausted from trying to "do it all" at home with more of the housework and traditional gender roles than she had expected. She was frustrated that Kirk did not seem to notice. . . . Larisa wondered about control issues and gently inquired if Melissa and Kirk had been fighting.

Melissa replied, "No, no fighting. He's just busy all the time."

Larisa added, "What about saying things to hurt your feelings or checking up on you during the day?"

Melissa shook her head. "No, I understand you're asking about abuse. It's not like that. It's just that he seems so distant compared to before."

Working with the partner during prenatal visits and labor and delivery may shed light for the provider on the partner's attitudes toward gender roles and suggest his degree of belief in men's authority over women. While Larisa has not previously wondered about abuse during the prenatal period with Melissa and Kirk, she knows that clinicians frequently miss abusive situations. Rigidity in gender roles, controlling behaviors, poor communication, and physical and emotional symptoms can all be indicators of a relationship in trouble and can alert the clinician to the possibility that the woman will find herself disempowered, isolated and therefore at risk for spousal and child abuse. Clinicians must have a high index of suspicion and must a priori establish the psychological, physical, sexual, and emotional safety of mother and child when considering the involvement of fathers in woman-centered care.

FATHERS IN THE POSTPARTUM PERIOD

When a clinician can be confident that abuse is not a concern, he or she can join with the family to promote a positive, woman-centered role for the father in the postpartum family.[78] Breastfeeding is an area where the attitudes of the partner are influential in success.[79-81] Moreover, a woman whose partner is not fully supportive of breastfeeding will have difficulty weathering the ups and downs of lactation. Not uncommonly, however, the father may feel excluded by breastfeeding and inadequate in not providing sustenance to the baby and not being able to soothe the baby as well as the mother seems able to. While having strong feelings of responsibility toward the baby, the new father of a breastfeeding baby can feel frustrated, disappointed, and inadequate.[82]

> Dr. Miller arrived to see Pat on her first postoperative day just as she was finishing nursing Madeline. Mike leaned over his wife, helping adjust the pillows to make her more comfortable, and then cradling the baby to bring her over to change her diaper. Dr. Miller took a moment to acknowledge Mike's partnership. "I knew what an expert dad you were going to be! All that work you did in prenatal care and labor, and here you are again – already figuring out what Pat and Madeline need for the breastfeeding to work."

The woman-centered provider will address the father's need for knowledge about breastfeeding and support him to develop skills in infant care. Exploring a father's thoughts and feelings fosters his ability to provide more physical and emotional support to his partner during the period of lactation. Emphasizing the importance of the father's role of support and the health benefits of breastfeeding may prevent his alienation from the process and mitigate the tendency for him to feel separate from the mother–baby dyad in the early infancy period.

Many men feel uncertain in the unfamiliar environment of clinical care of women and infants. Finding and honoring areas of competence is crucial to facilitating the partner's sense of pride in his ability to be a good partner and a good father. Just as in parenting, finding a way to "catch him doing something good" and praising that behavior is the best avenue to foster such behaviors. Men are often socialized to leave the work of childbearing, birthing, and childrearing to the mother. A practical example to counter such gender role patterning is to be sure that the father has the opportunity to change the baby's diaper during the newborn period. Fathers who engaged in very early infant contact in the newborn period were more likely to still be touching their infants three months later.[83,84]

> Larisa learned that Kirk was doing most of the diaper changes when he was home. Larisa commented, "I wonder whether you would be willing to put your obvious expertise in that to work at night, also, so that Melissa could get a bit more sleep." Kirk offered in addition to do one of the night-time feedings with pumped breast milk if Melissa agreed.

When the clinician takes the stance of assuming that the father can become competent in infant-related activities and provides on-the-spot suggestions to enhance that competency, he or she is fostering that father's participation and connectedness. Making suggestions that do not come across as condescending requires sensitivity and practice, but such opportunities boost the father's sense of competence and thereby his involvement in active parenting of the infant.

> After Larisa helped Kerry and Ron work out a way to have Ron stay involved in Erika's care, Ron lagged a minute after Kerry went out with the baby to thank Larisa. "You make me feel like a real dad."

In Melissa and Kirk's situation, pumping milk and allowing Kirk to take over one of the feedings would require that Melissa relinquish a portion of her role as the exclusive provider of feedings. A more involved father means that the mother cannot be completely in charge of the infant. Thus, the clinician can also remind the mothers that each parent develops his or her own strategy to accomplish routine tasks of childcare; the mother needs to be reminded to avoid the stance of "Let me show you how to do it right," as seen in Michelle and George's situation (*see* Part Three):

> Nathan, George and Michelle's first baby, was very fussy. Michelle had read that fussy and colicky babies liked to be wrapped tightly and carried around, so she used this strategy but quickly got discouraged when it did not work. She also wondered if something she was eating was making the baby colicky. George, who felt somewhat excluded from the breastfeeding duo, offered to help. He laid Nathan out on his forearm and jiggled him steadily while reading a book or the newspaper. Nathan responded to this treatment and calmed and finally fell asleep. Michelle seemed to disapprove of George's strategy because it did not match what she had read, but also felt that she could not do it alone. She wanted George to do it her way, but his way worked. She called their family doctor, Judith Peters, who asked what was working. Michelle admitted that George was able to calm the baby with his method. Judith advised Michelle that there was no magic answer to colic and that sometimes fathers found innovative ways to solve problems. She suggested, "If it works, by all means, keep doing it!" And, Judith added, "If you and George are really going to parent 50–50, you need let him do it the way it works for him." Deep down, Michelle knew Judith was right.

In the setting of talking about handling distress, the provider has the opportunity to raise a key issue for all new parents under stress – how sleepless parents and a constantly crying child can lead to anger toward the infant, even the potentially deadly shaking of a baby. A proactive discussion of the impulse to shake a baby may be a critical preventive measure. Giving this message to all parents (not just the mother) – beginning in the immediate postpartum period – is a concrete step that providers can make toward reducing this form of abuse. Parents with a history of maltreatment themselves during childhood are more at risk of mistreating a child if they are under age 21, have a history of depression or other psychiatric illness, or if another violent adult lives in the home.[85,86] When the genogram and the presence of any of these risk factors suggest that parents may be particularly at risk in their parenting skills, the clinician can offer more frequent visits, introduce additional supports, and be prepared for further interventions if necessary.

The woman-centered provider asks parents how they support each other and reminds them that they may not always agree. Acknowledging the stress of a new infant, the provider can explore marital stress and ask how the birth has affected their relationship. To foster the father's involvement, the clinician can remind him of his importance – that his role is not limited to being the breadwinner. Many resources are available to help clinicians support fathers (*see* http://nccic.acf.hhs.gov/poptopics/ fatherinvolvement.html). After determining his concerns and comfort with parenting tasks, the provider can encourage the father in taking on some specific task and in spending time alone with the infant. In this way the father can support the mother and decrease maternal stress. The provider can also suggest that he be on the lookout for symptoms of depression for either of them.

AFTER THE NEWBORN PERIOD

Not all maternity providers stay involved with families in the postpartum period beyond the postpartum visit, but providers such as family physicians, who offer care to whole families, may continue their relationships with fathers after the newborn period, even after the issues of contraception and breastfeeding have been addressed. Some midwives, likewise, may have longer range follow-up with families in their care. And pediatricians, especially if they are already involved with a family because of an older child, have a wide opportunity to foster engagement with fathers over the course of well-child care. The following section addresses working with fathers after the immediate newborn period.

The early experience of fathering a baby can often be rocky. Fathers enter the process with high expectations of the relationship, wanting emotional involvement and connection with the child.[82] Often fathers use the opportunity of pregnancy and early parenting to reflect on their relationships with their own fathers,[87] and many want to be different from their own fathers.[78] But as the reality of life with a new baby unfolds, they see that their expectations were unrealistic – no magical bond appears instantly, and the infant does not respond specifically to them as a nurturer the way the baby responds to the mother. After the first few weeks go by, fathers often realize that they will have to change their expectations and develop new strategies to create the fathering role for themselves. When infants start to respond more, usually around six to eight weeks of age, with smiling and social responsiveness, fathers start to feel more enjoyment and connection.[82]

The father's ability to provide practical and emotional support can counteract or buffer the effects of maternal postpartum depression.[88] Fathers want to offer such support, but often lack the skills and the role models for providing this help; without explicit encouragement from clinicians, fathers may lose the opportunity to reduce their partners' risk of postpartum depression.[89] Clinicians can encourage the partner to give the new mother some time alone – to shop, exercise, or just relax – when she does not have to be attending to the baby. Likewise, fathers can benefit from finding peer support in the postpartum period, apart from the mother of the baby. Through welcoming fathers and making their office schedules friendly to fathers' work schedules, clinicians who care for children can play a strong role in enhancing fathers' caregiving and increasing their involvement.[78]

Fathering is not without its challenges. Fathers, as well as mothers, experience significant distress and depression during the year of pregnancy and childbearing.[90] Their symptoms are highest during pregnancy with only a small improvement three months after the birth.[91] Postpartum depression in fathers is not uncommon; 10% of fathers are depressed at nine months,[90] twice as often as among adult men in general. Fathers are more likely to get depressed if they were depressed during the prenatal period,[92] and if the mothers have postpartum depression, when 25–50% of fathers will measure as depressed as well.[88] Paternal depression tends to start after maternal postpartum depression and be long lasting, with the highest level of distress at one year.[92] Fathers also feel that the sexual aspect of their relationship deteriorates after pregnancy as well as other quality of life measures such as recreation, job satisfaction, and sleep. Conventional measures may miss their depression or anxiety problems.[91] For different reasons, several of the fathers in the vignettes may be more vulnerable to depression – Mike, already anxious, with more responsibility; Danny, with his mother's sickness and dependency; Ed, working two jobs and now with Evelyn depressed and a premature infant (*see* Part Two); Kirk, inundated with work demands – each of these fathers merits clinicians' awareness that paternal depression might become an issue during the postpartum year.

Maternal and paternal distress are not isolated processes; when the partners of depressed mothers try to provide support, they experience an increase in the tension in the relationship; they get told they "can't do anything right."[93] Paternal depression also affects how the mother parents – for instance, she is less likely to tell stories to the child if the father is depressed.[90] Family physicians who care for both partners and the child(ren) are ideally poised to identify paternal depression and work to relieve it. Other clinicians, such as family-centered pediatricians or midwives working with well woman care beyond the postpartum period, will need to make use of referral networks to facilitate treatment of this condition and its sequelae.

Fathers are increasingly involved in childcare in developed countries, especially among families who are poor or where unemployment is frequent, when the parents are working part-time, and when the children are small.[94] Employed mothers *want* fathers to be providing childcare in these situations; indeed 53% of women identify the father of the baby as the person they most prefer to do childcare.[95]

> Rosa and José decided that they would share the childcare by working opposite shifts. Rosa would be home in the daytime with Eva and work evenings while José looked after Eva; José would work nights and sleep in the daytime. . . . José became very skilled at feeding and changing Eva and recognizing her needs. Once in a while the schedule worked for him to be the one bringing Eva for her morning well-child visits.

Marital status can influence how fathers of infants view their role. Unmarried fathers, who may not see marriage as essential, emphasize their importance in the baby's present life, whereas married fathers view their fathering as modeling supportive behaviors toward the mother and striving for work–family balance in the relationship.[96] In both instances, presence and role modeling are key. Whether married or unmarried, fathers want to serve and can serve as models and as teachers who can provide affection, nurturing, and comfort. Supporting paternal involvement for its own sake is important. Although parents may enter childbearing with the rosy illusion that having children will make their relationship stronger, ultimately 50% of unions dissolve, with particular rapidity for couples under age 20 and those without a high school education.[97] In such an unstable and unpredictable climate, the ultimate goal of promoting father/partner's involvement may not revolve around the mother's well-being or his relationship with the mother of the child. Rather the goal of partner involvement may lie in promoting lasting, healthy joint parenting when relationship is desired, and fostering safe, caring, effective parenting even if the parental relationship is not enduring. Thus the provider who works with teen parents can bring up the fragility of teen relationships and reinforce the importance of each parent continuing the connection with the baby even if the couple's relationship does not last.

Clinicians who care for the whole family and see fathers at well-child visits have the unique opportunity to help shape how fathers think about parenting. Creating a genogram with the partner helps the clinician gain an understanding of the role of men in his family, particularly in relation to childbirth and infancy. Eliciting information about his memories and feelings about his own parenting is an important step – a "parenting history."[78] "Do you want to be a father like your father?" is one of the most revealing questions. A father's own symptoms postpartum may relate to the parenting that he himself received.[92] Asking what he hopes to replicate from his own childhood and what he hopes to avoid allows the clinician to identify areas of risk and to initiate interventions to prevent problems in parenting. With the knowledge of both parents' genograms, the provider is well situated to encourage them about creating new patterns for their new family and not falling into distressing patterns from their families of origin.[78]

New mothers and their partners bring to their family life strongly held beliefs about how men and women should relate to each other and to their children. When the woman chooses to seek care for pregnancy, birth, and the postpartum period with her partner, the woman-centered clinician needs to find a way to build a partnership with the couple and to discover their values and beliefs. Likewise, clinicians need to be aware of their own personal, family, and cultural beliefs about the "best" kinds of spousal relations and ways to raise children so that they can provide care unencumbered by biases, prejudices, and discrimination. The challenges are great, as we have seen earlier: work with the teenage couple (Samantha and Jack), the couple in recovery from problematic substance abuse (Delia and Paco), the immigrant family (Rosa and José), the lesbian couples (Maria Isabella and Guadalupe, Susan and Geri), the academic couple (George and Michelle), the grieving couple (Nancy and Tam), the anxious couple (Pat and Mike), or the professional engineering couple (Melissa and Kirk), will require a wide range of skills and a variety of strategies to work with the partners in such different couples. Despite the differences in the structure and economics of medical care for parents around the world and despite the fact that these examples derive from a largely North American perspective, the kinds of problems these couples face are likely to have their parallels around the globe.

SUMMARY

In the work of maternity care, clinicians forge relationships with women, their partners, and their families – relationships based in continuity and constancy that attend to issues of power and trust and that incorporate compassion and caring into the minute-to-minute, hour-to-hour, day-to-day process of delivering care. The woman-centered character of such relationships takes into consideration the provider's self-awareness and knowledge of transference and counter-transference in the course of striving for a healing relationship. Such personal work runs counter to the trend of the increasingly technical and risk-based obstetrical attention available to women in many modern settings. Not surprisingly, the practice of relationship-based woman-centered care faces great challenges in today's media-driven, technology-dominated medical marketplace. The next part will address how the woman-centered clinician and his or her colleagues might realistically approach some of these challenges.

REFERENCES

1 Stephens GG. *The Intellectual Basis of Family Practice.* Tucson, AZ: Winter Publishing Co.; 1982.

2 Stephens GG. Reflections of a post-Flexnerian physician. In: White KL, editor. *The Task of Medicine: dialogue at Wickenberg.* Menlo Park, CA: The Henry J. Kaiser Family Foundation; 1988. pp. 172–89.

3 Gore J, Ogden J. Developing, validating and consolidating the doctor–patient relationship: the patients' views of a dynamic process. *Br J Gen Pract.* 1998; **48**: 1391–94.

4 Coughlan R, Jung KE. New mothers' experiences of agency during prenatal and delivery care: clinical practice, communication & embodiment. *J Prenat Perinat Psychol Health.* 2006; **20**: 1–25.

5 Reime B, Klein MC, Kelly A, *et al.* Do maternity care provider groups have different attitudes towards birth? *BJOG.* 2004; **111**: 1388–93.

6 Brown S, Lumley J. Changing childbirth: lessons from an Australian survey of 1336 women. *Br J Obstet Gynaecol.* 1998; **105**: 143–55.

7 Lamont JA, Woodward C. Patient–physician sexual involvement: a Canadian survey of obstetrician-gynecologists. *CMAJ.* 1994; **150**: 1433–9.

8 Kluft RP. Incest and subsequent revictimization: the case of therapist–patient sexual exploitation, with a description of the sitting duck syndrome. In: Kluft RP, editor. *Incest-related Syndromes of Adult Psychopathology.* Washington, D.C.: American Psychiatric Press; 1990. pp. 263–87.

9 Golden GA, Brennan M. Managing erotic feelings in the physician–patient relationship. *CMAJ.* 1995; **153**: 1241–5.

10 Nerum H, Halvorsen L, Sorlie T, *et al.* Maternal request for cesarean section due to fear of birth: can it be changed through crisis-oriented counseling? *Birth.* 2006; **33**: 221–8.

11 Henry MS. Uncertainty, responsibility, and the evolution of the physician/patient relationship. *J Med Ethics.* 2006; **32**: 321–3.

12 Winnicott DW. The theory of the parent–infant relationship. *Int J Psychoanal.* 1961; **41**: 571–95.

13 Kerber KJ, de Graft-Johnson JE, Bhutta ZA, *et al.* Continuum of care for maternal, newborn, and child health: from slogan to service delivery. *Lancet.* 2007; **370**: 1358–69.

14 Haggerty JL, Reid RR, Freeman GK, *et al.* Continuity of care: a multidisciplinary review. *BMJ.* 2003; **327**: 1219–21.

15 Olesen F. A framework for clinical general practice and for research and teaching in the discipline. *Fam Pract.* 2003; **20**: 318–23.

16 Saultz JW, Albedaiwi W. Interpersonal continuity of care and patient satisfaction: a critical review. *Ann Fam Med.* 2004; **2**: 445–51.

17 Baker R, Mainous AG, Gray DP, *et al.* Exploration of the relationship between continuity, trust in regular doctors and patient satisfaction with consultations with family doctors. *Scand J Prim Health Care.* 2003; **21**: 27–32.

18 Brown H, Smith H. Giving women their own case notes to carry during pregnancy. *Cochrane Database Syst Rev.* 2004; **2**: CD002856.

19 Bernstein PS, Farinelli C, Merkatz IR. Using an electronic medical record to improve communication within a prenatal care network. *Obstet Gynecol.* 2005; **105**: 607–12.

20 Handler A, Raube K, Kelley MA, *et al.* Women's satisfaction with prenatal care settings: a focus group study. *Birth.* 1996; **23**: 31–7.

21 Hicks C, Spurgeon P, Barwell F. Changing childbirth: a pilot project. *J Adv Nurs.* 2003; **42**: 617–28.

22 Oropesa RS, Landale NS, Kenkre TS. Structure, process, and satisfaction with obstetricians: an analysis of mainland Puerto Ricans. *Med Care Res Rev.* 2002; **59**: 412–39.

23 Hildingsson I, Waldenstrom U, Radestad I. Women's expectations on antenatal care as assessed in early pregnancy: number of visits, continuity of caregiver and general content. *Acta Obstet Gynecol Scand.* 2002; **81**: 118–25.

24 Ekstrom A, Widstrom AM, Nissen E. Does continuity of care by well-trained breastfeeding counselors improve a mother's perception of support? *Birth.* 2006; **33**: 123–30.

25 Williamson S, Thomson AM. Women's satisfaction with antenatal care in a changing maternity service. *Midwifery.* 1996; **12**: 198–204.

26 Davey MA, Brown S, Bruinsma F. What is it about antenatal continuity of caregiver that matters to women? *Birth.* 2005; **32**: 262–71.

27 Omar M, Schiffman R. Pregnant women's perceptions of prenatal care. *Matern Child Nurs J*. 1995; **23**: 132–42.

28 Leopold N, Cooper J, Clancy C. Sustained partnership in primary care. *J Fam Pract*. 1996; **42**: 129–37.

29 Scott KD, Klaus PH, Klaus MH. The obstetrical and postpartum benefits of continuous support during childbirth. *J Womens Health Gend Based Med*. 1999; **8**: 1257–64.

30 Waldenstrom U, Brown S, McLachlan H, *et al.* Does team midwife care increase satisfaction with antenatal, intrapartum, and postpartum care? A randomized controlled trial. *Birth*. 2000; **27**: 156–67.

31 Biro MA, Waldenstrom U, Brown S, *et al.* Satisfaction with team midwifery care for low- and high-risk women: a randomized controlled trial. *Birth*. 2003; **30**: 1–10.

32 Hodnett ED. Continuity of caregivers for care during pregnancy and childbirth. *Cochrane Database Syst Rev*. 2000; **2**: CD000062.

33 Homer C, Davis G, Cooke M, *et al.* Women's experiences of continuity of midwifery care in a randomised controlled trial in Australia. *Midwifery*. 2003; **18**: 102–12.

34 Green J, Renfrew M, Curtis P. Continuity of carer: what matters to women? A review of the evidence. *Midwifery*. 2000; **16**: 186–96.

35 Hundley V, Ryan M. Are women's expectations and preferences for intrapartum care affected by the model of care on offer? *BJOG*. 2004; **111**: 550–60.

36 Farquhar M, Camilleri-Ferrante C, Todd C. Continuity of care in maternity services: women's views of one team midwifery scheme. *Midwifery*. 2000; **16**: 35–47.

37 Freeman LM. Continuity of carer and partnership. A review of the literature. *Women Birth*. 2006; **19**: 39–44.

38 Fraser DM. Women's perceptions of midwifery care: a longitudinal study to shape curriculum development. *Birth*. 1999; **26**: 99–107.

39 Boss DJ, Timbrook RE, Fort Wayne Medical Education Research Group. Clinical obstetric outcomes related to continuity in prenatal care. *J Am Board Fam Pract*. 2001; **14**: 418–23.

40 Gill JM, Saldarriaga A, Mainous AG, *et al.* Does continuity between prenatal and well-child care improve childhood immunizations? *Fam Med*. 2002; **34**: 274–80.

41 Pistella CY, Synkewecz CA. Community postpartum care needs assessment and systems development for low income families. *J Health Soc Policy*. 1999; **11**: 53–64.

42 Hjortdahl P. Continuity of care: general practitioners' knowledge about, and sense of responsibility toward, their patients. *Fam Pract*. 1992; **9**: 3–8.

43 Stewart M. Continuity, care, and commitment: the course of patient–clinician relationships. *Ann Fam Med*. 2004; **2**: 388–90.

44 Schers H, van de Ven C, van den Hoogen H, *et al.* Patients' needs for contact with their GP at time of hospital admission and other life events; a quantitative and qualitative exploration. *Ann Fam Med*. 2004; **2**: 462–8.

45 Corke CF, Stow PJ, Green DT, *et al.* How doctors discuss major interventions with high risk patients: an observational study. *BMJ*. 2004: bmj.38293.435069.DE.

46 Elcioglu O, Kirimlioglu N, Yildiz Z. How do the accounts of the patients on pregnancy and birth process enlighten medical team in terms of narrative ethics? *Patient Educ Couns*. 2006; **61**: 253–61.

47 Bennett I, Switzer J, Aguirre A, *et al.* "Breaking it down": patient–clinician communication and prenatal care among African American women of low and higher literacy. *Ann Fam Med*. 2006; **4**: 334–40.

48 Teagle SE, Brindis CD. Perceptions of motivators and barriers to public prenatal care

among first-time and follow-up adolescent patients and their providers. *Matern Child Health J.* 1998; **2**: 15–24.

49 Gramling L, Hickman K, Bennett S. What makes a good family-centered partnership between women and their practitioners? A qualitative study. *Birth.* 2004; **31**: 43–8.

50 Woods JR, Rozovsky. *What Do I Say? Communicating intended or unanticipated outcomes in obstetrics.* San Francisco: Jossey-Bass; 2003.

51 Committee on Quality Health Care in America, Institute of Medicine. *To Err is Human: building a safer health system.* Washington, D.C.: National Academy Press; 1998.

52 Matlow A, Stevens P, Harrison C, *et al.* Disclosure of medical errors. *Pediatr Clin North Am.* 2006; **53**: 1091–1104.

53 Stewart M, Brown JB, Weston WW, *et al.*, eds. *Patient-centered Medicine: transforming the clinical method.* Thousand Oaks, CA: Sage Publications; 1995.

54 Campbell DA, Lake MF, Falk M, *et al.* A randomized control trial of continuous support in labor by a lay doula. *J Obstet Gynecol Neonatal Nurs.* 2006; **35**: 456–64.

55 McGrath SK, Kennell JH. A randomized controlled trial of continuous labor support for middle-class couples: effect on cesarean delivery rates. *Birth.* 2008; **35**: 92–7.

56 Pascali-Bonaro D, Kroeger M. Continuous female companionship during childbirth: a crucial resource in times of stress or calm. *J Midwifery Womens Health.* 2004; **49**: 19–27.

57 Gagnon AJ, Meier KM, Waghorn K. Continuity of nursing care and its link to cesarean birth rate. *Birth.* 2007; **34**: 26–31.

58 Fairhurst K, May C. What general practitioners find satisfying in their work: Implications for health care system reform. *Ann Fam Med.* 2006; **4**: 500–5.

59 Robinson WD, Priest LA, Susman JL, *et al.* Technician, friend, detective, and healer: family physicians' responses to emotional distress. *J Fam Pract.* 2001; **50**: 864–70.

60 Candib LM. What doctors tell about themselves to patients: implications for intimacy and reciprocity in the relationship. *Fam Med.* 1987; **19**: 23–30.

61 Candib LM, Steinberg SL, Bedinghaus J, *et al.* Doctors having families: the effect of pregnancy and childbearing on relationships with patients. *Fam Med.* 1987; **19**: 114–19.

62 McDaniel SH, Beckman HB, Morse DS, *et al.* Physician self-disclosure in primary care visits: enough about you, what about me? *Arch Intern Med.* 2007; **167**: 1321–26.

63 Morse DS, McDaniel SH, Candib LM, *et al.* "Enough about me, let's get back to you": physician self-disclosure during primary care encounters. *Ann Intern Med.* 2008; **149**: 835–7.

64 Gulbrandsen P, Hjortdahl P, Fugelli P. General practitioners' knowledge of their patients' psychosocial problems: multipractice questionnaire survey. *BMJ.* 1997; **314**: 1014–18.

65 Roter DL, Hall JA, Aoki Y. Physician gender effects in medical communication: a meta-analytic review. *JAMA.* 2002; **288**: 756–64.

66 Roter DL, Geller G, Bernhardt BA, *et al.* Effects of obstetrician gender on communication and patient satisfaction. *Obstet Gynecol.* 1999; **93**: 635–41.

67 Stoller DL. "I need your help" – stories of physician–patient collaboration. 17th Annual Family in Family Medicine Conference. Kiawah Island, South Carolina 1997.

68 Maharaj R, Talbot Y. Male gender role and its implications for family medicine. *Can Fam Physician.* 2000; **46**: 1005–7.

69 Choudhry NK, Fletcher RH, Soumerai SB. Systematic review: the relationship between clinical experience and quality of health care. *Ann Intern Med.* 2005; **142**: 260–73.

70 Shaller D. *Patient-centered Care: What does it take?* 2007 [cited October 23, 2009]. Available from: www.commonwealthfund.org/~/media/Files/Publications/Fund%20

Report/2007/Oct/Patient%20Centered%20Care%20%20What%20Does%20It%20Take/
Shaller_patient%20centeredcarewhatdoesittake_1067%20pdf.pdf

71 Lazare A. *On Apology.* New York: Oxford University Press; 2004.

72 Candib LM. The family approach at each moment. *Fam Med.* 1985; **17**: 201–8.

73 Midmer DK. Does family-centered maternity care empower women? The development of the woman-centered childbirth model. *Fam Med.* 1992; **24**: 216–21.

74 Whitridge CF. The power of joy: pre- and peri-natal psychology as applied by a mountain midwife. *J Prenat Perinat Psychol Health.* 1988; **2**: 186–92.

75 Norcross WA, Ramirez C, Palinkas LA. The influence of women on the health care-seeking behavior of men. *J Fam Pract.* 1996; **43**: 475–80.

76 Hedin LW. Postpartum, also a risk period for domestic violence. *Eur J Obstet Gynecol Reprod Biol.* 2000; **89**: 41–5.

77 Harrykissoon SD, Rickert VI, Wiemann CM. Prevalence and patterns of intimate partner violence among adolescent mothers during the postpartum period. *Arch Pediatr Adolesc Med.* 2002; **156**: 325–30.

78 Coleman WL, Garfield C, American Academy of Pediatrics Committee on Psychosocial Aspects of Child and Family Health. Fathers and pediatricians: enhancing men's roles in the care and development of their children. *Pediatrics.* 2004; **113**: 1406–11.

79 Arora S, McJunkin C, Wehrer J, *et al.* Major factors influencing breastfeeding rates: mother's perception of father's attitude and milk supply. *Pediatrics.* 2000; **106**: E67.

80 Bar-Yam NB, Darby L. Fathers and breastfeeding: a review of the literature. *J Hum Lact.* 1997; **13**: 45–50.

81 Pisacane A, Continisio GI, Aldinucci M, *et al.* A controlled trial of the father's role in breastfeeding promotion. *Pediatrics.* 2005; **116**: e494–8.

82 Goodman JH. Becoming an involved father of an infant. *J Obstet Gynecol Neonatal Nurs.* 2005; **34**: 190–200.

83 Kennell JH, Klaus MH. Bonding: recent observations that alter perinatal care. *Pediatr Rev.* 1998; **19**: 4–12.

84 Rodholm M. Effects of father–infant postpartum contact on their interaction 3 months after birth. *Early Hum Dev.* 1981; **5**: 79–85.

85 Dixon L, Browne K, Hamilton-Giachritsis C. Risk factors of parents abused as children: a mediational analysis of the intergenerational continuity of child maltreatment (part I). *J Child Psychol Psychiatry.* 2005; **46**: 47–57.

86 Dixon L, Hamilton-Giachritsis C, Browne K. Attributions and behaviours of parents abused as children: a mediational analysis of the intergenerational continuity of child maltreatment (part II). *J Child Psychol Psychiatry.* 2005; **46**: 58–68.

87 Campbell NR. *Adaptation to Emergent Fathering in a Prenatal Education Support Group.* Dissertation Abstracts International; 1992.

88 Goodman JH. Paternal postpartum depression, its relationship to maternal postpartum depression, and implications for family health. *J Adv Nurs.* 2004; **45**: 26–35.

89 Steinberg S, Kruckman L. Reinventing fatherhood in Japan and Canada. *Soc Sci Med.* 2000; **50**: 1257–72.

90 Paulson JF, Dauber S, Leiferman JA. Individual and combined effects of postpartum depression in mothers and fathers on parenting behavior. *Pediatrics.* 2006; **118**: 659–68.

91 Condon JT, Boyce P, Corkindale CJ. The First time Fathers Study: a prospective study of the mental health and wellbeing of men during the transition to parenthood. *Aust N Z J Psychiatry.* 2004; **38**: 56–64.

92 Matthey S, Barnett B, Ungerer J, *et al.* Paternal and maternal depressed mood during the transition to parenthood. *J Affect Disord.* 2000; **60**: 75–85.

93 Morgan M, Matthey S, Barnett B, *et al.* A group programme for postnatally distressed women and their partners. *J Adv Nurs.* 1997; **26**: 913–20.

94 Casper LM, O'Connell M. Work, income, the economy, and married fathers as child-care providers. *Demography.* 1998; **35**: 243–50.

95 Riley LA, Glass JL. You can't always get what you want – infant care preferences and use among employed mothers. *J Marriage Fam.* 2002; **64**: 2–15.

96 Garfield CF, Chung PJ. A qualitative study of early differences in fathers' expectations of their child care responsibilities. *Ambul Pediatr.* 2006; **6**: 215–20.

97 HealthyMarriageInfo.org. National Health Marriage Resource Center: Facts & research. 2007 [cited February 20, 2007]. Available from: www.healthymarriageinfo.org/facts/index.cfm

PART SEVEN

Being Realistic – an Uphill Battle

Lucy M. Candib and Sara G. Shields

What are the impediments to the vision of woman-centered care that we have outlined? This final part will first address the themes of time, teamwork, and wise stewardship of resources – in particular, the vast contribution of technology to modern medicine – that are key elements of being realistic in the practice of woman-centered care of pregnancy and birth. We will look at the concatenation of powerful forces working against woman-centered care and then identify the counter-forces working on behalf of woman-centered maternity care.

CHAPTER 1

Time and Timing

Larisa attended a series of workshops on the patient-centered method and is very interested in applying the method to her woman-centered practice. But at times it feels like an uphill battle. In the office she faces competing demands for her time and the expectation that her prenatal appointments will be brief checks; at the hospital she feels torn between the hospital and the office; in her call system she has to address how to achieve balance in between her desire to provide continuity to her own patients and her need for time for her own life – exercise, rest, relationships, and ultimately her own desires around childbearing.

While recognizing the benefits of the longitudinal framework of monthly prenatal visits, Larisa nonetheless finds that an occasional woman with a complicated personal history, for instance with a history of abuse, requires more time both in the office and during labor and postpartum to feel confident and safe with all the life changes.

TIME IN THE OFFICE

Will woman-centered care take Larisa longer during office visits? Many maternity providers use a model of short prenatal visits scheduled frequently. In primary care, even in such short visits, patient-centered care does not take more time than less patient-focused visits.[1-4] Innovations in prenatal care, like the CenteringPregnancy® group visit model (and the group visit concept in general), offer the possibility of more time in the same room with pregnant women, more opportunity for detailed health education and patient participation, reduced hierarchy between pregnant women and providers, and substantial interpersonal support for the mothers-to-be. The traditional definitions of visit time and "efficiency" change with group visits, where 8 to 12 women are seen together in a 1.5 to two-hour time span every two to four weeks. The time spent with the pregnant women is less repetitive, more positive, and more satisfying for them, in that they get 90 or more minutes with a provider at each group compared with 10 to 15 minutes in an individual visit. Such care is indeed more woman-centered in organization than prenatal care delivered in the customary one-to-one fashion and has already shown other beneficial biomedical outcomes, such as reduction in prematurity for high-risk African-American mothers.[5] For a clinician with a smaller practice, the exact replication of the CenteringPregnancy® model with groupings based on a minimum of six to eight women due in one month may not be realistic. However, modification of the group concept that maintain the goal of facilitated woman-centered empowerment may still provide benefits. For example, some practices have tried group care without reference to due date. (Sharon Rising, personal communication, May 16, 2008).

Time is important in a couple of other models of woman-centered care strategies in the office setting: first, teaching self-management to pregnant women and, second, having women carry a copy of their own prenatal records. Each of these simple strategies puts power back into the hands of the individual woman. Teaching women to take their own blood pressure or graph their weight on a chart during prenatal visits, for instance, may expedite the moment-to-moment care in the office after the initial time needed to teach accurate measurements. Medical assistants can show women the use of the scale and where to document their weight in their chart, and when reviewing this data with women the provider can talk about normal weight gain in pregnancy as part of teaching women to attend to how this month's weight compares to last month's. Giving women a copy of their own prenatal records can be a teaching tool as well as a time-saver within systems, especially around communicating between office and birth site;[6] giving women access to web-based patient records can be another avenue to tailor prenatal education to individual needs.[7]

Furthermore, the longitudinal nature of prenatal visits affords clinicians more time than in other aspects of care to engage in patient-centered care, especially prevention and health promotion. The relationship can develop over the course of multiple pregnancy-related visits, and the potential for common ground can emerge between clinician and pregnant woman, clinician and couple, and even clinician and extended family. The clinician has more opportunities to choose the ideal timing for raising concerns: for instance, he or she can bring up the possibility of domestic violence at multiple visits. Problems of smoking and substance abuse are important to address at the beginning of the pregnancy, but must also be the ongoing focus of later visits if the woman is to deal with the difficulties of her addiction to nicotine or other substances. Later visits also allow more time to bring up these issues with the partner. Discussing the future health of the baby and the family unit helps move health promotion and prevention concerns to the foreground in new ways.

Such longitudinal prenatal care happens quickly, over nine months, compared to long-term primary care relationships where a person with diabetes or hypertension may see their physician only a few times a year. This compressed time frame, along with the anticipation of the life-changing aspects of childbirth, may create more readiness for both the woman and the provider to reach levels of sharing different from non-maternity clinical settings. The woman-centered provider has "flexibility and a readiness to respond"[8:134] when the woman is ready to share more deeply; if this happens at a time when the provider is rushed or tired, the next prenatal visit is not far in the future for follow-up. Longitudinal care adds the dimension to the clinical relationship that the woman comes to know the provider as a real person – one who gets fatigued but also practices self-care when he or she is tired.

TIME IN LABOR

For generations, the most precious virtue in obstetrical care has been patience. Giving a woman time to labor in an emotionally safe environment, trusting that her own physiology will prevail in most instances, and exercising restraint in intervening in a natural process – this attitude appears antiquated in today's labor and delivery settings. In fact, the dominant medical perspective today views *time* itself as a highly structured entity in which medical language and thought places the woman within strict confines – by due date during pregnancy, and with a variety of countdowns at the end of pregnancy and during labor. Researchers have even gone to the length of "proving" that a rate of 12 contractions an hour (i.e. every five minutes) is associated with imminent cervical dilation or labor – confirming the time-honored advice "Call when the contractions are five minutes apart."[10] However, such clock-watching does not address the problem that bringing every woman to the hospital just by the definition of 12 contractions per hour may initiate a technological cascade. (This relationship between timing and the cascade of interventions was a comment from Michael Klein, September 27, 2007, on the Canadian multidisciplinary electronic listserve, Maternity Care Discussion Group at www.cfpc.ca/MCDGResource.)

Most of the time women and their maternity care providers would like labor to be shorter. Yet one of the few factors known to shorten labor, the uninterrupted presence of a supportive woman in the labor room, or a doula, does not play a central role in labor management in most hospital settings.[11] Clinicians in hospital settings often feel tremendous pressure to conform to institutional standards of care with regard to time. Deviations from accepted norms of length of pregnancy and length of labor are seen to require intervention, even if all indications are that mother and fetus are healthy. The impact of a woman's psychological state – her anxiety and fears with resulting biochemical and physiological effects that a doula's presence may alter – usually takes a back seat to the more mechanical measurements of centimeters and hours on the Friedman curve. In contrast, a woman-centered approach follows a more naturalistic view of time, less pegged to the limitations of "institutional time."

Clock-watching is not only an issue for the woman's progress in labor but also for the providers' shift work as well. For a variety of reasons related to the history of workers' rights in industrial society, modern work is demarcated by rigid time categories – for instance, hours, shifts, the 40-hour week, the eight-hour day, and overtime. The layering of this template on the institutions and practice of healthcare results in the organization of care into shifts. Increasingly, doctors, nurses, midwives, and other hospital personnel work in shifts, and people "go off" by the clock regardless of where a woman may be in the course of her labor, or the relationships the provider may have established with her and her family during the course of pregnancy, or of labor itself. Work-hour restrictions for residents in training in the USA and Canada[12] can *require* trainees to leave the hospital at the end of their shift or else incur reprimand for themselves and citation for their residency program. Occasionally, of course, a maternity provider in the hospital setting will stay with a woman about to deliver, simply for the sheer joy and connection of doing so, but this constancy is increasingly rare. Likewise, nursing care is subject to the same pressures. Switches, interruptions, and transfers of care can have deleterious effects – one study of nursing care on a maternity unit at a university teaching hospital showed that continuity with the same nurse for more than 33% of the labor was associated with a reduced risk of cesarean section, and each additional nurse involved increased the risk by 17%.[13]

TIME IN POSTPARTUM CARE

Larisa and her partners have decided that whoever is assigned to do hospital rounds each day will see all the new mothers and babies, rather than having the primary provider try to re-arrange office scheduling. On busy days, however, the rounding provider might have to juggle labor triage with postpartum rounds and an expectation that he or she will return to the office by late morning to see patients there. Wanting to promote breastfeeding and prevent postpartum depression, Larisa struggles to personalize her care within the time constraints of these clinical demands, as she recognizes that some women need very little advice and are ready to go home in a few hours, while others have endless questions and need three or four days and multiple support people to get comfortable with their new role.

These issues come up again once Larisa is seeing newborns in the office within the first week when she finds that many of the new mothers have already faced so much breastfeeding difficulty that they have stopped exclusively nursing. Some mothers at this visit have few needs, while others need extensive visits to fully address their lactation challenges and depression risks.

With flexibility and teamwork in meeting the diversity of women's and families' needs in the first days to weeks to months after childbirth, woman-centered postpartum care can fit realistically into a provider's busy schedule. The longitudinal nature of prenatal care, as noted previously, lays the groundwork for both assessment and education in these early postpartum times. With many families needing hands-on support (for instance, with breastfeeding, or with household support to relieve exhausted parents), Larisa and her group can establish connections with community support resources such as new mothers' groups, or breastfeeding groups such as La Leche League. Larisa can encourage the doulas with whom she works to provide at least a few postpartum visits for additional evaluation and counseling, ideally with the same mothers whose births the doulas have attended, again to foster continuity and longitudinal care. Providers may also choose both to help develop and then to utilize resources such as 24-hour hotlines ("Warm Lines" or "Milk Lines") for nurse-led evaluation of postpartum issues, usually around breastfeeding. Home-based nursing or midwife visits can offer some of these supports either to increase breastfeeding[14] or to improve postpartum mental health.[15] Breastfeeding duration also increases in at-risk women given home-based peer counselor support.[16,17]

TIME AND CALL

Time – measured in minutes, hours, days, weeks, years, and generations – has a complex relationship to the concept of continuity of care.

> Judith started her practice 30 years ago and still enjoys maternity care. In her recruitment letter to Larisa, Judith wrote, "When I choose to get up from sleep to attend the second delivery of a woman whose own birth I attended 30 years ago, I know I am participating in a rare and special aspect of the cross-generational relationship in family medicine. Even though I am confident in the care given by my partners, nothing short of being several hundred miles away would keep me from that birth."
>
> Larisa has to find an answer for her pregnant patients when they bring up the oft-asked question, "Will you be there when I'm in labor?" She realizes that careful explanation of her call coverage system is essential to woman-centered care. First she asks, "What are you expecting about who will see you in labor? How do you feel about my partner being there? How important is it to you that you meet the person ahead of time?" After learning how the woman feels about this issue, Larisa then can address her individual needs with an explanation of her call system, such as, "My partners and I take turns being on call, so that someone is always available to be with women in labor. If it is not my turn, my partner will see you and evaluate your labor. She will try to reach me to let me know what is going on, and if I am able to, I try very hard to come to my own patients' deliveries. However, I cannot always do that."

Although Judith is committed to extended continuity, other, equally woman-centered maternity care providers have devised call systems that allow them more personal time. Some abide by strict call systems and completely sign out all their patients when they are not on call. Others will maximize daytime continuity between provider and laboring woman or postpartum woman, using flexibility in office appointment systems. Some groups, including Woman-Centered Community Family Practice, do rely on rotational systems to cover rounding and daytime work when the provider is scheduled in the office. These needs and strategies often evolve over time as the clinicians themselves go through life-cycle changes – single, partnered, childbearing, with young children, then older children and teenagers, then children launched, and single or partnered at home again.[18] Likewise the size and composition of providers' call groups shift and change with the years, the hospital arrangements and consultation patterns, and the local obstetrical, midwifery, and family medicine cultures. An electronic discussion in 2007 of maternity care call systems on the Maternity Care Discussion Group (www.cfpc.ca/MCDGResource) reflected a wide variety of arrangements caregivers have devised to maximize what they most care about in maternity care, while still allowing adequate time for themselves both personally and professionally.

Many clinicians whose call groups cover deliveries will still commit to trying to attend deliveries of "their own" prenatal patients even when they are not on call, sometimes relying on the covering clinician until labor is well established. Other providers work toward a cohesive approach to labor and delivery among their call group that allows them to completely rely on their covering system when they are not on call and never come in for deliveries of their patients. Those maternity care providers who stay in the hospital for scheduled shifts ("laborists"), followed by blocks of time off, trade the continuity relationship for predictable sleep and family time. Whatever the arrangement, woman-centered clinicians seek to construct systems of clinical care that allow for continuity of patient care through the development of support for each other and shared commitment among providers to empowering the women whose births they attend. This discussion of the realities of time in relation to call responsibilities by definition is provider-focused, since it involves the arrangements in providers' lives. Nevertheless, the woman-centered approach to this problem incorporates the woman's right to understand how the call system works.

As discussed in Part Six, the midwifery literature suggests that women feel satisfied with the call systems in place in their location (country, region, etc.).[19] Women want "consistent care from caregivers that they trust," but continuity when defined as continuity in labor with a known caregiver may not be the highest priority for the woman herself.[20,21] Thus what seems most important about call systems is that they allow for both provider rest and for realistic clinical volume, so that the provider who is at the bedside has the energy and enthusiasm and time to stay woman-centered, whether or not he or she has a longitudinal relationship. With such an approach, woman-centered maternity care can simultaneously be both enormously time-consuming and enormously satisfying, although no one generalization about time and woman-centered care can capture the complexity and flux of so many variables.

> Larisa feels very compatible with the style of her three partners in delivering maternity care, but the practice is growing, and her partners would like to consider joining call pools with the local community health center (CHC) so that call would be every seventh night and every seventh weekend. Larisa feels ambivalent about the call merger because she is uncertain if the providers at the CHC fully share her woman-centered delivery practices. She is also uncertain if some of her patients will accept the possibility of a male provider during labor and delivery. Larisa also has mixed feelings about cross-covering the low income and immigrant population at the community health center – positive feelings because she enjoyed this interesting population during residency, but anxious because of the need for additional supports in social service and language. At the same time, despite her reservations about the call merger, Larisa is finding it challenging to be on call so often. She is not sure if in the larger call pool she would feel obliged to go to the hospital for "her own" patients and end up just as overcommitted as she is now in the every-fourth-night pattern.

Judith Peters and Simon Miller are old friends and colleagues. They had jointly worked on initiatives to foster progressive maternity care practices in the community and at the hospital. Both of them are looking forward to the call merger, as they have been doing every fourth night call for many years. Nevertheless, Simon confides in Judith that he worries that not everyone in her practice is as enthusiastic about refugee and immigrant care, and the non-English speaking population, as those at the CHC. Judith acknowledges this reality.

"What about setting up some cross-cultural sessions for our folks?" she proposes. "And what about the prison women? And the addiction program? We're going to need help learning to do right by those women as well."

"You're right – I can do some extra backup for those programs to help with the transition," Simon offers. "And we'll come up with some trainings – we could even invite the maternity nurses. Do Tuesday lunchtimes still work for you?"

Call systems always involve compromises. For Larisa to feel comfortable with a new arrangement, obviously the two practice groups need to sit down together and discuss the details of each member's delivery style and philosophy. Larisa's all-woman practice would also have to advise women and their families that their coverage system would include male providers; a change that may be difficult for some women, but may offer advantages to the men in her practice. Each provider would need to feel that the others in the call group agree on woman-centered attention to each pregnant woman's unique feelings, thoughts, expectations, and function. And the community health center physicians want to be sure that their often-disparaged patients will get women-centered care appropriate for their specific needs. Unfortunately, such conversations among covering colleagues are all too uncommon.

Regardless of what specific arrangements each maternity care provider chooses at any given moment, comfort and confidence in shared arrangements require the complete support of those at home, specific concordance in values about the importance of maternity care with their practice partners, and shared philosophy with the others in their maternity care call system. When these elements are in place, the woman-centered clinician can deliver the care she or he believes in, regardless of the specific details of the arrangement. Thus the most satisfying use – both personally and professionally – of the provider's time requires excellent communication and commitment to teamwork.

CHAPTER 2

Teamwork and Team Building

COMMUNICATION, COLLABORATION, AND TRUST

Communication is a cornerstone of teamwork in woman-centered maternity care. While the individual clinical relationship between provider and pregnant woman is a central aspect of woman-centered care, this relationship is often dependent on the smooth functioning of teams at various levels of care. A physician is not the only and often not even the primary person involved with the woman. In many countries, the primary provider during pregnancy may be a midwife or team of midwives, but teams involving nurses, nutritionists, social workers, and physiotherapists are essential.

Collaborative work with specialists around women with high-risk pregnancies further expands the kinds of teamwork that are essential to maintaining patient-centeredness. Some kinds of highly complex problems require the interventions of a multidisciplinary team: the drug or alcohol-using mother; the HIV-positive woman in pregnancy; the woman actively being abused; the woman with a fetal anomaly; the woman with a multiple gestation; or the woman with a chronic medical condition. Each of these clinical issues requires drawing on the expertise of others and implementing coordination of care that extends well beyond the usual services offered in a family medicine office, a community health center, or a private obstetrician's solo practice. Women carrying fetuses with fetal anomalies, for instance, may require the early and ongoing involvement of the pediatric medical and surgical specialties to guarantee the optimal timing and location of delivery; a team is necessary to convey the information to the family and support them during such difficult pregnancies. Knowing when to consult, when to refer, when to collaborate but continue to manage the care of the woman oneself – these choices require self-scrutiny by the primary provider as well as scrutiny of the available resources in the practice.

In community settings serving ethnic minorities, immigrants and refugees, the outreach workers or case managers may be the central figures for pregnant women. Particularly where much of what such workers do is language interpretation, the bilingual interpreter/advocate may be the only person with whom the woman feels comfortable in confiding her actual concerns, practices, and symptoms. For instance, a non-English-speaking multiparous Vietnamese woman with a prior cesarean in an actively abusive relationship might technically be appropriate for referral to the high-risk center, due to the practice agreements about trial of labor after cesarean, but this transfer would disrupt her relationship with the Vietnamese case manager who is the only person outside her family who knows about the abuse. Ongoing woman-centered communication and collaboration with the high-risk center becomes critically important to facilitate comprehensive, individualized care for women in such situations.

Problematic substance use in pregnancy is another example of an issue requiring dedicated teamwork (*see* Part Three). Successful programs to foster healthy pregnancies for drug and alcohol-abusing women require the involvement of a dedicated multidisciplinary team committed to working with this often-vilified population. In settings where all "high-risk" women are folded in together (diabetes, hypertension, substance abuse, multiple gestation, etc.), substance-abusing women may be deemed less worthy of attention than other high-risk pregnant women and may be openly or subtly treated in negative ways. All the team members, including the physicians, working with women with substance abuse need to share a commitment to this population, a common set of strategies, and a common vocabulary with the team to approach acute issues. When clinical care, such as consultation, comes from outside the team, the women can get differing messages and uneven care. Being realistic in this situation may mean developing consultation arrangements that are consistent with the team's philosophy.

> With consultants, Larisa's experience of teamwork is mixed. When Greg is on call as her consultant, he is able to join her smoothly in providing consultation in a woman-centered way, collaborating easily. Other obstetricians who help back him up, however, express annoyance: why is she consulting so early in labor? Or in antenatal care? Why is she consulting so late? Why is she consulting at all?

As discussed in Part Four, ideally woman-centered consultants recognize the importance of the caring clinical relationship constructed during prenatal visits between a woman and her primary provider, and make recommendations that buttress that relationship rather than dismantle it. However, more specialty-focused consultants may see the providers of routine prenatal care as inadequate for caring for complications and may unconsciously convey to the pregnant woman that they do not respect or value the primary caregiver. This unconscious undermining has a very destructive effect on the woman, the primary provider, and the entire system of care. If there is not excellent two-way communication to cement trust between the front-line provider of prenatal care and the referral consultants, many of the salubrious aspects of the healing relationship cannot take place because of the mixed messages, unalleviated anxiety, and uncertainty on the woman's part about whom she can trust. The ultimate goal in collaborative consultation is thus:

> Figuring out how to keep the woman well supported in the face of uncertainty, the other team members feeling as though we respect one another and can work

collaboratively, and looking after ourselves – to stay thoughtful, alert, compassionate, safe . . . that is the true skill that takes time and a great environment to nurture.

(Reproduced with permission from MCDG Resource, November 28, 2007.)

Teamwork takes on different forms in different settings. In talking about leadership and communication in the care team, Canadian midwife Vera Berard describes her understanding of a New Zealand approach to teamwork:

Lead professional is the term that is used in New Zealand where a woman can choose a midwife, GP or Obstetrician as her primary caregiver. It denotes the person responsible for coordinating a woman's care, although more than one caregiver may be involved. Midwives provide approximately 70% of NZ maternity services in collaboration with other practitioners . . . the maternity team can better support a woman's informed decision if the woman has been counseled by her primary caregiver and a consultant and that information, along with the woman's preferences, has been **relayed back to all members of the maternity team**. Sometimes the midwife/GP and OB who devised a care plan with a woman may not be available when the woman goes into labor. It's the primary caregivers and/or consultant on-call and the nursing staff who are likely to implement the woman's plan.

(Reproduced with permission from MCDG Resource, and Vera Berard, July 18, 2007.)

Berard has discovered in her region that the communication processes in place "will either enable effective care or not." She continues:

Egalitarian communication processes are key to collaborative maternity care that enable informed decision making, best practice and the development of a diverse, but respectful team – processes such as department meetings where members are **comfortable** discussing cases and differences in philosophy; perinatal care committees where care plans and best evidence are considered and perinatal morbidity and mortality rounds where expected and unexpected outcomes are dialogued and reflected upon.

(Reproduced with permission from MCDG Resource, and Vera Berard, July 18, 2007.)

Forums where generalists, specialists, nurses, and other staff can discuss communication problems in risk-free "protected" peer-review meetings offer the possibility to ameliorate these kinds of problems between the maternity care disciplines. Such safe and evidence-based peer review can focus on system problems, continuing education needs, and other objective measures rather than individual personalities.

Beyond individuals, small groups, and multidisciplinary teams, large-scale institutions must also agree on the need for communication among the clinicians common to the systems. In settings where inpatient and outpatient settings do not share a common computer network, or where telephone systems are mechanized or overly burdened, important communications can get lost. Seamless communication about important laboratory results would appear to be an obvious requirement of systems that involve laboratories, hospitals, and outpatient providers, but even in today's world of electronic medical records, email, and fax machines, outpatient providers may be left out of the loop. In Great Britain, for instance, 16% of primary care maternity care providers were unaware of serum test results and 28% were unaware of ultrasound reports suggesting a possible genetic abnormality.[22]

Low-income and vulnerable women are likely to be particularly at risk to experience difficulties with communications in the systems they use, perhaps because these settings may face constant crises in resources. Lack of coordination between hospital and clinic, poor communication between providers – including missing records – and poor telephone and transportation access combine to create major barriers to care for low-income women and their families.[23] For example, in Australia, where satisfaction with maternity care is generally high, women born in non-English-speaking countries are less likely to rate their care as good.[24] Non-English-speaking Latino patients in the USA may be particularly at risk of feeling that physicians and their office staff do not respect them and rush through visits.[25] If they are to be able to provide attention focused on the patient and not on the hassles of the system, providers in these settings must address such problems at a systems level, including the need for interpreters.

Systems need ways to scrutinize their usual modes of operation for patient-centeredness and explore mechanisms to correct communication glitches. As large healthcare systems implement quality-improvement programs, providers have the opportunity to insist that patient-centeredness be a central goal, requiring new strategies to correct problems in communication. The new focus on reducing errors within the medical system in the USA, when applied in the obstetrical area, has begun to address the importance of communication and the centrality of the mother–baby pair while reducing medical errors and failure of documentation.[26]

> . . . Idealized Design of Perinatal Care represents the Institute for Healthcare Improvement (IHI)'s best current assessment of the components of the safest and most reliable system of perinatal care. The four key components of the model are: 1) the development of reliable clinical processes to manage labor and delivery; 2) the use of principles that improve safety (i.e. preventing, detecting, and mitigating errors); 3) the establishment of prepared and activated care teams that communicate effectively with each other and with mothers and families; and 4) *a focus on mother and family as the locus of control during labor and delivery.*
>
> Reviews of perinatal care have consistently pointed to failures of communication among the care team and documentation of care as common factors in adverse events that occur in labor and delivery. They are also prime factors leading to malpractice claims. [Italics added.][26]

However, while addressing induction and augmentation of labor, the IHI recommendations do *not* address the misuse or overuse of technology in maternity settings. For instance, they do not speak to the fact that low-risk patients in tertiary care settings are more likely to undergo interventions – presumably unnecessary – in their care compared to equivalent low-risk patients in low-risk settings.[27] The attention to the technical aspects of care in points 1 and 2 above emerges from a model derived from ventilator care and applies it to birth. This focus diverts attention from the communication problems or the system's difficulty in putting the mother and family in control. Truly woman-centered promotion of satisfaction and communication with mothers and families is about highlighting the birth experience for women and less about the provider-centered issue of reducing risk of malpractice allegations.

Teamwork with intrapartum nurses is another key arena for woman-centered providers. The maternity care provider needs to make sure that the laboring woman's nurse, who usually has never met the woman before, is clear about the woman's goals. When the provider and nurse share a clear consistent viewpoint on maximizing these goals, including her sense of being in control, while maintaining both her and her baby's well-being, the woman is likely to feel supported in her labor and satisfied with her care. When provider and nurse are not congruent in their approach to the laboring woman, indirect communication and undercurrents of conflict may undermine the woman's care and adversely affect her safety and well-being.

> Larisa feels she has input at the office about who is hired to become part of the office team caring for patients, but at the hospital finds that expectations about teamwork vary widely in her work with nurses. On labor and delivery, sometimes she and the nurse engage easily in the joint task of facilitating a woman-centered birth, but at other times Larisa feels that the nurse is disapproving or critical and acting primarily to get her own required work done. Sometimes Larisa gets "vibes" that her woman-centered style is inconvenient, annoying or even interfering with nursing responsibilities (e.g. for the mother to hold the baby for an extended period after birth interferes with banding, footprints, vitamin K injection, hepatitis B immunization, administration of antibiotic eye ointment, and a host of other required nursing tasks immediately postpartum in the hospital environment). For their part, the nurses want to finish these duties before transferring the woman's care to the postpartum nurse, who will not have time to attend to such missing clinical care issues. Likewise, Larisa feels that not all staff on the postpartum floor or in the nursery are fully supportive of the Baby Friendly Initiative as she often finds formula bottles in the crib when a mother has been having trouble initiating breastfeeding. Again she worries that being woman-centered takes too much time for overextended nursing staff.

Unfortunately, woman-centered practice at the hospital level in many settings is often patchy. Hospital systems expect increasing amounts of documentation from nursing staff whose training and support around being woman-centered may itself be uneven, so that the emphasis on correct and complete documentation may override true woman-centered care. In general, hospital systems function to get hospital work done, and the work of each member of the staff is organized primarily around accomplishing in a timely way the work apportioned to his or her role. As Larisa noticed, support for breastfeeding – a highly intensive one-to-one process – often falls lower in priority than other required tasks for busy staff. At the same time, ways to get more support for women at low cost to the hospital itself, for instance, the training of lay doulas chosen by the pregnant woman herself,[28] get little systemic support from highly technical maternity settings.

Teamwork requires trust. Clearly, woman-centered care requires the healthcare team to work with the woman's goals, and also for the woman to trust the team to support her. Yet, is it realistic for women to trust maternity practitioners or the healthcare system? Many healthcare professionals in the USA recognize that the system is broken and even dysfunctional, even for them and their own families.[29,30] Such malfunction means that healthcare providers may need to prove themselves trustworthy for many patients who feel they have been harmed or betrayed by healthcare institutions or other systems of authority – within the family, like Delia, Chantel, and Mariluz, as we have seen earlier; or by police, school systems, or prior healthcare providers. In addition to instances of obvious error, which are frequent and costly whenever measured – wrong patient, wrong dose, wrong surgery, wrong medication[31] – other systematic errors are common and not measured: excess use of technology, (e.g. daily labs in the hospital, repeated tests ordered because multiple providers are not communicating with each other, routine CT scans in the emergency room as defensive strategy, too long a wait for a call back, too much intervention, poor communication such that the patient takes wrong dose or does not take it at all, and so on). Thus, unquestioning trust in the system and in individual practitioners within it may not be safe for patients; being woman-centered means *encouraging* a woman or her family to ask questions about her care and *joining* with them when they question or challenge standard operating procedures. While, realistically, many patients are unable to challenge the system – perhaps because of lack of education, lack of psychological preparedness, passivity in the face of authority, or sickness itself – those who do question the system run the risk of being labeled difficult.[32] (Also, Michael Klein, personal communication, October 30, 2007.)

Providers also face a challenge around trust. Obstetricians are likely to endorse the statement "birth is only normal in retrospect" and therefore do not trust women's bodies to have healthy outcomes. The pathology-focused viewpoint typical in highly technical obstetrical settings denies the normality of physiological birth. This technocratic position, while increasingly typical in hospitals around the world, contrasts starkly with humanistic and holistic approaches to childbirth.[33] Many kinds of practitioners (doctors, nurses, midwives, traditional birth attendants) attend women during pregnancy and delivery with philosophies that derive from very different traditions quite remote from the technocratic model. The hospital specialist, embedded within the technocratic model, cannot see that his or her vision is skewed not only by the selected sample of patients in high technology settings, but also by not recognizing that the hospital itself makes interventions that affect the normality of birth

– bedrest, medication in prodrome, etc., even before the cascade of technical interventions. A generation of trainees is seeing that as many as one-quarter to one-third of births "require" cesarean section – not surprisingly, these trainees are unlikely to view birth as normal.[34]

For providers, the issue of trust also connects to fears of allegations of malpractice. Those in the USA, in particular, have been repeatedly exposed to litigation and therefore do not trust women and their families not to retaliate in the event of a bad outcome. They fall back to the defensive position of always assuming retaliation will take place in the form of litigation and that preventive intervention with cesarean section is preferable to running the risk of litigation. This practice is a version of the *maximin strategy*, "the prevention or adequate management of the rare disaster rather than the optimal conduct of the many normal cases"[35] which we will discuss further in Chapter 3. Thus mistrust on both sides exacerbates the interventional cascade: women do not trust the system because they do not feel heard or respected; litigation is their recourse. And providers do not trust women not to litigate. Fear of lawsuits and of huge financial judgments against clinicians has resulted in many providers always choosing the "safe" option in any management decision, regardless of the expressed wishes of the woman or her family. At the beginning of the 21st century, this choice usually means increasing use of technology, including more ultrasounds, more electronic fetal monitoring, more epidurals, and earlier cesarean sections. With more claims and higher judgments come rising insurance premiums – spiraling costs in Canada and the UK, as well as the USA, that affect clinicians' decisions to provide such care.[36-39]

Thus neither women nor providers feel safe. Only mutual transparency has the potential to loosen this deadlock. Malpractice reform must go beyond prevention of "frivolous" suits, limits on monetary awards and lawyers' fees, and controlled costs of insurance, but must also include ways to keep women safe. In systems with good communication, when mistakes happen, patients want full disclosure, apologies, and some kind of commitment toward preventing such errors in the future. Consistent application of a woman-centered strategy in all contacts between the woman and her clinician, from diagnosis, through prenatal care, and into labor and delivery offers human – rather than interventional – protection against litigation. In labor, a woman-centered approach to this crisis in trust would promote more human rather than technical contact: strategies of active but non-technologic labor support using massage, relaxation techniques, music, movement, bathing, and family involvement. Exploring the feelings, ideas, and expectations in every conversation between clinician and patient builds a basis of communication that fosters trust and shows commitment. Solutions to the malpractice crisis are complex and beyond our scope, but one thing is clear: prevention of malpractice suits begins with woman-centered communication.[40]

THE RISK SOCIETY

Contemporary society's obsession with risk aversion is part of the issue of trust. Such a preoccupation is a social phenomenon of the so-called risk society.[41] Modern society's emphasis on the prevention or minimization of risk has transformed how childbearing women, and society in general, have come to think differently about childbirth compared to previous generations.[42,43] Applying this concept of risk to childbirth, Possamai-Inesedy cites the insidious and invisible nature of the risks affecting childbearing women today, in contrast to the stark life and death risks of childbirth previously.[43] Despite the increasing safety of birth in the last half century, paradoxically women are both increasingly fearful and yet more accepting of the impossible responsibility for protecting their fetuses from all the myriad risks around them. Women planning their deliveries in various settings (private hospital, midwifery birthing center, and home births) all engage in "constant speculation and negotiation of the potential risks they [feel] confronted with on practically an everyday basis."[43:413]

The medical system itself, does not, of course, view itself as a risk to patients, except in the event of medical error. Yet the normal working of medical systems can be a hazard. For instance, a system designed to decrease medical risk – the regionalization of obstetrical care of rural Aboriginal women – actually poses risks for them. Requiring women to deliver distant from their homes and their communities means that they must leave their children, their lands, and their support systems for as long as four weeks just to be able to deliver in a hospital. Yet this dislocation creates **increased risk** by leaving their children, their homes, and their livelihoods unattended, and disrupts their relationship to the land and their husbands' relationships to the babies.[42] Likewise in Laos, for women traveling a distance to deliver at a hospital, "the 'safety' of hospital birth did not outweigh the other risks associated with hospital stays for birthing."[44]

CHAPTER 3

Wise Stewardship of Resources

Time, trust, teamwork, and questioning risk aversion all relate to the question of how best to use limited healthcare resources for the betterment of maternity care. Resources are important: the provider integrates both public health strategies of prevention, with evidence from both the population and the individual level, and a focus on the unique pregnant woman. During prenatal care, appropriate interpretation of evidence-based studies and woman-centeredness can theoretically work together to foster the wise and fiscally responsible use of resources. However, many conjoining forces are working *against* the wise stewardship of resources.

RUNAWAY TECHNOLOGY

Patient demand

Many women with technical sophistication want every possible test to determine or verify their baby's normality. For example, discussion of first-trimester screening for neural tube defects and congenital anomalies increasingly dominates early interactions – as for Melissa and Kirk – between the woman and her provider in the initial prenatal visits. Likewise women and their partners want early ultrasounds to see and connect with the fetus and later ultrasounds to determine the sex of the baby. Such patient demand for what technology can offer – in this case multiple ultrasounds and videos for the sheer pleasure of seeing their baby – far exceeds the medical necessity for ultrasounds in pregnancy. Such a market for ultrasounds with photos, albums, and videos has now caused a controversy over the non-medical use of ultrasound, the profits to be had, and the potential risks of ultrasound by non-medical commercial vendors.[45]

> During labor, a woman's expectations of a painless childbirth where she feels in control and has a beautiful television-style birth, smiling, may lead to her surprise at the painfulness of early labor and then to her insistence on an early epidural with its likely sequelae of interventions. Even for women who originally did not want an epidural, but become overwhelmed by the reality of labor, the constant availability of epidurals means that many women get them who, with a bit more waiting and much more support, might not have needed them.
>
> (Reproduced with permission from MCDG discussion list, November 26, 2007.)

So the question comes up: does being woman-centered in maternity care mean giving the pregnant woman whatever technical intervention she asks for? Providers know that not all interventions are appropriate and that spiraling technologies may carry unknown risk (three ultrasounds with a total exposure of three minutes do not seem to cause measurable harm but what about 100 ultrasounds or 100 minutes of exposure? Or more?)[46] Other women are preoccupied with the potential risks of technology and interventions and choose low-intervention settings such as out-of-hospital birth centers and home births, opting for certain risks over others. They are more likely to refuse even indicated interventions. Woman-centeredness must therefore attend to the woman's values first and then interpret and explore her demands from within the values framework, conveying as accurate a picture of risk as current data permit, in language that women can understand.[47] This task requires that the provider himself or herself be comfortable with a certain level of uncertainty and not let his or her own anxiety overwhelm the pregnant woman.

Monetary interests

Fetal monitors are big business both nationally and internationally. As "standard practice" in hospitals in the USA, practitioners have to ask for them to be removed, as opposed to asking for their use. Most women coming into a hospital in labor in North America have electronic fetal monitoring unless the individual woman refuses. In that case, an obligatory period of monitoring followed by periodic electronic monitoring, or intermittent auscultation, might be the alternative practice. Students, nurses, midwives, residents, and supervising physicians all attend to the monitor strip and are expected to describe the tracings in their chart notes. Centralized EFM, also becoming increasingly available in hospitals, is a mechanism that allows hospitals to employ fewer nurses since one nurse can watch multiple monitors from a central station, permitting an individual nurse to "follow" a woman's labor from outside the room.

Despite the evidence from systematic reviews about the lack of superiority of EFM in maternal infant outcomes, and the increasing rate of cesarean sections when monitoring is universal, intrapartum use is routine both in industrialized countries and increasingly in the developing world. Changing this culture of intrapartum technology faces profound barriers. For instance, in a Canadian study to introduce nationally approved guidelines for fetal health surveillance, adoption for low-risk women of the alternative method of monitoring fetuses, intermittent auscultation, met diffuse opposition.[48] With no experience in using intermittent auscultation with fetoscopes or hand-held Dopplers, recently trained nurses in a tertiary care hospital were reluctant to follow women with this method, despite nursing administration support for the intervention. Possibly because of malpractice concerns, physicians and anesthetists also opposed the change.[48] Nurses were hesitant to abandon the electronic monitor technology for which they had been trained, and settings lacked the cheaper technology (portable Dopplers) that would have facilitated the intervention. The other low-technology labor care strategy of these guidelines, using one-to-one labor support, found even smaller increases in frequency (6%) in the tertiary care site, no improvement in the community hospital site, but a disturbing and significant 7% decrease in one-to-one labor support in the control community hospital, suggesting worsening erosion of personal nursing care on maternity floors.[48] Thus the integration of EFM machinery and depersonalized central monitoring into standard practice is complete, even without evidence for an improvement in outcome, and personal labor support is waning. Attempts to reverse this trend, even with administrative and guideline support, were largely unsuccessful.

Furthermore, efforts to publicize the negative findings of systematic reviews of EFM have met with forceful opposition from the health technology industry in the form of personal attacks on researchers. Industry has sought court injunctions to prevent publication of technology assessment unfavorable to the further dissemination of EFM.[49] In fact, the whole area of technology assessment is constantly in conflict with industry in a healthcare system where costly innovations diffuse widely into practice without adequate evidence-based assessment.

Beyond the profit for the manufacturers and reduced nursing costs for hospitals, fetal monitoring, given its position as "standard of care," is often cited as a key element in malpractice defense. Monitor tracings are customary pieces of evidence in peer review settings and in malpractice trials. However, there is some argument that the monitor may actually expose obstetricians to increased liability.[50]

Provider enthusiasm and access

Some providers are gadget-oriented, and like new technology, especially if it makes them appear modern and up-to-date. Others are more suspicious of new machinery, particularly if using it requires any extensive training in application or interpretation (e.g. fetal pulse oximetry). On the whole, however, those providers with convenient access to technology – such as 24-hour epidural availability – are more likely to use it than those with more limited access.[27] Not surprisingly, when maternity care providers are surveyed, as a group, obstetricians favor technology more than family doctors or midwives.[51] With fewer family doctors doing obstetrics, and a relatively slow increase in midwifery care, an increasingly technological approach is likely to prevail.

RUNAWAY INTERVENTIONISM

Being realistic means recognizing that technology has a dynamic of its own. Hospital-based deliveries, as well, have a dynamic of resource use that is difficult to control. The current reality of obstetrics in North America suggests that increasing technical and surgical resources are likely to be sought by both pregnant women and providers in the future. Even for pregnant women with no identifiable risk, a group that should have a stable cesarean rate, the rate is steadily climbing in both the USA and Canada.[52-54] With a 31.8% cesarean section rate in the USA in 2007,[55] and a 26% rate in Canada in 2005, and with more than two-thirds of deliveries occurring under epidural anesthesia in the USA and 56% in Canada, (but varying greatly by region)[54-56] the preferences of both consumers and practitioners continue to be dominated by resource-intensive and expensive strategies. In this context, the wise stewardship of resources will remain an ongoing challenge.

Being realistic means trying to understand the multiple causes at work pushing expensive intervention and technology forward. Apart from the economics of sales, and the appeal of technology itself, a specific approach to decision-making in obstetrics ties to interventionism. Contributions from game theory and complexity science can help us understand the self-perpetuating nature of the problem of escalating technology and interventions in obstetrics that limit our ability to control resources. More than 25 years ago Brody and Thompson described how modern obstetrical practice exemplified the "maximin" strategy – an approach from game theory in which the player chooses "the alternative that makes the best of the worst possible outcome, regardless of the probability that that outcome will occur."[35:977] (The maximin strategy in obstetrics parallels that kind of military approach that advocates striking out

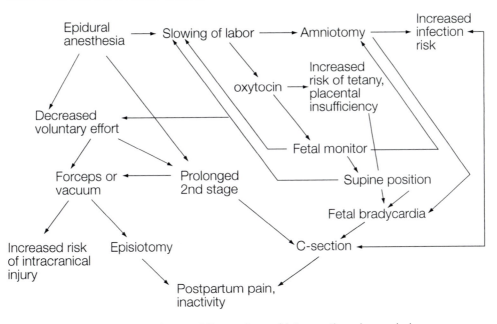

FIGURE 7.1 Interconnectedness of the system of interventions in maximin obstetrics[31]

(Adapted with the kind permission of Dowden Health Media.)

with maximum power in the event of even minimal risk.)[57] Brody and Thompson recognized several assumptions underlying the "maximin" strategy that are equally relevant today (*see* Figure 7.1). The arrows show how each intervention leads to greater risk and possibly requires subsequent interventions.

They point out that the maximin strategy applied to obstetrics actually *does change* the outcome, and that the interventions themselves form an interconnected system "with one intervention leading to additional risk factors or additional data gathering needs, which in turn require new interventions."[35:978]. For instance, the rate of maternal hyperthermia for nulliparous women in labor with an epidural ranges from 24% to 33%, compared to 5% to 7% for women with intravenous opioids for analgesia.[58,59] Subsequent to maternal fever, the following interventional cascade often occurs:

➤ Neonatal specialists attend the delivery.
➤ The infant is immediately transferred to the hands of the neonatologists instead of into maternal arms (interfering with immediate bonding and sometimes breastfeeding).
➤ Many infants undergo a sepsis evaluation (CBC and blood cultures at a minimum).
➤ Many infants receive intravenous antibiotics for 48 hours, requiring at least a 48-hour nursery stay to be sure of negative cultures.
➤ Increased parental and medical anxiety about infant with intravenous line on antibiotics who requires additional blood work.

➤ Increased promotion of microbial resistance to antibiotics in the infant, the family, the hospital, and the community because of high frequency of use.

These undesirable secondary outcomes derive from the physiologic effect of the epidural itself, but since maternal fever in labor cannot be ignored *in case* it represents sepsis, the cascade is invoked. Brody and Thompson offer a diagram just as relevant today as it was in 1981 – reproduced as Figure 7.1. The image suggests some of the multiple effects of epidural anesthesia in obstetrics. Although vacuum-assisted deliveries have replaced forceps, and our later understanding of the impact of epidurals on fetal descent is not included in the diagram, the cascade of events is still applicable. These multiple interventions synergistically produce effects requiring further interventions, ultimately increasing the rate of cesarean sections; and in the instance of the common side-effect of maternal fever, a further cascade of interventions affecting the infants.

This analysis of the maximin strategy is rooted within the events specifically occurring in labor and does not delve into either the underlying physiology or the social and political context of the woman, the doctors, or the institutional culture of the hospital. A more multi-layered analysis of dysfunctional labor in first-time mothers by Lowe[60] examines multiple interacting factors that contribute to the rising rate of

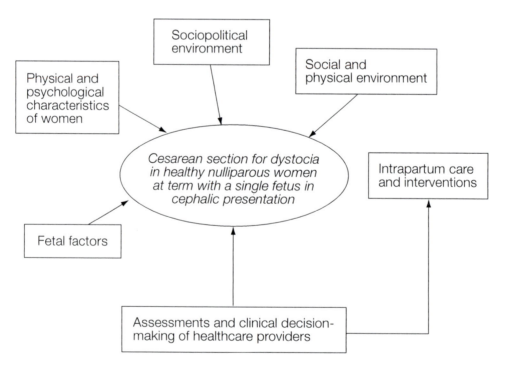

FIGURE 7.2 Conceptual model of factors affecting the occurrence of cesarean section for dystocia in healthy nulliparous women[60]

(Reproduced with the kind permission of Elsevier.)

cesareans among nulliparous women (*see* Figure 7.2). Lowe categorizes these factors into six different areas:
1 maternal physical and psychological issues
2 fetal factors
3 intrapartum care and interventions
4 provider issues about clinical care
5 environmental issues, both social and physical
6 sociopolitical issues.

Maternal obesity with subsequent fetal macrosomia risk, the so-called maternal request for cesarean demand, and provider liability are commonly publicized as major reasons for the dystocia and cesarean epidemics, with less recognition given to the other areas that may in fact be more significant contributors.[60] For instance, few women receive continuous labor support early in labor when it may be especially important in helping labor progress.[61-3] Furthermore, those few institutions that regularly engage in evidence-based practice improvements – e.g. auditing outcomes such as induction rates or cesareans done for dystocia – have been able to maintain lower cesarean rates.[56,64-7] Lowe's dissection of the issues in this one specific area – dystocia in first-time mothers – fits squarely within an understanding of the rapid increase in cesareans as a *syndemic*.

INTERVENTIONISM AS A SYNDEMIC

The acceleration in the rate of cesarean sections and the proliferation of this intervention around the world fit the characteristics of a syndemic – a complex and widespread phenomenon in population health produced by multiple reinforcing conditions.[68] Syndemic can refer to a synergistic interaction of two or more diseases multiplying the burden of disease,[69] and also to the interaction of complex factors – genetic, physiological, psychological, familial, social, economic and political – coalescing to accelerate disease.[70,71] The study of syndemics helps us see that we need a broader screen to understand the brief local events in which we participate every day, in this case the increasingly technological approach to childbirth with a 30% cesarean section rate in many US hospitals and rates of 50–63% in some hospitals in Greece, Brazil, and Mexico, as well as multiple other countries in Latin America. This problem has multifactorial causes, a historical trajectory, and no simple answers. Viewing the accelerating rise in cesarean sections as a syndemic allows us to think more widely about the causes and about the potential responses that would be needed at multiple levels in multiple locations to begin to reverse the tide.

Attempting to depict graphically the multiple forces at work in promoting interventionism in maternity care makes it clear how extensive and complex are the factors involved. Figure 7.3 represents an attempt to make a two-dimensional visual representation of this complexity.

Leading to an **increasingly technological environment** are: market forces pushing products: drugs, monitors, ultrasound machines, etc., with competition for promoting the latest gadget; the inherent appeal of new technology as part of progress; the popular appeal of technology to "see" the baby and predict normality.

Leading to **increased inductions** are: the popular appeal of choosing the timing of delivery (connected to women's work and family life); preferred daytime deliveries, lifestyle issues for maternity providers; and increased professional preoccupation with risk of post-dates or other conditions identified by technical means.

Leading to **increased rates of epidural anesthesia** are: the popular appeal and widespread promotion of "painless" childbirth with its illusion of control; decreased acceptability of pain of labor as part of a normal physiologic process; increased public acceptance of intervention overall; widespread availability of 24-hour anesthesia on call in obstetrical settings; widespread acceptance in obstetrical circles of a faulty meta-analysis supposedly showing a lack of relationship between epidural anesthesia and cesarean section;[102,103] recent anesthesia recommendations for "early" epidurals in women with complications like obesity or pre-eclampsia.[104]

Leading to **increased perception of risk** by providers are: threat of litigation, magnification of risk of previously acceptable strategies (VBACs, vaginal breech deliveries), decreased exposure to such strategies for trainees (resulting in a workforce that relies on operative delivery for any deviation from routine), increased rates of obesity among childbearing women leading to increased gestational diabetes; the self-fulfilling prophecy of obese women's increased need for operative delivery predisposing obstetricians to perform more cesareans on this group; and the concentration of deliveries by obstetricians with an absent or reduced cadre of professionals trained in normal deliveries (midwives and family physicians) leading to a perception that deliveries are a surgical procedure.

Women's increased perception of risk to the fetus relates to women delaying childbirth and having smaller families, thus wanting perfection and searching for ways to guarantee normality of the fetus; this increases acceptance of interventions to assess or measure fetal status, and acceptance of surgical and emergency environment of hospital as necessary to decrease risk.

Joining these factors are: **the profit motive**, resulting in increased cesarean sections all over the world (particularly in private hospitals); **the maximin strategy**, fostering the most aggressive response regardless of the low frequency of a given risk; **decreased continuity of care by providers, nurses and residents**, resulting in unfamiliarity and increased intervention; **decreased perception of risk of hazards from cesarean section** for mother and infant (by both professionals and lay people) despite well-known complications in later pregnancies, and internationally documented higher maternal and neonatal mortality and morbidity.[94-8] All these forces conjoin to create an environment in which one in three, or more, deliveries occur by cesarean section in the USA, and rates upwards of 50% in private settings around the world.

Finally, **the rising rate of obesity** around the world (itself a syndemic)[70] is a small but real biological contribution to the increase in cesareans, but cannot account for the extent of the syndemic.

The study of syndemics fits into an appreciation of complexity science, a relatively

Key to Figure 7.3

Intellectual Environment

1 Faulty EBM: see Part One, Chapter 10.
2 Failure to follow up on newer evidence disputing risk of intervention, such as from breech delivery: See Part One, Chapter 10.
3 Failure to implement low-tech EBM: See Part One, Chapter 10.[48,72]
4 Faulty EBM denying increased risk of cesarean section from early epidurals: See Part One, Chapter 10.
5 Faulty EBM denying benefit of walking in labor: see Part One, Chapter 10.
6 Publication bias in favor of devices, drugs, and intervention.[73-7]

Economic Environment

7 Profit motive in private hospitals.
8 Costs of malpractice litigation.
9 Hospitals depend on NICU and surgery for revenue.
10 Increased reimbursement for surgical management.
11 Market forces pushing products – drugs, machines, tools – all putting birth under more technological control.[78,79]
12 Costly interventions have become standard practice without evaluation.[49,80-2]
13 Industry opposition to EBM that does not support their product.[49,83,84]
14 Funding bias pushing products and research: drugs, machines, tools.[76]

Provider Environment

15 "Maximin" strategy: see Part Seven.
16 Faulty interpretation of EBM: See Part One, Chapter 10.
17 Preoccupation with post-dates and need for induction; EBM on this issue is inconclusive.[85,86]
18 Risk magnification: relative vs. absolute.[87,88]
19 Birth reinterpreted as a surgical procedure.[78]
20 Decreased continuity of care of nursing.[13]
21 Staffing patterns for nurses.
22 Lifestyle issues for maternity care providers.[89,90]
23 Work hour rules for residents limiting continuous participation with laboring women.
24 Decreased continuity for residents.
25 Time pressures lead to preferred daytime deliveries.[91-3]
26 Procedural skills more valued than expectant care for normal birth.
27 Fewer trainees in midwifery and family medicine programs – providers who are more likely to pursue normal births.
28 Fewer normal births to witness and learn from.
29 Fewer practitioners (midwives and FPs) available to attend normal births.
30 Threat of malpractice litigation.

31 Increased preoccupation with risk by obstetricians.
32 Decreased perception of risk of cesareans despite known increased later complications for mother and more NICU admissions for infants.[94-8]
33 Magnification of risk from VBAC and vaginal breech deliveries.
34 Increasing rate of cesareans in past 25 years results in increased complications from prior cesareans requiring increased cesareans.
35 Increased belief by obstetricians that obese women will need cesareans, leading to self-fulfilling prophecy when obese woman is in labor.
36 Decreased rate of VBAC and vaginal breech delivery leading to trainees not acquiring the relevant skills.

Consumer Environment

37 Increased women's acceptance of increased obstetrical intervention overall.[99,100]
38 Increased perception of risk to fetus leads to increased acceptance of intervention.[43,100]
39 Inherent appeal of new technology as part of progress.
40 Desire for "perfect baby."[101]
41 Increased detection of possible abnormalities during increased use of ultrasound and other testing in normal pregnancies.
42 Birth viewed as emergency.
43 Increasing rate of obesity among childbearing women.
44 Increased consumption of fast food, decreased time for exercise.
45 Increased gestational diabetes and increasing macrosomia.
46 Older women with more chronic medical problems having children.
47 Isolation of women from extended family and community.
48 Media portrayal of childbirth.
49 Popular appeal of painless childbirth.
50 Popular appeal of timing of delivery.

Hospital Environment

51 Increased rate of epidural anesthesia.
52 Central monitoring reduces bedside nursing support.
53 Women staying in bed (horizontal) resulting in dystocia.
54 Requirement for 24-hour anesthesia staffing (to offer VBAC).
55 Increased rate of inductions.
56 Image of technology to promote hospital as most advanced, desirable.[78]
57 Hospital birth setting increasingly surgical and increasingly focused on emergencies.

recent approach to frame how we think about highly complex and often unpredictable phenomena in medicine, public health, sickness, and the human body. Obstetric interventionism with its worldwide increase in the rate of cesarean sections even in resource-poor settings is an excellent target for the tools of complexity science. The technological vision of birth with the resulting lack of woman-centered attention in maternity care is clearly a complicated interaction of individuals, organizations, and wider social, political, economic, and belief systems. The woman's body, the woman herself, her family and social setting, her culture including the media, her ethnic and national identities and her belief system interact with medical care providers, institutions, scientific advancements, technical developments, commercial interests, legal environments, and wider cultural beliefs about life, death, pain, disability, and meaning to create the intricate and enormously complicated web of modern maternity care.

Complexity science tells us that these systems are dynamic. They can influence each other in unpredictable ways – a small change in one area can have enormous influence in another location in the web through amplification effects. The wide variation in cesarean section rates for nulliparous women across hospitals, across states, and across nations shows that non-clinical issues are critical in determining the rate of obstetric intervention, not women's biology.[65,105] How to induce change in dynamic systems is an active discussion among those interested in complexity science. "Neither illness nor human behaviour is predictable and neither can safely be 'modeled' in a simple cause and effect system."[106] For this reason, "Command and Control" management will be an ineffective strategy to address the international syndemic of cesarean sections.[107] Taking on the rapid increase in cesarean sections requires first an analysis of the syndemic nature of its causes, and second, a multilevel, nuanced approach in many sectors of health, science, and public life. At the practical, day-to-day level, given that low intervention settings have lower cesarean rates without an increase in maternal or fetal morbidity,[108-113] finding out what works to keep rates low and propagating these practices is clearly a strategic approach. Certain aspects of clinician style and healthcare systems appear to prevent labor dystocia and resultant cesarean section, including caregiver continuity during the assessment of early labor,[114] encouraging a "pro-physiologic" cultural attitude toward natural childbirth,[105] requiring consultation with a second clinician prior to non-emergent cesarean deliveries for dystocia,[105,115] and providing regular feedback to clinicians regarding their cesarean delivery rates.[64,116,117]

An example of complexity science at work is the debate in family medicine about the "preventive" induction of labor to decrease the rate of cesareans. In a project known as AMOR-IPAT, Nicholson advances the idea that since certain risk factors at 40+ weeks are associated with cesareans, induction of labor earlier than 40 weeks may prevent cesareans in women with a constellation of these factors.[118-120] The evidence for the utility of this strategy is under vigorous and heated argument within both family medicine and obstetric circles.[120-122] On the one hand, cautious practitioners remember that the field of obstetrics has been historically prone to functioning according to authority and myth, for instance in long promoting routine episiotomy to prevent later pelvic floor prolapse despite lack of evidence to defend this practice.[123,124] Thus any new drive to advocate an intervention to prevent a later complication requires careful and adequate prospective study. Aggressive induction of a woman with an unripe cervix is not an innocent intervention, especially for woman-centered maternity providers with a deep respect for the normality of the physiological process of birth. This approach also may not work as well in the general obstetrical milieu without combining it carefully with an individualized, personalized approach that includes woman-centered assessment throughout pregnancy and options for labor support, alternatives in labor analgesia, and other care practices associated with lower cesarean rates.[122] On the other hand, the steep rise in cesareans is clearly an epidemic, and multiple other related epidemic factors – obesity, use of epidurals, poor nutrition, etc. – already interrupt normal physiological processes. As with any health epidemic, woman-centered providers need to seek all reasonable, evidence-driven efforts to address root causes and possible solutions, with preliminary retrospective data from Nicholson's work deserving further study along with interventions to address these other epidemic risks.

CHAPTER 4

Where Do We Go From Here? Strategies to Promote Wise Stewardship of Resources

During maternity care, evidence-based medicine and woman-centeredness can theoretically work together for the wise and fiscally responsible use of resources. But demand for what technology can offer – for example, prenatal videos of the fetus – will exceed the medical necessity for such technology.[125] Hospital-based deliveries, as well, have a dynamic of increasingly interventive use of resources. Current trends in obstetrics in North America suggest that increasing technical and surgical resources will be sought, even demanded, by both women and providers in the future. The culture surrounding birth conveys the impression that "no cost is too great" for the pain-free delivery experience and for the healthy baby. Being realistic means recognizing that despite the benefits of modern obstetrics, a runaway technology has a dynamic of its own. In the context of highly technical and commercialized birth, the wise stewardship of resources in the interest of patient-centeredness will remain an ongoing challenge. Options to address that challenge follow.

Syndemic thinking posits that change in a syndemic such as obstetric interventionism requires actions at multiple levels involving many different kinds of people: gathering forces, taking stock of the problem, using mathematical models and simulations to project the process forward and to map the implications of change efforts onto these projections. Individual practitioners in hospital settings struggling to keep birth as technology-free as possible may have limited effect on population outcomes, especially given the culture of hospitals and the litigious environment that pushes providers toward increasing interventions. Those working in birthing settings outside of hospitals (home births or alternative birthing centers) by choice are unlikely to influence the trend in hospital births or the overall population outcomes given that relatively few births occur in such settings in the North America and Europe (with the exception of the Netherlands). The upsurge in midwifery in hospitals in Canada is an important exception to this trend. Many people, many institutions, and many organizations will be required to implement change.

PATIENT EMPOWERMENT

Encouraging women to understand and take charge of their own health and illness is a key strategy in health promotion (*see* Part Five). Woman-centered maternity education is central to good nutrition, avoidance of harm, and preparation for birth and lactation. For a woman to take charge of her maternity care and make choices about her birth, she needs to clarify her values for a healthy pregnancy and birth in a highly technical environment. When possible she needs to choose providers who share her values, or at least are willing to do everything possible for her to realize the birth she hopes for. Values clarification then allows further discussion of the risks and benefits of her various choices, including the newest technology. While the benefits of the newest technology may seem readily apparent to them, when women and their families clearly understand the risks of those same technologies, they may make different choices.

Empowered women and their family members may be the first to identify and even prevent medical error in the hospital setting. While some providers may fear increased provider liability from patient empowerment that leads to patients' discovery of errors, woman-centered providers seek any possible strategies for error prevention, including teaching patients and families to track and report such problems. While organizations such as the American College of Obstetricians and Gynecologists officially endorse partnership with patients in decisions and discussion about "any aspect of their care,"[126] woman-centered care encourages a more explicit discussion of ways to teach patients to recognize and report errors. Another step toward a woman-centered approach to medical error includes the movement toward disclosure and apology, again recently endorsed by ACOG.[127]

Patient empowerment continues even when obstetric emergencies happen. Obstetrics is unpredictable: even in the least interventive settings, 10% to 15% of births require cesareans. The much higher numbers in most settings today appear as emergencies, and often may in fact be emergencies, but are tied to the cascade of interventions described above. And some are not emergencies but are portrayed as such. For the woman (or woman and her partner) making choices in moments of emergency is usually not in their power. When experts present a situation as endangering the life of the woman or the baby, even empowered lay people are unlikely to be able to make a "choice" that would challenge the professionals' recommendations.[128] Thus patient empowerment has to include not only anticipating but also correctly defining emergencies.

WOMAN-CENTERED DECISION-MAKING

Part of patient empowerment also involves identifying and using tools that will help make decisions centered around the pregnant woman's values. The field of decision analysis has shown that patients' (and providers') decision-making is strongly influenced by how the choice is situated and phrased. Women may understand words to describe the frequency of a complication – e.g., two in a thousand – better than percentages like 0.2%. Similarly when providers frame numbers by focusing on success, patients are more inclined to accept the risk.[88] For instance, saying, "199 VBACs out of 200 will have no emergency" is a more optimistic frame than saying "1 in 200 VBACs will have a uterine rupture." Clinicians can thus influence women's decision-making in subtle ways without explicitly stating their recommendation. A more balanced approach gives the woman both the positive and negative outcome statistics, leaving her the opportunity to look at it both ways. Drawing on these understandings, patient educators have constructed tools that make complex risk assessments understandable to lay decision-makers. A further step is the development of tools that incorporate patients' values into the instruments. An example of woman-centered decision-making is exemplified by the use of a decision aid for women trying to decide about a trial of labor after cesarean (TOLAC). (*See* www. aafp.org/online/en/home/clinical/patiented/counselingtools/tolac.html for a tool designed to both inform and help women make this decision.) Clearly, providers need tools understandable to lay people to make decisions about common pregnancy decisions such as whether to undertake first-trimester screening, how to understand the quadruple screen, or how to consider Group B Streptococcus (GBS) screening. These decision tools become even more essential at very difficult clinical moments – for instance, how to make decisions about extremely premature infants on the border of viability.

PRIORITIZING HUMAN OVER TECHNICAL SOLUTIONS

Prenatal group visits, training women's friends or family members as lay doulas, putting doulas in the labor room with every woman, exploring and addressing fears about vaginal birth prior to labor, engaging and educating partners to support breast feeding – all these strategies, if systematically implemented, have the potential to decrease interventions. Here again professionals, health educators, and women's health activists, joined by advocacy organizations and by women themselves, create the possibility of envisioning another kind of birth, not just for a few educated or stubborn women, but for all who want their baby's birth to be their delivery, not the system's delivery. The new book, *Our Bodies, Ourselves: pregnancy and birth*,[129] by the Boston Women's Health Book Collective, puts this message into language accessible and available to women.

MOBILIZING CONSUMERS

Organizations such as the Boston Women's Health Book Collective (www.ourbodies ourselves.org/) exemplify the power of women's health advocacy at a consumer level to work toward woman-centered decision-making. In the United Kingdom, activists have developed a website to encourage women's choices around where to deliver: www.birthchoiceuk.com/BirthChoiceUKFrame.htm. Another UK organization is the Association for Improvement in the Maternity Services (www.aims. org.uk/) whose goal is to foster normal birth by providing information to women to support their decision-making. In North America, the Childbirth Connection (www.childbirthconnection.org/home), formerly the Maternity Care Association, has a long history of educating women for normal births and is now creating a long-term national program to promote evidence-based maternity care, offering "research translation" of evidence-based information into language women and their families can use to make empowered decisions. With this goal of educating consumers, professionals, and the media, the Childbirth Connection takes as its explicit mission "promoting safe, effective, and satisfying maternity care" and is a voice for the needs and interests of childbearing families.[130] To this end the Childbirth Connection performed a systematic review about cesarean section and made the results available in lay language as a booklet, published as *What Every Pregnant Woman Needs to Know About Cesarean Section*.[131] An independent voice, not tied to specialty or trade interests, carries the potential to speak loudly and clearly in a way that will help women make choices rather than accept whatever they are told.

Other consumer organizations such as La Leche League seek support for normal birth and breastfeeding and exist wherever women have gained enough empowerment to educate themselves and make demands. Likewise, healthcare professionals from a variety of disciplines, including obstetricians, are making international linkages to foster normal birth. When these organizations join forces and pool their resources and exert influence in the halls of public health and fiscal decision-making for health internationally, when these forces exert an impact on consumer understandings of the risks of interventionism, and when these forces begin to shape trainees' understanding of the excesses of interventionism, normal birth will regain its proper place as a goal of maternity care.

NATIONAL AND INTERNATIONAL RECOGNITION OF THE PUBLIC HEALTH COSTS OF TECHNICAL SOLUTIONS

While improvement of infant and maternal mortality in developing countries requires access to emergency cesareans by trained providers, accelerating rates of cesareans in urban centers of countries like Mexico and Brazil are clearly expenses that those countries can ill afford. Action by international health and funding organizations to promote physiologic birth with emergency backup rather than imitation of North American surgical birth is a strategy to focus attention on the unnecessary costs of technology in the developing world. In Brazil, publicizing the fact that most women do not want cesareans, that it is doctors who have been pushing surgical births, and making the high rates of intervention a public scandal have been effective strategies in changing the Brazilian culture of childbirth.[132] Denying government reimbursement to hospitals with excess cesarean section rates has been a part of creating that change in Brazil.[132] The recent WHO survey of cesarean sections in Latin America, where rates in private hospitals have climbed as high as 51%, reveals the increased morbidity and mortality of both mother and infant when women whose fetuses are in cephalic presentations have cesarean section.[94,133] Promulgation of this information among those attempting to stretch limited budgets for health in Latin American countries has the potential for putting brakes on the accelerating rates of surgical delivery in that region.

PROMOTION OF PRIMARY CARE MATERNITY PROVIDERS

Primary care maternity care providers (midwives and family doctors) appear best situated to practice wise stewardship in obstetrics: "By acting as an appropriate filter for high-technology care, primary care helps ensure that it is appropriately applied, a major determinant of outcomes."[134] Enkin *et al.* in their comprehensive text on childbirth, *A Guide to Effective Care in Pregnancy and Childbirth*,[135] place primary care maternity providers at the center of care of women with normal pregnancies:

> As technical advances have become more complex, in many countries care has come to be increasingly controlled by, or even carried out by, specialist obstetricians. The benefits of this trend can be seriously challenged. It is inherently unwise, and perhaps unsafe, for women with normal pregnancies to be cared for by obstetric specialists, even if the required personnel were available. Because of time constraints, obstetricians caring for women with both normal and abnormal pregnancies have to make an impossible choice: to neglect the normal pregnancies in order to concentrate their care on those with pathology, or spend most of their time supervising biologically normal processes. Midwives and general practitioners, on the other hand, are primarily oriented to the care of women with normal pregnancies, and are likely to have more detailed knowledge of the particular circumstances of individual women. The care that they can give to the majority of women, whose pregnancies are not affected by any major illness or

serious complication, will often be more responsive to their needs than that given by specialist obstetricians. Industrialized countries in which midwives are the primary caregivers for healthy childbearing women have more favorable maternal and neonatal outcomes, including lower perinatal mortality rates and lower cesarean delivery rates, than countries in which many or most healthy women receive care from obstetricians during pregnancy.[135]

(Reproduced with the kind permission of Oxford University Press.)

Clearly, many different patterns or organizations of maternity care are possible around the world, and the promotion of midwifery and general practice obstetrics for normal delivery care holds the promise of limiting the spiraling technology.[51,136] Countries promoting this solution need to address the problem of fewer and fewer people providing obstetrical care in rural areas. Fostering an increase in the number of rural practitioners requires attention to the selection and recruitment of trainees in healthcare beginning in the high school years, with attention to service and geographical commitment over test scores, specialization, science orientation, and income goals.[137-139]

CLOSING THOUGHTS

Woman-centered maternity care faces enormous challenges in today's highly technological birth environment. Practitioners like Larisa must be creative in how they manage time to promote best practices in care. They need to work collaboratively with many kinds of caregivers – doulas, midwives, nurses, obstetricians, nutritionists, lactation consultants, physical therapists, to mention only the most obvious – in teams with a flexible approach to the many different kinds of women who seek their services. The woman-centered clinician will also engage in teamwork with the woman and her support system to help make her delivery the fulfilling experience that she hopes for. And all of this must take place within a technical, hierarchical and sometimes even hostile atmosphere that has come to characterize today's obstetrical settings. Fortunately, many voices and hands together have the potential to foster the delivery of woman-centered care one birth at a time, and to join with the many kinds of practitioners and consumers also working for woman-centered maternity care. In all the larger arenas – hospitals, educational settings, and national and international organizations involved with maternal well-being – clinicians, scholars, researchers, educators, and policy-makers can be found who work tirelessly for this goal. The task is daunting, the future uncertain, and the obstacles enormous. Nevertheless, Larisa and those of us like her, with the daily experience of taking part in woman-centered birth, know that the goal, as with childbirth itself, is well worth the struggle.

REFERENCES

1 Arborelius E, Bremberg S. What can doctors do to achieve a successful consultation? Videotaped interviews analysed by the 'consultation map' method. *Fam Pract.* 1992; **9:** 61–6.

2 Greenfield S, Kaplan SH, Ware JE, Jr., *et al.* Patients' participation in medical care: Effects on blood sugar control and quality of life in diabetes. *J Gen Intern Med.* 1988; **3:** 448–57.

3 Henbest RJ, Fehrsen GS. Patient-centredness: Is it applicable outside the West? Its measurement and effect on outcomes. *Fam Pract.* 1992; **9:** 311–7.

4 Marvel MK, Doherty WJ, Weiner E. Medical interviewing by exemplary family physicians. *J Fam Pract.* 1998; **47:** 343–8.

5 Ickovics JR, Kershaw TS, Westdahl C, *et al.* Group prenatal care and perinatal outcomes: a randomized controlled trial. *Obstet Gynecol.* 2007; **110:** 330–9.

6 Brown H, Smith H. Giving women their own case notes to carry during pregnancy. *Cochrane Database Syst Rev.* 2004: **2.** CD002856.

7 Shaw E, Howard M, Chan D, *et al.* Access to web-based personalized antenatal health records for pregnant women: a randomized controlled trial. *J Obstet Gynaecol Can.* 2008; **30:** 38–43.

8 Stewart M, Brown JB, Weston WW, *et al.*, eds. *Patient-centered Medicine: transforming the clinical method.* 2nd ed. Oxford: Radcliffe Medical Press; 2003.

9 Simonds W. Watching the clock: keeping time during pregnancy, birth, and postpartum experiences. *Soc Sci Med.* 2002; **55:** 559–70.

10 Pates JA, McIntire DD, Leveno KJ. Uterine contractions preceding labor. *Obstet Gynecol.* 2007; **110:** 566–9.

11 Declercq E, Sakala C, Corry M, *et al. Listening to Mothers: Report of the First National U.S. Survey of Women's Childbearing Experiences.* New York: Maternity Center Association; 2002 October.

12 Woodrow SI, Segouin C, Armbruster J, *et al.* Duty hours reforms in the United States, France, and Canada: is it time to refocus our attention on education? *Acad Med.* 2006; **81:** 1045–51.

13 Gagnon AJ, Meier KM, Waghorn K. Continuity of nursing care and its link to cesarean birth rate. *Birth.* 2007; **34:** 26–31.

14 Sikorski J, Renfrew MJ, Pindoria S, *et al.* Support for breastfeeding mothers. *Cochrane Database Syst Rev.* 2002: CD001141.

15 MacArthur C, Winter HR, Bick DE, *et al.* Redesigning postnatal care: a randomised controlled trial of protocol-based midwifery-led care focused on individual women's physical and psychological health needs. *Health Technol Assess.* 2003; **7:** 1–98.

16 Kistin N, Abramson R, Dublin P. Effect of peer counselors on breastfeeding initiation, exclusivity, and duration among low-income urban women. *J Hum Lact.* 1994; **10:** 11–15.

17 Morrow AL, Guerrero ML, Shults J, *et al.* Efficacy of home-based peer counselling to promote exclusive breastfeeding: a randomised controlled trial. *Lancet.* 1999; **353:** 1226–31.

18 Carroll JC, Brown JB, Reid AJ. Female family physicians in obstetrics: achieving personal balance. *CMAJ.* 1995; **153:** 1283–89.

19 Hundley V, Ryan M. Are women's expectations and preferences for intrapartum care affected by the model of care on offer? *BJOG.* 2004; **111:** 550–60.

20 Green J, Renfrew M, Curtis P. Continuity of carer: what matters to women? A review of the evidence. *Midwifery.* 2000; **16**: 186–96.

21 Farquhar M, Camilleri-Ferrante C, Todd C. Continuity of care in maternity services: women's views of one team midwifery scheme. *Midwifery.* 2000; **16**: 35–47.

22 Statham H, Solomou W, Green JM. Communication of prenatal screening and diagnosis results to primary-care health professionals. *Public Health.* 2003; **117**: 348–57.

23 Gramling L, Hickman K, Bennett S. What makes a good family-centered partnership between women and their practitioners? A qualitative study. *Birth.* 2004; **31**: 43–8.

24 Brown S, Lumley J. Changing childbirth: lessons from an Australian survey of 1336 women. *Br J Obstet Gynaecol.* 1998; **105**: 143–55.

25 Tandon SD, Parillo KM, Keefer M. Hispanic women's perceptions of patient-centeredness during prenatal care: a mixed-method study. *Birth.* 2005; **32**: 312–17.

26 Cherouny P, Federico F, Haraden C, *et al. Idealized Design of Perinatal Care. IHI Innovation Series white paper.* Cambridge, Massachusetts: Institute for Healthcare Improvement; 2005.

27 Carroll JC, Reid AJ, Ruderman J, *et al.* The influence of the high-risk care environment on the practice of low-risk obstetrics. *Fam Med.* 1991; **23**: 184–8.

28 Campbell DA, Lake MF, Falk M, *et al.* A randomized control trial of continuous support in labor by a lay doula. *J Obstet Gynecol Neonatal Nurs.* 2006; **35**: 456–64.

29 Chen FM, Feudtner C, Rhodes LA, *et al.* Role conflicts of physicians and their family members: rules but no rulebook. *West J Med.* 2001; **175**: 236–9; discussion 40.

30 Chen FM, Rhodes LA, Green LA, *et al.* Family physicians' personal experiences of their fathers' health care. *J Fam Pract.* 2001; **50**: 762–6.

31 Committee on Quality of Health Care in America. *Crossing the Quality Chasm: a new health system for the twenty-first century.* Washington, D.C.: Institute of Medicine, National Academies Press; 2001.

32 Klein MC. Too close for comfort? A family physician questions whether medical professionals should be excluded from their loved ones' care. *CMAJ.* 1997; **156**: 53–5.

33 Davis-Floyd R. The technocratic, humanistic, and holistic paradigms of childbirth. *Int J Gynaecol Obstet.* 2001; **75**(Suppl. 1): S5–23.

34 Klein MC, Eftekhary Shirkoohy S, Asrat G. *Obstetrics and Gynecology Residents: who are they and what do they believe about childbirth?* North American Primary Care Research Group. Vancouver, BC 2007.

35 Brody H, Thompson JR. The maximin strategy in modern obstetrics. *J Fam Pract.* 1981; **12**: 977–86.

36 Anonymous. Cost of malpractice insurance set to rise in Canada. *BMJ.* 2000; **320**: 602e–.

37 Godwin M, Hodgetts G, Seguin R, *et al.* The Ontario family medicine residents cohort study: Factors affecting residents' decisions to practise obstetrics. *CMAJ.* 2002; **166**: 179–84.

38 Wiegers TA. General practitioners and their role in maternity care. *Health Policy.* 2003; **66**: 51–9.

39 Xu X, Siefert KA, Jacobson PD, *et al.* The impact of malpractice burden on Michigan obstetrician-gynecologists' career satisfaction. *Womens Health Issues.* 2008; **18**: 229–37.

40 Sibbald B. SOGC sounds ALARM on legal pitfalls facing ob/gyns. *CMAJ.* 1999; **161**: 565–6.

41 Beck U. *Risk Society*. London: Sage Publications; 1992.

42 Kildea S. Risky business: contested knowledge over safe birthing services for Aboriginal women. *Health Sociol Rev*. 2006; **15**: 387–400.

43 Possamai-Inesedy A. Confining risk: choice and responsibility in childbirth in a risk society. *Health Sociol Rev*. 2006; **15**: 406–14.

44 Eckermann L. Finding a 'safe' place on the risk continuum: a case study of pregnancy and birthing in Lao PDR. *Health Sociol Rev*. 2006; **15**: 374.

45 Watts G. First pictures: one for the album. *BMJ*. 2007; **334**: 232–3.

46 Tanne JH. FDA warns against commercial prenatal ultrasound videos. *BMJ*. 2004; **328**: 853 ff.

47 Lyerly AD, Mitchell LM, Armstrong EM, *et al*. Risks, values, and decision making surrounding pregnancy. *Obstet Gynecol*. 2007; **109**: 979–84.

48 Graham ID, Logan J, Davies B, *et al*. Changing the use of electronic fetal monitoring and labor support: a case study of barriers and facilitators. *Birth*. 2004; **31**: 293–301.

49 Banta HD, Thacker SB. Electronic fetal monitoring. Lessons from a formative case of health technology assessment. *Int J Technol Assess Health Care*. 2002; **18**: 762–70.

50 Lent M. The medical and legal risks of the electronic fetal monitor. *Stanford Law Rev*. 1999; **51**: 807–37.

51 Reime B, Klein MC, Kelly A, *et al*. Do maternity care provider groups have different attitudes towards birth? *BJOG: An International Journal of Obstetrics and Gynaecology*. 2004; **111**: 1388–93.

52 Declercq E, Menacker F, Macdorman M. Maternal risk profiles and the primary cesarean rate in the United States, 1991–2002. *Am J Public Health*. 2006; 96: 867–72.

53 Declercq E, Menacker F, MacDorman M. Rise in "No indicated risk" Primary caesareans in the United States, 1991–2001: Cross sectional analysis. *BMJ*. 2005; 330: 71–2.

54 CIfHI. Giving birth in Canada: Regional trends from 2001–2 to 2005–6. 2007 [cited January 10, 2009]. Available from: http://secure.cihi.ca/cihiweb/dispPage.jsp?cw_page=AR_1106_E

55 Hamilton B, Martin J, Ventura S. Births: preliminary data for 2007. *Natl Vital Stat Rep*. 2009; **57**(12): 1–23.

56 Caesarean Section Working Group. *Attaining and Maintaining Best Practices in the Use of Caesarean Sections: an analysis of four Ontario hospitals*. Ontario Women's Health Council; 2000.

57 Declercq E, Norsigian J. The folly of 1% policy. *Boston Globe*. 2007 August 6.

58 Goetzl L, Rivers J, Evans T, *et al*. Prophylactic acetaminophen does not prevent epidural fever in nulliparous women: a double-blind placebo-controlled trial. *J Perinatol*. 2004; **24**: 471–5.

59 Sharma SK, Alexander JM, Messick G, *et al*. Cesarean delivery: a randomized trial of epidural analgesia versus intravenous meperidine analgesia during labor in nulliparous women. *Anesthesiology*. 2002; **96**: 546–51.

60 Lowe NK. A review of factors associated with dystocia and cesarean section in nulliparous women. *J Midwifery Womens Health*. 2007; **52**: 216–28.

61 Jackson DJ, Lang JM, Ecker J, *et al*. Impact of collaborative management and early admission in labor on method of delivery. *J Obstet Gynecol Neonatal Nurs*. 2003; **32**: 147–57; discussion 58–60.

62 Janssen PA, Iker CE, Carty EA. Early labour assessment and support at home: a randomized controlled trial. *J Obstet Gynaecol Can*. 2003; **25**: 734–41.

63 Janssen PA, Still DK, Klein MC, *et al.* Early labor assessment and support at home versus telephone triage: a randomized controlled trial. *Obstet Gynecol.* 2006; **108**: 1463–69.

64 Main EK. Reducing cesarean birth rates with data-driven quality improvement activities. *Pediatrics.* 1999; **103**: 374–83.

65 Main EK, Bloomfield L, Hunt G. Development of a large-scale obstetric quality-improvement program that focused on the nulliparous patient at term. *Am J Obstet Gynecol.* 2004; **190**: 1747–56; discussion 56–8.

66 Robson MS, Scudamore IW, Walsh SM. Using the medical audit cycle to reduce cesarean section rates. *Am J Obstet Gynecol.* 1996; **174**: 199–205.

67 Ontario Women's Health Council. *Ontario Women's Health Council Caesarean Section Best Practices Project: impact and analysis*; 2002.

68 Singer MC, Erickson PI, Badiane L, *et al.* Syndemics, sex and the city: understanding sexually transmitted diseases in social and cultural context. *Soc Sci Med.* 2006; **63**: 2010–21.

69 Singer M, Clair S. Syndemics and public health: Reconceptualizing disease in bio-social context. *Med Anthropol Q.* 2003; **17**: 423–41.

70 Candib LM. Obesity and diabetes in vulnerable populations: reflection on proximal and distal causes. *Ann Fam Med.* 2007; **5**: 547–56.

71 Marshall M. Carolina in the Carolines: a survey of patterns and meanings of smoking on a Micronesian island. *Med Anthropol Q.* 2005; **19**: 365–82.

72 Wood SH. Should women be given a choice about fetal assessment in labor? *MCN: Am J Matern Child Nurs.* 2003; **28**: 292–8.

73 De Vries R, Lemmens T. The social and cultural shaping of medical evidence: case studies from pharmaceutical research and obstetric science. *Soc Sci Med.* 2006; **62**: 2694–2706.

74 Tatsioni A, Zarin DA, Aronson N, *et al.* Challenges in systematic reviews of diagnostic technologies. *Ann Intern Med.* 2005; **142**: 1048–55.

75 Bekelman JE, Li Y, Gross CP. Scope and impact of financial conflicts of interest in biomedical research: a systematic review. *JAMA.* 2003; **289**: 454–65.

76 Bodenheimer T. Uneasy alliance – clinical investigators and the pharmaceutical industry. *N Engl J Med.* 2000; **342**: 1539–44.

77 Rennie D. Fair conduct and fair reporting of clinical trials. *JAMA.* 1999; **282**: 1766–68.

78 Wendland CL. The vanishing mother: cesarean section and "evidence-based obstetrics". *Med Anthropol Q.* 2007; **21**: 218–33.

79 Lewin T. Despite criticism, fetal monitors are likely to remain in wide use. *New York Times.* 1988 March 27.

80 Johri M, Lehoux P. The great escape? Prospects for regulating access to technology through health technology assessment. *Int J Technol Assess Health Care.* 2003; **19**: 179–93.

81 Hoerst BJ, Fairman J. Social and professional influences of the technology of electronic fetal monitoring on obstetrical nursing. *West J Nurs Res.* 2000; **22**: 475–91.

82 Hartling L, McAlister FA, Rowe BH, *et al.* Challenges in systematic reviews of therapeutic devices and procedures. *Ann Intern Med.* 2005; **142**: 1100–11.

83 Hailey D. Scientific harassment by pharmaceutical companies: time to stop. *CMAJ.* 2000; **162**: 212–13.

84 Hemminki E, Hailey D, Koivusalo M. The courts – a challenge to health technology assessment. *Science.* 1999; **285**: 203–4.

85 Wei S, Fraser WD. Induction of labour post-term or expectant management with serial fetal monitoring had similar neonatal outcomes. *Evid Based Med.* 2007; **12**: 174.

86 Menticoglou SM, Hall PF. Routine induction of labour at 41 weeks gestation: nonsensus consensus. *BJOG.* 2002; **109**: 485–91.

87 Malenka DJ, Baron JA, Johansen S, *et al.* The framing effect of relative and absolute risk. *J Gen Intern Med.* 1993; **8**: 543–8.

88 Gigerenzer G, Edwards A. Simple tools for understanding risks: from innumeracy to insight. *BMJ.* 2003; **327**: 741–4.

89 Xu X, Siefert KA, Jacobson PD, *et al.* Malpractice burden, rural location, and discontinuation of obstetric care: a study of obstetric providers in Michigan. *J Rural Health.* 2009; **25**: 33–42.

90 Fondren LK, Ricketts TC. The North Carolina obstetrics access and professional liability study: a rural–urban analysis. *J Rural Health.* 1993; **9**: 129–37.

91 Goodman MJ, Nelson WW, Maciosek MV. Births by day of week: a historical perspective. *J Midwifery Womens Health.* 2005; **50**: 39–43.

92 Lerchl A. Where are the Sunday babies? Observations on a marked decline in weekend births in Germany. *Naturwissenschaften.* 2005; **92**: 592–4.

93 Curtin SC, Park MM. Trends in the attendant, place, and timing of births, and in the use of obstetric interventions: United States, 1989–97. *Natl Vital Stat Rep.* 1999; **47**(27): 1–12.

94 Villar J, Carroli G, Zavaleta N, *et al.* Maternal and neonatal individual risks and benefits associated with caesarean delivery: multicentre prospective study. *BMJ.* 2007; **335**: 1025.

95 Tita ATN, Landon MB, Spong CY, *et al.* Timing of elective repeat cesarean delivery at term and neonatal outcomes. *N Engl J Med.* 2009; **360**: 111–20.

96 Signore C, Klebanoff M. Neonatal morbidity and mortality after elective cesarean delivery. *Clin Perinatol.* **35**: 361–71.

97 Rossi AC, D'Addario V. Maternal morbidity following a trial of labor after cesarean section vs. elective repeat cesarean delivery: a systematic review with metaanalysis. *Am J Obstet Gynecol.* 2008; **199**: 224–31.

98 Ramachandrappa A, Jain L. Elective cesarean section: its impact on neonatal respiratory outcome. *Clin Perinatol.* **35**: 373–93.

99 Banta HD, Oortwiin W. Health technology assessment and screening in the Netherlands: case studies of mammography in breast cancer, PSA screening in prostate cancer, and ultrasound in normal pregnancy. *Int J Technol Assess Health Care.* 2001; **17**: 369–79.

100 Harris G, Connor L, Bisits A, *et al.* "Seeing the baby": pleasures and dilemmas of ultrasound technologies for primiparous Australian women. *Med Anthropol Q.* 2004; **18**: 23–47.

101 Remennick L. The quest for the perfect baby: why do Israeli women seek prenatal genetic testing? *Sociol Health Illn.* 2006; **28**: 21–53.

102 Klein MC. Does epidural analgesia increase rate of cesarean section? *Can Fam Physician.* 2006; **52**: 419–21, 26–8.

103 Kotaska AJ, Klein MC, Liston RM. Epidural analgesia associated with low-dose oxytocin augmentation increases cesarean births: a critical look at the external validity of randomized trials. *Am J Obstet Gynecol.* 2006; **194**: 809–14.

104 American Society of Anesthesiologists Task Force on Obstetric Anesthesia. Practice guidelines for obstetric anesthesia: an updated report. *Anesthesiology.* 2007; **106**: 843–63.

105 Leeman L, Leeman R. A Native American community with a 7% cesarean delivery rate:

does case mix, ethnicity, or labor management explain the low rate? *Ann Fam Med.* 2003; **1**: 36–43.

106 Holt TA, ed. *Complexity for Clinicians.* Oxford: Radcliffe Publishing; 2004.

107 Cooper H, Geyer R. *Riding the Diabetes Rollercoaster: a new approach for health professionals, patients and carers.* Oxford: Radcliffe Publishing; 2007.

108 Butler J, Abrams B, Parker J, *et al.* Supportive nurse-midwife care is associated with a reduced incidence of cesarean section. *Am J Obstet Gynecol.* 1993; **168**: 1407–13.

109 Hueston WJ. Site-to-site variation in the factors affecting cesarean section rates. *Arch Fam Med.* 1995; **4**: 346–51.

110 Hueston WJ, Applegate JA, Mansfield CJ, *et al.* Practice variations between family physicians and obstetricians in the management of low-risk pregnancies. *J Fam Pract.* 1995; **40**: 345–51.

111 Hueston WJ, Lewis-Stevenson S. Provider distribution and variations in statewide cesarean section rates. *J Community Health.* 2001; **26**: 1–10.

112 Reid AJ, Carroll JC, Ruderman J, *et al.* Differences in intrapartum obstetric care provided to women at low risk by family physicians and obstetricians. *CMAJ.* 1989; **140**: 625–33.

113 Rosenblatt RA, Dobie SA, Hart LG, *et al.* Interspecialty differences in the obstetric care of low-risk women. *Am J Public Health.* 1997; **87**: 344–51.

114 O'Driscoll K, Meagher D, Robson M. *Active management of labour: the Dublin experience.* 4th ed. Edinburgh; New York: Mosby; 2003.

115 Althabe F, Belizan JM, Villar J, *et al.* Mandatory second opinion to reduce rates of unnecessary caesarean sections in Latin America: a cluster randomised controlled trial. *Lancet.* 2004; **363**: 1934–40.

116 Flamm BL, Berwick DM, Kabcenell A. Reducing cesarean section rates safely: lessons from a "Breakthrough Series" Collaborative. *Birth.* 1998; **25**: 117–24.

117 Liang WH, Yuan CC, Hung JH, *et al.* Effect of peer review and trial of labor on lowering cesarean section rates. *J Chin Med Assoc.* 2004; **67**: 281–6.

118 Nicholson JM, Kellar LC, Cronholm PF, *et al.* Active management of risk in pregnancy at term in an urban population: an association between a higher induction of labor rate and a lower cesarean delivery rate. *Am J Obstet Gynecol.* 2004; **191**: 1516–28.

119 Nicholson JM, Parry S, Caughey AB, *et al.* The impact of the active management of risk in pregnancy at term on birth outcomes: a randomized clinical trial. *Am J Obstet Gynecol.* 2008; **198**: 511 e1–15.

120 Nicholson JM, Yeager DL, Macones G. A preventive approach to obstetric care in a rural hospital: association between higher rates of preventive labor induction and lower rates of cesarean delivery. *Ann Fam Med.* 2007; **5**: 310–19.

121 Caughey AB. Preventive induction of labor: potential benefits if proved effective. *Ann Fam Med.* 2007; **5**: 292–3.

122 Klein MC. Association not causation: what is the intervention? *Ann Fam Med.* 2007; **5**: 294–7.

123 Grimes DA. Technology follies. The uncritical acceptance of medical innovation. *JAMA.* 1993; **269**: 3030–3.

124 Klein MC, Gauthier RJ, Jorgensen SH, *et al.* Does episiotomy prevent perineal trauma and pelvic floor relaxation? *Online J Curr Clin Trials.* 1992; Doc No 10.

125 Leff B, Finucane TE. Gizmo idolatry. *JAMA.* 2008; **299**: 1830–2.

126 ACOG. ACOG Committee Opinion. No. 286: Patient safety in obstetrics and gynecology. *Obstet Gynecol.* 2003; **102**: 883–5.

127 ACOG. ACOG Committee Opinion No. 380: Disclosure and discussion of adverse events. *Obstet Gynecol.* 2007; **110**: 957–8.

128 Crossley ML. Childbirth, complications and the illusion of 'choice': a case study. *Fem Psychol.* 2007; **17**: 543–63.

129 Boston Women's Health Book Collective. *Our Bodies, Ourselves: pregnancy and birth.* New York: Simon and Schuster; 2008.

130 Childbirth Connection. Vision, mission and beliefs. 2008 [cited May 16, 2008, 2008]. Available from: www.childbirthconnection.org/article.asp?ck=10253

131 Childbirth Connection. What every pregnant woman needs to know about cesarean section. Second revised edition. 2006 [cited July26, 2009]. Available from: www.childbirth connection.org/article.asp?ClickedLink=279&ck=10164&area=27

132 Wagner M. *Born in the USA: how a broken maternity system must be fixed to put women and children first.* Berkeley, CA: University of California Press; 2006.

133 Villar J, Valladares E, Wojdyla D, *et al.* Caesarean delivery rates and pregnancy outcomes: The 2005 WHO global survey on maternal and perinatal health in Latin America. *Lancet.* 2006; **367**: 1819–29.

134 Ferrer RL, Hambidge SJ, Maly RC. The essential role of generalists in health care systems. *Ann Intern Med.* 2005; **142**: 691–9.

135 Enkin MW, Keirse MJNC, Neilson J, *et al. A Guide to Effective Care in Pregnancy and Childbirth.* New York: Oxford University Press; 1995.

136 Janssen P, Ryan E, Etches D, *et al.* Outcomes of planned hospital birth attended by midwives compared with physicians in British Columbia. *Birth.* 2007; **34**: 140–7.

137 Bowman RC. The world of rural medical education. 2006 [cited April 22, 2007]. Available from: www.ruralmedicaleducation.org/physician_workforce_studies.htm

138 British Columbia Perinatal Health Program. *Caesarean Birth Task Force Report 2008.* British Columbia Perinatal Health Program; 2008.

139 Department of Health and Ageing. *Improving Maternity Services in Australia: a discussion paper from the Australian government.* Department of Health and Ageing; 2008. Report No.: 1-74186-693-6.

Complete Vignettes:
The Women and the Providers

THE WOMEN
Alexandra

Alexandra was a 16-year-old who did not want her mother to find out when she started having sex but who did want some kind of reliable birth control. She told her provider, Helen the midwife in Judith's practice, that she and her boyfriend would probably have sex at his cousin's house. After hearing about her various options and seriously considering an IUD, Alexandra ultimately chose the injection of depot medroxyprogesterone.

The next year, Alexandra and her boyfriend broke up. Not planning to be sexually active again for a while, she decided not to stay on "the shot." However, she then became involved briefly with a new partner and used condoms at first. One night the condom broke, and she called the health center the next day looking for emergency contraception, but became frustrated by how long she had to wait on the phone and the attitude of the busy nurse who finally took her call. Alexandra gave up, hoping not to get pregnant, but she missed her period the next month and started to have morning sickness. When she told her new boyfriend the news, he was angry, blaming her and refusing to acknowledge that he was the father. Facing this lack of support, Alexandra reluctantly told her older sister about the pregnancy, fearing that her mother would be furious. Her sister encouraged her to keep the pregnancy and helped her tell their mother. She was able to get an appointment with Helen to start prenatal care within a few weeks.

After this, her pregnancy was uncomplicated. Although she was 19, Alexandra had always seemed to Helen to be very "young," but she asked good questions, came to every prenatal appointment, and participated in the school-aged pregnancy program. Helen was somewhat skeptical about Alexandra's specific request for natural childbirth and no epidural, but was open to helping her pursue these goals.

Helen came in to the hospital on her day off when she got the call that Alexandra was in labor at term and found her to be actively laboring at 6 cm. Helen was pleased to meet in the labor room Alexandra's two older sisters, both of whom worked as medical assistants in a local medical office. With these sisters' ministrations, Alexandra's labor flourished beautifully, and she proceeded without anesthesia or pain medication to full dilation and delivery of a healthy baby girl, Jasmine, within a few hours. One sister brought out her camera just as the baby was born and followed the baby to the warmer snapping photos, while the other sister held Alexandra's hand during delivery of the placenta. Helen encouraged the maternity nurse to allow an extra family member into the delivery room so that Alexandra's mother and third sister could come celebrate the new arrival. Watching them gather around both Alexandra and Jasmine, Helen began to appreciate Alexandra's role as the "baby sister" who was especially treasured in her family. While examining baby Jasmine, Helen talked with all these family members in the room, commenting on this new daughter's place in a family of strong women. Helen found out that all of Alexandra's sisters had breast-fed at least short term, even though their mother had not. She asked Alexandra's oldest sister to help bring Jasmine back to the new mother and talk to her about the first breastfeeding.

On postpartum rounds on her first day after delivery, Alexandra was breastfeeding well but told the resident working with Helen that she was having a lot of pain in her lower abdomen when she tried to sit up, stand up, or move around at all. Her sister pressed the resident, "What's wrong? I never had this problem after my babies." When the resident examined Alexandra, her uterus was not tender, but she winced with midline pressure over her lower abdomen. The nurse reported that Alexandra had not been out of bed except with help and that she was limping, doubled-over, to the bathroom only with assistance. The resident, who had seen Alexandra first, told Helen that he thought Alexandra's problem was due to not getting out of bed enough postpartum. Helen, knowing Alexandra and the family, doubted this conclusion. She re-evaluated Alexandra with the resident present and saw that even with both sisters helping, Alexandra's discomfort was beyond the usual. On her exam Helen found the pain to be located in the pubic symphysis not in the abdomen and pointed out this difference to the resident. She diagnosed pubic symphysitis and arranged for a physical therapist to see her since Alexandra lived in a third-floor apartment and would need to manage stairs to be discharged. The therapist agreed with the diagnosis and arranged for daily sessions in the hospital for three more days until Alexandra could tolerate stairs with the use of a special girdle and enough pain medication. Alexandra wanted to avoid too much medication while she was breast-feeding but was also frustrated with the long hospital stay and with the continued pain. Helen had to carefully document all of these findings to justify the longer stay to the insurance company.

Alicia

Alicia became pregnant when she was a shy, overweight, stay-at-home 16-year-old, who could articulate little about her vision for her future except that she hoped to be a good mother. She had immigrated from Mexico when she was nine and lived in a small house with her parents, siblings, and various extended family members. She entered prenatal care at the local community health center where the staff enrolled her in a Spanish language prenatal group; she was both the youngest and the only bilingual participant. In the group, 12 women due in the same month received care together in a series of 10 two-hour meetings. Alicia quickly learned how to check and chart her own weight, blood pressure, and urine sugar and protein, and was soon enjoying helping the other women do these tasks. In the group discussions, she learned from the older women about being pregnant and being a parent and did reflective self-assessment exercises that asked her to look seriously at her resources and aspirations. She began to reflect honestly about ways to realize her goal of being a good mother. She had said she could not attend school because of not having her required vaccines; soon after joining the group, she asked for and kept an appointment for the immunizations that could be safely given in pregnancy such as tetanus, polio, influenza, or hepatitis B. She completed the first year of a high school equivalency academic program before delivering a healthy baby girl, Jennifer. She was so inspired by the pregnancy and birth experience that she decided to become a nurse, quickly finishing her high school equivalency degree and enrolling in the associate degree nurses' aide program at the local community college.

By this time her prenatal group had transformed into a well-child care group, in which Alicia continued to be a great support to the others. For instance, she visited with Maria, another young and isolated recent immigrant who was able to overcome a very profound postpartum depression with the group's and Alicia's support. Carefully observing the babies at the group, Alicia was the first to notice subtle motor delays in her own daughter, facilitating an early referral to the tertiary care center and enrollment in weekly multidisciplinary therapeutic interventions. As baby Jennifer grew increasingly skilled and engaged, Alicia blossomed into a very busy, motivated and loving young mother, who consciously tended to both her daughter's and her own development. Alicia played on a soccer team, held a job in a welding shop, and had almost finished with the nursing program. Now a volunteer assistant at the clinic's prenatal care groups, Alicia was considering working at the clinic as a nurses' aide or continuing her education to become a midwife, or a doctor.

Amanda

Amanda was a 28-year-old G3P2 office manager who connected strongly with her primary midwife, Helen. Helen worked part-time doing prenatal and postpartum work including home visits and relied on the coverage system on the nights she was not on call to be able to have time at home with her family. Amanda was a bit disappointed that Helen could not guarantee being at the delivery but liked that Helen was a mother herself. Amanda tried hard to have all her prenatal appointments with Helen, even if it meant that Amanda had to change her own work schedule to be available on the days Helen was in the office. At her 39-week visit, Amanda was having some cramping and requested a cervical exam, which showed her to be 2 cm dilated and partly effaced. Helen predicted that Amanda might go into labor before her next visit, and they joked about how the baby might thus share a birthday with Helen's daughter in two days. Amanda did go into labor the next evening and gave birth to baby Kate on the predicted day; they went home from the hospital the following day, and Helen visited them later that week at home where they shared birthday stories.

Anjana

Anjana was a 32-year-old Tamil-speaking woman from South India who was pregnant with her first child. Though she and her husband Ram, along with both sets of their parents, had immigrated almost two years ago when Ram was offered a long-term job in computer engineering, Anjana had continued to live a largely Indian lifestyle. She cooked and cleaned for her parents and in-laws, did not drive or go out alone, and had few friends outside of family contacts. Because of Ram's job, they had excellent insurance and chose Woman-Centered Community Family Practice because they saw Dr. Usha Rao's name on the list of potential maternity providers, and they hoped she would be able to speak Tamil. As it turned out, Usha spoke only a few words of Tamil as her family came from North India and spoke Hindi, Urdu, and English at home. For Tamil, Usha needed to rely on a telephone interpreter. At each office visit for prenatal care with Usha, Anjana's mother or her mother-in-law accompanied her, but Ram was unable to attend, as he was too busy to take time off from work.

Anjana's pregnancy was relatively uncomplicated, though Usha had difficulty getting her to talk about any specific issues, such as nutrition or plans for breastfeeding. Even with the telephone interpreter, Anjana did not volunteer much information. Her only request, at every visit, was that her blood be tested. Anjana's shyness reminded Usha of the recently immigrated Indians she has met through her family, and she felt distressed that they could not communicate better with each other.

At 36 weeks during a routine prenatal visit Anjana's blood pressure was 152/92. Usha rechecked the BP three times, with the same result. When she asked Anjana about any symptoms – including headache, blurry vision, or abdominal pain – Anjana reported none. Usha explained that increased blood pressure late in pregnancy might be a sign of pre-eclampsia and needed to be watched carefully. She recommended blood work, a 24-hour urine collection, and a return visit in three or four days for a recheck of her BP. To be certain that Anjana understood, Usha asked the telephone interpreter to have Anjana to repeat back the instructions in Tamil to the interpreter. Anjana stayed in the waiting room until results of her stat blood work, which were all normal, were complete. Usha talked Anjana's care over with Greg, the obstetrician consultant, who thought her plan was appropriate. But Usha continued to worry and asked her parents on the phone that night if they would have done anything differently.

Forty-eight hours later, when Usha checked the lab tests, the 24-hour urine results were not yet ready. When she tried to contact Anjana on the phone to follow-up, an older man who spoke no English answered. The phone number given for Anjana's husband at work had also been changed. Usha sent the local visiting nurse association to the home, but their nurse found no one at home. Three days later, Usha received a phone call from University Hospital in the city 50 miles away letting her know that Anjana had presented to the Emergency Room with a severe headache earlier that day, after being taken there by ambulance from a suburban shopping mall. After waiting three hours to be seen, Anjana was transferred to the labor suite.

There, while the nurse struggled with Anjana to get an IV started, she had an eclamptic seizure. The nurse reached for the emergency button on the wall to notify the "crash" team for delivery, and tried to keep Anjana from getting hurt. When the obstetric and neonatal teams arrived, the nurse was already moving Anjana, still seizing, to the operating room. The attending obstetrician ordered magnesium sulfate and had the resident start to scrub but waited to see what effect the medication had. When the fetal heart tracing continued to show prolonged bradycardia, the doctor opted to begin an emergency cesarean. Since she was unable to get consent from Anjana, she asked the nurse to attempt to contact her husband while the surgery began. Before Anjana's husband arrived at the hospital, and with no consent obtained, Anjana underwent surgery, which fortunately went smoothly.

Ann

Ann was a 26-year-old woman married for a year and wanting to get pregnant. However, she developed perplexing symptoms of joint pains, facial rashes and fatigue, and eventually after multiple medical visits and tests was diagnosed with lupus, with kidney complications. As she and her husband Joe struggled with adjusting to this chronic illness, they wondered about their plans for pregnancy and parenting. The nephrologist was worried about how active her disease seemed to be and recommended that before conceiving she meet with a perinatologist in consultation to discuss the risks in pregnancy and the potential fetal risks of her various medications. Ann herself felt guilty that she could not be the wife and mother that Joe had hoped for, and became quite depressed; their primary care internist recommended both individual and couples' counseling with Joe to address the strain on their marriage that such issues caused. When Ann's symptoms finally abated on treatment, she felt strong enough to cope with parenting, but she was worried about having to stop her medication because of fetal risk while trying to get pregnant. She had also heard about a significant rate of miscarriage and fetal demise during pregnancy, and a risk of her disease worsening postpartum. She and Joe decided not to risk pregnancy and began considering their adoption choices.

Beverly

Beverly was a 31-year-old African-American biochemist at a research lab in a pharmaceutical company. Her husband, Carleton, was a successful investment broker. They postponed their pregnancy until Beverly had finished her postdoctoral training and had secured a high-level research position in a competitive lab. They prepared for the baby by attending childbirth classes, decorating the nursery, and reading books on parenting. Both sets of grandparents lived within a day's drive, and Beverly's mother planned to stay with her for a few weeks after the birth. Although both Beverly and Carleton worked long hours, Beverly planned to cut back in the lab for her first six months after the baby's birth.

Beverly decided to get her obstetrical care at Dr. Diamond's small practice at the

University Hospital in the city. Tall and thin, Beverly gained exactly 25 pounds with the pregnancy and hoped to regain her figure quickly postpartum. Her pregnancy was uncomplicated except for a few elevated blood pressures in the last few days before she went into labor, but her tests did not suggest significant pre-eclampsia.

Beverly went into labor after a 24-hour prodrome that allowed her mother plenty of time to arrive to support her in labor. She had planned to try for an unmedicated childbirth, and her mother strongly supported her in this goal. Carleton was nervous about Beverly's health and did not want her to suffer, but felt that the choices about pain control were up to Beverly. He was also somewhat frightened by the hospital environment, but felt that all would be under control in the tertiary care hospital attached to the medical school.

Beverly's labor was difficult. After remaining at 7 cm for several hours, she had an IUPC inserted, and oxytocin begun. At this point, exhausted and discouraged, she asked Dr. Diamond and the nurse Laura for an epidural. She proceeded slowly to full dilation, but did not feel an urge to push; as the head was descending slowly, Dr. Diamond suggested that she rest to allow more descent before she began pushing. After two hours, she felt the contractions more strongly and wanted to push. Carleton and the nurse worked with her in the different positions that she could move into with the dense epidural, and finally after two hours, the baby's head began to crown. Dr. Diamond, not expecting any issue with the delivery without any of the usual risk factors for shoulder dystocia, noticed that this penultimate stage seemed to take longer than usual and wanted to alert the nurse to the possibility of dystocia, but also did not want to alarm Beverly or her husband as she was working so hard to finish pushing.

"C'mon, Beverly, the head is almost out, that's it!" he said as the baby's nose and mouth finally emerged but then retracted slightly, making it hard for him to assess for a nuchal cord or suction the baby's mouth. "Okay, take a breather and let's get your legs back as far as you can. Tell me when you're ready to push again."

Beverly took a sip of water and then nodded and gasped, "Okay, let's do this finally!" Dr. Diamond attempted gentle traction on the baby's head but was not able to move the anterior shoulder. As he adjusted his hands to try alternate maneuvers for the shoulders, he looked Beverly in the eye and urged her, "Okay, Beverly, let's work together. I need you to help make more room for your baby. Push again while I do this. Carleton, hold her leg even further back – think about trying to get your heels to your ears, and Laura will push down right here on your pubic area. We also need to get some others in here to help."

Beverly kept pushing with Carleton, looking on worriedly, moving her legs back and urging her on. Dr. Diamond still did not feel the shoulders budge, and he looked back directly at Beverly. "Okay, you're doing great. I need to put my hand in here now and may need to do a few other things that may be uncomfortable, but we need to get the baby out. Bear with me, and keep working with me." Another obstetrician and the perinatal team arrived to help as finally, after repeating the Woods' maneuver, with the nurse on a stool applying suprapubic pressure, Dr. Diamond was at last able to extract the posterior arm. "Here he is, great work!" he told Beverly as baby

Jackson emerged at last, limp and not yet crying. While Dr. Diamond clamped the umbilical cord and offered the scissors to Carleton to cut it, he added quickly, "I can feel that he's got a solid heartbeat, but needs some help to breathe. Take a look while I let our newborn team take over."

The pediatric team was in the delivery room for the birth and received the baby who responded quickly to stimulation and blow-by oxygen. But when Dr. Diamond peeked in between the nursery staff to see the baby in the warmer, he recognized the brachial palsy immediately. While he felt relieved that the baby was finally out, he also noted in himself the usual complex feelings that come with a complication: guilt mixed with anxiety – the knowledge that there would need to be long discussions with this couple and the grandparents about the palsy. He said softly to the neonatal team, "Let me tell them about the arm."

Taking a deep breath, Dr. Diamond walked over to Beverly, and looked at Carleton and Beverly together, and began, "Your baby is doing fine – he's breathing well, has lots of oxygen, his heart sounds good. But there is a problem – he's not moving his arm. We see this sometimes after a hard delivery when the nerve to the arm gets stretched as we get the baby out. I'll bring him over in a minute so you can hold him. He's fine otherwise."

"What does this mean? Is he going to be paralyzed?" shot out Carleton, fearing the worst.

"To be honest, we don't know yet whether this problem with the arm will last – sometimes the nerve recovers fully and sometimes it doesn't. The injury is called a brachial nerve palsy. The whole arm is not paralyzed, but with this palsy the hand and arm can't do some movements controlled by that nerve."

"Is he going to be all right?" asked the grandmother.

"Overall, the baby is fine, but we can't say about the arm yet," Dr. Diamond repeated. "Here, let me show you." By this time the nursery staff had begun to leave, and Dr. Diamond picked up baby Jackson in some blankets and brought him over to Beverly and Carleton. He carefully pointed out the baby's good color and tone, and then showed how the baby did not move his right arm.

Everyone looked frightened, and Dr. Diamond realized that he had perhaps jumped too far ahead. "You are all tired and Beverly must be exhausted. Let's take a little time to hold Jackson and feed him and wonder at him, and we can talk about the arm later. Let's just welcome him for now." The nurse stepped in and helped Beverly position him next to her on the bed, pointing out all his newborn features and encouraging them to look at his hair and toes and eyes. Gradually, the atmosphere in the room relaxed as the nurses completed their postpartum routine. Dr. Diamond stepped out of the room, pointedly telling the nurse that he would be back after completing his notes.

After Beverly had a chance to nurse the baby, she slept awhile, and then remembered about Jackson's arm. She felt anxious about it but just wanted to have a chance to be with the baby and hold him and love him, and did not want to think about it all the time. She trusted Dr. Diamond, and did not think he was to blame. But she also knew that her mother, who could be militant about any adverse event, might start talking about whose fault it was. Beverly really did not want "to go there."

During the subsequent 48 hours, Dr. Diamond reviewed over and over in his mind how the labor had gone and what had happened during the delivery. He knew that the family was wondering about whether he should have done a cesarean section. Even though he felt anxious about bringing it up, he decided to address it directly when he came to see her for discharge on the second postpartum day. Carleton was there helping prepare for going home.

After his usual postpartum care discussion and exam, Dr. Diamond added, "I would like to talk to you now about what happened with the delivery. I think now is a good time if you are okay with that, since you both here." Beverly and Carleton nodded their assent.

Dr. Diamond proceeded to pull up a chair and began, "I am really sorry about Jackson's arm. I am guessing that you both may be wondering whether we should have done a cesarean section to get Jackson out . . ." He paused, and Carleton admitted that he had been thinking about that.

Dr. Diamond continued, "Let me share with you my thinking about this. We do cesareans usually when the baby shows sign of distress, or when the baby won't come out. In Beverly's situation, although the labor was progressing slowly, we had no advance warning that there would be a problem with the birth – the baby was not especially big, and Beverly has normal bone size."

He paused again, and Beverly, holding Jackson in her arms, nodded again. Dr. Diamond went on, "Could we have done a cesarean? Sure, but what would I have been telling you then? That maybe the baby wouldn't fit? That there's a chance of a complication? All that would have been true, but I couldn't know it for sure. This is one of the big uncertainties. Sometimes we can't know until the birth itself. We did what we thought best at the time."

He waited, watching their faces, and then went on, "Think about it for a while. I know it's hard that your baby isn't perfectly normal. I know that you or your family may want to blame someone. I take full responsibility for allowing you to have a vaginal delivery, and this injury is a complication of that delivery. I still hope it will completely resolve, but there is no way to know in advance. You will be the first to know. In the meantime, most parents want the babies to be seen by a pediatric neurologist, but to be honest there is nothing to be done right now to change how it will come out. . . . I am so sorry about this complication – I know it must be very hard for you."

Three months later Jackson was still not moving his right arm. While Beverly's mother still thought that the doctor should have performed a cesarean and prevented the nerve injury to his arm, Beverly and Carleton were more ambivalent and felt that although they did not understand the risks in advance of an injury from a vaginal delivery, they were disinclined to begin a lawsuit against Dr. Diamond or the hospital. They had heard about some surgery to move a muscle in the arm to enable the baby to move the hand and arm more normally, and they wanted to look into it when Jackson was a bit older. Beverly was fond of telling Carleton, who loved tennis, that Jackson could still be a champion left-handed tennis player.

Chantel

Chantel was a 21-year-old African-American woman arrested on a parole violation when police raided a house where she was present during a drug deal. They took her initially to a local jail facility where her urine tested positive for pregnancy, as well as opiates and cocaine. Because of the positive pregnancy test, the jail staff transferred her to the emergency room for evaluation of possible withdrawal symptoms. Later they sent her to the regional correctional facility where on-site medical staff could continue observation for drug withdrawal, initiate methadone maintenance therapy and begin prenatal care.

When interviewed by a nurse on admission to the prison infirmary, Chantel gave a history of significant substance abuse dating back to her early teenage years. She had begun to smoke both cigarettes and marijuana at age 13, and then progressed to using cocaine within a few years. Although she did not disclose more of her life history initially, Chantel herself felt that her earliest drug use began in response to her feelings of loss and depression after her mother died of a sudden cardiac event when she was 12. Since her father was uninvolved with the family, Chantel was separated from her two younger brothers and went to live with an aunt who was the single mother of her two older cousins. Her aunt tried hard to raise all three girls "right" but worked two jobs and was not around the house much; the two older cousins were already experimenting with drugs and made them available to Chantel at that time. Chantel's aunt had a boyfriend who was an unemployed alcoholic who made frequent attempts to fondle Chantel when he was intoxicated. He would threaten that if she told her aunt about this, he would personally see to it that she was thrown out of the house and put in foster care.

One of Chantel's older cousins introduced her to Jason, 18, who initially seemed genuinely interested in Chantel and treated her with kindness and respect. Anxious to get away from her aunt's house whenever possible, Chantel spent more and more time with Jason and began to have sex with him. Within three months she was pregnant. When Jason found out about the pregnancy, he stopped calling or coming to see her. Certain that Jason would return once she had the baby, Chantel decided to continue the pregnancy. She gave birth to a healthy term baby boy with one of her cousins and her aunt present as labor support. Because of her age of 14, and the fact that she tested positive for marijuana at delivery, the child protection agency became involved with the baby's disposition in the hospital. After interviewing her aunt, who said that she would not be able to closely supervise Chantel's parenting, the social worker from child protective services placed the infant in temporary foster care and told Chantel that she might be able to have the infant back if she either entered a residential teen parenting program or entered foster care herself with the baby. Uncertain of what these options meant, Chantel initially refused to do either. After leaving the hospital without her son, Chantel quickly sank into a profound postpartum depression, but got no formal evaluation or treatment.

Chantel continued to smoke marijuana and began experimenting with cocaine on the advice of one of her cousin's friends who told her it would help her stop crying and sleeping so much. She did not follow through on the suggested treatment plans, and was not able to gain custody of her son. During this time, Chantel's cocaine use escalated even further, evolving into a major crack addiction. She began to trade sex for drugs in order to support her crack habit, and was thrown out of her aunt's house after she stole money from her. She quickly got pregnant again, this time without knowing who the baby's father was. At 25 weeks gestation she went to the hospital for abdominal pain. She underwent an emergency cesarean delivery for placental abruption of another baby who died at two days of age of complications of prematurity. Chantel had no clear recollection of the events surrounding the birth of this second son, except remembering that the hospital staff treated her with disdain and disapproval. She received the clear message from them that because of her crack use, she had killed her baby. The staff did not encourage her to see or hold the baby and by their actions implied that she did not deserve any of the care and support that would usually be offered to a mother who experienced the loss of a baby. Chantel never found out what happened to his remains. After her discharge from the hospital, Chantel intentionally overdosed on the narcotic given to her for post-operative pain leading to admission on the psychiatric floor. When the psychiatric team thought she was stable, they sent her to a publicly funded residential program for "troubled" teens.

Feeling overwhelmed by the enormity of her losses over the preceding years, Chantel was unable to engage in either substance abuse or mental health treatment offered at the residential teen program. She ran away, and spent the next several years using drugs and prostituting, acquiring a serious heroin habit in addition to her ongoing cocaine addiction. She had two pregnancy terminations during those years, feeling that she would be unable to bear the loss of another baby. The police arrested her for prostitution at age 20 and eventually paroled her to a substance abuse treatment program where she received methadone briefly before returning to the streets. Since remaining in the program and drug-free for six months was a condition of her parole, her second arrest became inevitable.

Chantel was able to disclose her personal history to a supportive obstetrical nurse practitioner, Amy, in the state correctional facility where she stayed for the rest of her pregnancy. Initially, she was unable even to decide whether she wanted to continue the pregnancy. She felt overwhelmed by her past life issues, complicated by apprehension, shame and guilt over being in prison again. Amy was able to listen to Chantel's fears of being unable to stay drug-free during the pregnancy and of losing another baby. She worried that the state child protection agency would inevitably take this baby, too, and that even if she gained custody of the baby, her depression would be too profound to parent. Chantel knew that under stress, and given the opportunity, she would often choose to use drugs in an attempt to buffer her feelings of sadness and isolation from her missing family and children. Amy helped Chantel clarify her feelings about the pregnancy. Despite all her concerns, Chantel was finally able to say that she really wanted to keep the pregnancy, deliver her baby, and keep her baby and parent her child when she was released.

Once Chantel had decided to continue her pregnancy, Amy did a full obstetrical intake, in conjunction with the supervising physicians. They treated a newly diagnosed chlamydia infection and arranged a colposcopy for an abnormal Papanicolaou (Pap) smear. Chantel found out that she had a hepatitis C infection, a new diagnosis for her, but she was relieved that her HIV test was negative. After adjustment of her methadone dose, her withdrawal symptoms resolved. Concern about her significant mental health and substance abuse histories led her obstetrical providers to refer Chantel to the mental health team on site who assigned her a therapist and planned a psychiatric evaluation. Chantel began to work with the social worker who looked for a residential substance abuse treatment program where Chantel could go after her release, hopefully with the baby as well.

Chantel tried to engage with the team members working on her behalf, but admitted to feeling irritable and impatient with her life at the correctional facility. She got in trouble for arguing with some of the other inmates and correctional officers; such behavior threatened to prevent her release from prison to another less restrictive setting.

Chantel's mental health therapist, Rhonda, and Amy continued to work closely with Chantel around her lashing out at other inmates and officers. They empathized with her about how hard it was to be pregnant and incarcerated, and worked with her to get some items to increase her comfort at night and help her sleep. As it was unclear whether Chantel would be able to go to a residential substance abuse treatment program prior to delivery, Amy reviewed what would happen if Chantel delivered her baby while incarcerated. The prison social worker discussed the importance of self-control and of conforming to the rules of the correctional facility so that potential treatment programs would view her favorably. Chantel still expressed much predictable frustration with her situation, but with ongoing encouragement was able to avoid disciplinary action during her imprisonment.

Chantel had difficulty joining into group sessions on addiction, as she felt self-conscious about her drug use in pregnancy and current methadone maintenance. When some other inmates criticized her for being on methadone, she felt accused of making her baby into an "addict." Rhonda, her mental health therapist, encouraged her to continue attending these sessions, reminding her that abstaining from illicit drugs and protecting her fetus from opiate withdrawal by taking methadone were brave actions that should make her proud. Chantel was still shy about defending herself in the group setting, but did begin to write in a journal about her struggle to stay sane in prison, which she was able to share during individual counseling sessions. A portion of the journal was written as a letter to her unborn child, expressing Chantel's fervent hopes for her baby's health and strong desire to stay with her baby after delivery.

Chantel went to court in the third trimester of her pregnancy where the judge sentenced her to one year in prison. He left open the possibility of transfer to a supervised residential substance abuse treatment program. He did not offer parole as an option, due to her prior parole violation. If she left an assigned treatment program, she would be re-incarcerated immediately for the duration of her sentence. The social worker continued to look for open programs, but many hesitated because of Chantel's history of leaving a previous residential program. One program that did accept Chantel did not have a bed immediately available and did not know if one would open up prior to her delivery. Chantel did not have any family members or friends who were willing to provide temporary custody for the baby. She began to panic over the possibility that she would have to place her infant in foster care after delivery.

Despite attending weekly psychotherapy visits, Chantel's depression began to worsen to the point that she was not sleeping or eating regularly, and she struggled to participate in the required group sessions on her unit. Amy called a multidisciplinary meeting of the mental health and social work staff working with Chantel. The team recommended antidepressant medication. Although she had previously declined medication because of fears of its effects on the baby, Chantel now accepted this option. Her psychotherapist also worked more intensively with Chantel about what it would mean to have to give up another infant, at least temporarily. After three weeks on medication, Chantel's mood stabilized. Although she still worried about the disposition of her baby after delivery, she managed to focus on an interim plan.

A discussion was undertaken to determine whether Chantel wanted to have a trial of labor after cesarean section or an elective repeat cesarean section, and she chose to try to have a normal delivery. She went into spontaneous labor at 39 weeks' gestation, and was transported to the University Hospital by guards. The guards stayed right outside her labor room. The obstetrical residents, none of whom she had ever met before, and whose names she never learned, attended her labor. She was not restrained in labor, but could not have any family or friends present. She had an uncomplicated vaginal birth after cesarean (VBAC) delivery of a normal healthy baby girl, and was discharged back to prison 48 hours after delivery.

After several weeks in the hospital for neonatal opiate withdrawal, Chantel's baby daughter, Iris, went to foster care while Chantel remained incarcerated. Within three months, Chantel was able to transition to an available bed at a residential treatment program. The child protection services agency placed Iris in Chantel's physical custody there, still under the agency's legal supervision, but in her mother's care for as long as Chantel met the requirements of her substance abuse treatment plan. The program was comprehensive in its approach, recognizing that training for other life skills was essential in reducing the rate of repeat offenders, so Chantel was also able to enroll in a high school completion class and to begin to attend a series of lectures on parenting.

Delia

Delia was a 25-year-old G4P3 who had been on methadone since the birth of her last child. Delia's first stepfather repeatedly fondled Delia from age 8 to 12, culminating in a rape at the time of her first period. Delia never revealed the abuse because her stepfather told Delia he would kill her mother if she disclosed. Delia believed him because he kept a loaded gun at the bedside. After the rape, Delia used an excuse of proximity to school to go live with her grandmother. Shortly after the sexual assault her stepfather was arrested and jailed for killing a pedestrian while driving intoxicated.

During his incarceration, Delia confided the abuse to her mother, who wanted Delia to come home, but also hoped that her husband would return once released from prison. Delia chose to stay with her grandmother; ultimately her mother broke off the relationship with her stepfather and soon started a relationship with a very strict but non-abusive new partner.

Delia returned home at 14, but was already dating and having sex with boys in her school. Her first boyfriend, Junior, who was 17, was the father of her first child. He initiated Delia into marijuana use, and later into cocaine. Delia used these two substances alternatively to calm her down and give her pep. She enjoyed Junior's attention and compliments and for once in her life felt special. Junior was so important in her life that Delia got a tattoo of his name on her neck. Her mother and new stepfather were furious when they saw the tattoo and began limiting her freedom. Delia retaliated by staying out all night. She began associating with heavy drug users and started using heroin on an intermittent basis. Within a month of her first use, she was not only hooked but pregnant.

Junior was angry about the pregnancy, and began assaulting her and withholding drugs. When Delia told her parents about the pregnancy, they threw her out, saying that if she wanted help, she should get it from Junior. Because of shame and fear of what they would do to her, she did not tell them about the drug use or the physical abuse. With the help of her friend Angela, she made an appointment for prenatal care at the local hospital, and put on a "good girl" face for most of her appointments. Although they asked her about physical abuse and drug use at the first visit, she denied these, and no one asked her again after the intake. Delia was only able to break off with Junior by attaching herself to an older boyfriend who used and pushed drugs. He sometimes used Delia to move drugs or forced her to have sex with others as part of drug deals.

Delia went to the hospital in labor accompanied by Angela, her long-term and steadfast teenage friend, who was also dealing with a substance use disorder. The hospital staff refused to allow Angela to support Delia during labor because she was not family. When Delia complained of ongoing severe pain even after a shot of Demerol, one nurse suggested she was drug-seeking and would not call the on-call physician for further orders. The delivery was uneventful except that the baby girl was admitted to the neonatal intensive care unit for initial monitoring due to the substance use. During labor Delia tested positive for marijuana, cocaine, and heroin, mandating the involvement of social services. Delia did not have a chance to hold her daughter, whom she named Angelica. Once the baby was stabilized in the NICU, child protective services took Angelica into custody. The hospital staff did little to ease Delia's sense of loss. No one inquired if Delia was safe on her discharge from the hospital.

Delia was soon back on the streets staying with friends or living in derelict buildings and within 10 months was pregnant again. She made attempts to change her life and even attended an outpatient rehabilitation center, but found that men dominated the meetings. She felt too intimidated to speak up. She could not stay clean. During this second pregnancy, Delia spent four months in the regional detention center for shoplifting. While in prison, she received methadone treatment, but was also able to "score" cocaine and marijuana through friends. This pregnancy ended with her second child, another girl, named Janine Ivette, also taken into custody because of her chaotic lifestyle and ongoing addiction to heroin. She had no ongoing contact with the two girls and received no information about their well-being or whereabouts.

After the second pregnancy, motivated by support from Angela and other non-using friends, Delia went through a 28-day inpatient rehabilitation program and successfully initiated methadone maintenance therapy. Delia made a strong connection with the social worker in the program and revealed to her the details of her past history of victimization during childhood as well as during adolescence.

Delia's revelation to the social worker of her childhood sexual abuse facilitated a deeper connection than she had previously ever made with a clinician, and she was able to voice her anger, without relapsing. She found a part-time job as a cashier at a grocery store and entered into a stable relationship with a new partner, Paco, a welder. Paco, also a former drug user, had been on methadone for the last two years. They met at Narcotics Anonymous meetings and tried to support each other in staying clean. During Delia's third pregnancy and delivery, Paco, who was very involved as a new father, supported her emotionally and financially. His presence at prenatal appointments and during labor impressed the staff who perceived Delia differently, and provided more compassionate care. In the course of her prenatal care Delia talked with her provider about getting an intrauterine device placed postpartum since she did not want any more children in the near future. She was planning on doing this after her postpartum visit, but she never made it back to the appointment.

Under close surveillance by child protective services, she and Paco were allowed to take home her third baby, Jeromey. They both smoked cigarettes, but tried to do so outside their apartment as part of the plan to make their home safe for Jeromey. Delia's mother and stepfather became supportive grandparents, babysitting when Delia was at work. Staying drug-free was a requirement for her keeping custody of Jeromey. Child protective services kept her case open on a long term basis sending in a caseworker biweekly, making Delia feel very anxious. She continued to obtain methadone from the local drug treatment program, and was stable for almost one year, thus allowing her to "carry" methadone home so she only needed to attend the pharmacy three times a week. This arrangement made Delia happy.

A year later Delia found out that she was pregnant with her fourth child. Delia had seen multiple providers at the health center over the years and did not have a good connection with anyone except for one of the nurses, Maureen, whom she would call for a variety of needs – to make an appointment, get a letter for housing, or when she or Jeromey had an acute illness. At visits, Jeromey appeared clean and well-fed and much attached to his mother. Delia knew she did not want to get pregnant, but contraception and getting an IUD placed had never seemed to be a priority during her visits. When Delia discovered she was pregnant again, Maureen was the first person she told. Maureen suggested Delia talk to one of the providers about her options with this pregnancy. Delia was not sure she wanted another child. However, after meeting with Dr. Adelle Epps and talking about having an abortion or having another child, Delia decided to continue with the pregnancy.

Maureen then arranged for Delia to have her prenatal intake visit at the health center with the obstetrical nurse practitioner, Harmony Lott. Harmony's unassuming and welcoming attitude helped Delia feel more connected to the prenatal program. Delia denied current drug use at her intake prenatal visit and agreed to a routine urine toxicology screen at that appointment. The urine drug screen was positive for marijuana. Discussing this result, Harmony and Maureen reviewed Delia's multiple needs and wondered whether she would be better served by the Perinatal Team specializing in problematic substance use in pregnancy at the hospital across town. Delia was averse to leaving the safety of the clinic and the support from Maureen and went to the Perinatal Team with reluctance.

When she arrived at the new clinic, the office staff greeted Delia warmly. They asked her to complete a short questionnaire in the waiting room. The first visit included a general introduction to the services available and an opportunity to meet some of the providers. The staff asked questions in a sensitive manner, and Delia was relieved that she had not been "interrogated." A second appointment was scheduled for the following week. At this visit the intake nurse completed a comprehensive assessment and raised the issue of her positive urine screen for marijuana. Delia admitted to smoking a few joints with Paco and, after being counseled about the benefits of reducing or abstaining from drug use, she decided to stop using altogether. She returned for a visit two weeks later and admitted that she slipped and shared a joint with Paco on one occasion. The nurse treated her admission respectfully and praised her for cutting down on her drug use. Delia left with increased resolve to stop her use altogether.

Evelyn

Evelyn was a 29-year-old G2P1 who had a young toddler at home and also worked as a night shift nurses' aide in order to supplement her husband Ed's income as a taxi driver. They juggled childcare and jobs, so that it was easiest for her to have early morning appointments for prenatal care on her way home from her night work while Ed was at home with their daughter before leaving for his day job.

During her pregnancy, Evelyn was overwhelmed by her schedule. She was sleeping poorly during the day while her toddler, Marilyn, was with her mother. Ed was working longer hours to keep up with their financial needs. They were arguing about childcare and household chores. Evelyn found herself crying easily and being easily distracted, forgetting what tasks she had each day; she was feeling guilty that the baby would be affected by her stress and that she was not enjoying her pregnancy but rather dreading having to juggle even more duties with a newborn at home. At her 20-week visit her weight was down a few pounds, and she looked noticeably tired; when Dr. Rosen mentioned this, Evelyn burst into tears, saying, "I'm really having a hard time."

Dr. Rosen, pausing, offered her tissues and gently touched her arm in sympathy. "I'm really glad you're able to let me know this. You're brave to share this. Let's talk through a few other possible symptoms." He asked about Evelyn's sleep patterns and used a depression screening tool that took about five minutes to complete. Evelyn revealed that in her late teens she was in treatment for major depression, and her mother had also been treated for anxiety and depression. Dr. Rosen commented, "It's really helpful that you can make a connection between depression in your family and in your teenage years with the way you feel now. I'm impressed by how well you've done since then and the strengths that you have had along the way." He asked if there might be any way for Evelyn and her extended family to consider additional help so that Evelyn could get a bit more rest. They discussed the options of cutting back her work hours and considering some brief counseling, as well as the possibility of medication. Evelyn did not want to take anything that might hurt the baby, but was willing to try some counseling if the scheduling worked around her childcare, work, and sleep issues. Dr. Rosen congratulated her, "It's great that you're being so thoughtful about your options. I can see that you already know that treatment for you is going to be helpful for your baby in the long run, too."

Evelyn began weekly visits with a social worker whose office was near her house. She arranged for her mother to take her toddler one afternoon a week so that she could sleep a bit longer on that day. Her husband continued to work long shifts but asked his sister to help out with one meal a week. Evelyn's mood stabilized, and by 26 weeks she had fewer depressive symptoms and was starting to look forward to the baby's arrival and her maternity leave, which she planned to start with the baby's birth, working up until her due date.

The night after her 27-week mark, however, Evelyn was at work and noticed a gush of fluid out of her vagina. She began feeling nauseated and dizzy. She called Dr. Rosen's answering service and was told to come to the hospital. Evaluation there revealed that she had in fact ruptured membranes but did not appear to be dilated or contracting yet. Dr. Rosen and the perinatologists recommended hospitalization for medical treatment to prevent infection, promote fetal lung maturity, and to attempt to delay such a preterm delivery. For the next 10 days, Evelyn remained in the hospital at bedrest. Ed brought Marilyn to visit after work, and then left her with Evelyn's mother overnight. Evelyn worried about how they were coping and about what would happen to her job. She also worried about the baby's prematurity and was willing to do whatever the doctors said might help, even though she was uncomfortable lying in bed for a long time. During the daily testing with the fetal monitor, she found it reassuring to hear the baby's healthy heartbeat and hear from the doctors that all seemed well for now.

After 10 days of hospitalization at bedrest, Evelyn awoke late one night needing to go to the bathroom and noticed both further leaking of fluid and uterine cramping. She rang for her nurse and went into the bathroom, where she felt a particularly strong cramp and an odd sensation in her vagina. As the nurse came in, they both realized suddenly that the umbilical cord was coming out of the vagina. The nurse urged, "Evelyn, you need to lie right down while I put the head of the bed way down and call the doctors. This is an emergency. Your job is to take slow deep breaths of this oxygen so your baby gets as much as possible." Evelyn felt very scared but tried to do what the nurse said as the on-call obstetrical team rushed into the room.

The chief obstetrician saw the cord and came immediately to the head of the bed to talk to Evelyn. "The umbilical cord is coming out first. It has a good pulse, which is good. You are going to need an emergency cesarean right now. Until we get you in the operating room, you need to be upside down like this and one of us needs to put a hand in to hold the baby's head off the cord to keep it from being squeezed. It all feels weird, but stay with us."

Several other nurses and doctors were readying her hospital bed for moving quickly to the operating area, so Evelyn behind the oxygen mask just nodded, wide-eyed and asked if someone could call Ed to alert him. As they pushed her bed down the hall, the chief doctor was asking Evelyn to sign the surgical consent form, saying, "I apologize in advance that we'll have to put you to sleep for this surgery. That's safest for the baby." The doctor who was holding the cord kept Evelyn posted, "Your baby has a nice strong heart rate. You're doing a great job breathing oxygen for the baby."

Once in the operating room, Evelyn felt overwhelmed by all the rush but then remembered nothing after taking some more deep breaths until she awoke in the recovery room with Ed at her side, telling her about their 1100 gram son, David. The obstetrician came in to tell her, "You did such a great job working with us in all the crazy rush. The surgery happened as fast and as well as we could have hoped for. David was vigorous at first, breathing well at first on his own but then getting a bit tired as we expect for a baby his size." Evelyn, exhausted and astonished by the emergency cesarean and anxious about David's condition, held Ed's hand tightly and nodded wordlessly.

Although David had done well at first given the emergent nature of his delivery, breathing spontaneously, he soon developed respiratory distress and needed intubation so was already in the intensive care nursery. Evelyn, in pain from her unexpected surgery, was too tired and uncomfortable to visit David or to start pumping her milk in the first day.

Once she had recovered enough to be discharged herself, Evelyn tried to spend as much time as possible at the hospital with David, continuing to rely on her mother to help with Marilyn. At first when he was still on the ventilator she was nervous about all the machinery and about touching him, and fearful that he might die. The day nurses, while kind and obviously competent, were busy, and Evelyn was shy about interrupting their work or the doctors on rounds to ask for more information. She still felt tired and sore with walking or climbing any stairs, and she wondered how she would ever feel capable of caring for David when he got well enough to come home. She preferred visiting in the evenings when she did not have to worry so much about Marilyn and when she felt more included in David's moment-to-moment care by the nurses.

In the course of juggling her toddler's needs, her return to work, and her husband's work schedule, Evelyn's depression symptoms flared again. She continued to have frequent crying spells, including tears at Dr. Rosen's office for her postpartum check-up.

Farhiyo

Farhiyo was a 25-year-old Muslim Somali woman who fled her war-torn homeland at the age of 15. She spent the next six years in Pakistan. Since her mother died in childbirth and her father was killed in the war, Farhiyo functioned as the surrogate parent for her four younger brothers, keeping house and cooking meals for them and making sure the youngest had what he needed for school. When she first met Dr. Adelle Epps, Farhiyo was working as a certified nursing assistant and going to school to become a registered nurse.

During Farhiyo's first pelvic examination, Dr. Epps noted the evidence of prior genital mutilation – a small stump where her clitoris should have been and a small vaginal introitus indicating that the inner labia had been sewn together. Building on the trust already in the relationship, Dr. Epps asked Farhiyo if she could tell her more about her experience of genital mutilation. Farhiyo said she had been about eight years old at the time, and had only few memories of the event. When Dr. Epps asked about current symptoms, Farhiyo said that she did not now feel pain and that she did have sexual sensations in the area. Still, she was certain that she would not want any future daughter to go through this procedure, but she worried about the consequences. Would a daughter be able to find a suitable Somali husband if she was not properly cleansed and "made" into a true Somali woman?

Over time, Farhiyo began to address her own sexuality. She asked Dr. Epps for articles on FGM and wrote a paper on it for a class in nursing school. Despite knowing that her family would disapprove, she became sexually active with a non-Muslim man. Dr. Epps viewed her as a remarkably reflective young woman and was not surprised when Farhiyo told her that she wished she "had the bravery" to confront her family and culture. When Dr. Epps asked her if she would like more support to work through these conflicts, Farhiyo readily agreed. Dr. Epps referred her to a supportive therapist and continued to see her regularly.

Felicity

Felicity was a 20-year-old woman in her next-to-last year at a vocational high school when she became pregnant with her third child. She had grown up in a home with her mother, four siblings – all of whom had different fathers – and the father of her youngest sister, whom her mother had recently married. Her grandmother, mother, aunts, and two sisters all became pregnant as teenagers. Felicity's first pregnancy occurred at age 16 with Tony, her first serious boyfriend. She had hoped to have a lasting relationship with him and named the baby after him. However, Tony left Felicity during her pregnancy for another girlfriend, also pregnant, and had since remained only peripherally involved in parenting his namesake via court-mandated assistance. Since that first pregnancy, Felicity lived in turn with her mother, aunt, two friends, and most recently with her boyfriend Rafael, the father of her daughter and the third child she was now expecting. During this most recent pregnancy, Felicity transferred from vocational high school to the school-age mothers program where she continued in the same grade. School attendance was quite difficult for her, not only due to demands of pregnancy care and maternity absences, but also due to her other chronic medical conditions (low-back pain exacerbated by obesity, depression and anxiety, and almost-daily migraine headaches). Despite difficulties with attendance, Felicity maintained the goal of high school graduation. Though in the short term she planned to focus on parenting, she occasionally spoke of resuming vocational training to become a beautician. She now had stable housing with Rafael and the three children. Help with childcare came mostly from Felicity's mother and older sister (herself with four children). Rafael, though present, struggled with his own chronic medical issues; within the relationship, Felicity took the majority of the responsibility for parenting as well as caretaking for Rafael.

Felicity began her third pregnancy more than 50 pounds heavier than her postpartum weight after the birth of her second child. Always heavy, she attributed this most recent weight gain to the use of hormonal contraception. However, she also admitted eating fast food several times a week with the children, doing no exercise apart from walking, and snacking late at night. Without a car she found it difficult to get from the public housing project to a supermarket where she might buy cheaper fresh fruits and vegetables than were available at the corner store. Her mother, grandmother, and sisters were also all heavy.

Felicity disliked how the staff at the community health center insisted on her getting weighed in the hall. She felt criticized by the medical staff for her weight and found the word *obese* very demeaning. At her initial nurse visit for this pregnancy, the nurse reminded her that "obese women" have more risk of cesarean section and other complications. Felicity felt that this harping on her weight was particularly judgmental since she could not do anything about her weight at that moment. Apart from the negative experience of being publicly weighed at each prenatal visit, Felicity actually felt less self-conscious about her weight during pregnancy. Her prior pregnancies had been times when being "big" felt normal, and pregnancy gave her permission to eat "for two" without need for dieting or an expectation of weight loss. Felicity hoped that Harmony Lott, the new obstetrical nurse practitioner who did her first prenatal exam, would continue to be her prenatal provider and would not nag her about her weight. Harmony was an African-American woman who herself was overweight.

Harmony ordered a routine ultrasound when Felicity appeared to be about 16 weeks to help confirm her due date, since Felicity was not sure of the date of her last period. Rafael, her boyfriend and the father of her daughter, accompanied Felicity to the ultrasound office, eager to see a picture and learn if this time it was a boy. The technician silently did the ultrasound and then told them that she would be calling in the supervising ultrasound doctor to discuss the results further with them. Felicity, seeing her solemn face, felt her heart sink, and asked worriedly, "What's wrong?" but the sonographer without looking her in the eye replied only, "I need to talk to the doctor who can then talk with you."

Rafael, not having been with Felicity for their daughter's ultrasound, was puzzled, thinking this was the routine, but Felicity said, "This didn't happen before," and gripped his hand nervously while they waited. Finally, the ultrasound doctor arrived and told them that the fetus appeared to have a "space in the heart," which was sometimes a marker for Down syndrome. She mentioned the term, "echogenic cardiac focus."

Felicity asked, "What do you mean? Is the baby's heart okay? Oh my god . . ." The doctor answered, "I'm sorry. You didn't expect to hear this. It's supposed to be such a happy time to see your baby, and now I'm telling you something is a bit out of the ordinary. There's a lot of complicated information to share about what all this means for you and your baby. Would you like a minute to gather yourself? Then you can either get dressed and come out into the office to talk more comfortably, or we can stay in here to look at the ultrasound together."

The ultrasound doctor asked what Felicity and Rafael already knew about both her risk of having a fetus with Down syndrome and the further options for diagnosing it, and then offered written information and Internet resources for them to explore further. The doctor also told Felicity that she would notify her primary provider at the health center so that Felicity could have a prompt appointment to review options including a consultation with the genetic counselor to have more time to discuss the option of amniocentesis.

Felicity's initial feelings of shock and dismay about her baby's potential cardiac issue were tempered as she learned more about the prognostic significance and opted not to take the risk of amniocentesis. However, knowing that something about her baby was "different" stayed with her for the rest of the pregnancy. She found herself worrying privately about the baby's health and about each minor pregnancy symptom. Even though subsequent ultrasounds turned out to be normal, she doubted their accuracy, convinced that something would be wrong when the baby was born. At each prenatal visit she outwardly joked with Harmony about how well she was doing and how this strongly kicking baby kept her up all night, but inwardly she found herself even more focused than with the other pregnancies on whether the heartbeat sounded normal when Harmony listened during office visits.

Rafael was much less overtly worried than Felicity about the minor abnormality on her ultrasound, focusing instead on Harmony's reassurances and wanting to get on with things during the pregnancy. He came to most but not all the later prenatal visits, when his work schedule allowed, and commented more than once during these visits when Felicity was anxious about the Doptone, "Man, Felicity, you need to chill out or the baby's gonna feel your nerves inside." Harmony did not pay much attention to this comment the first time Rafael said it, but at the next visit when Rafael said, "All this stress is making you get fat, Felicity," Harmony noticed Felicity flinch at this and decided to acknowledge the remark. "Sometimes tensions build up during pregnancy, and no one wants to talk directly about what's going on. You two seem a little tense with each other."

When labor finally began just after supper one night, Felicity wanted to finish cleaning the kitchen, putting the kids to bed, and folding up some new baby laundry before deciding to go to the hospital. She felt torn between going right away to hear the fetal monitoring and staying at home as long as possible to avoid learning any bad news from the monitoring. When baby Omar was finally in her arms looking healthy and normal, Felicity at last felt relieved.

With her other babies, Felicity had chosen formula feeding from the beginning and liked having someone else feed the baby at night or when she was at school. She thought her breasts were too big and did not like to expose them either in public or in front of anyone in her family. During this pregnancy, worrying about the baby due to the abnormal ultrasound, she decided with Harmony's encouragement to at least try breastfeeding. She remembered that her milk had come in with her other babies a day or two after her discharge from the hospital, and expected that to happen this time, too, so she envisioned no real issues with breastfeeding. But baby Omar, while healthy, was not that interested in breastfeeding at first. Felicity attended the hospital's daily breastfeeding class and got help with positioning from the daytime nurse. She had a hard time imagining that the few drops of colostrum that seemed to come out were really enough for the baby and asked lots of questions about how to tell the amount of breast milk that Omar was receiving, especially when he suckled only a few minutes at a time. While her postpartum nurses were kind and concerned, they had responsibility for caring for several women at a time and once they got Omar positioned at the breast could not stay to help further. When Omar fell asleep yet again at the breast his first evening, and the evening nurse verbalized concern about whether he had enough wet diapers, Felicity decided to give him a bottle, which he readily took. She then agreed that the next time he was hungry that night, he could get a bottle, and she would try nursing again the next day. She left the hospital doing both, with Rafael eager to help however he could. Two days later, she became so engorged that she could not figure out how to get Omar to latch on, and they all were frustrated. It felt a lot easier to satisfy Omar with a bottle. Within a few days, Omar was mostly bottle-feeding, and by the time of his two-week visit in the office, Felicity's milk supply had dried up. She reported matter-of-factly to Harmony, "I didn't have enough milk again. He was too hungry, and I couldn't keep up."

Jackie

Jackie was a 36-year-old G5P3 African-American woman whose first three children were born eight, 10 and 12 years ago. She became pregnant this time unexpectedly from a brief reconciliation with her children's father, but they were no longer in a relationship. She was a foster mother for three other children and was very active in her church. She also worked part-time as a nurses' aide. Her mother had diabetes, and her father had hypertension and had had a stroke at 55 years old. Jackie was very overweight (body mass index [BMI] of 40) and had a lot of back pain even when she was not pregnant. So far she had not had diabetes or hypertension diagnosed herself, but she had severe fatty food intolerance. She had been avoiding getting a gallbladder ultrasound, as she was afraid of surgery. Although she took her children to her family doctor, Judith Peters, for regularly scheduled appointments, Jackie avoided care for herself. At these well-child visits, Judith tried to remind Jackie about getting her own healthcare as well. Jackie began prenatal care at four months of pregnancy.

After examining Jackie at the first prenatal visit, Judith was concerned about Jackie's large fundal height, her late presentation to care, and her advanced maternal age. She wanted Jackie to have the maternal serum marker screening, see the genetics counselor, and get a detailed ultrasound. Jackie did not see the logic in these evaluations, as she would not consider abortion. She was annoyed that Judith did not remember that she would never consider an abortion so "why should I have these tests anyway?" Judith nonetheless encouraged Jackie to keep the appointments.

Judith also referred Jackie to the obstetrical specialists for her multiple risk factors, but Jackie returned from this consultation saying she would not see them any more because they only talked about how fat she was and did not deal with her concerns about her back pain and her gallstones that appeared on her ultrasound. She felt that they were prejudiced against her because she was black as she felt interrogated about substance abuse and because they immediately brought up the possibility of cesarean and sterilization without asking her if she would want more children after this pregnancy.

At about five months of pregnancy Jackie was not tolerating many foods as "everything" gave her right-sided abdominal pain, and she was having a lot of back pain. Although she wanted the baby very much, she was angry about feeling sick all the time, and kept pushing Judith to "do something." She called the office regularly with symptoms and was often given a squeeze-in appointment so that Judith could assess her in person.

At 28 weeks, Jackie had a one-hour glucola challenge of 160 mg/dl (8.9 mmol/l) but postponed the glucose tolerance test (GTT) for two weeks, which, when she finally was able to come in fasting, showed all four values to be abnormal. While upset about this diagnosis of gestational diabetes (GDM), Jackie was actually not surprised. She had checked her blood sugar with her mother's glucometer after a big family meal and knew that it was running high. Judith talked with her about the implications of gestational diabetes both for her and for the baby. Jackie took diabetes very seriously because of her mother's history and committed herself to following a strict diet, something she had never done before, even though this plan meant preparing separate meals for herself from those for her children, which was a difficult task given her work schedule. She obtained her prescription for a glucometer, and saw the diabetes nurse educator and the dietician at the hospital.

The African-American nurse in Judith's office found a reference on the Internet to an interactive educational DVD about gestational diabetes for women of color. She asked Judith about purchasing it, and they found some extra money in their supply budget to get a copy. The nurse called Jackie to see if she could come in early for her next appointment to view the DVD; Jackie said she would need to bring her kids along, so together they all watched the DVD and responded to its interactive format.

At first her blood sugars remained high, and Judith worried aloud that she might need to start insulin and transfer her care to a specialist. Hearing that, Jackie tried harder to deal with portion sizes and snacks, and within the next week proudly showed Judith her more normal blood sugar numbers. She admitted with frustration that the strictness of the diet was really difficult, especially given her continued intermittent abdominal pain; she wanted to stop checking her blood sugar so many times a day because her fingers hurt.

At about 33 weeks, with her blood sugars just under control, Jackie's blood pressure at her prenatal visit was high. Judith evaluated her for other signs and symptoms of pre-eclampsia, and all were normal, but she asked Jackie to return in three days to recheck her blood pressure. At that visit it was even higher, and Judith recommended hospitalization to evaluate more closely given her diabetes and preterm status. Jackie had to find childcare overnight but agreed reluctantly to come to the hospital "as long as you're the one in charge of my care." She stayed overnight for monitoring and testing. With her BP normalizing, Judith discharged her the next day, but recommended further close follow-up and modified bedrest. Jackie asked for a note for her employer to confirm her need for sick time, and wondered how she was going to handle her foster children's needs.

At about 35 weeks, Jackie's blood pressure remained high, with all other evaluations for pre-eclampsia risk still normal. Judith wanted additional consultation with the maternal and fetal medicine specialist. Jackie, after her prior experience, was very opposed to this idea but finally agreed to see one specific consultant who had worked closely with Judith in other situations. This consultant agreed to co-follow Jackie with alternate visits with Judith for management of her blood pressure. At 37 weeks, the consultant suggested considering induction of labor since Jackie's blood pressure while stable remained elevated. Jackie needed to wait until her sister could arrive from out of state to help her with childcare so they arranged an induction plan for a few days later.

Jackie's induction began with cervical ripening but everyone in her family anticipated that the process would not take long, given that this was Jackie's fourth baby and her other labors were relatively quick. Hospital policy allowed only two people in the room to be with Jackie. She chose her best friend and her mother to accompany her. The ripening drug set off uncomfortable, frequent contractions but did not cause much cervical change, and by the next day Jackie was exhausted and frustrated that her cervix was still only 2 cm dilated and not effaced in spite of frequent, tiring contractions. Judith suggested a brief rest but then continuing with an induction, given her blood pressure. The labor progressed arduously – Jackie's blood pressure edged up and she started dipping 3+ protein in her urine, leading Judith to start magnesium therapy to prevent eclampsia, which made Jackie feel miserable. She eventually insisted on an epidural, even though her other children's births were medication-free. Finally, she was fully dilated, but pushed for two hours without much descent even after trying position changes.

During the pushing, before evaluating Jackie's cervix and the baby's descent, Judith watched her through a contraction and asked, "You look like you're working really hard with that contraction. Tell me what you were feeling with that." Jackie shook her head in frustration, "Man, this baby was supposed to come easy, like his sisters did! Everyone's right that these contractions hurt more than regular labor, but they're not working the same." Judith nodded her head. "Yes, other women who have had both spontaneous and induced labors talk about that. It is frustrating that this labor has not been as smooth as your other labors were. We were assuming your strong body would do the same this time. . . . With all that you juggle so well in your life with work and being such an experienced parent, you know both that each child is different from the beginning, and that sometimes things do not go just as planned."

As Jackie neared the two-hour mark of pushing, the baby's heart rate started to become abnormal, and Judith decided a cesarean was likely to be imminent. She asked the consultant to see Jackie in case there was a possible chance of an assisted delivery. The consultant evaluated Jackie and agreed that the baby was posterior and too high to safely attempt an assisted vaginal delivery and recommended a cesarean section.

Jackie wanted her mother with her during the birth. The labor nurse prepared Jackie's mother before they went into the operating room and encouraged her to praise Jackie's hard work and endurance. The mother sat by Jackie's head and whispered to her daughter how proud she was of her.

Judith accompanied Jackie into the operating room to do the initial care for baby Joshua, who was vigorous and healthy. She encouraged Jackie to hold him right away, even while the consultant was still closing her abdomen, and to try nursing as soon as possible in the recovery area. Jackie was not sure she could cope with the immediate post-operative pain and still breastfeed but knew how good that could be for his health so kept trying.

Although Joshua's initial Apgars were stable in the delivery room, by about six hours of life he developed mild respiratory distress and needed to stay in intensive care for a couple of days. In the immediate postpartum period, Jackie was still hypertensive with proteinuria to the point that Judith and the consultant both recommended antihypertensive medication and staying on magnesium sulfate for 24 hours. Judith was careful to reassure Jackie that the medicine for blood pressure that she chose was safe with breastfeeding. The long induction, these medications, and her post-operative pain all left Jackie feeling drugged, exhausted, and unable to cope with breast-pumping or visiting Joshua much in the neonatal intensive care unit. Her postpartum nurse reminded Jackie to pump at least every four hours; each time the nurse came to record vital signs, she brought fresh pre-labeled bottles for the electric pump that stayed at Jackie's bedside. The nurse then stored the milk so that Joshua could have it when he was ready to eat. The intensive care nursery was on a different floor of the hospital, which made the trip even harder for Jackie. Finally, by the middle of the second day, her pain was better and her intravenous medications were finished, so she could spend a bit more time with Joshua, but she still was not able to start nursing him directly until he was over 72 hours old. At the time of discharge from the postpartum floor, Jackie was still hypertensive to the point that Judith recommended continuing antihypertensive medication at least until her check-up.

Postpartum, Jackie's blood pressure remained up past her six-week check-up visit. At that visit she was very proud to still be breastfeeding; she was supplementing with formula to give herself a break when she was dealing with all the other kids, but she liked that she had been able to keep up with the nursing longer than with any of her other birth children. Her daughters, delighted with their new baby brother, accompanied their mother to this visit to help with Joshua, and Judith noted that the girls were overweight also. She suggested that Jackie have a screening test for Type II diabetes and that the whole family work with the nutritionist about weight issues. The doctor also recommended that Jackie continue to take an antihypertensive medication with a plan for follow up to reconsider the medication over the next several months. Jackie continued to breastfeed with bottle supplementation at home for many months after her delivery, which helped her lose weight and lowered her blood pressure.

Six months after Joshua's birth, Jackie returned for a visit to check her blood pressure. She had struggled to fit exercise into her daily routine with her new baby and her other children; the winter months were the hardest given the short days, but she tried to walk with the baby. She had returned to her pre-pregnancy weight, and Judith confirmed that she felt Jackie would be able to wean off her antihypertensive medications.

Judith also remembered that Jackie had never decided on a birth-control method after Joshua's birth and asked her about that. Jackie replied that at this point in her life she did not want to have any more children, but she also did not want to have more surgery, and she was unsure if she may want to have children in the future. She did not want a method that might interfere with sexual spontaneity, nor one with hormones. After discussing her options, Jackie decided on an intrauterine device. Judith asked her to come back the following week to have it placed.

Jen

Jen was a 17-year-old student who knew she was pregnant but had not told her mother because she was sure she would be thrown out of the house. She missed school to go to the city where she had scheduled a prenatal visit at the hospital she had heard was the best. There she had an intake visit with the nurse and was scheduled to come back for her first appointment with the doctor. After missing that appointment, Jen finally came in for a visit with Dr. Mary Thibeault at 19 weeks because of a bad cold. She had not gained much weight and had not been taking her prenatal vitamins as directed. She looked very tired. And, in fact, she had started smoking. Dr. Thibeault scolded Jen, and in a reprimanding tone, asked her why she had missed her appointment, why she started smoking, why she was not taking her prenatal vitamins, and why she was not taking care of herself. Jen just shrugged her shoulders and smiled in a defeated way, providing no satisfactory answer. She left the office verbally agreeing to keep her next appointment.

At seven months of pregnancy when her mother found out about the pregnancy, Jen moved to live with her aunt. During prenatal visits with her new provider, Larisa, she hinted that something bad had happened causing her to move to her aunt's town, but even with gentle probing, she steadfastly refused to discuss whatever it was. "I don't want to talk about it." Larisa anticipated that labor would be difficult for Jen because she was skittish about pelvic exams and jumped when she was touched.

Jen presented to labor and delivery at 35 weeks in extreme pain, seemingly in active labor and almost ready to push. Upon examination, Larisa found that she was in fact not even 1 cm dilated. Larisa appreciated that Jen was overwhelmed by pain, and was reacting to it with tears and agonized cries.

After several hours of observation and reassurance by Larisa, Jen's contractions subsided. Much calmer, she agreed to go home. Larisa scheduled a follow-up visit for the next morning, where she hoped to unravel Jen's previous experiences and discuss ways to help Jen cope with the fear of pain and labor. Without an explicit awareness of Jen's likely experience of some kind of sexual violence, the labor and delivery team caring for her was unable to anticipate her feelings of helplessness and being out of control. Although Jen had not made any explicit connection between her abuse and the pain of having a baby, her overwhelming sense of victimization had permeated the atmosphere surrounding her presentation.

After Jen's presentation with "false labor," Larisa knew that she needed a better understanding of what happened to Jen to cause such panic. She was sure that Jen had gone through some kind of frightening event that continued to trouble her. Larisa decided to be very direct: "Jen, I know that you don't want to tell me what happened to you before you moved here, but now it is starting to get in the way of your having a safe and trouble-free delivery. I don't know what happened to you, but I do know that someone did something to harm you and that those events still bother you a lot. Whatever happened, I know it was not your fault and you did not deserve it."

In response to this opener, Jen dissolved in tears. Chokingly, she related the story that the previous fall she had gone with a girlfriend to her first cousin's fraternity house, even though her mother had told her she could not go. She drank what was offered her and passed out, waking up to find a boy on top of her and others indicating that they had had sex with her too. Word got back to her high school. When she turned out to be pregnant, kids started to call her "a slut." She started skipping school but pretended to her mother that everything was normal, wearing baggy sweatshirts to hide her belly. Yet she knew she needed to take care of herself and even kept some of the prenatal appointments she had made in the city. When the pregnancy became obvious, her mother, a single mother who worked as a secretary in the grammar school office, felt very ashamed and insisted that Jen leave town for the rest of the pregnancy. Jen never told her mother about the gang rape at the fraternity house.

After Jen told Larisa about this rape, they talked more about how Jen could handle labor and who she wanted to support her in this. Jen admitted that every vaginal exam was excruciatingly difficult for her. They discussed that she would need some further vaginal exams once labor truly started, but that Larisa or other providers would try to minimize these. Jen asked about getting an epidural earlier rather than later in labor since she imagined that not being able to feel the exams would help her immensely.

Kerry

Kerry, now at 23, had begun dating Ron in college. She had wanted foolproof contraception as she had career plans and a vision of their future. When she went then to her primary care doctor, she was pleased that the doctor started the visit with a discussion of confidentiality – how she recognized that it was a small community and that she knew how important it was for Kerry to receive medical care in a place that respected and protected her private decisions. She presented Kerry with several options, helping her imagine how each one would work with her lifestyle and her need to keep her sexual activity hidden from her parents and family. Kerry wanted a very effective method, since she did not believe she could have an abortion if she got pregnant accidentally. She chose to take the pill, since her doctor had explained that she would be able to get refills if she just called the office, which was easier than coming in to the office for an injection, and since she did not want anything like an IUD that would stay inside her body.

She was the oldest of four children – she had always entertained her younger sisters and brother and often looked after the neighborhood children as well. Kerry majored in early childhood education and took a job right away after college as a preschool teacher, marrying Ron soon after. Kerry and Ron lived in the same community nearby both sets of parents who were all awaiting their first grandchild. Having postponed starting a family until Ron finished building their first house, Ron and Kerry were now eagerly awaiting their first pregnancy. Right after Kerry had stopped the birth control pill, she missed her period. Kerry was excited that her period was late. She bought a home pregnancy test and waited till she and Ron were both home to do the test. They were ecstatic when it came out positive. He picked her up and swung her around. They could hardly wait to phone their parents, but decided to wait until they had a chance to celebrate alone by going out to dinner. Kerry carefully avoided any alcohol because now she knew she was pregnant.

As happy as she was to be pregnant, at her first prenatal visit with Larisa, Kerry looked and felt tired and wan. She reported multiple episodes of vomiting for the last week and only holding down small amounts of liquids. She had expected to feel nauseated but was unprepared for the vomiting. She also felt fatigued, arriving home after work feeling that she needed to go to bed right away. She had tried to go to work, but had to leave the classroom several times to throw up. Although she had not wanted to take any medications during her pregnancy, she was now willing to "do anything" not to feel so sick. Usually, Kerry did most of the cooking as she arrived home earlier than Ron, but that week she had been too nauseated and tired, so Ron had stepped in to do the cooking. Kerry left the office visit with multiple suggestions: vitamin B6, ginger capsules, ginger ale, nausea bands, morning crackers, and a word of caution to call if she was not urinating in normal amounts or if she felt weak and dehydrated.

The following week Ron called Larisa's office saying that Kerry seemed more nauseated than ever and he wondered about dehydration. Indeed Kerry had ketones in her urine when she came to the office, and readily accepted the offer of hospitalization for hydration and medication to try to control her nausea. Ron confided to Larisa while Kerry was at the lab that he wondered if he had done anything wrong to make Kerry so nauseated – that maybe she was really upset about something, although he did not know what. Later when Kerry was alone with Larisa she confided that she hated the nausea so much that if it were just up to her, she would just have an abortion. She also felt terribly guilty that she felt this way, since she and Ron really wanted a baby, and she knew that Ron was going to be a great father, but she was hating the process so much she would like to "get rid of it." She hated herself, as well, for these feelings.

After five days in the hospital, with intravenous hydration and metoclopramide, Kerry was finally able to tolerate some small frequent bland meals. Ron agreed to continue doing all the cooking until the nausea resolved, and Kerry took off a few weeks from work. Larisa assured Kerry and Ron that the nausea did not have emotional origins, and would usually improve with the treatment and with time. Over the course of the five days and nights, Kerry had a chance to talk frequently with the nurses on the maternity floor who assured Kerry that such bad feelings about oneself and the pregnancy were temporary reactions to the nausea and did not have anything to do with how competent a mother she would be. Kerry hoped they were right, but was not convinced. Kerry finally left the hospital able to keep down very small amounts of a very bland diet although still pretty nauseated.

Kerry came for her next prenatal visit at 12 weeks, finally feeling better after her hospitalization. Larisa acknowledged first, "I'm so glad to see you are well enough now to be seeing me in the office," then said, "I have a few things I'd like to discuss today, but, first, do you have any questions for me?" Kerry wondered how her weight was today and whether she really still needed to try to take the prenatal vitamins that made her nausea worse. Larisa reviewed her weight gain and her normal hemoglobin results, and asked Kerry to lie back on the exam table to listen for the heartbeat while saying, "Your weight has stabilized so I am hopeful that you are past the worst of the nausea and vomiting now. You are not anemic, which is great, but let's talk more about your nutrition needs now so that we can decide together if you need to take the vitamin still." Kerry described what she had been able to eat over the last week, and Larisa showed her an easy-to-read pamphlet that summarized the expected needs for iron, protein, and other nutrients at this point in pregnancy. She mentioned that some women tolerated a chewable vitamin without iron better, and suggested that Kerry try this until she was tolerating a more regular diet.

Kerry's nausea finally dissipated as she neared 16 weeks' gestation. During lunch breaks, her fellow teachers offered her frequent advice about what to eat, and her mother-in-law, hearing of Kerry's new craving for certain foods, remembered her own pregnancy cravings with Ron and was convinced this meant that the baby would be a boy. At last past the unrelenting nausea, Kerry slowly began to put on weight and feel renewed energy. She enjoyed sharing stories with the other teachers at work about their prenatal experiences. As she entered her fourth month, her friends asked, "What are you having?" and "When is your ultrasound?" They showed her their baby books with the first pictures of ultrasounds prominently displayed. Kerry and Ron went together after work to their scheduled ultrasound. Ron was allowed into the room, but the screen faced away from them until the sonographer had finished all the measurements and then took time to show them a few views. Kerry, who had not yet felt any fetal movement, was surprised by how much the fetus was moving on the ultrasound screen.

In the early third trimester Kerry's weight increased a bit faster than expected, and she suddenly felt big and immobile. She was having more trouble sleeping. She headed into the final two months of pregnancy with more frequent symptoms such as heartburn, urinary frequency, and back pain. Ron was working extra hours now in order to have some financial cushion to be able to take time off after the baby's birth. He was not around home much to help with some of the chores that were becoming harder for Kerry to do, such as laundry, or even to help when by 36 weeks she had trouble bending over to tie her shoes.

Kerry planned to work up until she went into labor, but as her due date approached, she was deluged by calls and inquiries about when she would have the baby. At her baby shower, several friends told their birth stories, most of which revolved around long labors or dramatic deliveries.

Kerry and Ron began childbirth classes weekly for a month starting at 34 weeks and enjoyed meeting some of the other couples also expecting their first baby. Before the class was over, one of the women had already delivered and brought the baby to the last class. Kerry was bothered by heartburn at this point but mostly just felt big and bloated, and while holding this newborn was all the more eager and anxious to give birth herself. She and Ron received almost daily phone calls from the rest of their family inquiring about her symptoms, but she had had no signs of labor as her due date approached. At her 40-week visit, Kerry's mother came to the prenatal visit. She was particularly nervous about how much longer until the baby arrived. Larisa acknowledged Kerry's mother's upcoming change in status as a new grandmother and her concern for her daughter. Larisa reassured everyone that Kerry was already a bit dilated and that the baby was healthy. They discussed the plan for monitoring her over the next one to two weeks.

At just past 41 weeks, Kerry awoke with painful contractions just after midnight. Ron called the on-call provider, who suggested that they wait at home as long as they could. Within a couple of hours, however, Kerry found the contractions too uncomfortable, and Ron called again. They decided to go to the hospital, where the night nurse examined Kerry and found her only 1 cm dilated. After discussion with the on-call provider over the phone, they opted to return home and contact the office once the contractions were stronger. At home, Kerry took a warm bath and tried to sleep, but by breakfast time she again felt too uncomfortable, and Ron drove her to the office for the first morning appointment. Larisa had a full schedule already but evaluated Kerry quickly and reported that she was still "just" 2 cm dilated and not yet effaced much. She and Ron were discouraged and tired but agreed to return home to try to sleep some. Finally, at supper-time Kerry felt even more exhausted and unable to cope, but she did not want to go back to the hospital only to find out that she was still not dilating. Ron, feeling helpless, finally called the answering service again at around 10 p.m. Just as they were deciding that maybe Kerry should return now, she reported from the other room that she thought her waters had broken, so they went back to labor and delivery. There, about 24 hours after she first woke with contractions, the nurse found Kerry to be 3 cm dilated and 90% effaced. Finally, Kerry was admitted to the hospital.

Although glad to be making progress, Kerry was still exhausted after 24 hours of prodromal labor and discouraged that labor still had so far to go. The nurses encouraged her to walk and take a shower; after waiting as long as she could, Kerry requested an epidural around 3 a.m. when she was at last 4 cm dilated. Once she had this anesthesia, she slept briefly and so did Ron, after phone calls from the eagerly waiting grandparents.

At around 8 a.m. Kerry felt like she needed to have a bowel movement, so the nurse checked and found that Kerry was indeed fully dilated. Larisa, Ron and the nurse all worked together to help Kerry with different pushing positions. At first Kerry did not want to push much with everyone watching her because she did not like the idea of passing stool in front of the nurse. She was also embarrassed about the grunting noises she made with the pushes that the nurse said were the best ones. The nurse cleaned the bed frequently and let Kerry know that dealing with stool was a normal part of her job and that lots of noises were healthy parts of the pushing process. With Larisa and the nurse encouraging Kerry's efforts, after two hours of pushing in different positions, Kerry gave birth to baby Erika.

After an uncomplicated hospital stay, Kerry, Ron, and Erika went home with both their families visiting and helping out. Kerry had planned to take three months off and return only to substitute teaching, to stay home longer with the baby. She found, however, that she missed both the classroom and the adult companionship of her fellow teachers, and by six weeks negotiated a half-day position at her old school where she could still be home in the afternoon with baby. Ron's mother had offered to help with childcare. Ron, proud of his wife and baby, accompanied Kerry to her postpartum visit to help with Erika while Kerry had her pelvic exam. They mentioned to Larisa that Ron's new business had finally taken off. However, he was incredibly busy, leaving before dawn and arriving home exhausted at dark, with little energy left for Kerry or Erika. Ron was feeling guilty but did not remember his own father doing much of the small child fathering, and did not really know how to be different. Larisa, remembering their prenatal conversation, reminded Ron what he was able to do to help out before his work got so busy, and suggested that maybe they could figure out a way to work around Erika's sleeping and feeding schedule and Ron's morning hours. They decided that Ron could take the baby after her morning nursing, dress her and prepare her for daycare before he left; Kerry could take her in to daycare on her way to work, with Ron then picking her up baby on his late lunch break to bring her to Kerry at her school just as she was finishing up. Both liked the feel of this plan. Ron lagged a minute after Kerry went out with the baby to thank Larisa. "You make me feel like a real dad."

After Erika's birth, Kerry worried that with her busy schedule she would miss doses of oral contraceptives. She was glad to hear that other hormonal options were possible even while breastfeeding. She knew Ron was anxious to have another child soon. After discussing her choices, she opted for the hormone-infused vaginal ring, deciding that even though the manufacturer listed this as "safety unknown" during lactation, the hormones in this were the same as standard birth control pills.

Lisa

Lisa was a 28-year-old married Anglo woman expecting her second child. Her first child, Abigail, now three years old, was healthy after an uncomplicated pregnancy and birth, so Lisa was not anticipating any problems with this planned pregnancy.

She had left her job as an administrative assistant when Abigail was born and had done part-time home-based sales work since then to allow her to spend more time at home. She looked forward to the routine ultrasound that her primary provider, Dr. Usha Rao, ordered, wanting to know this baby's sex. However, the ultrasound showed likely gastroschisis, an abnormal formation of the fetal abdominal wall. She and her husband Randy reeled with this news as the perinatologist briefly discussed what it meant.

After their initial brief meeting with Dr. Rao following the abnormal ultrasound, Lisa and Randy juggled their schedules and childcare for Abigail to go to the regional high-risk perinatal center to meet with the obstetrical and neonatal specialists. The doctors discussed with them a plan for both prenatal care and immediate newborn surgery, and sent an initial consultation report to Dr. Rao. The obstetrical specialist was hopeful that Lisa would make it to term.

After the initial grief at the diagnosis at 20 weeks, Lisa struggled with worrying about the baby's prognosis and yet feeling so healthy herself and noticing all the normal symptoms and fetal movements she remembered from her first pregnancy. She was not sure she wanted to name the baby now as they had done at six months with Abigail's pregnancy, but Randy in his worry wanted that connection with his unborn son. Lisa told her friends from a mothers' group about the baby's problem; several offered immediately to do whatever they could for childcare and other home support. One of her closest friends was also expecting a second child due around the same time. Lisa used to want to get together with her frequently to share their experiences, but now found it awkward to talk about things like delivery plans and sibling adjustment. When she encountered strangers at the supermarket who smiled at her obvious pregnancy and asked how she was, Lisa was never quite sure how to answer as she thought about her son's illness. She now had to go to the regional center for prenatal appointments every other week, and decided after one round trip with her daughter that taking Abigail along was too much to handle so left her with one of these friends. At the 28-week visit, the perinatologist at the regional center noticed that she appeared anxious and tired and asked her about plans for support. When her tears welled up, he made a call to the perinatal social worker Reina who spent the next half hour with Lisa. Reina suggested that both Lisa and Randy come to the next appointment so that they could talk to her as a couple. She began meeting regularly with Lisa (and Randy when he could make it) after her prenatal appointments to provide emotional support.

The perinatologist emphasized at each visit his hope that Lisa would make it to term, but at 34 weeks, Lisa's waters broke while at her appointment in the regional center. Randy was back home with Abigail and quickly arranged for their neighbor to stay with her so that he could get to the hospital in time. Just after he arrived, Lisa was taken to the operating room for a cesarean because of fetal distress. She barely got to see baby Anthony before he was taken for emergency neonatal surgery.

Both sets of grandparents lived out of state and although they had planned to come near her due date were not emergently available when Anthony was born prematurely. Randy went to the pediatric operating room waiting area while Anthony was undergoing surgery. The surgeon promised to come out and talk to him immediately after the surgery. During those few hours, Reina came up to the delivery floor to spend a little while with Lisa. She asked her if she would be interested in talking with another mother whose child had a gastroschisis. Lisa took the woman's phone number and hoped to call her within a few days.

Lisa had breastfed Abigail for nearly a year and expected to breastfeed with this second pregnancy even with the anticipated complications of gastroschisis. After her preterm cesarean, however, she was groggy and in pain. When she obtained a breast pump, all the parts felt awkward to put together, the cold plastic was uncomfortable, and she had forgotten how sore her nipples and breasts would feel at first, especially with using a machine. Lisa was also discouraged by getting only a few drops of colostrum at a time. Meanwhile after surgery, Anthony remained intubated in intensive care, unable to eat. Even after he had been slowly weaned from the respirator, he was unable to have anything by mouth until his intestines were more healed. After her own discharge at four days, Lisa juggled her surgical recovery with caring for Abigail, traveling to visit Anthony and continuing to pump and store milk. She tried various herbal remedies and medications in hopes of increasing her milk supply, but to no avail. Trying to be helpful, Randy and Lisa's mother, who was staying for a few weeks to help, both thought that Lisa was not getting enough rest and encouraged her to sleep through the night rather than wake to pump. Lisa felt that they did not understand how important it was for her to make milk for Anthony. The lactation consultant from the intensive care nursery worked with Lisa several times, both in the hospital and after discharge when she was able to come back to see Anthony. Finally, Anthony could eat, but between his prematurity and the long intubation, he suckled too weakly to get much milk directly from her breasts and gave up quickly while gulping readily from a bottle. Lisa tried a tubing device attached to her nipple to give Anthony the sense that he was getting some milk but found this also quite awkward and time-consuming. She was exhausted and saddened that she could not fulfill what she saw as her most important motherly role.

Mai Yer

Mai Yer was an 18-year-old high school student known to Dr. Miller as a quiet, intelligent and respectful daughter in a Hmong family. She sought Dr. Miller's help for infertility. He learned that she had irregular periods every one to two months, had never used contraception, and had been sexually active with the same boyfriend for two years. He asked, "Do you want to have a baby now before you graduate from high school?"

Mai Yer replied, "Not really. It would be hard to juggle school and a baby."

Dr. Miller responded, "Hmmm, so can you tell me about why you don't want to wait until high school is over?"

"I am afraid I can't get pregnant," Mai Yer admitted. "And if I can't, then my boyfriend won't want to marry me, or his family won't allow him to marry me. So, I just want to know that I can get pregnant."

Dr. Miller considered his cross-cultural ethical dilemma in the context of being a woman-centered physician. Should he impose his cultural and ethical values of valuing school over pregnancy and refuse to prescribe medicines? Or should he defer to her experience as a recent refugee balancing both traditional cultural norms of the importance of fertility for a Hmong woman with new personal options to succeed academically? Or should he help her explore how traditional cultural values might be influencing her self-worth so strongly that they could be limiting her bright academic future?

Dr. Miller suggested an alternative. "If you can postpone getting pregnant for one year, I will help you get pregnant after you finish high school."

Mai Yer shook her head. "No, I need to know now if I can get pregnant," she asserted again.

So he suggested another alternative approach, to approach her fear directly, "I can do a pelvic exam and draw some blood today. Then I can explain how you can monitor your body for three months. When you return to see me in three months, I will use this information to help you understand your fertility."

She thought for a minute, and then said, "If this helps me know I can get pregnant without being pregnant, then I would be glad to try it. But if not, then I want to use your fertility medicine."

Dr. Miller smiled at her tenacity and felt that they had found common ground.

Six months later, Mai Yer returned. She asked the nurse for a pregnancy test, which was positive. When Dr. Miller told her the news, he also asked, "How do you feel about being pregnant?"

She smiled back at him, "I couldn't be happier. This is what I have always wanted."

Dr. Miller responded, "And tell me, what happened?"

Mai Yer explained how her family was so concerned about her that they did a shaman ceremony for her. Since then she had not had a period. Dr. Miller asked about her school plans.

"My boyfriend and I will get married, and my mother-in-law will help with my baby until I finish high school and when I go to college next year," Mai Yer explained without hesitation. "I have already received a scholarship to college, and my husband's parents don't want me to lose it. They really know that going to college will help me and my family."

Dr. Miller made a mental note of the strength of this family's adaptation to this new country with their valuing of both fertility and education.

When Mai Yer planned her delivery, she hoped that many of her family members could be present during her labor and birth. Besides her husband and her mother-in-law (traditionally the people who attend births), she wanted to include her mother, her two sisters, and her paternal grandmother (who was the shaman who had done her ceremony). Anticipating that the nursing staff might object to more than two support people, she and Dr. Miller developed a birth plan to allow her family to attend and Dr. Miller discussed with the head nurse on the delivery floor to allow this exception when the time came.

The postpartum nurse, had difficulty administering routine postpartum practices to Mai Yer, because her mother and grandmother objected to vigorous uterine massage, a cold drink to quench her thirst, and an ice pack on her swollen perineum. To the postpartum nurse, these were important practices to prevent postpartum hemorrhage and to provide relief. To Mai Yer's mother and grandmother, these practices endangered her short-term postpartum recovery and long-term health and fertility. Mai Yer did not know whose advice to follow or which practices were best. She found herself caught between two cultures while actively learning about both.

Dr. Miller, with the assistance of a hospital interpreter, asked the family about their concerns. Mai Yer's mother explained that blood must flow out of the uterus for the uterus to recover and be fertile in the future. However, cold water, food, and air could congeal the blood in the uterus and prevent its flow, which would impair recovery. And vigorous massage could directly harm the uterus. The doctor asked what practices they wanted for their daughter, and the mother said they needed hot water, hot food, warm air, gentle massage, and an abdominal binder.

Dr. Miller replied, "Thank you for explaining that to me. We can easily accommodate your needs. And then, if the uterus hemorrhages, what should we do?"

The mother said not to worry, it would not. Recognizing that Mai Yer was at low risk for hemorrhage and had not had any concerning signs or symptoms yet, Dr. Miller decided not to push that point, but rather asked Mai Yer's mother to help monitor the blood flow, particularly when Mai Yer first got up to the bathroom after delivery.

As Dr. Miller and the interpreter left the room, the grandmother said to her daughter, "I don't know why the doctors and nurses don't know this. How can they be so educated and yet be so ignorant?"

Mai Yer chose to bottle-feed because her mother-in-law would be the primary daytime caregiver while she attended school.

Maria Isabelle

Maria Isabelle was a 30-year-old multiparous woman from Mexico City who came to Dr. Jonathan Rosen for prenatal care. She had left her husband several years ago and immigrated to look for work. Maria Isabelle's first two children stayed with her parents and sister in Mexico. When Jonathan asked about the father of her current pregnancy, Maria Isabelle stated that her boyfriend left her when he found out she was pregnant. She worked in housekeeping for a local hotel, and was grateful for the medical assistance she would receive during pregnancy. Maria Isabelle lived with "a friend" and told Jonathan that her friend would help her during labor.

Maria Isabelle's pregnancy was a healthy one, only complicated by some low-back pain made worse by her housekeeping work. When Maria's contractions started at 39 weeks, her friend Guadalupe brought her to the hospital to be checked. She was 5 cm dilated.

When Jonathan walked into the room he greeted Maria Isabelle, and then introduced himself to Guadalupe, who was actively supporting her friend during contractions. Over the course of the next few hours it became clear from their interactions that Guadalupe and Maria Isabelle were very close friends. Maria Isabelle invited Guadalupe to make decisions for her as the contractions became stronger. Guadalupe stayed physically close and to Jonathan's eye seemed quite affectionate at times. Jonathan learned that Guadalupe and Maria shared an apartment since Maria had moved here a few years ago and that Guadalupe was to be very involved in the child-rearing of this soon-to-be-born child.

Jonathan hypothesized that the two women were in a committed relationship that they chose to keep secret from the hospital system, and probably many others as well (family, friends, neighbors). Jonathan's own sister was partnered with a woman and raising two children, and he wanted to show explicitly his acceptance of a same-gendered partnership to these women as soon as possible. He chose, however, not to address these issues directly in the context of the labor and delivery area, but rather to focus on involving Guadalupe in the birth to the extent that Maria and Guadalupe desired ("no" to cutting the cord, "yes" to holding the baby soon after birth). Later, when he discharged Maria Isabelle and her baby, Jonathan invited Guadalupe to come to future well-child appointments.

Jonathan was somewhat aware of the different realities and cultural meanings in other countries for women who partner with women and imagines that that these women may not self-identify as "lesbian", even when their relationship may look like a lesbian relationship to many people in the USA.

Mariana

Mariana was a 30-year-old Brazilian immigrant. She was the youngest child of four and the only daughter. She had been married for two years to Roberto and finally became pregnant. Her mother-in-law was able to visit from Brazil during her pregnancy and accompanied her to several of her prenatal visits. She had no medical risks and was having a medically uncomplicated pregnancy, but was quite anxious about the body changes, particularly around weight gain and stretch marks. Both she and her mother-in-law asked at every early visit about when she could have an ultrasound to know the baby's sex.

Her pregnancy remained otherwise uncomplicated until 38 weeks' gestational age when her blood pressure reached 140/90 and she had protein in her urine. Dr. Miller, her provider, suggested hospital admission to evaluate her pre-eclampsia and make a delivery plan. Her husband and his mother (for whom this was the first grandchild) anxiously accompanied her and confronted Dr. Miller about her care. They talked in Portuguese, expecting Mariana to translate for them. Dr. Miller obtained a telephone interpreter, and heard the family's concerns. They particularly demanded to know why Mariana was not being offered an immediate cesarean section. Dr. Miller carefully explained the options for care, including a cervical ripening agent, oxytocin, and fetal monitoring. As they continued to be alarmed, and demand a cesarean section, Dr. Miller asked them, "What happens in Brazil?"

Mariana's mother-in-law replied, "In Brazil, a cesarean is the safest, most modern, and best delivery method for people who can afford it. Anyone who can pay for it gets a cesarean."

Mariana then interjected, "She is worried that you won't give me a cesarean because we can't afford to pay for the C-section here. They think you are trying to save insurance money." She smiled, a bit embarrassed, and continued, "And I think they are worried about me and the baby. Whenever there is any problem in Brazil, they do a cesarean."

Then understanding their perspective, Dr. Miller explained, "In this country, vaginal deliveries are usually the safest birthing method for a woman with pre-eclampsia. But if something changes and I think you need a cesarean section, I will recommend one. What kind of insurance you have won't make any difference."

Mariana asked Dr. Miller to wait until her mother arrived the next day from Brazil, to have her assistance if the family had to decide between medical options. Dr. Miller agreed to wait because her pre-eclampsia had stabilized, so he felt comfortable delaying the plan for cervical ripening. Once her own mother had arrived, Mariana agreed to go ahead with induction, and after a night of prostaglandin gel and a day of oxytocin, she delivered a healthy daughter, Veronica, without further complications.

The first few times Mariana tried to nurse baby Veronica, she struggled to position the baby comfortably, and found that the initial suckling was intensely painful. Her nipples felt cracked and dry after the first couple of feedings. She worried that Veronica was not satisfied and wondered how else to comfort her. When Dr. Miller visited on the first postpartum day, Mariana asked about supplementing, saying she was not sure she could handle the nipple soreness and that she thought the baby needed more milk.

Dr. Miller discussed lactation physiology with her briefly. He suggested that Mariana try breastfeeding while the nurse was there so that she could observe and help problem-solve. While Mariana was working to position Veronica, the nurse asked, "Okay if I help with getting her to latch by touching your breasts? I'll try to be gentle. Let me know if it's too uncomfortable."

On the day of discharge Dr. Miller arrived to see Mariana when both her mother and her mother-in-law were in her room waiting to take her home. He invited questions from the grandmothers about how both Mariana and Veronica were doing and learned that neither grandmother had breastfed her children. Dr. Miller with the interpreter's assistance again reviewed lactation and invited further questions.

The family went home with plans for daily home visits by a nurse and an office visit five days later. The home nurse's written report arrived at Dr. Miller's office on that appointment day, and noted that breastfeeding was going well with mother pumping for one bottle a day. At the office visit, with Roberto and both grandmothers present along with Mariana, Veronica was alert and vigorous, and had regained her birth weight. Mariana's mother helped Veronica get positioned to nurse, and Roberto's mother had packed the diaper bag and knew where to find everything. Mariana focused on breastfeeding while everyone else peppered Dr. Miller with lots of questions about the baby's mild facial rash, her yellow stools, and her sneezing.

Dr. Miller, observing how Mariana cradled her daughter closely and how her mother was cooing back at the baby's wide-awake eyes, commented, "Veronica seems to know how lucky she is to have all of you caring for her. You are already an expert at comforting her, Mariana." He reviewed normal newborn issues and added, "Moms and dads often have lots of worries and concerns about the baby in these first few days and weeks. Let's talk about some of the ways Veronica can communicate with you, even at this age, and about how you can figure out when to call to get more help." He further acknowledged that taking care of a newborn could feel overwhelming even with experienced grandparents around. He commented on how well Mariana was able to focus on Veronica's needs in the midst of this and how involved each grandmother was in ways that supported Mariana's healthy choice of breastfeeding. They talked about the immediate concerns but also about ways for both Mariana and the rest of the family to find answers to future questions in between appointments.

Mariluz

Mariluz was a 23-year-old mother of three with a troubled life. Mariluz's doctor, Dr. Burman, had been her doctor since she was born (in fact, she had attended Mariluz's mother in childbirth) and was still the doctor for Mariluz's immediate and extended family. Dr. Burman cared for Mariluz in all her previous pregnancies and births. Dr. Burman knew well the story of Mariluz's harsh childhood: her mother, Carmen, drank a lot and frequently hit the children. All four children had been placed in foster care several times during Mariluz's school years. Although Carmen stopped drinking and found a stable partner, the impact of her children's experiences persisted in their lives.

Mariluz became pregnant from a single apparently consensual sexual episode when she was 14; her mother raised this son, José. José was only four years younger than Mariluz's youngest brother, and he was raised as another child in her mother's household. Mariluz moved out as soon as she could when she was 17 with Rocky, who because of his job stability and income seemed like an ideal partner.

However, when Mariluz became pregnant, he began to be possessive and accused her of seeing other men when he was at work. He called her countless times during the day to check on her whereabouts, and hassled her if her clinic visits were longer than expected. He subsequently became increasingly abusive. His jealousy turned into threats to kill anyone he caught her with. He became physically aggressive, pushing her and knocking her to the ground on one occasion when he was intoxicated. The next day he apologized and promised that it would not happen again. In addition to the stress from the changes in Rocky's behavior, this second pregnancy was also difficult for Mariluz physically. She had frequent exacerbations of her asthma, severe fatigue, and debilitating back pain.

Mariluz became more fearful as the pregnancy progressed and Rocky's abuse accelerated, but she thought maybe he would get better after his child was born or if he found a new job. She felt ashamed about the abuse and felt that the problem was her own fault. Her mother had warned her not to get involved with Rocky, and Mariluz was embarrassed to admit that the relationship was in trouble.

At six months, Dr. Burman found Mariluz more anxious and asked her about the home situation. She gradually revealed what was going on with Rocky. Dr. Burman convinced Mariluz to come in more frequently and sent her home with the plan for visits, normalizing it so that Rocky did not become suspicious. Over the next few visits, Dr. Burman helped Mariluz identify her strengths: she was very careful about her medical care and kept all her appointments, she took good care of her asthma, she was able to make strong connections with women friends and relatives, especially her sister Beatriz and her friend Evie, and she was good at predicting Rocky's reactions and anticipating when he would "lose it" or "blow up." Dr. Burman encouraged Mariluz to make a safety plan in case Rocky's violence escalated further before delivery. Together, they figured out that Beatriz and Evie would be good supports in the delivery room, and each woman agreed to be there when Mariluz went into labor. Mariluz thought it would be hard for her to feel safe and to manage pain with Rocky present in the room, but did not feel she could keep him out. Mariluz decided with Dr. Burman that she would try to indicate if and when, during labor, she wanted Rocky to leave and to communicate that to her labor support people. Dr. Burman investigated the security protocols at the hospital and planned to inform the charge nurse on the day of delivery of the potential need to ask for Rocky to be removed.

On the night that Mariluz went into labor, Rocky was out with his drinking buddies. Mariluz called Evie and Beatriz, asking them to meet her at the hospital. When Rocky arrived, loud and inebriated, at the nursing desk in the labor area while Mariluz was in labor, the charge nurse called hospital security, and Rocky was escorted out of the hospital. Because he then got into a car and started to drive away, the town police were alerted and arrested him for driving under the influence. After delivery, Mariluz worked with the hospital social worker to take steps to be safe. She decided to file a restraining order against Rocky and to enter an anonymous shelter with the baby to be able to get back on her feet without having to worry about staying safe from Rocky. Dr. Burman encouraged her in her plan and again underscored her strengths. They discussed ways that she could keep follow-up visits without alerting Rocky to her whereabouts. Despite these well-laid plans, within a few weeks, Mariluz was back with Rocky, who promised that he would not drink and that he would never hit her again. He bought the baby a very expensive stroller with a removable car seat.

Rocky was pleased with the birth of Rocky Junior but began to be increasingly physically abusive again as time went on. Mariluz was reticent about acknowledging the abuse, but as she became increasingly symptomatic from her asthma, fatigue, and musculoskeletal complaints, Dr. Burman began pushing her to be open about what was really going on. Finally, when Rocky Junior was two years old, Mariluz obtained a restraining order and moved out from Rocky, temporarily doubling up with one of her sisters. Although Rocky was furious, he did not want to jeopardize his job and income by an arrest, and he did not pursue Mariluz except with abusive phone calls.

After almost a year of homelessness, Mariluz finally found a place of her own and lived on her own with Rocky Junior for a year before she met Louie. She quickly became pregnant with Louie and had an uncomplicated pregnancy, delivering Louis Junior with no difficulty. However, soon after this third pregnancy, Mariluz's other medical issues worsened: poorly controlled asthma requiring frequent urgent visits, intermittent depression, and ongoing heartburn and chronic low-back pain. She needed letters to keep her electricity and phone connected as she had fallen far behind in her bills. Mariluz's lifetime relationship with Dr. Burman meant that many aspects of the history were familiar to Dr. Burman, but it also meant that if Mariluz arrived for a visit for herself with any of her children in tow, she usually hoped Dr. Burman would also see them for their illnesses rather than sending them to urgent care. Most of the time Dr. Burman could accommodate Mariluz's needs for continuity of care, but at times, superimposed on Mariluz's own medical problems and intermittent depression, the expectation was a burden. For the most part, however, they were able to balance these demands based on their long history together. Mariluz kept every appointment for her children, and their immunizations were always up to date. Louie was supportive and helpful, and she was now pregnant again with him, hoping for a girl after three boys, but swearing that this would be her last child.

Toward the end of this pregnancy Mariluz began having severe pain in her back on walking and found it difficult to manage her young children at home. She seemed demanding in a passive kind of way, sitting without apparent inclination to end the visit until something was decided. Using a cane and taking pain medications had not really relieved the situation. She could not bear to think she had four more weeks to go. "I can't sit, I can't stand, I can't clean my house, I can't do my kids. It just hurts ALL THE TIME," she finally blurted at one visit in tears.

"Oh, Mariluz, you are hurting so much!" responded Dr. Burman, hearing finally how much Mariluz's back pain was restricting her life. At this point, Dr. Burman offered the option of inducing the birth when the pregnancy reached 38 weeks, discussing the minimal risks of lung problems for the baby and the likely success of induction. Mariluz finally felt attended to and was able to go through the next 10 days of the pregnancy without any extra visits.

Mariluz presented to the labor floor with irregular contractions at 37½ weeks a few days before her scheduled induction for her severe back pain. Unfortunately, Dr. Burman was out of town. The resident on call found Mariluz to be 3 cm dilated and −3 station, and her cervix did not change after an hour of observation. The resident discussed her with the on-call attending, and they agreed to send her home. Mariluz was clearly upset and begged to stay. She tried to tell them that this was how her labor started and that she was going to have her baby that night, but they told her that she could return if the contractions became stronger or more frequent. Once back home, her labor progressed rapidly, and she called the ambulance to return to the hospital, but it was too late – she gave birth in the ambulance en route back to the hospital, with her friends not allowed to accompany her for support. When the delivery floor received the call that a woman had delivered in the ambulance, the resident rushed to the ER to find Mariluz on the stretcher with her baby wrapped in ambulance blankets and the placenta still inside her uterus with the umbilical cord hanging out. The resident approached her to deliver the placenta, but Mariluz snarled at her, "Don't you touch me. I told you I was in labor." The resident had to call in the attending to the hospital to deliver the placenta.

At her two-week follow-up visit with Dr. Burman, Mariluz was depressed, and when Dr. Burman asked her about her childbirth experience, Mariluz collapsed into tears. Despite the fact that they had discussed the possibility that Dr. Burman would not be available and that she had been introduced to the doctor who would fill in for Dr. Burman, Mariluz was very disappointed that Dr. Burman was not there, that the covering staff had not listened to her, and that the ambulance staff had not allowed her friends to come with her. In the hospital environment Mariluz felt she had very little control and was forced to rely on people she did not know. As she began to talk about her delivery, Dr. Burman could tell that Mariluz blamed Dr. Burman for not "being there" for her. She knew that her unavailability during Mariluz's hour of need replicated childhood issues of betrayal and lack of protection by her mother.

Dr. Burman decided that a clear, deliberate, and focused apology would be appropriate. She took Mariluz's hands and looked directly at her, stating, "I am so sorry I wasn't able to be there for you. I really wish I could have been. You must feel so disappointed and angry. Let's try to work really hard on these feelings and see if we can help you feel better."

Martha

Martha was a 39-year-old West African woman who entered prenatal care for this pregnancy at five months of gestational age. She had a history of two prior normal vaginal deliveries, 10 and 8 years ago in her country; one child was alive, but the second baby had died of an infection shortly after birth. The father of this baby – who was not the father of her prior children – was still in her country, and she was living with cousins. Recently arrived, she did not have legal immigration status but found out that she could obtain prenatal care through a local program. Martha spoke some English, but her provider, Dr. Epps, found her accent difficult to understand. Dr. Epps brought up the topic of screening for HIV by saying that in this country doctors recommended that all pregnant women get screened for HIV because the spread of the infection to infants can be prevented if mothers receive treatment during pregnancy and delivery. Martha nodded but started to cry. Dr. Epps was not sure what this meant. She asked Martha what was the matter, but received no answer. Realizing that the visit was going to be much longer and more complicated than the allotted time, Dr. Epps left the room to get help to arrange her later patients. When she re-entered the room, she found Martha standing with her coat on, preparing to leave. She asked Martha to sit back down and again tried to open the topic of necessary blood tests, but she felt Martha did not fully understand or could not process the information. She asked Martha if she would like an interpreter in her native language, and Martha nodded.

Dr. Epps called the telephone interpreter service and within a few minutes had a bilingual native speaker of Martha's language on the phone. She explained her recommendation for HIV testing and then Martha talked at great length with the interpreter; she became very animated and appeared upset. By speakerphone, the interpreter explained that Martha understood that Dr. Epps thought that she had HIV and that her prior baby died of HIV and now they wanted to treat her for HIV. Dr. Epps was initially stunned at the confusion and then apologized for having confused Martha. She patiently explained via the interpreter that HIV testing is a routine practice in this country and that she had no reason to think that Martha's baby had died from HIV. She went on to say that every woman who has sex is at risk for HIV, so Martha had risk like everyone else and should be tested. She did not mention that HIV is more prevalent in Africa as she felt that going in this direction would just make matters worse. Martha settled down as the three-way conversation proceeded and agreed to the HIV testing and to scheduling an ultrasound to see about the size and dates of the baby. Dr. Epps thought to ask Martha if she would like to bring her cousin with her at the next visit to interpret, and Martha responded that she did not want her cousin to know about the HIV testing. They agreed that Dr. Epps would use the telephone interpreter again at the next visit.

Martha arrived at the hospital's birth center in active labor at 37 weeks and told the nurse that she already felt an urge to push. The nurse examined her and quickly notified the on-call provider, Dr. Jonathan Rosen, that Martha was already almost fully dilated. Jonathan arrived as the nurse was preparing for the baby, and within minutes Martha had spontaneous rupture of membranes with bloody fluid followed within a contraction by the baby's head. Jonathan barely had his gloves on in time to catch the newborn and deliver the placenta soon after. The nurse cared for the healthy baby while Jonathan turned to deal with Martha's heavy bleeding. Martha, uncomfortable when he tried to do bimanual uterine massage to slow the hemorrhage, tried to push away Jonathan's hands but was able to nod when he urged, "Martha, look at me. You are bleeding heavily. I will need to press here on your womb to help you stop bleeding. The nurse will give you medicine too. I am sorry this may hurt, but I need to do this to keep you from bleeding too much. Tell me if I am hurting you."

Melissa

Melissa was a 38-year-old married software engineer who was a team leader in a highly competitive company. She worked 12-hour days and had no time for exercise or relaxation. She and her husband, Kirk, also an engineer, had been trying to get pregnant for the last eight months. They had scheduled intercourse on the thirteenth and fifteenth days of her regular cycle without success. Sex now seemed like work, and Melissa just wanted to get it over with. When she married five years earlier, she felt her sex life was satisfactory with no difficulty with interest or orgasm. She was unclear about how a baby might change her life. At the same time she was starting to panic that she was not yet pregnant. She read online about infertility and lifestyle issues and was careful to cut down on caffeine and alcohol. She was only a bit overweight. She did not smoke and had always tried to eat a healthy diet. She was very frustrated that none of this effort seemed to help, and found herself in tears each time her period began. She was particularly frustrated with the frequent advice that stress could cause infertility and should be avoided, as this seemed impossible to her, and also made her feel as if she was the cause of the problem.

One month her period did not come, and both she and Kirk hoped that this meant she was pregnant, but the home pregnancy test they used after five weeks was negative. Still hoping at six weeks, they visited her doctor, Larisa Foster, and requested the most sensitive test available but again had their dreams dashed when it, too, was negative. The next day Melissa's period started.

They scheduled another visit to meet with Larisa about the infertility, not wanting to wait a full year, since Melissa was already over 35. After eliciting their medical and reproductive history, Larisa took a few minutes to express her empathy for their feelings of fear and frustration. She also explained that half of all couples who have not conceived in the first six months of trying will conceive in the following six months. Melissa was skeptical that these statistics applied to her, as she had been so careful in tracking her ovulation. Furthermore, a 50:50 chance of conception without intervention was unacceptable to Melissa and Kirk, who had read that fertility declines with age and thus felt anxious to find what they assumed was a problem and to fix it right away.

While Melissa and Kirk had not really considered the possibility of male infertility, they readily agreed to semen analysis. Kirk expressed some relief when the result was normal. They next bought an ovulation test kit and began using it. The next two cycles showed a definite LH surge on day 13, but did not result in pregnancy. Melissa's blood tests for thyroid hormones and prolactin were normal, and a midluteal phase progesterone level confirmed ovulation.

At their next office visit, Larisa discussed options for further evaluation. They all agreed that a hysterosalpingogram and hysteroscopy to evaluate for tubal infertility factors was important and a referral was arranged to a gynecologist who could perform these tests. Melissa and Kirk also faced a brief but frustrating delay caused by an insurance company rule limiting coverage to those couples who had been seeking pregnancy for at least a full 12 months. Melissa and Kirk were also unhappy to learn that many infertility tests such as post-coital examination of cervical mucus and timed endometrial biopsy were quite limited at predicting eventual success or at pointing toward a clear treatment strategy. Larisa, hearing the expressions of anger and frustration, asked about what it was like to live with so much uncertainty, and Melissa began to cry.

Larisa asked Melissa about her fears and encouraged her to think through the worst-case scenarios. As they talked, it became clear that Melissa was confident that even if she did not succeed in having a baby, she and Kirk would become parents through adoption. She did not believe that Kirk would in any way reject her, but she did believe that lack of a biological child would be a deep disappointment to both Kirk and to her mother, and that she would feel responsible and guilty. She viewed her body as defective. She also felt responsible for having made things worse by delaying childbearing. She certainly could have tried to have a baby before she got to this age. Kirk could have chosen a different wife. Hearing Melissa voice this preoccupation prompted reassurance from Kirk that this situation was not her fault. While he was also very disappointed by the infertility, he did not see Melissa as a vessel for his babies and wanted to be with her no matter what. They were both able to say that it was very hard to give up the hopes that they had talked about – that their baby would have his musical talents, her brown eyes, and the genetic components of their intelligence that had been so important to both of them.

Eventually, the hysteroscopy and hysterosalpingogram were normal, although Melissa found the experience of undergoing these tests in a room full of strangers and big machines exceedingly unpleasant. Melissa and Kirk thus found themselves coping with "unexplained infertility" – something they had thought did not exist in the high-tech medical system. When they learned that clomiphene could sometimes help as a treatment for unexplained fertility, they talked over the risk of multiple gestation and agreed to go ahead. They were action-oriented people and felt relieved to be finally doing something that might help.

It worked! This time when she missed her period, Melissa waited a few extra days and then did a home pregnancy test with Kirk in attendance reading the instructions. They were astonished and thrilled that it was finally positive. They called the on-call doctor that night with several questions about what would come next in the care plan. The on-call doctor reassured them that they could make a first prenatal appointment with Larisa sometime in the next few weeks. They felt that they could not wait so long but also needed some time to adjust both their work schedules to fit in the prenatal appointments.

At the first and subsequent prenatal visits, Kirk peppered Larisa with many questions about what might happen and what the possible consequences were. Each visit was longer than average, as Melissa and Kirk found the waits and the unpredictable part of pregnancy very problematic and always had long lists of questions and concerns. They occasionally became demanding with office staff. They wanted every possible test to gain the most certainty about her pregnancy. Larisa felt frustrated with their need for certainty and schedules, and tried to explain that this was just the beginning of unpredictability in their lives, but they did not hear that.

At the 10-week visit, Melissa and Kirk pulled out the brochure in their standard prenatal packet that discussed the pros and cons of the various methods for maternal serum screening for neural tube defects and chromosomal disorders. They had researched this question extensively on the Internet and were ready to talk about the decision to have first-trimester screening. Larisa then referred them to the local perinatal center for this testing, and the next week Melissa and Kirk were back in Larisa's office to discuss the abnormal results. They felt panicked about the possibility of Down syndrome; Melissa was tearful while Kirk was trying to keep a stiff upper lip. Larisa planned a long visit and calmed them with a description of the statistical uncertainties of the testing. They discussed the options of chorionic villous sampling or waiting a few more weeks to have an amniocentesis as early as possible by the perinatologist who came to their town once every two weeks for consultation. They decided on the latter option to minimize risks. Larisa arranged this and alerted the specialist to the couple's high anxiety level. Although Melissa had some cramping immediately after the test, she tolerated it, but then they faced the waiting period for the final results. They both poured themselves into their work during this time to avoid having to worry too much. Finally, the results returned normal.

In preparing for the intrapartum and postpartum period and looking for sources of support for Melissa, Larisa sketched out a brief genogram with her. Melissa was the oldest daughter of three in a family where her father drank heavily and ultimately became an invalid after a car accident where he was driving drunk. Her mother became the sole breadwinner and moved back in with her parents when Melissa was 12. Her grandfather began touching her in increasingly invasive ways when no one else was around, but Melissa had never felt she could tell her mother who often expressed being indebted to her parents for taking them in after the accident. Melissa stayed late at school and took after-school jobs that kept her out late throughout high school to be at home as little as possible, but the sexual abuse went on until she left home for a distant engineering school. She now had little contact with her family except for her mother. Five years ago she married Kirk, whom she met in school. She had not previously discussed her history of abuse with him.

However, the process of doing the genogram led to Melissa revealing the past abuse to both Kirk and Larisa. Larisa had not anticipated either this history or Kirk's lack of knowledge of it. Melissa's disclosure had the effect of releasing visible non-verbal empathy and support from Kirk, and they left the office holding hands. Melissa and Kirk's connection with Larisa was perceptibly warmer and more engaged and trusting after the genogram visit. Larisa was able to begin working with them at subsequent visits about the fact that sexual abuse survivors often feel difficulty trusting providers and trusting their own bodies. She discussed how feeling out of control of an intimate event like a birth where her body would be exposed had a possibility of provoking anxiety for Melissa as a survivor of childhood sexual abuse. Melissa and Kirk began talking about ways that he could help her feel safe during labor. Larisa encouraged them to write down some ideas about how Melissa envisioned labor to be, how those around her could be helpful to her, and how she might cope if things did not go according to plan. Kirk focused again on worst-case scenarios but from the perspective of having Melissa think through how he could help her through such possibilities.

Melissa worked full-time until 40 weeks when her membranes ruptured without her going into labor. She and Kirk dutifully walked around the hospital for several hours trying to get contractions going, but ultimately she needed to have labor augmentation. She did well until about 6 cm with Kirk's support, but at that point asked for an epidural. She reached full dilation and began pushing.

Larisa watched Melissa push as she entered the second hour of second stage. As the contraction ended, Melissa groaned and closed her eyes, saying, "He's just not coming!" Larisa asked, "From what I see, you are working really hard with some good pushes. Why do you think the baby is not coming?" Melissa replied, "I just don't know. Maybe he won't fit. I really don't want to tear, either." Larisa reminded her, "Holding the baby in won't help that." She also reminded Melissa of the normal length of second stage with a first baby, and described how her perineal tissues would begin to stretch out as the baby's head descended further. After the next contraction, Larisa also reminded her that they had discussed in prenatal care different options for preventing perineal lacerations.

Melissa pushed for four hours with her dense epidural but ultimately required Larisa to perform a vacuum assist to deliver a healthy boy, Martin, who weighed 3.5 kg (7 pounds 12 ounces) with Apgars of 8 and 9, which Kirk was very certain to ascertain! Melissa felt too exhausted to hold Martin immediately but briefly admired his vigorous cry before the nurse took him to the warmer. Kirk reminded the nurse that Melissa had asked not to have the eye medications given right away so that she and Martin could look wide-eyed at each other after Melissa's perineal laceration was repaired. Martin had a significant cephalohematoma that preoccupied Melissa in the first few days; she felt very guilty that she had to have the vacuum delivery and this sequela. Larisa reassured her and commented on how eagerly Martin rooted at Melissa's breast in spite of his difficult start.

Melissa was surprised how tender her nipples felt at first, and worried about how to keep them from hurting so much. Kirk helped her find extra pillows to prop herself more comfortably, and took on the diaper changing after each feeding. She worked with the nurses over the first few days on different breastfeeding positions and other nipple care routines, with Kirk paying close attention to the instructions and assisting her. She and Martin left the hospital with an excellent pattern of nursing.

At the two-month well-baby visit with Larisa, Melissa was red-eyed and upset, and within a few moments broke down into tears. She said, "There's no way I could possibly return to work full-time in another month. I cry every night nursing him, thinking about it." She added that she had had no idea that she would want to keep breastfeeding, and would feel so connected to this small person. She felt exhausted from trying to "do it all" at home with more of the housework and traditional gender roles than she had expected. She felt frustrated with Kirk that he did not seem to notice. She was also nervous about not having started the childcare search yet. Whenever she brought it up with Kirk, he had lots of strong opinions about what kind of childcare they should find, but he did not offer to leave work earlier to check out any daycare possibilities. Kirk's job demands had escalated so that he could not take time off to come to this visit but had sent a list of questions along with Melissa and had agreed to be available by phone at the time of the visit.

Larisa remembered how involved Kirk was with prenatal visits. She wondered about control issues and gently inquired if Melissa and Kirk had been fighting.

"No, no fighting. He's just busy all the time," replied Melissa.

Larisa continued, "What about saying things to hurt your feelings or checking up on you during the day?"

Melissa shook her head. "No, I understand you're asking about abuse. It's not like that. It's just that he seems so distant compared to before."

Larisa reviewed Kirk's list of questions and had Melissa phone him from the exam room. In discussing one of Kirk's concerns about Martin's stool patterns, Larisa learned that Kirk still did most of the diaper changes. Larisa commented, "I wonder whether you would be willing to put your obvious expertise in that to work at night, also, so that Melissa could get a bit more sleep." Kirk offered in addition to do one of the night-time feedings with pumped breast milk if Melissa agreed. Larisa asked Kirk to come to Melissa's postpartum visit in a few weeks so that they could follow up on these issues.

While Larisa finished examining Martin, she asked Melissa a few screening questions specifically about postpartum depression. The screen that she usually used scored Melissa as moderately depressed. They talked more about her work choices, and about counseling options or medication. Melissa voiced her idea that the issues revolved around her return to work; she did not think depression treatment was needed. She decided to call her work supervisor to discuss options to delay her return, to do some work from home, and to return to work part-time. Melissa felt guilty about abandoning her colleagues for so long, but also felt completely unable to consider leaving Martin yet. Aware of her past history of sexual abuse, her harsh criticism of herself for needing a vacuum-assisted delivery, and her strong need for being in control, Larisa thought the postpartum conflicts might push her into a more significant clinical depression. She asked Melissa to call in about a week to discuss what happened with the work plans and to review her symptoms further.

Melissa's supervisor was happy to hear from her but acknowledged that it would be difficult for her to be gone from the team for too much longer. They agreed that she would do some work from home for her third month postpartum, could work part-time the following two months, but then would have to return to work full-time at six months postpartum.

Michelle

Michelle, 39, and her husband George, 45, were both university professors. George's parents had both died, and Michelle's elderly parents lived at a great distance. They had no close family in their university town but had a rich social network and many friends, mostly other university couples who already had children. They felt very fortunate to have had excellent family daycare for their first baby, Nathan.

Nathan had been a very fussy baby. Michelle had read that fussy and colicky babies liked to be wrapped tightly and carried around, so she used this strategy but quickly got discouraged when it did not work. She also wondered if something she was eating was making the baby colicky. George, who felt somewhat excluded from the breastfeeding duo, offered to help. He laid Nathan out on his forearm and jiggled him steadily while reading a book or the newspaper. Nathan responded to this treatment and calmed and finally fell asleep. Michelle seemed to disapprove of George's strategy because it did not match what she had read, but also felt that she could not do it herself. She wanted George to do it her way, but his way worked. She called their family doctor, Judith Peters, who asked what was working. Michelle admitted that George was able to calm the baby with his method. Judith advised Michelle that there was no magic answer to colic and that sometimes fathers found innovative ways to solve problems. If it worked, by all means, keep doing it. And, Judith added, if Michelle and George were really going to parent 50–50, she had to let him do it the way it worked for him. Deep down, Michelle knew Judith was right.

Michelle and George both worked full-time in the year after Nathan's birth, allowing them both to continue their full teaching schedules and academic work. They both believed strongly in sharing all the household roles and split the cooking, cleaning, childcare and household maintenance equitably with a minimum of gender-stereotyped activities.

Michelle and George had chosen to have an amniocentesis with their first pregnancy because of their fears about an abnormal child. When they became pregnant with a much-desired second child, they mutually decided not to have another amniocentesis. They felt that if there were a genetic abnormality such as Down syndrome, they would still keep the pregnancy. When asked what had changed since their first pregnancy that led them to this decision despite an actual increase in risk, they answered that if their first child had been abnormal they felt the defect would have been a huge assault on their "ego." Now that they were accomplished parents of their first child, they felt they could "handle" the potential impact of an abnormal baby.

With the birth of their second child, Michaela, now four years later, they jointly decided that one of them would need to work part-time at least for a few years. Michelle thought that the first year she should be the more at-home parent to be more available for breastfeeding; George agreed and worked on a plan for him to be part-time the second year. To save on childcare costs, they planned part-time nursery school for Nathan and part-time daycare for Michaela.

After Michelle had been home with both children on maternity leave for five months after the birth of Michaela, she found herself doing almost all the cooking and cleaning as well as most of the childcare and child transportation. George "helped out" in the evening by doing the evening dishes and bathing Nathan and putting him to bed. Michelle became increasingly irritable and worried that her brain was "shriveling." She knew that George was a "great father" and that he would keep up his end of the bargain for Year Two, but she could not see beyond the next 24 hours. She had a month left before the end of her formal maternity leave, but had been too tired to prepare any of her work for the part-time schedule coming up, much less do the reading to keep up in her field. After stewing about her increased assumption of parenting and "housewife" roles while George remained the "breadwinner," Michelle finally confronted him with the way their roles had become gender-stereotyped. She became very tearful; George wondered about postpartum depression. After talking half the night, they decided to make some changes in their plans: Michelle would remain part-time this year, but they would resume full-time childcare to enable her to continue her academic work.

Nancy

Nancy Nguyen, a 22-year-old G2P1 Vietnamese-born woman who spoke English, came in for a regular prenatal visit at 32 weeks having felt decreased fetal movement for a few days. Dr. Burman was unable to hear the heartbeat and walked her over to the ultrasound suite where no heartbeat was visible. Dr. Burman quietly said, "The baby has no heartbeat," and let the words sink in. She called the Vietnamese perinatal advocate who quickly joined them and began talking to Nancy in Vietnamese and helped her to call her husband and family. A few days later Dr. Burman assisted Nancy in delivering her stillborn baby girl after an eight-hour induction. Nancy and her husband Tam chose not to see or hold the baby after the birth. The nurses took a photo of the baby for Nancy to look at when she was ready.

The morning after the delivery, Dr. Burman found Nancy subdued and tearful; Tam was present along with their two-year-old toddler, Amy. Nancy said she was not yet ready to look at the picture and that she wanted to wait until Amy was not present. Dr. Burman talked to Nancy and Tam about how husbands and wives may grieve differently and show their grief differently. She noted that often spouses do not talk with each other about how sad they feel because they do not want to upset the other, with one result being real loneliness in their loss. Dr. Burman emphasized how normal it is to cry and to feel empty and sad, and that these feelings might linger for a few months, and might be different for each of them. Nancy and Tam decided that Nancy would stay in the hospital one more night to feel stronger.

When Dr. Burman visited Nancy and Tam on the day of discharge, she asked how they were doing with the sadness and saying goodbye to the baby. Nancy reported solemnly, but with an edge of pride, that Tam had held the baby. She had still not even looked at the picture. Tam said he had wanted to see and hold the baby. It was clear that he did this for both of them, and that Nancy felt together with him in this process. The doctor commented how Tam's action showed how he could be strong for Nancy, just as she was strong in sustaining the delivery. Dr. Burman recognized that Tam's choice to claim the difficult and painful role of seeing and holding their dead baby, which Nancy did not feel she could do, was a way in which he strengthened their relationship and their recovery.

Pat

Pat, age 17, was in her last year of high school; her mother had died earlier that year after a long battle with cancer. Pat's relationship with her boyfriend deteriorated over the course of her mother's illness and during her mourning; they broke up just before graduation. Pat's period had always been irregular, so she did not think much of its delay later that month. When she could not keep food or drink down at all one hot summer weekend, even after trying some of the anti-nausea medicine still in the house from her mother's chemotherapy, she called her family doctor's office where the on-call doctor recommended remedies for gastroenteritis and an appointment the next day if she were not better. At that appointment Pat was stunned when the doctor suggested a pregnancy test and then burst into tears when the results came back confirming that she was indeed pregnant.

Pat's family doctor, knowing about her recent loss, touched her hand gently as she reacted to the pregnancy test results. "Pat, I know this is a tough time for you, and this is unexpected news."

As Pat began to suppress her tears, she blurted out, "I can't tell my father about this. He would be so devastated."

The doctor responded, "Is there someone in your life right now who might be able to help you think through this? When you leave here, who do you think you'll be able to call to talk this over with?"

"I guess I could tell my aunt. She got pregnant in college. She could help me without my father having to know."

They discussed a plan for Pat to get back in touch with the doctor after talking with her aunt, but Pat opted for an abortion and did not return to see the doctor.

A decade later, Pat was again unexpectedly pregnant. She and her current partner, Mike, had been together for two years. Although they had not planned to start a family at that time, the pregnancy news was welcome and crystallized their decision to marry. Pat had a few friends who were already mothers and called them for advice when the initial excitement of the positive pregnancy test passed and she started feeling nauseated and tired. She called the health center to get an appointment for her first prenatal visit. At her first visit with Dr. Miller, Pat had lots of questions about treatment and about possibly dangerous exposures from the dental x-rays she had had before she knew she was pregnant. She called a few times before the first visit to ask about additional concerns about her pregnancy's progress; the office nurse reassured her.

At about seven weeks, Pat had some vaginal spotting in the middle of one night and panicked, calling the on-call doctor who tried to reassure her that this was a relatively common symptom. After she hung up the phone, she and Mike decided to go to the emergency room anyway. There she waited several hours to be seen but eventually had an ultrasound that showed a pregnancy, but it was too early to definitely see a heartbeat, and her blood work showed a level of human chorionic gonadotropin (HCG) that was compatible with the early gestation. She was told to follow up with her doctor. Pat called later that morning when the office opened and insisted on being seen that day, accompanied by Mike. The covering doctor, Dr. Rosen, was rushed due to the added visit and quickly reviewed her chart but did not yet have the final ultrasound result. He told Pat and Mike, "Don't worry, almost one-third of women have some early bleeding and more than half of them go on to have a normal pregnancy," and left the room.

Pat felt convinced that she was going to miscarry because of her exposures early in pregnancy. She took a few sick days off of work and rested at home, without any further spotting until a week later, when she awakened in the middle of the night with some vague lower abdominal cramping and again noted some blood on her underwear. She wakened Mike in a panic, and they decided again to call the on-call doctor, who advised them to stay at home and come in to the office in the morning. They spent a nervous few hours and again called promptly when the office opened. The same doctor, Dr. Rosen, saw her early in the day, knew that she had called earlier, and this time after reading in her chart about her prior calls, took more time during the exam to ask about how Pat was handling all of this. After a pelvic exam, he initially reassured her that her cervix was closed, but offered to arrange an emergent ultrasound later that day. He also asked her to have another HCG level done. He checked his office schedule for the rest of the day and asked if Pat and Mike could return directly from the ultrasound, explaining that he would like to review the results in person with them whatever it showed.

Later, with the report of the ultrasound showing a gestational sac but no embryonic development, also known as a "blighted ovum," and with the report in hand of a non-rising HCG, Dr. Rosen patiently and gently explained this to Pat and Mike, who looked stunned. He asked before proceeding if they were okay with further discussion right away or wanted some time together. They asked for more information, and he explained the likely natural course of the non-developing pregnancy, and the choices of expectant care, medication to induce miscarriage, or surgical evacuation.

Once he realized that the pregnancy was no longer viable, Mike wanted to get everything over with as soon as possible, but Pat was too shocked to decide, and was not sure she wanted any kind of surgery. Mike was nervous about her choice but agreed to go home with careful instructions about warning signs. He felt torn between leaving her at home and returning to work where his boss had been warning him about missing too much time. Mike wondered about asking the doctor for a note for work. Later that day Pat had more cramping and heavier bleeding, and called Mike at his office. Her symptoms frightened Mike, who insisted that they go back to the emergency room, where Pat passed several clots and tissue while waiting to be seen. By the time the doctor was ready to see her, her cramping was better and the bleeding had diminished. She declined further testing or ultrasounds, feeling like she had reached her limit. The emergency room physician gave her a prescription for pain medication, which she decided not to fill, and a plan for follow-up with her family doctor, Dr. Miller. Mike returned to his office but had a hard time concentrating on his work.

Pat and Mike went together to see Dr. Miller two weeks later. Her pain and bleeding were gone, and she reported that her spirits were fine. They were moving ahead with plans to get married. They felt ready to have a baby and showered the doctor with questions about when they could try again to conceive.

Six months later, when Pat's home pregnancy test was positive, she and Mike were both delighted and scared. They decided not to tell anyone right away, but called Dr. Miller begging for an ultrasound as soon as possible to be able to see that this time the baby was okay. He explained that it was still too early to tell, and offered a visit in a couple of weeks for blood work and physical exam. At that visit, because of her anxiety, he agreed to an early ultrasound. Pat wanted to book it at a time that Mike could be there, too. In the waiting room of the ultrasound office, she suddenly felt sweaty with palpitations and a dry throat. Going into the darkened room with the somber technician made her even more nauseated, and waiting for the silent technician to show them any of the images caused Pat's head to pound. Finally, the technician turned the screen to show them the tiny embryo and its heartbeat. Although reassured for the moment, both Pat and Mike continued to be anxious about a variety of symptoms, including vaginal discharge and palpitations, with frequent calls to the health center.

Now in the third trimester of this pregnancy, they brought to each visit a long list of questions and concerns about possible exposures, illnesses, and symptoms. They worried about all the unusual outcomes mentioned in the popular books on pregnancy and childbirth. One of these books mentioned writing a birth plan, and they came to their 32-week visit to discuss this further with Dr. Miller. One part of the plan they felt strongly about was having their own provider for visits as much as possible, and meeting ahead of time anyone who might be on call when Pat actually started labor. Dr. Miller was curious about why Pat and Mike, two healthy adults, had so many medical anxieties. In reviewing Pat's genogram, he learned that her mother died when she was a teenager from cancer that the family felt the doctors did not diagnose on time. Mike also felt distrustful in medical settings because of some high school sports injuries that he felt never healed properly.

Pat had several visits between 34 and 36 weeks because of frequent contractions and discharge and swelling, all of which made her panic about preterm labor, ruptured membranes, or pre-eclampsia – all problems she had read about. Dr. Miller tried to reassure her but also wanted her to report any danger symptoms. The office nurse triaged most of her calls and squeezed her in for visits if Pat reported anything concerning, such as decreased fetal movement or watery leaking. Pat insisted on these visits being as much as possible with Dr. Miller, even if it meant waiting longer to see him. At one of these visits, both she and Mike asked about getting another ultrasound "just to make sure the baby is okay." At her 38-week visit, both she and Mike were stressed to hear that her Group B Streptococcus screening test was positive. They had lots of questions about what this meant about the baby's risk of infection.

The night of her 38-week prenatal visit, Pat noticed a trickle of fluid after she awoke to go to the bathroom, but this time did not think much of it since the other times she had these symptoms and saw Dr. Miller, he had reassured her. When she arose a second time a few hours later, more fluid was leaking out, however, and she wakened Mike and headed into the hospital. The resident on call confirmed that her bag of waters had broken, but she was not contracting or dilated yet. Pat wanted to talk to Dr. Miller, who would be in later that morning, before starting any induction of labor, but was worried about the Group B strep infection so agreed to start an antibiotic. Once Dr. Miller arrived, they discussed the various choices for induction, and Pat and Mike decided that they wanted whatever the doctor thought would work fastest and most safely for the baby. They wanted to try as long as they could without pain medication as well, and had also read about the risk of infection if Pat had too many vaginal exams, so they also asked for as few as possible of those. Dr. Miller agreed but noted that he would need to make some regular assessment of how labor was progressing in order to determine the best induction method for them.

The initial prostaglandin started Pat's labor, enabling her to progress to 3 cm of dilation after just one dose with her own contractions coming regularly and strongly. To help her cope with the pain, she and Mike found different positions with her ambulatory monitor attached, and also brought out their own music and pillow and Pat's favorite old nightgown and slippers. After a few hours, her contractions spaced out, and Dr. Miller suggested starting oxytocin to re-invigorate her labor. Once the contractions became more regular, her cervix still did not progress beyond 4 cm, and the doctor recommended an intrauterine pressure monitor (IUPC). Pat and Mike were hesitant since they wondered about increased infection risks, and Pat started thinking that everything was going in the wrong direction (induction, IUPC, what next?).

While Pat and Mike were thinking about the doctor's suggestion, Dr. Miller was called away to evaluate another woman in labor and returned to Pat's room after the nurse reported, "She's really not coping very well right now." Dr. Miller observed that while previously Pat had been blowing and moaning rhythmically through each contraction with Mike holding her hand, she was now tightening her brow immediately with each contraction and shaking Mike's hand away. Dr. Miller, recalling the intensity of Pat and Mike's prenatal anxiety, wondered how this might impact her labor now and asked, "I'm remembering how much you worried about your baby's health during the pregnancy. What are you thinking right now about the baby and how this labor is going?"

Pat and Mike voiced their concerns about infection, and Dr. Miller reassured them that Pat did not show any signs of infection. They decided to proceed with the intrauterine monitoring, and over the next several hours the oxytocin was increased until the contractions appeared to be strong and regular with the internal monitor. Nevertheless, her cervix stopped dilating beyond 5 cm and was starting to thicken, with the baby's head still not engaged and starting to have molding; Pat also had a low-grade fever. Pat was getting tired, but had not yet wanted any anesthesia. Dr. Miller recommended a cesarean section, but she and Mike were reluctant to proceed with this yet, wondering if there is anything else still to try.

Dr. Miller sat down with them and reminded them of their individual past histories – how difficult it was to trust doctors, and how frightening medical settings and especially complications could be. He asked if they would like to speak with the obstetrical consultant first, before any decision is made, and they agreed.

Dr. Miller was pleased that the day's obstetrical consultant was an old friend, Greg Diamond, with a very warm and reassuring style. He reviewed the obstetrical case with Greg, but also reviewed the couple's personal difficulties with trust. Greg spent 20 minutes with Pat and Mike, and after some time by themselves, they agreed that they would like to move ahead with the cesarean.

As Pat was wheeled into the operating room, Mike reiterated to Dr. Miller that one of the points in their birth plan was Pat's desire to have immediate skin-to-skin contact with the newborn, in hopes of promoting breastfeeding. "Is there a way to do this for her even with a cesarean section?" Mike wondered. "We read somewhere about trying to do that in the operating room. Of course, only if the baby is okay," he added. Dr. Miller nodded and agreed to ask the surgeon and the nurses about this. While Pat was being prepped on the table, he discussed this plan with the rest of the medical and nursing team and offered to assist with the infant's care however he could to make this happen.

Mike accompanied Pat into the operating room and was able to help Pat hold baby Madeline skin to skin right away while the doctors were finishing her surgery. Pat immediately felt a bond but was also quite nauseated and uncomfortable while still in the OR. In the recovery room, she felt that all the various tubing for intravenous lines and blood pressure monitors made it hard to move around, let alone hold Madeline comfortably. Her sore incision also made it hard to get comfortable breastfeeding. Moving around in the bed at first, and later trying to get out of bed for the first time was difficult even with Mike's help and encouragement.

Knowing about Pat's experience of loss of her mother as a teenager, and her anxieties about medical care, Dr. Miller was sorry to have to conclude that she needed a cesarean. He had really wanted her to have the delivery she had dreamed of, and felt sad to have to transfer her care, even though he had total confidence in Greg, the consultant. Even though he had maximized Pat and Mike's control over the decision-making, he still knew she would be disappointed and might feel that she herself had somehow been inadequate to the challenge. Leaving the hospital that night, after staying to greet and examine nine-pound (4 kg) baby Madeline, he found himself relieved to know that such a big baby would not have fit through Pat's pelvis even if he had pushed her to labor for more hours. He thought hard about how best to address her likely disappointment and decided to focus on this couple's strengths when he saw them the next morning after the cesarean.

Dr. Miller arrived to see Pat the next day just as she was finishing nursing Madeline. Mike leaned over his wife, helping adjust the pillows to make her more comfortable, and then cradling the baby to bring her over to change her diaper. Dr. Miller took a moment to acknowledge Mike's partnership. "I knew what an expert dad you were going to be! All that work you did in prenatal care and labor, and here you are again – already figuring out what Pat and Madeline need for the breastfeeding to work."

After further admiring baby Madeline and reviewing how their first night had gone, Dr. Miller reflected out loud to Pat and Mike, "You know, I have to hand it to you all. You made a really good decision on having the cesarean when you did. She would never have fit through your pelvis, and if you had labored another six or eight hours, you would have had very little left to give her today. What's more, you two showed fabulous teamwork as a couple all day yesterday, and amazing flexibility in coming to the decision around the c-section. Teamwork and flexibility – those are what it takes to be great parents, and you two really have it. Madeline is a lucky little girl!" Dr. Miller hoped this would be a successful approach to what he thought might be a tough postpartum recovery.

Getting out of bed the first day was difficult even with Mike's help, and Pat remained sore. They were both anxious about Madeline's breathing and skin in spite of reassurance from the nursing staff. The third postpartum day, Dr. Miller took a moment to ask Pat what she knew about her own mother's deliveries. Pat looked sad and said she did not know. Dr. Miller encouraged her to call her aunt in another state to find out if her aunt remembered about her mother's deliveries.

On the third postpartum day, Dr. Miller also began to talk with Pat and Mike for discharge planning. He reviewed what they had discussed prenatally about postpartum birth-control options. He nodded when Pat and Mike both said, "Wow, after all we just went through, having sex again seems a long way off." He asked, "What are your thoughts about when you want to be ready to have sex again?" As they discussed this, he also inquired, "What do you expect from each other about this? What do you think about birth control that will work for you?"

Neither parent felt ready for the planned discharge on the fourth day. Pat had trouble with continence, and walking around the hospital room made her uncomfortable, so she was not sure how she could get up the stairs to their apartment. Her milk was just coming in and her breasts hurt, especially as Madeline latched on. The nurses and doctors reassured her that everything was healing appropriately, but she and Mike were dubious. They wanted to stay another night in the hospital to see the hospital lactation consultant another time. Dr. Rosen (who remembered this couple's heightened anxiety from before), who was seeing the hospital patients that day, decided to call Dr. Miller, back in the office seeing patients, and patched the call to their hospital room to discuss a discharge plan further. Dr. Miller listened to their concerns, reminded Pat and Mike of how challenging trust was for them, and offered to both call the next day to see how everything was going and to arrange for an experienced postpartum visiting nurse to see them at home within the next two days.

Ramona

Ramona was a 28-year-old Latina woman whose first child was born six years ago in her home country by cesarean section. She waited to get pregnant again because it took her a long time to recover from her first delivery, and because she immigrated and tried to further her education, including learning English. When she came for her first prenatal visit, she told Dr. Burman that her first labor lasted for two days but that the reason for the operation was that the baby, who weighed seven pounds (3.2 kg), had problems with his heartbeat that made the doctors decide to do the cesarean when she was almost ready to push. She also told Dr. Burman that she really wanted to avoid a cesarean, because of how exhausted the surgery and the new baby made her feel. Dr. Burman briefly discussed the choices and referred Ramona to her obstetrical colleague, Dr. Rosen, for consideration of a trial of labor after cesarean.

Ramona and her husband, who also spoke some English, came to the consultation appointment scheduled late in the day after work, after the interpreters had left, and met with Dr. Rosen without an interpreter. Dr. Rosen discussed the risks and benefits of vaginal birth after cesarean. Ramona brought the operative report from her country. She and her husband felt certain that this would be their last child, and thus asked if she needed to have a repeat cesarean in order to get a tubal ligation. Although Ramona felt like she understood enough English to comprehend all the issues that Dr. Rosen raised, she nonetheless wondered to herself if he might be more eager to perform a cesarean in order to be paid more for the delivery as was typical in her country.

After this consultation, Ramona came to her next appointment with Dr. Burman uncertain about what she would ultimately choose. She said her husband became nervous about the risks of uterine rupture and wanted her to have another surgery. She was not ready to give up on her body yet and dreaded the exhaustion of another post-operative course. Her cousins and friends described complications of repeat cesarean making her anxious about these, and other possibilities, as well. She and Dr. Burman agreed that they would continue to discuss her choices throughout the pregnancy.

By the time Ramona was eight months' pregnant, she started remembering the difficulty of waiting and wondering, and the long induction of labor. She and Dr. Burman discussed what would happen if her pregnancy went past her due date as she had with her first pregnancy. She decided that if she went into labor on her own, she still certainly wanted a trial of labor, but if she had little chance of doing that by her due date, she would like a repeat cesarean after all.

Roberta

Roberta Runningbear was a 32-year-old Ojibwa woman who visited Dr. Miller for a pregnancy test; she had missed her period, despite using birth-control pills, and was afraid of being pregnant. She had had two previous pregnancies. Her first infant was born at 36 weeks with induction because of pre-eclampsia and oligohydramnios; he was a low-birth weight infant and had spent several weeks in the neonatal intensive care unit; now he was a small three-year-old boy. Her second infant was born prematurely at 28 weeks and after two months in a NICU and multiple operations for necrotizing enterocolitis, had died at home in her arms.

When the pregnancy test came back positive, Roberta became quiet. Dr. Miller asked about her feelings about the pregnancy and waited for her response. Finally, she answered, "I would love to have a healthy pregnancy and a healthy infant, but I am afraid of having another pregnancy with serious complications." She cried quietly for a while and then continued, "How come I have so many difficulties when I am pregnant? I don't drink alcohol or take drugs or even smoke cigarettes." She sighed, adding, "I have a good job, enough money to keep up my own car, and I keep all my appointments. I don't understand. . . . How can I keep this pregnancy and be able to face any problems that might arise?" After a few more minutes, she wondered out loud, "And if I had another premature baby? I don't know if I could cope with another long terrible ICU stay . . . especially if the baby might die."

After a pause of silence, Dr. Miller asked Roberta what options she was considering. She slowly replied, thinking about each and every word, "I would have to consider having an abortion. It's never anything I thought I would do, but life brings challenges and one's options change. I know my husband would support me; he, too, is afraid of having another premature baby. But my mother would be upset. She is a strong Catholic and raised us as good Catholics . . . although now I go to a sweat lodge more than church. My mother would accept all of God's children as gifts, but I don't know that I can. But I don't know that I could disappoint her, either; she's helped me so much with my sick babies. And I don't know that my parents' parents or my parents' grandparents would agree with my being selfish, and considering my own needs over the baby's needs. I was always raised that we should think about how our actions influence the future, and our descendants, seven generations from now." She was silent for a long time. "I just don't know what I would do."

Dr. Miller reassured her that they would share this journey together, whatever she decided, and suggested she come back next week, alone or with her husband, whichever she preferred, to share her thoughts and feelings. Roberta smiled a little and agreed to return.

Rosa

Rosa was a 22-year-old undocumented Guatemalan immigrant with a third-grade education who lived with her husband José and several other friends and family in a small apartment. She had her first baby at home with a midwife in her village when she was 16 and left that child in her native country with his father's family to come north with José. She was working on an assembly line at a plastics company when she got pregnant.

At most of her prenatal visits, Rosa smiled pleasantly and denied questions or symptoms, saying "Sí, Doctor," when Dr. Jonathan Rosen described any pregnancy instructions such as nutrition, scheduling prenatal visits, or how to access the call system. She was assigned to Lupe, a Mexican-born bilingual case manager who had worked for the local perinatal program for the last decade. Lupe helped Rosa and José find baby clothes and a crib through a local church program. When Rosa learned she was pregnant, her co-worker friend told her that the fumes from the plastics might affect the baby. She asked Lupe about this, who interpreted for Dr. Rosen.

During her first prenatal visit, Dr. Rosen took a brief family history and learned that Rosa's mother has been ill. Watching Rosa's quiet, respectful demeanor answering his questions, he paused and asked through the interpreter, "How is that for you being here and thinking about your mother and your new child?" Rosa looked very sad as she acknowledged how torn she felt but knew that she would put herself and her fetus at risk if she went home and then tried to make the arduous and uncertain migration journey over again. When Dr. Rosen asked for details of her first birth, Rosa also appeared sad in talking about the son she had not seen in several years.

When Rosa came for her 16-week visit, Dr. Rosen asked if she had any questions about the quadruple screen that was explained in a Spanish patient education handout in the prenatal packet. Rosa smiled in reply, "No, doctor." Filling out the lab order form, Dr. Rosen then asked if anyone in Rosa's family had had any babies with birth defects for which the test screened. Rosa hesitated a bit, but again answered no. He next asked if Rosa would want an amniocentesis if the test were abnormal. Rosa looked blankly at him and said in Spanish, "I don't understand." Dr. Rosen decided to find Lupe to help describe the possible next steps of the test in Spanish. Rosa on hearing that one step was to have a needle in her uterus looked astonished, and began to shake her head "no," once Lupe, translating for Dr. Rosen, mentioned also the choice that some women make to have an abortion if the testing did prove abnormal. Rosa looked a little perplexed when Dr. Rosen then asked, "Do you want this blood test today?" since she thought that any blood test the doctor was offering must be necessary and not by choice. Lupe asked him to help clarify why Rosa had a choice about having the test, unlike the other blood work she had earlier in pregnancy. Dr. Rosen realized that he had to explain that some women who know they do not want to abort choose not to have this particular blood test so that they do not have to worry throughout the pregnancy about the possibility of any abnormalities it might find. Still a little puzzled, Rosa eventually chose to have the screen done. The results were normal.

Later in the pregnancy, Rosa's fundal height started to lag behind her pregnancy's gestational age, so Dr. Rosen ordered sequential ultrasounds to confirm that the baby was growing normally. When her due date neared, Dr. Rosen and Lupe spent much of each visit describing the various hospital routines such as electronic monitoring and the options for pain medication during labor. Rosa tried to follow all the providers' prenatal recommendations, but did not really understand much about the tests that Dr. Rosen ordered. She also was concerned about all the appointments she needed since she had to take time off of work for these and did not get any paid sick time. She missed a couple of appointments as a result.

José accompanied Rosa to a couple of her prenatal visits when he could fit his two-job work schedule around them. He nodded nervously when Dr. Rosen asked if he would be coming into the labor room.

When labor ensued, Rosa first called Lupe to provide translation and support in labor. Lupe notified the on-call physician and met Rosa at the hospital. She was well along in her labor. Lupe translated for the hospital staff and showed Rosa how to find comfortable positions while the nurse checked the fetal heartbeat. Although Rosa had already had ultrasounds and fetal monitoring antenatally, she was not expecting to have to stay attached to a monitor during active labor. She worried that even though the labor felt a lot like her labor at home in her country, this baby must have something wrong with it to need all this monitoring. José, having accompanied her to the hospital where he had never been before, was not quite sure where he was supposed to go while the nurses were settling Rosa into a room. He spoke a bit of English but was uncomfortable watching Rosa in pain and remembered to ask the nurse to have Lupe help with translation.

Rosa cried out in severe pain and thrashed about in bed during her strong contractions. Sofia Khan, her nurse, having previously discussed the possibility with Dr. Rosen, offered Rosa pain medication, but she declined, stating she wanted to deliver the baby naturally, as she had done in Guatemala. As the labor intensified, Ms. Khan thought that Rosa's anxiety might be slowing her progress and again offered her pain medication, using Lupe as the interpreter. Rosa replied, with Lupe translating, that she did not know what to do. Ms. Khan wondered what factors were important in her decision, and so asked her, "What are you thinking?"

Lupe translated Rosa's response: "I am afraid something is wrong. Why can't this baby come as easily as my first baby?"

Ms. Khan explained through Lupe that Rosa's labor was very strong but that it was proceeding normally.

Rosa wondered, "If I take the medication, will you then have to cut the baby out?" Lupe interpreted this question for the nurse.

Ms. Khan responded that medication would let her relax some but would not increase the need for a cesarean section, that Dr. Rosen would consider surgery only if the baby had difficulties and could not be born vaginally. Reassured by Lupe translating these words, Rosa accepted the medication and was able to relax between contractions.

Sofia came from a Pakistani family where women do not cry out in childbirth. She herself had had three unmedicated deliveries. She admired Rosa's desire for a natural childbirth, but also thought her thrashing and wailing were unproductive. She also knew that other nurses on the floor would think that the patient was making too much noise and should get an epidural. She was glad when Rosa calmed down and had better "control."

On preparing to examine Rosa, Dr. Rosen noticed José sitting in the back of the room quietly. Dr. Rosen asked him how he was feeling, and José replied that he was upset seeing his wife in pain. "A lot of dads feel that way," Dr. Rosen commented, offering to show José some ways to help relieve his wife's pain. But José declined to hold Rosa's hand or hold her legs while she pushed. When the birth became imminent, José left the room, unable to tolerate staying to watch the birth.

Soon after, Rosa proceeded to full dilation and quickly delivered a 5 pound 11 ounce girl, Eva, without any further pain medication. After delivering the placenta and assuring Rosa that she had no tears and no need for stitches, Dr. Rosen stepped out of the room to invite José back in. The nurses were busy cleaning up Rosa. Dr. Rosen brought José over to the warmer and scooped the baby up in a blanket and put her in José's arms. She looked right up into his face. José melted into a huge smile. Even the nurse commented, "Look how happy she is in her daddy's arms."

Lupe stayed on, translating and helping Rosa get Eva to the breast while the nurse was finishing paperwork. During the postpartum hospital stay, Lupe came in for one session of discharge teaching and helped with making the necessary postpartum appointments. She also taught Rosa how to use a manual breast pump.

When Rosa and Eva came to the baby's one-month visit, Eva was thriving, but Dr. Rosen noticed that Rosa was giving a bottle in spite of her leaking breasts. When he inquired about this, Rosa said that she was planning to return to work the next day. He mentioned that Rosa could pump milk for the baby, but Rosa looked at him blankly. He called Lupe for help, and she reminded him that Rosa was not eligible for extended parental leave. She worked in a setting where there were no facilities for privacy to pump, and (as an undocumented immigrant) her limited insurance coverage for the pregnancy and delivery did not cover the cost of a breast pump or rental.

Rosa had planned that her sister-in-law, Lilia, who was living in their apartment, would watch the baby when she returned to work. However, Lilia had just found full-time work and would not be available. Rosa and José decided to share the childcare by working opposite shifts. Rosa was home with Eva in the daytime and worked evenings; José looked after Eva in the evenings, worked nights, and slept in the daytime. Although exhausting, this arrangement enabled them to save money on childcare. José became very skilled at feeding and changing Eva and recognizing her needs. Once in a while the schedule worked for him to be the one bringing Eva for her morning check-ups. Rosa found that she was still able to nurse Eva a few times a day and when she arrived home from work. Even though her milk supply was not enough for exclusive breastfeeding, she felt great pleasure knowing that Eva still wanted her breast milk.

Ruth

Ruth and Lewis were recent college graduates who lived in a commune and worked in community development programs. They were pregnant with their first baby and had decided for a home birth with a midwife. Lewis's father was a psychiatrist in another state and his mother had been a midwife many years ago; Ruth's mother was a counselor. Ruth and Lewis did not want technological interventions in the pregnancy (use of Doppler, use of ultrasound) nor specific genetic screening such as quadruple screen, but they did want standard laboratory monitoring (blood and urine tests). They were aware of the small but real risk of an obstetrical emergency with the potential for a bad outcome for either mother or baby but preferred that risk to what they perceived as the risk of unnecessary technological intervention and early separation from the newborn in the hospital environment. All the grandparents supported their decision.

Their provider, Judith, an advocate of low intervention in the hospital setting, supported their overall plan but worried about the negative experience they might undergo if Ruth needed to be transferred to the hospital in labor, or if the baby required hospitalization. Judith also worried that the hospital specialists would be critical of her for "allowing" her patients to plan a home birth.

Judith explained that because of hospital politics she would be unable to take care of Ruth if she were to develop complications and needed to come to the hospital in an emergency situation in labor. Ruth and Lewis clearly articulated that what they wanted from Judith was appropriate prenatal screening blood work initially and at 28 weeks, and physical exams, including a late-pregnancy exam to be sure all was normal and a Group B Streptococcus screening at 36 weeks. Both parties agreed that they could live with this care plan.

Ruth started having contractions one afternoon while at work. Ruth continued working at her job to finish up details of an important project. Later that evening, she checked in with the midwife, calling her again just after midnight when her waters broke. As the contractions quickly intensified, she alternated between the rocking chair and the shower, with Lewis and the midwife nearby offering frequent sips of water and juice and massage. By noon she entered transition with the peak of each contraction almost overwhelming her. "I'm never doing this again!" she told Lewis. "I can't do this!" The midwife reassured her, and reminded both of them that this was what they had talked about ahead of time, of what hard work this stage of labor would be and how these feelings of hopelessness and endlessness were common. She suggested staying focused on each contraction one at a time, and suggested different options for coping. Ruth wanted to stay mostly in the shower until she felt like pushing. The midwife also reminded her how healthy she had been throughout her pregnancy, and reiterated, "This baby is doing great, thanks to all your hard work keeping yourself so healthy."

After a couple of hours of squatting, lunging, and kneeling, Ruth gave birth, with the midwife placing the baby right onto Ruth's chest so she and Lewis could greet the baby and then be the first to see that it was a boy. After a few minutes, Lewis cut the umbilical cord, and Ruth put Zachary to the breast right away. The placenta delivered easily, and the midwife prepared to repair Ruth's second-degree perineal laceration. It was not bleeding much, so the midwife offered Ruth the option of waiting until she was done nursing. The midwife reminded the new parents about their desire to take some early photos, and then Lewis held Zachary while the midwife sutured Ruth's tear, helped clean up the various supplies, showed them the placenta, and then examined the baby now back in his mother's arms.

After phone calls to family, Ruth was ready to eat, surprised by how hungry and thirsty she felt. While Zachary rested in the bassinette they had prepared, Lewis prepared a light meal, and the midwife helped Ruth to the bathroom. She felt a lot of symptoms suddenly: her legs were wobbly, her stitches stung, her uterus was cramping, and she wondered if her vaginal bleeding was heavier than it should have been.

Ruth breastfed Zachary for 18 months, then she and Lewis decided to conceive again, with the same plan for midwifery care and home birth. Ruth's periods were somewhat irregular while she was breastfeeding, so that when she began to have tender breasts and morning nausea and confirmed her pregnancy with a home test, she thought she might already be a few months' pregnant. When she returned to Judith for the same prenatal monitoring that she had with her first pregnancy, Judith suggested an ultrasound to confirm her dates. As with her first pregnancy, Ruth and Lewis were reluctant to do this and declined. When they returned to Judith at 28 weeks, Ruth's fundal height was lagging significantly, and she reported that her midwife had been noticing the same finding, along with less weight gain than expected. Ruth's explanation was that this pregnancy was somewhat more difficult for her, with a busy toddler and juggling work schedules. She and Lewis agreed to get the ultrasound, which showed a smaller fetus than expected for her presumed dates. The ultrasound report recommended follow-up ultrasounds and consideration of antenatal monitoring for possible intrauterine growth retardation. Ruth and Lewis came back to Judith with the report to discuss the findings. They continued to be very reluctant about doing a lot of monitoring, thinking that this would be just a slippery slope to interventions and hospital birth that they so much did not want, and yet they were worried that maybe something really was going on with the baby.

Judith knew how strongly Ruth and Lewis felt about the possibility of technical intervention, and proposed a compromise: Ruth would cut her work hours in half and increase her caloric intake. Judith would see Ruth weekly, in addition to her midwifery visits. Judith believed that if the baby turned out to be growth-restricted over the next few visits, Ruth and Lewis would recognize the slower fundal growth and at that point would agree to further evaluation. They agreed to Judith's plan, which they felt took their concerns into account but still paid attention to the concerns raised on the ultrasound. Fortunately, Ruth's fundal height continued to grow during her weekly assessments.

Sabrina

Sabrina was a 26-year-old Haitian woman who began prenatal care at nine weeks of gestation at the University Hospital obstetrical clinic. She lived with her husband, father-in-law, aunt, and younger sister. Her parents had both died in Haiti since she migrated three years ago. Her husband worked full-time, and Sabrina stayed home with her family who "helped take care of her." She had no primary care physician and used the emergency room when she was ill. Both Sabrina and her husband reported no history of tobacco, alcohol, or drug use, and no history of physical or emotional abuse. Her husband related that Sabrina witnessed her brother's death in Haiti. They both attended church "unless she's sick." According to her husband, Sabrina spoke English and Creole, but he did all the talking during the interview.

The resident working at the ob clinic, Dr. Mary Thibeault, through an interpreter was able to learn more of Sabrina's medical history. In Haiti they had lived too far from a doctor to get medical care. Since immigrating, Sabrina reported, "I take some pills for my sugar." Her husband recalled that "she had some infection in the last two years that caused her to cry, yell, and scream at us," and required a brief hospitalization in the local hospital two to three times. On discharge from the hospital, she was given medication, but they did not now recall the name. She stopped taking the medication once she started to feel better.

Dr. Thibeault suspected that Sabrina had uncontrolled diabetes, among her many other problems. She sought help from Dr. Greg Diamond, the clinic supervisor that day, with her worries about the complexity of Sabrina's issues. He supported her plan to get screening blood tests, but pushed her to consider the strengths that Sabrina and her family brought to this situation.

Dr. Thibeault suggested that Sabrina have some specific prenatal testing done. The results showed the following:

> Random blood glucose 256 mg/dl (14.22 mmol/liter)
> HbA1c 11.0% (average blood glucose 314 mg/dl or 17.5 mmol/l)
> Creatinine 1.0 mg/dl (88.4 μmol/l)
> Blood type: O negative
> HIV: negative
> Tuberculin skin testing: negative
> Hemoglobin electrophoresis: Hgb AS

When Dr. Thibeault told Sabrina that the blood test showed she had uncontrolled diabetes and an abnormal hemoglobin screen, she became very anxious. This increased tension made her family more fearful that her mental problems might recur either during or after the pregnancy. Nonetheless, with the assistance of the public health nurses and advocates, Sabrina kept all her appointments with Dr. Thibeault.

Sabrina had had five years of primary education and could read numbers and dates and simple instructions. Her husband had the required documentation to work, but Sabrina did not have legal resident status. Nevertheless, she was open to developing a relationship with Dr. Thibeault who assured her that keeping these appointments would give her the best chance to stay healthy herself and have a healthy baby. Sabrina liked the fact that Dr. Thibeault had a French name even though she did not speak French. For her part, Dr. Thibeault was pleased that Sabrina came for all her appointments, smiling and looking happy. Coming to the clinic, the resident decided, was one of Sabrina's strengths. But Dr. Thibeault worried about how to follow up on Sabrina's many problems. Dr. Diamond suggested that Dr. Thibeault involve the perinatal team in the high-risk clinic who could provide a comprehensive approach to diabetic education, nutrition counseling, and social work, and could facilitate genetics and psychiatric consultations, all assisted by the French Creole interpreter.

Although Sabrina's diabetes control improved, her HgbA1c remained around 8.0. An ultrasound at 38 weeks showed her baby weighed almost 8.5 pounds (3.86 kg). After talking with Dr. Diamond, Dr. Thibeault called the interpreter to help her explain the risks of a big baby at delivery, and Sabrina agreed to go ahead with delivery. After a short induction, Sabrina, assisted by Dr. Thibeault, delivered a nine-pound (4 kg) boy, Josue, with mild hypoglycemia that resolved with feeding. The staff encouraged her to breastfeed and explained that this would help lower her blood glucose. Sabrina and her family were happy with the good outcome and appreciated all of the team's efforts. As Dr. Thibeault was going off call after the delivery, the family presented her with a painting from Haiti.

The morning after delivery, the nursing staff paged the obstetrical team because Sabrina began yelling and throwing utensils at the visitors and staff and shouting at her husband. Dr. Thibeault could not calm her down either, and she called the hospital psychiatrist to evaluate Sabrina for risk of harm to herself or to her baby. Dr. Thibeault had never seen a woman with an immediate postpartum psychosis – it was more frightening to her than many obstetrical emergencies that she had seen and managed. She was greatly relieved when the on-call psychiatrist came immediately. The resident was also worried that Sabrina's behaviors might jeopardize her ability to take the baby home with her. Dr. Thibeault knew that placing the baby in foster care would be an emotional catastrophe for Sabrina and her family.

The psychiatry consultant suggested antipsychotic and antidepressant medication, and, within 24 hours, Sabrina no longer appeared to be a risk to herself or the baby. The nurses called the social worker to assess whether the baby would be safe at home. The social worker advised Dr. Thibeault that the team had already notified the child protective services of the need for a home evaluation. After an additional day of observation, Sabrina's milk came in, and her psychological status stabilized. Dr. Thibeault talked directly with Sabrina's husband about watching her carefully for any further changes in her thinking or behavior and emphasized strongly the importance of her medication to keep her mind healthy. Sabrina went home with her family on postpartum day four with plans to follow up with Dr. Thibeault, the behavioral health team, and the public health team. The immediate plans included ongoing diabetes care, management of depression, parenting education, newborn education, postpartum education (including risk associated with short interval pregnancies), and contraceptive counseling. Dr. Thibeault felt very reassured to know that so many team members would be working with the family over the coming weeks. Baby Josue was scheduled for a visit within three days to assess breastfeeding, and weight gain, and maternal and family adjustment.

Samantha

Samantha was 16 years old and struggling to stay in school. She lived with her mother and stepfather and two younger brothers. She had never gotten along well with her stepfather and argued with her mother about the stepfather's role in the home. She had started spending more time out of the house at her part-time job at a fast-food restaurant where she met Mark, her 22-year-old boyfriend. At her check-up with her family doctor, she admitted to having sexual intercourse but did not want to use any method of birth control other than condoms.

One night after a few drinks, Samantha and Mark had intercourse but did not use a condom. Two weeks later Samantha noticed some funny vaginal discharge instead of her usual period. When the discharge continued and her period still did not come after another month, she found her way to the local family planning clinic for a pregnancy test because she did not want to tell her mother or Mark. The nurse practitioner there confirmed that Samantha was pregnant and also diagnosed a chlamydia infection.

The nurse practitioner reviewed Samantha's options and gave her an antibiotic and a referral to a maternity care provider. Later that week, Samantha pulled Mark aside after their shift at work to tell him the news. He was shocked and angry and denied paternity. Their breakup devastated Samantha. She could not at first bring herself to talk to her mother about the pregnancy. Her mother was a high school dropout who had given birth to Samantha at the age of 16 and had always loudly and disparagingly talked about the mistakes of "girls who get into trouble." The only time she ever talked about sex with Samantha was to say, "If you ever get pregnant with that guy your father will kill him." Samantha did not want to go to the family doctor because she worried that the doctor would have to notify her mother of the pregnancy. She delayed getting care, and was able to keep her nausea and her weight gain secret from her mother as she struggled with what to do. Finally, one day at school at about 20 weeks along she was feeling too tired to cope, and went to the school nurse. The nurse asked a few questions and then gently inquired about the possibility of pregnancy. Samantha confessed, and together they made a plan to have her mother come to school where they would tell her together.

Samantha's mother was furious as expected, and told Samantha not to come home. Samantha called her 25-year-old cousin Alice who had two children herself but who offered to let her stay with them for a while, and the school nurse arranged for her to get prenatal care through a school mothers program and its connection to a prenatal clinic at the hospital. The doctors there were busy and harried, and Samantha did not like going there or talking to them about her family or the baby's father. She had a hard time figuring out the bus schedule from Alice's apartment to the clinic and thus missed a few appointments. As an alternative strategy, the school nurse arranged for her to transfer her care to the community health center where she would have one main provider, Dr. Adelle Epps.

Rushing to catch the bus to get to the after-school appointments not too late, Samantha usually stopped to grab a quick meal at the local fast-food place. One afternoon, the school nurse saw her finishing French fries and sipping soda, and asked about her meal habits. Samantha admitted that she usually skipped breakfast although had been trying to at least drink some juice on the way to school; she had a hard time remembering to take her prenatal vitamins. The nurse called Dr. Epps to discuss Samantha's weight gain (only 10 pounds (4.55 kg) by 30 weeks) and nutrition habits. At the next visit, Dr. Epps asked about her favorite foods, her understanding of prenatal nutrition, and her access to food coupon programs or food stamps. Samantha had not had time to do the paperwork for those programs but was interested in them. She agreed to try to eat a piece of fruit and drink one small glass of milk each morning when she was helping Alice feed her cousins. She asked for chewable vitamins.

Samantha also worked with the social worker at the health center to get some baby supplies and to attend some childbirth classes with other teen mothers. She started dating Jack, the older brother of one of these new friends, and he promised to support her through the labor and postpartum period. The nurse and social worker tried unsuccessfully to encourage Samantha to reconcile with her mother.

By about 37 weeks, Samantha started to have painful regular contractions, but without cervical change. She called the on-call service and the office several times and came in for several labor evaluations. At each one, the provider (who was a different provider each time) told her that this was not truly labor and that she did not need to be admitted to the hospital yet. Samantha was frustrated to be sent home several times when the feelings in her body were so intense.

The day after a midnight labor check at the hospital, Samantha came into the office for a labor check with Dr. Epps. Her cervix was now 1.5 cm and 90% effaced and anterior with the vertex at 0 station. Clearly frustrated, Samantha blurted out, "I thought I'd be in labor this time. How long is this going to last? What's wrong that it's taking so long? How do I know when I'm really in labor if this already hurts so much?"

Dr. Epps responded, "You must be exhausted. Being up all night and going back and forth with no sleep! But guess what? You really are making progress. I know hearing 1.5 cm again sounds discouraging, but compared to last night, your cervix is all thinned out. Last night it was thick as a winter coat, and now it is as thin as your sweater. And, remember how we had to reach way in the back to get to it? Now it is all the way up front with the baby's head lower. So this is REAL PROGRESS. Your body is doing some great preparation that is going to make it much easier when you get to the hospital. I am really pleased with how well this is going."

"Really? I'm so wiped out. And it feels like it will never end."

"Some of that discouragement is from feeling exhausted. Who's at home today who can help you? Let's think together about things you can do to get some rest, and who can help you with that. Your baby's doing wonderfully. Everything is going in a very good direction."

With Samantha's fourth visit to the hospital for false labor, the on-call doctor asked the hospital doula service to advise Alice and Jack how they might support her. The doula on call made some very specific and helpful suggestions that helped Samantha to manage at home until she just could not bear it any longer. With this fifth trip to the hospital, the same doctor on call shared Samantha's relief that at last her cervix was 4 cm dilated and well effaced. Her labor nurse praised her ability to cope with labor and offered her the shower to help with the pain. When she got out of the shower, the teen was already 7 cm dilated and started to panic with the intensity of the contractions. Alice, remembering her own natural labors, helped Samantha with back massages and cool facecloths and softly reassured her that everything was OK. The staff encouraged her, "You've been able to get this far in labor. You don't need to feel scared of how it is going to happen or that it will never end. You just need to keep doing what you are doing."

Dr. Epps arrived to relieve the doctor on call. She entered the room and knelt by the bed, looked directly at Samantha and asked how she was feeling and then reassured her that she was coping very well. Dr. Epps initiated a discussion of options for labor including anesthesia and amniotomy. Samantha was uncertain what was best. Alice and Jack asked if those options were necessary if the labor was progressing normally. Dr. Epps asked Alice and Jack about their prior experiences with labor and reassured them about Samantha's normal progress so far. Samantha opted with Alice and Jack's assistance to continue with physiologic techniques and delay the amniotomy. The nurse, Alice and Jack worked together with Samantha encouraging breathing and massage and position changes.

Samantha tried the shower again before her water broke spontaneously at 9 cm dilation. Then the pushing urge became overwhelming, but being in the hands–knees position helped that sensation, and she eventually started pushing in that position even though it felt unusual and was not what she remembered her friends talking about for this part of labor. After 20 minutes the baby's head was crowning, and Samantha resisted pushing because of the overwhelming burning sensation. She began to panic again and was about to scream when Dr. Epps praised her stamina and strength and asked her to focus right on the doctor's voice, coaching the teen through easing the baby's head out with gentle short pushes so that her perineum did not tear. Baby Kyle was vigorous at birth, and went straight into Samantha's arms while Jack cut the umbilical cord.

Because Samantha was an adolescent mother, she received maternity care coordination with Shereen, a postpartum case worker. Shereen visited Samantha while she was still staying at her cousin Alice's house one week after Kyle was born to check on them. Samantha was tired, but doing well and still seemed on a "high" about having a new baby. She had wanted to breastfeed, but did not feel that she had enough milk, and Alice had suggested that she give the baby formula too which she had been doing. Samantha believed this was helping Kyle sleep better and be less hungry and fussy.

Shereen asked Samantha if she felt that Kyle was happy and healthy. Samantha replied, "I think he may be too skinny." She wondered if this might have been her fault because she had not gained much weight and had smoked throughout pregnancy. She added, "I don't think my milk is 'rich' enough for him." She also admitted that at this point she pretty much was doing what Alice told her to do because she had been so helpful to her through the pregnancy.

Shereen weighed Kyle and explained that he was already very close to his birth weight and that most babies lose some weight in the first week and then gain it back. She watched Samantha breastfeed and gave her a few pointers for positioning and latching on. While doing this, she talked about Samantha's diet and encouraged her to drink enough herself. Shereen could see Alice in the kitchen listening in, and invited her to come watch Kyle nurse and hear his swallowing. They talked a bit about Alice's own breastfeeding experiences, which were short-lived due to her perception of a limited milk supply. On the way out, Shereen thanked Alice for all she was doing and her important role in Samantha and Kyle's lives.

At four weeks, Samantha came to the clinic with Kyle for his first well-baby exam in the office. Without her own car, she nonetheless maneuvered her donated car seat and diaper bag into a local taxi and was proud of herself for arriving "put together" and on time. She still felt tired and anxious, and to calm herself she reached for a cigarette outside the clinic door, and then regretted this. Samantha knew Dr. Epps disapproved of her smoking and had encouraged her to quit the whole pregnancy, but somehow she just could not. But now, when holding Kyle after smoking, Samantha thought not only about her health but also the harm her habit might have on his health. She decided to ask Dr. Epps for help with quitting smoking for good.

Kyle had gained a pound (4.55 kg) since Shereen had gone out for the home visit, and was thriving. Samantha proudly talked about still breastfeeding. Dr. Epps talked to her about lots of things – what it is like to be out of school with a baby, any symptoms or concerns about postpartum depression, plans for using condoms if she became sexually active again, and basic baby care issues. At the end of the appointment, Dr. Epps asked if she were still smoking, and Samantha sheepishly said, "Well, yes, but now I really want to quit." Dr. Epps reminded her that it was never too late to quit, that it could take a few tries, and that there were major health advantages for both her and Kyle. They reviewed specific interventions, like identifying smoke-free spaces at home and avoiding trigger situations. Dr. Epps asked if she would come back and talk about this again in a month, and also asked when Shereen would make another home visit to check on her. Together they set a complete quit date for one month later. Samantha was relieved to be able to talk about her smoking and have a plan, and agreed that what they had outlined sounded like a good plan.

Two months later, Samantha had returned to school and had moved out on her own. However, the busy schedule of juggling school, newborn, and new apartment led Samantha to neglect her own health in spite of this careful smoking plan and reminders from the school nurse and social worker. She delayed her next visit until Kyle was more than three months old.

At her postpartum visit, Samantha was shocked to learn that she was pregnant again. She and Jack had already been having unprotected sex. Harmony, the nurse practitioner who worked with Dr. Epps, gave Samantha information about pregnancy options and encouraged her to make her own decision with follow-up in a week. Samantha went to talk with the nurse at the school mothers' program who reminded Samantha of the healthy, responsible choices she made in labor with the help of her support system and how those choices reflected her ability to make adult decisions. . . . Samantha ultimately decided to go to the Planned Parenthood in the city where she met with a counselor and received medication and instructions for a medical abortion.

Siobhan

Early in their relationship Siobhan and Danny used condoms the majority of the time, and emergency contraception for the few times they had not. They chose to use condoms with emergency contraception as a backup method after Siobhan's medical provider had talked with her about making choices that worked for her. Siobhan felt that the counselor at the family planning clinic was non-judgmental when she said, "It's hard to use condoms all the time; maybe you should have a back-up method just in case." Siobhan told Danny that the counselor had even used the metaphor "that people buy car insurance without planning to drive into a tree," and so everyone should have post-coital contraception at home, "just in case we need it." Danny felt that was a good plan, and appreciated that no one was blaming him for their occasional contraceptive lapses. After five years together, they decided they felt ready to start a family. Although she did not have regular healthcare to get a pre-conception visit, Siobhan found some information on the Internet about getting pregnant and started taking multivitamins.

She attended a hospital outpatient department for prenatal care, but did not have a specific physician assigned to her. Her pregnancy was uncomplicated, but her labor was long and tiring, with painful prodromal contractions for about two days and several frustrating visits to the hospital with intense discomfort but no cervical change. Siobhan did not have any specific birth plan and was never asked about that by the obstetrical staff in the outpatient department. When she finally entered active labor she felt quickly overwhelmed and asked for an epidural, which had to be placed twice and gave her only partial relief. She had found pushing particularly uncomfortable and remembered having yelled grouchily at her nurse and other people in the room. She had not met the doctor who delivered her baby, and felt no connection to him. She had not been able to hold Danny Jr. immediately after the birth because of meconium. She was so tired that she did not mind getting some rest and asked the nurse to give him a bottle. Siobhan tried to breastfeed for a few days but stopped when she became frustrated over her inverted nipples and apparent lack of milk. She had thought she could adjust to breastfeeding in front of others, but when she had to add the nipple shield (and then the additional tubing), it became too much for her.

After Danny Jr.'s birth, Siobhan never returned for her postpartum visit. She had irregular bleeding in the first few months. She and Danny continued to use condoms for contraception as they had for many years. Danny Jr. was sick with a respiratory infection when he was two months old, and during his first winter needed hospitalization twice and then ongoing nebulizer treatments. In addition, Danny's mother became very ill and was in a coma for several weeks. Siobhan had lost some weight after delivery, but soon began to gain again. She was too busy with family responsibilities to think much about her changing shape. When Danny Jr. turned nine months old, Siobhan realized that she could no longer attribute her abdominal sensations to gas – she was pregnant again and had been feeling fetal movement for some time. She had been responsible as a teenager, avoiding pregnancy, alcohol, and drugs, and now she was spending so much energy on caring for her baby and mother-in-law that she had neglected herself. She was embarrassed to be pregnant again and did not want to return to her prior physicians.

It took another month before she worked herself up to call a new doctor to establish care. She first called an office recommended by a friend, but was told that they could not accept her as a patient because she had waited so long. This added to the guilt she was already feeling. She called the community health center and was relieved to speak with an understanding staff member who scheduled an urgent appointment with the nurse practitioner the next week. The day after her first prenatal appointment, her ultrasound indicated that she was further along in pregnancy than she had thought – she had already completed 34 weeks of pregnancy.

Danny accompanied Siobhan to the next visit with Dr. Miller, their new primary doctor. Danny felt awkward to be in an office full of pregnant women and wished he could become invisible. At the same time he was worried that Siobhan had begun prenatal care so late. He was afraid that there might be a problem with the baby since she had not been taking prenatal vitamins or eating the way she would have if she had known that she was pregnant.

When Dr. Miller came into the exam room, he immediately approached Danny and shook his hand. "Danny, isn't it?" he asked. Danny was impressed that the doctor knew his name. After reviewing the normal ultrasound results with both of them, Dr. Miller turned to Danny and asked him how he was doing with the pregnancy. Danny surprised himself by confiding how worried he was about the baby and about Siobhan. He talked about how busy Siobhan had been trying to look after his mother, as well.

The doctor said, "I am really glad you came today and let me know that. Even though it is late in pregnancy, everything looks fine. I know you have a lot going on now with your mother being sick and all, but I want you to know that you're always welcome at visits here." He further explained to them that with ultrasound dating this far into pregnancy, the due date could be off by a few weeks either way, so they would wait for her to go into labor naturally. Siobhan began weekly visits.

Danny and Siobhan decided that they really liked this new doctor, and Danny made an extra effort to attend the next prenatal visit. Again Dr. Miller called Danny by name and asked him how his mother was doing. Danny was touched by his interest.

At the 36-week visit, Dr. Miller finally had time to ask Siobhan about her prior labor experience. She described her story and commented, "Wow, I hope it doesn't take as long this time. I really was tired. I pushed forever."

Dr. Miller responded, "It sounds like it was a tough first birth for you. Second births often don't take as long because your body has been through this before. What do you think would help you with this labor? Other than how long it took before, is there anything else you would like to be different?"

They discussed a few options, and then Dr. Miller turned to Danny.

"Tell me about how the first delivery was for you," he asked.

Danny replied, "Well, after the long labor, the delivery itself was pretty fast because the baby had pooped in the water, and they had to rush him over to a bunch of doctors, but I did get to cut off the extra cord from his belly button."

"Well, let's hope the water's nice and clear this time so that you can both hold the new baby right away and you can cut the cord again."

At the 37-week visit, Danny and Siobhan questioned Dr. Miller carefully about the anticipated due date, since they were going to have to arrange for Danny's out-of-town brother to come help care for Danny's sick mother and for Danny Jr. when Siobhan went into labor.

With her second pregnancy, even though she was late to care, Siobhan considered again her breastfeeding options and wanted to try again, especially once she had connected with Dr. Miller. He encouraged her at each of her prenatal visits, discussing a care plan to help with the inverted nipple issue.

Siobhan's waters broke the next day, and she called Dr. Miller, who advised her to come to the hospital. Shortly after settling in to her room, Siobhan began having regular contractions. Dr. Miller arrived and examined her to confirm that her water had broken, but she had not yet dilated. They talked about a care plan, including intermittent monitoring and pain-management choices. Siobhan, at ease with this now familiar doctor, joked, "I thought the baby would come right now, since you're already here!" She talked about how awful the pain was for her with her first labor and was emphatic that this time she wanted more help with that, no matter how fast the labor progressed. Dr. Miller asked her to specifically guide him and the nurse about what to do to help her cope.

After a few hours of alternately resting, walking, or rocking, with the doctor in and out of the room offering encouragement, Siobhan asked for pain medication as she was more uncomfortable and now 3 cm dilated. Dr. Miller spent time between contractions reviewing again her choices. Siobhan had brief relief from a parenteral narcotic, and two hours later asked for an epidural. She had dilated another 2 cm. After the anesthetic took effect, Siobhan was so comfortable that she slept for an hour. Stronger contractions and an urge to push wakened her, and Dr. Miller checked her and found that she was fully dilated. After about 10 minutes, Siobhan gradually pushed out baby Katie with gentle pushes guided by Dr. Miller, who passed her directly to Siobhan's belly while Danny Sr. cut the cord. Siobhan, smiling and laughing throughout the delivery, felt amazed by the difference between her two labor experiences less than one year apart.

Within minutes of baby Katie's birth, Siobhan put her to breast, with the nurse and Dr. Miller offering suggestions about her nipples. Over the first 24 hours, Siobhan's postpartum nurses taught her to use breast shells between feedings and other techniques to evert her nipples. Katie's vigorous suckling was still more painful than Siobhan expected, and she really did not want to end up with all the tubing and gadgets that she had briefly tried with Danny Jr. Using the pump hurt, too, but she kept trying while in the hospital.

On the morning of Siobhan's discharge from the hospital, Danny came in with the car seat. At just that moment Dr. Miller came in to do her postpartum check. He greeted Danny with a big smile and said, "Well, perfect timing. Now that I have you both here, let's talk about the important thing – sex!" Siobhan and Danny both laughed.

"So what were you two planning to do this time?" the doctor asked, still smiling.

"I guess condoms didn't work so well, this last time around," said Danny.

"I was thinking about an IUD," offered Siobhan. "I'm afraid of gaining weight with the shot."

"Can't you feel that thing if it's in there?" asked Danny. "I mean, couldn't *I* feel that thing?" he added sheepishly.

"Good question," responded Dr. Miller, proceeding to explain about IUDs and their strings. After a brief discussion, the couple agreed that Siobhan would use progesterone-only oral contraceptives until she could have an IUD insertion at her postpartum exam.

On the first night at home with Katie, Siobhan was in tears each time she tried to nurse, and Danny Sr. tried to reassure her but wondered if this just was not going to work. They ended up trying a bottle so that Siobhan could sleep. Two days later, at the early office newborn visit, Dr. Miller's nurse noted both Siobhan's tears and Katie's loss of weight and pointed this out to the doctor just before he entered the room. He reviewed what Siobhan had tried and how Katie was otherwise well; Siobhan was ashamed to admit that they had already supplemented with a bottle, feeling that she had let down herself and the doctor. As he re-examined her breasts and watched the stress of feeding, Dr. Miller commented, "You've worked really hard another time to make this work. That's one of your strengths as a mom – you don't give up easily in situations where many women would give up sooner. One of your other strengths is to recognize when things aren't going well, when other options are needed. You're not a failure if you switch to formula."

Susan

Susan was a 36-year-old nurse practitioner and athlete who ran 40 miles a week and regularly competed in half-marathons and triathlons. She made an initial appointment for well-woman care at a family practice that had a strong orientation toward women's health. She felt comfortable at her initial visit with her family physician, Judith Peters (whom she chose for her reputation for woman-centeredness), who inquired in an open way about her sexual orientation. Susan freely told Judith that she was in a long-term committed relationship with Geri, a woman who taught at a local college. They were thinking about getting pregnant in the near future.

A few months later Susan and Geri came in for an appointment to talk more about getting pregnant. Susan had decided to be the one to try to get pregnant. Through their lesbian community they learned quite a bit about sperm banks and other related issues. Susan kept records of her menstrual cycle and finally one month was able to detect her luteinizing hormone (LH) surge using an ovulation predictor kit. They felt ready to pursue getting pregnant. Judith referred them to a colleague in the city who did donor insemination as part of her practice, and invited Susan to return for prenatal care once she became pregnant.

Susan and Geri considered using a sperm bank that had "identity release donors," but eventually decided that they would use a particular anonymous donor because they preferred the physical characteristics of that donor. Susan and Geri thought carefully about whom to tell regarding their efforts to get pregnant, and decided to tell Susan's sister and Geri's parents, who responded with the enthusiasm that Susan and Geri had anticipated.

It took eight cycles for Susan to get pregnant, longer than they were expecting, and somewhat longer than average. During that time they found resources about the emotional strain of dealing with infertility, as well as the support of lesbian mothers who had struggled with the process. Susan worried that her athletic training might be impacting on her fertility. Just before she decided not to train for the next local marathon she finally became pregnant. She returned to Judith's practice for ongoing prenatal care, and appreciated the acceptance that she and Geri experienced from the staff, as well as Judith and the other providers.

In the first few weeks of her pregnancy Susan felt tired enough that she cut down on her total running, but continued to run shorter distances several days a week and to do yoga to stay flexible. By about seven weeks she started having more morning nausea. She kept a sports drink and crackers next to her bed to eat before she arose, but most days still ended up vomiting after any more breakfast. She tried ginger tea and acupressure bands in hopes of feeling better.

By the time she was 16 weeks pregnant, however, Susan was slowing down a bit, noticing her growing uterus now halfway up to her umbilicus, and feeling somewhat uncomfortable with pelvic pressure while running. At her prenatal visit at this time, Judith asked about exercise and encouraged Susan to continue with whatever level felt comfortable to her. They agreed on a screening ultrasound for a fetal survey.

When Susan registered by phone for the ultrasound, the hospital clerk became very flustered when Susan offered a "second mom" to list, rather than "father of baby." The phone clerk put Susan on hold and called her supervisor. When the supervisor came to the phone he apologized, saying, "The clerk didn't know what to do because the computer doesn't have that category."

Susan and Geri gradually told their family and friends about the pregnancy. Susan was relieved to get support from her parents, whom she feared would react the way they did when she first came out to them 10 years ago. In fact, after Susan told her mom, her mother wept happily about the prospects of being a grandmother and embraced Geri for the first time. As expected, Geri's brother reacted by sending Susan a letter with quotes from the Bible to justify his disapproval.

As her body revealed her pregnancy more and more, Susan also had to decide when to come out to strangers and colleagues who casually asked how her husband was doing with the pregnancy. She realized that she would likely face the same kind of assumptions in the future when she was out in public with her baby. She decided to confer with some of her lesbian mom friends to hear how they handled such situations in front of their children.

Once past the first-trimester nausea, Susan felt much stronger and more comfortable, but then in her early third trimester started noticing that she felt short of breath with slight activity. When she reported this at her routine prenatal visit, Judith asked her both about potential danger signs such as chest pain or leg swelling, and also framed the evaluation within a knowledge of Susan's experience. Judith knew that Susan was an athlete for whom physical endurance was especially important and who was not expecting to feel physically challenged by the changes of pregnancy. Susan worried that her breathing symptoms meant that her physical stamina would take longer to return after pregnancy. Knowing this, Judith addressed her frustrations and fears directly: "You sound frustrated by not being able to do as much as you would like to or are used to, because you get short of breath. Are you worried that this means something more serious or more permanent than this current stage of pregnancy?"

Judith also further described the problem by sharing further information about how she thought through possible diagnoses. "Certainly when women have trouble breathing during pregnancy, I think about both common issues such as the ways that pregnancy hormones change your breathing patterns or how the growth of your uterus makes it harder to take a deep breath. I also think about serious illnesses such as pneumonia, asthma, a heart problem, or a blood clot. At this point, based on what you are telling me about other related symptoms, my sense is that your breathing symptoms are related to the normal changes of pregnancy."

Susan also found the late-trimester weight gain and other physical changes of pregnancy especially hard to tolerate. The stretch marks made her feel ugly, and she worried that she would not be able to lose the weight after the baby was born. She liked that Judith did not overemphasize her weight at each visit, encouraged her overall healthy eating habits, and referred her to a pregnancy-related yoga class. But when her feet started to swell at 36 weeks, so that her favorite shoes no longer fit, she wondered if she would ever see her ankles again.

In the final two months of her pregnancy Susan decided to ask Judith to refer her for a primary caesarean section. Her main expressed fear was incontinence which, she worried, would compromise her running. She had read the literature on pelvic floor relaxation and incontinence and did not want to take any chances. She had tightly controlled her diet during the pregnancy in order to avoid gaining too much weight or having a big baby. She had never had major surgery and was a bit nervous about the anesthesia, but would rather run that risk than be incontinent.

When at the 32-week visit she first mentioned this request for an elective cesarean, Judith began asking more details about her past medical and social history. Eventually, with careful, gentle inquiry, Judith elicited that Susan had a past history of childhood sexual abuse, and was fearful of what would happen to her in labor, feeling exposed and out of control. Judith supported Susan's insight into her own fears and took seriously both Susan's fear of incontinence and fear of being out of control in labor.

Hearing Susan's request, Judith thought back to her own obstetrical experience many years ago, which left her with significant stress incontinence; a persistent but minor annoyance in her busy and physically active life. She considered sharing this fact with Susan – who herself was a nurse practitioner – but thought the better of it. Susan, she decided, had enough on her mind. "What good would it do Susan to hear from me that incontinence is something you can live with? She would probably get even more fixated on a cesarean!"

Instead, Judith listened to Susan's fears and then with her wrote down a list of possible options and outcomes. They discussed trying to prevent macrosomia and perineal tears and trying to start Kegel exercises early postpartum. Judith suggested that Susan start doing perineal massage regularly until delivery and encouraged her to hire a doula for labor support. They talked about how different labor and delivery positions might decrease the risk of perineal laceration.

Judith offered to strip her membranes regularly after 37 weeks in hopes of preventing a post-dates labor and to consider induction by 39 to 40 weeks if Susan had not started spontaneous labor by then. Susan agreed to try a vaginal delivery under these conditions, and with Judith's help found a doula, Rachel, to assist with labor support. Susan and Geri met with Rachel and formed a strong attachment to her. At 39 weeks with her cervix already 2 cm/50% Susan came to the hospital for an oxytocin induction, with Rachel and Geri accompanying her in labor.

The labor nurse encouraged Susan to use the telemetry fetal monitor that allowed her to walk and move around more. Rachel offered numerous techniques to relieve Susan's back labor: positioning, heat, massage, the lunge,[1] and the labor ball. Susan's labor progressed steadily, but as she entered transition at 7 cm of dilation, her back labor was particularly intense and starting to overwhelm her. Judith suggested the injection of sterile water around the sacrum as an option.[2-4] Judith did this procedure while Rachel stood at Susan's head and helped her stay focused on Geri during the stinging of the injections. After half an hour, Susan's waters broke spontaneously, and she felt a strong urge to push. Judith asked permission to examine her and found that her cervix was not quite fully dilated. Rachel helped her find more comfortable positions and blow through a few more contractions until the anterior lip finally disappeared. After 40 minutes of pushing, during which time Rachel used warm compresses and helped Susan blow through the crowning stage to stretch the perineum better, Maxwell was born, with Susan having no perineal tears.

Susan chose to go home on her first postpartum day, feeling confident about breastfeeding and about home support. She was surprised to find that climbing the stairs to her bedroom the first day home was more tiring than she expected, and she spent most of the first few days letting Geri bring her meals and getting out of bed just to rock the baby or use the bathroom. Every time she coughed, sneezed, or lifted even the baby, she involuntarily leaked urine; the leaking made her feel particularly desperate since she she it had been her main preoccupation about vaginal birth to begin with. The visiting nurse who came to check her and the baby recommended that she start doing Kegel exercises right away. She continued to feel stiff and sore with stair climbing but was anxious to get back to some physical exercise so by one week postpartum tried to go out for a short walk with the baby briefly each day.

Sylvie

Sylvie was a 25-year-old Albanian woman in her first pregnancy. She and her husband Viktor came in for an urgent visit where Dr. Mercedes Burman, her family doctor, found Sylvie crying. "I have lost my baby," she murmured as tears rolled down her cheeks. Viktor explained that she had missed her period for two months and then, two days previously, she had lot of cramping and bleeding, and "lost the baby."

Knowing that miscarriages could be significant loss events, equivalent to the death of a child, Dr. Burman wondered how their cultural background might affect their interpretation of the pregnancy and their experience of its loss. Might Sylvie or Viktor blame themselves for the loss? Might they fear they couldn't get pregnant again? Dr. Burman knew from previous visits that Sylvie felt disrespected by her in-laws and wondered how the miscarriage might affect her status in the family. After consoling Sylvie for a few minutes, Dr. Burman said, "Losing a pregnancy is very, very sad. And hard, too, in different ways. Can you tell me what is the hardest part of losing the baby for you?"

Sylvie dried her eyes and replied, "The hardest part? "I am a failure . . . I can not even have a baby for my husband." She began to cry again. Viktor put his arm around Sylvie and murmured to her in Albanian.

After a few moments, Dr. Burman provided some factual information about miscarriages, and then said, "Sylvie, I don't think you are a failure. You came to a new country and learned English and got a job. You have lived very far away from your family with only Viktor's support. You got pregnant and then handled a miscarriage at home when many women would not have been able to do that. You are a very strong and competent woman. You will get through this and then a baby will come." Sylvie offered a small smile back.

Over the next year, Sylvie's self-esteem suffered because Viktor's family had made it clear that they did not think she was good enough for him. When she became pregnant again, she was relieved that she carried her healthy second pregnancy to term, but progressed slowly when she went into labor. Despite analgesia, oxytocin, epidural anesthesia, and adequate contractions, the baby did not descend. Sylvie was exhausted, and Viktor was fearful. He wanted his wife safe and wanted the doctors to do something. Dr. Burman recommended a cesarean section, and Dr. Diamond, the obstetrical consultant, agreed. Just as they were all readying to enter the operating room, Sylvie's bilingual cousin Anna arrived, and Sylvie asked the nurse if Anna could also be in the operating room to help translate. The nurse discussed this with the consultant who agreed to have both Viktor and Anna in the OR as long as they kept out of the anesthesiologist's way. The surgery was uncomplicated, and a healthy baby girl, Elisabeth, was delivered. Anna held Sylvie's hand while Viktor stood near the newborn table to watch his daughter.

The next day Dr. Burman reviewed for both parents the need for the cesarean. She framed it as the problem of a small Albanian woman who ate a good American diet having a baby too big to fit through her bones that had developed when she lived in a country with less food. Sylvie quickly established a good breastfeeding pattern and recovered from the surgery without incident. On the day of discharge, Dr. Burman underscored her strength and resilience in labor, her excellent lactation, and her good healing. She commented to Viktor in Sylvie's earshot, "What a strong and powerful wife you chose!" They both beamed.

A few months later, they took Elisabeth back to Albania, where Sylvie experienced the emotional glow and social status of successful motherhood.

Tonya

Tonya Butler was a 28-year-old G4P3 African-American woman with a high school education who came for her first prenatal visit at 14 weeks to her newly assigned provider, Dr. Simon Miller. Dr. Miller noted that Tonya was smoking almost a pack a day. Her previous obstetrical history revealed that her first baby, born at term, weighed six pounds (2.7 kg); her second was born at 35 weeks weighing three pounds (1.4 kg) and then died of sudden infant death syndrome at four months. Her third child was born at 37 weeks weighing five pounds (2.3 kg). Dr. Miller thought that Tonya was again at risk for a preterm birth and possibly a small-for-gestational-age (SGA) infant. The only modifiable risk factor that he knew of was her smoking.

Dr. Miller asked Tonya if she thought she might want to use the prenatal period as a good time to give up smoking since it was harmful to the fetus.

Tonya said, "All you doctors are on my case about the smoking. I smoked for all three of my pregnancies. After all the stuff I went through, it's no wonder I smoke. They tried to say my baby died of SIDS because I smoke. But my other two babies were fine."

Dr. Miller was unsure how to respond to this and did not want Tonya to think that he, too, blamed her for the SIDS death. He felt dismissed by Tonya; he also felt that she did not trust him. He also saw why she seemed so distrustful.

He decided to take on this issue of trust directly. "Look, I know it must be hard to have to switch to a new provider; and I know doctors nag a lot about cigarettes, so it's no surprise to me that you might find it hard to trust me. I will try hard to earn your trust and to be here for you. What kinds of things are important to you in your prenatal care?"

This was the first time anyone had ever asked Tonya this question and she was astounded. "What do I care about? Me? Well, for one thing, I hate waiting. I want to get in, get checked, and get out. No sitting around waiting for hours. That's what's important for me." Dr. Miller said he would make that his first priority and, after the visit, made a notation for Tonya to have the first prenatal slot each month so that she would have the least likelihood of waiting.

She came promptly for all her visits and by seven months was measurably more open toward him.

"I've been thinking about what you said – about the smoking."

"Yes?" inquired Dr. Miller.

"Well, my other kids are nagging me and my boyfriend wants me to stop, too, so I have been thinking about it," Tonya replied.

"Would you like some help with that?" Dr. Miller offered.

"Yeah, do you have some ideas for me?" Tonya asked.

Dr. Miller reviewed some of the specific behavior changes that Tonya could do to decrease her smoking, and Tonya thought a few of them might be worth trying. She said she would make some attempts before the next visit.

Tonya slowly learned to trust Dr. Miller through working on smoking cessation, although she still had her doubts about doctors and institutions. She told him at the beginning of the third trimester that she wanted her epidural with the first contraction. He tried to talk about other options for pain relief, but she interrupted him, saying, "C'mon Dr. Miller, you've never had a baby, I don't want any pain. I got enough to deal with in my life."

He acknowledged, "Yes, you've had a lot of painful stuff in your life. Tell me about how you dealt with pain in your other labors."

She reported that in her first labor she had been induced for pre-eclampsia and had found the pain of "that contraction medicine" unbearable from early on because she had to stay in the hospital bed; the epidural had let her sleep even though she agreed that it probably made her labor somewhat longer. For her second pregnancy her water broke at 35 weeks without labor, and she had to get induced again. She recalled getting her epidural around the same time the oxytocin started. Her third labor came on quickly at 37 weeks, her waters breaking at home with strong pains coming quickly after that, so that by the time she arrived at the hospital she was "too late" to get the epidural and then had to push without it and felt "I just barely survived that." She said now, "I'm coming with the first contraction this time. I don't want to feel anything."

Dr. Miller knew that Tonya was likely to have a short labor and with support could easily have another delivery without an epidural. However, he recognized how strongly Tonya felt about getting an epidural for this birth. Part of really listening to her, and hearing her, was accepting this choice even though it was not the one he would recommend. He recognized that Tonya's ability to control this issue, like having control over waiting at the office, gave meaning to what "woman-centered" meant in caring for Tonya. Contrary to his usual practice, he smiled and suggested to her, "You'd better come in right away this time so we can get that epidural started as soon as we are sure that it's labor."

Zoë

During her second week in practice, Larisa encountered a 17-year-old woman Zoë who had decided she wanted to have an abortion. The teen chose Larisa over the older partners in the practice as she thought the young doctor might be more supportive of her decision. During medical school, Larisa always thought she would be a family physician who would offer medication abortion to her patients as part of her general primary care practice. She enjoyed an opportunity to see abortions covered by national health insurance in Canada during an elective rotation in women's health in Toronto. But she became caught up learning so many other things during residency and never found a mentor to help her figure out how to integrate abortion care into her practice. In her new practice, Larisa learned quickly about the problems that women faced in her community around reproductive choice. Her practice was in a conservative county where the school board had consistently opposed sex education in the schools. The area was 50 miles from a metropolitan area where abortion was available, in a state with strict laws about teenagers and parental consent and with a state legislature considering even stricter regulations about abortion in the future. Larisa learned that teenagers were concerned about confidentiality in obtaining birth control at local pharmacies, had trouble getting to the city for birth control or abortion services, and lacked solid understanding of their contraceptive choices. Uninsured patients were unable to afford either medication or surgery for abortion and had few options. Larisa spent a long time trying to figure out how to help Zoë with the unwanted pregnancy. Although she could not yet offer the service in her practice, she was able to share what she did know about abortion with Zoë.

THE PROVIDERS

Woman-Centered Community Family Practice:
Larisa Foster, M.D.
Judith Peters, M.D.
Usha Rao, M.D.
Helen McSweeney, C.N.M.

Obstetrician Consultant:
Greg Diamond, M.D.

Community Health Center:
Simon Miller, M.D.
Jonathan Rosen, M.D.
Mercedes Burman, M.D.
Adelle Epps, M.D.
Harmony Lott, N.P.

University hospital in urban setting where Larisa trained:
Mary Thibeault, M.D., Family medicine resident

Other practitioners:
Maureen
Shereen
Sofia Khan
Amy

Woman-Centered Community Family Practice

Dr. Larisa Foster is a family doctor who has just finished her residency and is joining Woman-Centered Community Family Practice (WCCFP). She entered residency with a focus on women's health and empowerment but has since learned that many women live in areas where they have little control over options in contraception and abortion. Larisa trained in high-tech interventional obstetrics but worries that she has not learned how to pay attention to the woman herself during prenatal care, labor, delivery, and the postpartum period. She is not sure she really understands about women's issues in lactation, and has not yet had children of her own so cannot refer to her own experience. She wonders how to be woman-centered with women from different cultures and women whose life experiences are as different from each other as a pregnant 16-year-old who has run away from home and a married professional woman having a baby in her thirties. Larisa is looking for help in forming her own personal strategies in working with women now that she is out of training and can shape her own practice pattern.

During her second week in practice, Larisa encountered a 17-year-old woman Zoë who had decided she wanted to have an abortion. The teen chose Larisa over the older partners in the practice as she thought the young doctor might be more supportive of her decision. During medical school, Larisa always thought she would be a family physician who would offer medication abortion to her patients as part of her general primary care practice. She enjoyed an opportunity to see abortions covered by national health insurance in Canada during an elective rotation in women's health in Toronto. But she became caught up learning so many other things during residency and never found a mentor to help her figure out how to integrate abortion care into her practice. In her new practice, Larisa learned quickly about the problems that women faced in her community around reproductive choice. Her practice was in a conservative county where the school board had consistently opposed sex education in the schools. The area was 50 miles from a metropolitan area where abortion was available, in a state with strict laws about teenagers and parental consent and with a state legislature considering even stricter regulations about abortion in the future. Larisa learned that teenagers were concerned about confidentiality in obtaining birth control at local pharmacies, had trouble getting to the city for birth control or abortion services, and lacked solid understanding of their contraceptive choices. Uninsured patients were unable to afford either medication or surgery for abortion and had few options. Larisa spent a long time trying to figure out how to help Zoë with the unwanted pregnancy. Although she could not yet offer the service in her practice, she was able to share what she did know about abortion with Zoë.

Larisa trained at a family medicine program where her prenatal and obstetrical training took place at a large public tertiary hospital with over 3000 births a year, mostly attended by obstetricians, with a small group of family physicians including Larisa's residency program faculty also offering intrapartum care. Larisa's experience with the obstetricians involved a model of care in which most of the intrapartum care was done intermittently by busy nurses in an understaffed environment. The labor triage area had one room with several beds separated by curtains where women were assessed before admission. Virtually all laboring women received continuous electronic fetal monitoring once in active labor. The hospital offered around the clock anesthesia coverage with separate obstetric anesthesia staff and residents, reaching a 90% epidural rate. The overall cesarean rate for low-risk women was 25% and climbing. When Larisa entered her new practice after residency, she chose a community hospital known for its lower intervention rates, but was surprised there to learn that the hospital was about to stop offering a trial of labor after cesarean due to risk-management concerns. In her new practice, Larisa consciously chooses to go back to basics and adopt a woman-centered approach to normal pregnancy. She hopes that choosing woman-centeredness as her principal value will enable her to develop the finest care for her patients.

During her residency, Larisa structured her prenatal and postpartum care using standardized protocols in her residency clinic. These prompted her to give anticipatory guidance during the last few weeks of prenatal care about specific postpartum issues such as breastfeeding and postpartum depression. Her clinic's routine was to see newborns within one to two weeks of hospital discharge and to see mothers back for routine postpartum care at about six weeks after delivery. She is interested in finding ways to increase breastfeeding duration and in doing better screening for postpartum depression.

Larisa and her partners have decided that whoever is assigned to do hospital rounds each day will see all the new mothers and babies, rather than having the primary provider try to re-arrange office scheduling. On busy days, however, the rounding provider might have to juggle labor triage with postpartum rounds and an expectation that he or she will return to the office by late morning to see patients there. Wanting to promote breastfeeding and prevent postpartum depression, Larisa struggles to personalize her care within the time constraints of these clinical demands, as she recognizes that some women need very little advice and are ready to go home in a few hours, while others have endless questions and need three or four days and multiple support people to get comfortable with their new role. While recognizing the benefits of the longitudinal framework of monthly prenatal visits, Larisa nonetheless finds that an occasional woman with a complicated personal history, for instance with a history of abuse, requires more time both in the office and during labor and postpartum to feel confident and safe with all the life changes. These issues come up again once Larisa is seeing newborns in the office within the first week when she finds that many of the new mothers have already faced so much breastfeeding difficulty that they have stopped exclusively nursing. Some mothers at this visit have few needs, while others need extensive visits to fully address their lactation challenges and depression risks.

Larisa finds that she can join an electronic discussion group (mcdg@list.cfpc.ca) that brings together hundreds of North American maternity care providers who are questioning the "evidence." With members of this group, she learns to re-examine the individual studies that make up the meta-analyses – in order to determine if study conditions match her clinical reality. Otherwise, she fears that uncritical incorporation of the results from meta-analyses will continue to push her clinical practice into increasingly technical interventions.

One of Larisa's friends from residency joined the Indian Health Service (IHS) and provided comprehensive care at one of their hospitals. When Larisa went to visit on vacation, she found that whole extended Native American families came to the hospital for births in their family, and that a sizable group of family members were allowed into the delivery room. Larisa wondered why this more flexible policy was not available to her for the families in her practice. She decided to find out how to change the policy at her hospital. Larisa attended a series of workshops on the patient-centered method and is very interested in applying the method to her woman-centered practice. But at times it feels like an uphill battle. In the office she faces competing demands for her time and the expectation that her prenatal appointments will be brief checks; at the hospital she feels torn between the hospital and the office; in her call system she has to address how to achieve balance in between her desire to provide continuity to her own patients and her need for time for her own life – exercise, rest, relationships, and ultimately her own desires around childbearing.

Larisa has to find an answer for her pregnant patients when they bring up the oft-asked question, "Will you be there when I'm in labor?" She realizes that careful explanation of her call coverage system is essential to woman-centered care. First she asks, "What are you expecting about who will see you in labor? How do you feel about my partner being there? How important is it to you that you meet the person ahead of time?" After learning how the woman feels about this issue, Larisa then can address her individual needs with an explanation of her call system such as, "My partners and I take turns being on call, so that someone is always available to be with women in labor. If it is not my turn, my partner will see you and evaluate your labor. She will try to reach me to let me know what is going on, and if I am able to, I try very hard to come to my own patients' deliveries. However, I cannot always do that."

Larisa feels very compatible with the style of her three partners in delivering maternity care, but the practice is growing, and her partners would like to consider joining call pools with the local community health center (CHC) so that call would be every seventh night and every seventh weekend. Larisa feels ambivalent about the call merger because she is uncertain if the providers at the CHC fully share her woman-centered delivery practices. She is also uncertain if some of her patients will accept the possibility of a male provider during labor and delivery. Larisa also has mixed feelings about cross-covering the low-income and immigrant population at the community health center – positive feelings because she enjoyed this interesting population during residency, but anxious because of the need for additional supports in social service and language. At the same time, despite her reservations about the call merger, Larisa is finding it challenging to be on call so often. She is not sure if in the larger call pool she would feel obliged to go to the hospital for "her own" patients and end up just as overcommitted as she is now in the every-fourth-night pattern.

With consultants Larisa's experience of teamwork is mixed. When Greg is on call as her consultant, he is able to join her smoothly in providing consultation in a woman-centered way, collaborating easily. Other obstetricians who help back him up, however, express annoyance: why is she consulting so early in labor? Or in antenatal care? Why is she consulting so late? Why is she consulting at all?

Larisa feels she has input at the office about who is hired to become part of the office team caring for patients, but at the hospital finds that expectations about teamwork vary widely in her work with nurses. On labor and delivery, sometimes she and the nurse engage easily in the joint task of facilitating a woman-centered birth, but at other times, Larisa feels that the nurse is disapproving or critical, and acting primarily to get her own required work done. Sometimes Larisa gets "vibes" that her woman-centered style is inconvenient, annoying, or even interfering with nursing responsibilities (e.g. for the mother to hold the baby for an extended period after birth interferes with banding, footprints, vitamin K injection, hepatitis B immunization, administration of antibiotic eye ointment, and a host of other required nursing tasks immediately postpartum in the hospital environment). For their part, the nurses want to finish these duties before transferring the woman's care to the postpartum nurse, who will not have time to attend to these clinical care issues. Likewise, Larisa feels that not all staff on the postpartum floor or in the nursery are fully supportive of the Baby Friendly Initiative, as she often finds formula bottles in the crib when a mother has been having trouble initiating breastfeeding. Again she worries that being woman-centered takes too much time for overextended nursing staff.

Dr. Judith Peters is a family doctor who established a woman-centered family practice and began providing maternity care in that setting over 30 years ago. She raised her family in this community and is tightly connected to many families in the practice. She has made choices along the way – to continue obstetrics, to offer comprehensive birth control to all women, including teenagers, to make home visits, to stop practicing full-time in order to teach in the local family medicine residency. She is eagerly looking forward to a new generation of family doctors to join her in practice. With her experience comes a calmness that leads the nurses at the hospital to respect her low-tech approach, even in a very high-tech environment. In her recruitment letter to Larisa, Judith wrote, "When I choose to get up from sleep and attend the second delivery of a woman whose own birth I attended 30 years ago, I know I am participating in a rare and special aspect of the cross-generational relationship in family medicine. Even though I am confident in the care given by my partners, nothing short of being several hundred miles away would keep me from that birth."

Judith Peters and Simon Miller are old friends and colleagues. They had jointly worked on initiatives to foster progressive maternity care practices in the community and at the hospital. Both of them are looking forward to the call merger as they have been doing every fourth night call for many years. Nevertheless, Simon confides in Judith that he worries that not everyone in her practice is as enthusiastic about refugee and immigrant care, and the non-English-speaking population, as those at the CHC. Judith acknowledges this reality.

"What about setting up some cross-cultural sessions for our folks?" she proposes. "And what about the prison women? And the addiction program? We're going to need help learning to do right by those women as well."

"You're right – I can do some extra backup for those programs to help with the transition," Simon offers. "And we'll come up with some trainings – we could even invite the maternity nurses. Do Tuesday lunchtimes still work for you?"

Dr. Usha Rao is a second-generation Indian-American both of whose parents were obstetricians in India. They migrated to a rural area in Canada where they continue to practice obstetrics with a low-income population. Usha grew up hearing her parents' conversations about obstetrics and also absorbing their commitment to service. She had thought she would become an obstetrician as well, but when she got to medical school decided that she liked taking care of children and teenagers, too, and decided to go into family medicine incorporating obstetrics. She was eager to join Woman-Centered Community Family Practice with its supportive environment and woman-centered focus. She is married to a neurologist and is balancing her practice with raising two small children.

Helen McSweeney is an Australian-trained nurse midwife who migrated to the USA because of her partner and who practiced at an alternative birthing center (ABC) before joining Judith at WCCFP. She has 10 years of experience attending births and brings many skills in non-pharmacological pain relief to labor management. She has some anxiety about returning to the hospital environment, but wanted a larger call pool so that she would have more day time with her children, an opportunity to teach, and the hope of establishing an ABC near to the hospital. She is a lesbian and lives with her partner Tami and their three children. She is delighted when Larisa decides to join their practice.

Obstetrician Consultant

Dr. Greg Diamond is an obstetrician with 15 years of experience who consults for WCCFP. He comes from a family where his father was a family doctor and his mother a nurse in a small rural town. He has great respect for what family doctors do and has enjoyed his role as the obstetrical educator in the family medicine residency at the hospital. He is proud of the quality of obstetrical care delivered by family doctors in the community, many of whom he trained, and he is also proud of the collaborative relationships that have slowly grown up between the obstetricians and family physicians who now engage in a far more collaborative approach to consultation than they did when he arrived at the hospital. Greg spent time in the Peace Corps in Africa where he met his wife Edith, a British-born psychiatrist. Greg is well versed in both the possibilities for natural birth and the risks of obstetrical catastrophe for women in the Third World, and women coming from poverty settings in North America. He is involved with the international health program affiliated with the family medicine residency and has done consulting work with the World Health Organization about maternity care internationally.

Community Health Center

Dr. Simon Miller is an experienced family doctor who has worked for nearly 20 years at the community health center across town from Woman-Centered Community Family Practice. He has had a long interest in cross-cultural medicine and has worked hard to make sure that immigrants coming to the health center get culturally competent care. He has also been concerned about the extent of violence and victimization he sees in women's lives. In recent years he has become interested particularly in addiction issues and has chosen to become involved with obstetrical care at the state prison and with an innovative substance abuse program for pregnant women that follows them inside and outside the prison system.

Dr. Jonathan Rosen is a family doctor who decided after two years in practice to pursue an obstetrics fellowship so that he could perform cesarean sections, tubal ligations, dilation and curettage procedures, and abortions for the women in his care. He came to the community health center with the goal of joining a practice caring for under-served families and providing woman-centered care. His sister is a lesbian in a long-standing relationship, and he has a special interest in gay and lesbian health issues. His residency training and obstetrics fellowship also emphasized finding and applying evidence to his clinical care of patients. While reading the medical literature, he learned to look for ratings of a study's strength of evidence. In his office now, he can search quickly in the Cochrane Database of Systematic Reviews to find the latest meta-analysis of many common obstetric issues. He has learned to rely on such searches to make decisions on the spot in his busy clinical schedule. He teaches regularly in both the local community hospital family practice residency and in continuing education programs about how to read journal articles and how to stay on top of the latest evidence.

Dr. Mercedes Burman is an Argentina-born family doctor who emigrated to the USA as a teenager with her family during the troubles in Argentina in the 1970s. She chose to do a family medicine residency with a focus on family systems because of her interest in family dynamics. She kept up her obstetrical work because the population she was committed to serving, Latino immigrant families, was a young cohort busy bearing and raising children and trying to hold their lives together in the face of ethnic discrimination and economic stress.

Dr. Adelle Epps is an African-American family doctor from Chicago. Both her parents were teachers; their roots are in South Carolina where her grandparents were born. She trained in an urban family medicine program in Toronto and, because of a long-standing interest in African women's health, including female genital mutilation, did advanced obstetrical training at a hospital in Toronto where many African immigrants deliver. She is active in the local Academy of Family Physicians and hopes to become a leader in a national family medicine organization.

Harmony Lott is an African-Caribbean obstetrical nurse practitioner. Her grandmother had been a lay midwife in Jamaica. She went to nursing school in Jamaica and then, after her children were teenagers, immigrated to the USA and went back to school to become a nurse practitioner with a focus on obstetrics. She would have liked to do deliveries, too, but did not feel that her health would permit her being on call and withstanding 24 hours without sleep. She has high blood pressure and is overweight. Her daughter is a pastor in the local church, and she moved to town and joined the CHC practice to be closer to her grandchildren.

University Hospital Family Medicine Residency

Dr. Mary Thibeault is a third-year family medicine resident. She is uncertain whether she will include maternity care in her future practice. She believes that patients should take responsibility for their own health. She would like to work with an educated population in a private practice because she feels that patients in that setting will be more likely to take care of themselves than the low-income and immigrant patients she sees in the clinic at the university hospital. Her supervisors have worked with her to be less judgmental but when she is tired and stressed she falls back into being critical of others.

REFERENCES

1 Simkin P. *The Labor Progress Handbook: early interventions to prevent and treat dystocia.* 2nd ed. New York: Blackwell; 2005.

2 Anderson FWJ, Johnson CT. Complementary and alternative medicine in obstetrics. *Int J Gynaecol Obstet.* 2005; **91**: 116–24.

3 Huntley AL, Coon JT, Ernst E. Complementary and alternative medicine for labor pain: a systematic review. *Am J Obstet Gynecol.* 2004; **191**: 36–44.

4 Labrecque M, Nouwen A, Bergeron M, *et al.* A randomized controlled trial of nonpharmacologic approaches for relief of low back pain during labor. *J Fam Pract.* 1999; **48**: 259–63.

Contributors

Louise Acheson, M.D., has practiced family medicine, including maternity care, since completion of her family medicine residency at the University of Washington in 1979. She has birthed and helped to raise two daughters. She has remained involved with free-standing birth centers, first in small group family practice in Seattle, then as an advisor for the Amish birth center in Middlefield, Ohio. For the past 25 years, Louise has taught family medicine and women's health at Case Western Reserve University School of Medicine. She is now a professor working on research to develop and study the use of computerized family history tools for cancer prevention. She also enjoys a position as one of the founding Associate Editors of the *Annals of Family Medicine*.

Pamela Adelstein, M.D., has worked in urban community health centers in central and eastern Massachusetts since graduating from medical school in 1997. She speaks Spanish, Portuguese, and some French with her patients. She completed a 300-hour Acupuncture for Physicians course at Harvard University in 2007–8, and incorporates acupuncture into her patient care. She also enjoys teaching, and was previously the Assistant Residency Director for the University of Massachusetts Family Medicine Residency Program. Currently Pam precepts residents and medical students from Boston University School of Medicine. She is also grateful to have experienced woman-centered maternity care from the patient's perspective, having birthed two beautiful daughters at home.

Katharine Barnard, M.D., is a family doctor practicing in Worcester, Massachusetts. She trained at the University of Massachusetts, graduating from residency in 2003. She is currently the medical director of a small clinic providing care in a predominantly Hispanic, low-income, urban neighborhood of Worcester. Her clinical interests include women's health including maternity care, care of multigenerational families, and providing culturally competent care to Latino patients. Katharine is also an Assistant Professor at UMass-Worcester, teaching family medicine to residents and medical students.

Joan M. Bedinghaus, M.D., graduated from Harvard Medical School in 1982 and completed a family practice residency at Cleveland Metropolitan General Hospital. She taught in residency programs at the University of Massachusetts and Case Western Reserve University. At the Medical College of Wisconsin in Milwaukee, where she currently teaches and practices family and community medicine, she was a member of the Genetics in Primary Care Initiative of the Human Genome Project, which designed curricula to incorporate advances in genetics into everyday practice.

Ambareen A. Bharmal, M.D., graduated from the New Jersey Medical School, UMDNJ, in 2003. She then completed her residency at the Worcester Family Medicine Residency Program, University of Massachusetts, in 2006. Since then, she has been working as a family medicine physician with under-served communities in a community health center setting. Her first position was in Wilmington, Delaware as a general practitioner, during which time she practiced full-scope family medicine including maternity care. For the past year, Ambar has been working for an under-served community in Harlem, New York City. In addition to continuing with her primary care responsibilities, she also serves as the Associate Medical Director for the Helen B. Atkinson Health Center, a federally qualified health center with the organization Community Healthcare Network.

Martha Carlough, M.D., M.P.H., is a family physician with additional training in both clinical and public health aspects of maternal and child health and over 10 years' experience in international health and development work. She currently serves as the Program Director for the Maternal Child Health Program at University of North Carolina Chapel Hill Department of Family Medicine, is the Medical Director for the Women's Birth and Wellness Center (the only free-standing birth center in North Carolina), and works part-time at IntraHealth International, where she serves as the Safe Motherhood Clinical Advisor. Martha is passionate about safe and gentle childbirth worldwide, the formation of new families, and the role of the family physician in making this possible. She loves teaching in a wide variety of situations, including: training skilled birth attendants in Africa and Asia, teaching global health to UNC medical students, and training family medicine residents in clinical settings.

Kathleen A. Culhane-Pera, M.D., M.A., is a family physician with a master's degree in anthropology. She is the Associate Medical Director of West Side Community Health Services and Adjunct Professor in the Department of Family Medicine and Community Health, University of Minnesota. As a faculty member in a family medicine residency program for 14 years, she has extensive experience in multicultural curriculum development, implementation, and evaluation. As an anthropologist and researcher, she has worked with the Hmong community in St. Paul since 1983 and has focused on improving diabetes management in the Hmong community since 2000. She is co-editor of a multicultural case story book on culturally responsive care, *Healing by Heart: clinical and ethical case stories of Hmong family and Western providers.* She lives in St. Paul, Minnesota with her husband and two teenage children.

Lori DiLorenzo, M.D., received her undergraduate degree in Neurobiology and Behavior from Cornell University in 1994, and her M.D. from the University of Pennsylvania in 1998. She completed her family medicine residency at the Lawrence

Family Medicine residency program in Lawrence, MA in 2001, where she received the Glenn O'Grady Award for her work in residency curriculum development. In 2001, she began working clinically at the Great Brook Valley Health Center in Worcester, MA. Her interests in teaching led her to share coordination of the obstetrical rotation for the University of Massachusetts Family Medicine Residency Program from 2002 to 2006, and to be an instructor for the Patient, Physician, and Society course at the University of Massachusetts Medical School. Lori is currently in clinical practice at a community health center in Gardner, MA, where she is working to develop prenatal curricula for the community and to promote breastfeeding education.

Debra Erickson-Owens, C.N.M., Ph.D., a nurse-midwife, has supported women in labor, both in-hospital and in a birth center setting, for more than 20 years. Debra has also been a midwifery educator at Georgetown University, the United States Air Force Midwifery Program in Washington, D.C., and the nurse-midwifery graduate program at the University of Rhode Island. Recently, she completed her doctoral studies and conducted a randomized controlled trial examining the effects of umbilical cord milking at the time of planned cesarean section. Currently, she is a research co-investigator of a National Institute of Nursing Research (NINR) funded grant examining the protective effects of delayed cord clamping in very preterm infants.

Krista Farey, M.D., M.S., is a Clinical Assistant Professor of Family Medicine at the University of California, Davis. She graduated from the University of California San Francisco-University of California Berkeley Joint Medical Program in 1984, and the University of Massachusetts Family Practice Residency in 1987. Krista practices and teaches family medicine and obstetrics at Richmond Health Center and Contra Contra Regional Medical Center, a county hospital in California with a family practice residency. Krista has served as medical staff president at CCRMC, and as the president of the California Physicians' Alliance. She is co-author of the text *Physiological Medicine – a clinical approach to human medical physiology* (McGraw Hill, 2000). She has been the Centering Pregnancy Program Director at Richmond Health Center since 2001.

Colleen Fogarty, M.D., M.Sc., completed her family medicine residency in 1995 at University of Rochester in Rochester, NY. During her entire career, she has practiced family medicine in community health centers in both rural and urban settings. After serving five years as Director of Psychosocial Medicine at Boston University Department of Family Medicine, Colleen returned to Rochester where she now serves as Assistant Program Director of the family medicine residency. She maintains her clinical practice at Brown Square Community Health Center, an urban clinical site, where she serves as Residency Site Director. Colleen has published empirical work on domestic violence and primary care mental health. Her creative writing includes poetry and prose, and has been published in the *Journal of Family Practice*, *Family Medicine*, and *Families, Systems, and Health*.

Josephine Fowler, M.D., M.S., FAAFP currently serves as Vice President of Academic Affairs/Chief Academic Officer at John Peter Smith (JPS) Health Network in Fort Worth, TX. She completed her residency at the Medical College of Virginia/ Blackstone Family Practice in Richmond, VA, and did fellowship training in Maternal and Child Health at Brown University, including a master's degree in community health with focus on epidemiology and biostatistics. She also completed the Executive Faculty Development program at Morehouse School of Medicine. Josephine currently serves on the Board of Directors for two community organizations, the United Way of Tarrant County as Co-Chair of the Kids Council and the Fort Worth Dallas Birthing Project as Secretary. Her community efforts in Tarrant County continue to be focused on improving the lives of under-served families and children. She has received numerous community service awards for her leadership: the Urban League's Medicine Award for Southeastern Massachusetts, Citizen of the Week by the La-Vida News, the Eminent Citizen Award from the National Sorority of Phi Delta Kappa, Inc., and the YWCA Tribute to Women in Business award.

Marji Gold, M.D., is a family physician in the Department of Family and Social Medicine at Albert Einstein College of Medicine/Montefiore Medical Center in the Bronx, NY. She has had an active full-spectrum continuity practice in a community health center for 35 years, and teaches medical students, family medicine residents, and fellows at that site. Marji is the co-coordinator of the women's health rotation for the family medicine residents. She is also the director of the Family Planning Fellowship, and was a past director of the Faculty Development Fellowship, both at AECOM.

Cathy Kamens, M.D., graduated from Mount Holyoke College, the University of Connecticut School of Medicine, and University of Massachusetts Worcester Family Medicine Residency and, in 2000, joined the faculty at University of Texas Southwestern Medical Center at Dallas, where she taught medical students and family practice residents, and coordinated the obstetrics teaching program. She moved to Toronto, Canada, with her husband and took several years off to birth and care for their children. Cathy resumed clinical practice in 2006 at Sunnybrook Health Science Center, Women's College Campus, where she continued to practice family-centered maternity care and teach residents and medical students. She has currently returned to her roots in Connecticut where she is in part-time practice at St. Francis Hospital, with maternity care and teaching at University of Connecticut School of Medicine in family medicine.

Tracy Kedian, M.D., graduated from McGill University in Montreal and the University of Massachusetts Medical School. She did her family medicine training at UMass as well and since graduation has been a member of the family medicine faculty at UMass and the Tufts University School of Medicine. Tracy practices the full breadth of family medicine including care to all ages in the hospital and health center. She serves a diverse urban population, speaking English, Spanish, Portuguese and French with her largely immigrant patients from all over the world. She particularly enjoys maternity care and teaching care of families to medical students and residents. Her research focuses upon working with medical students experiencing academic difficulty.

Clara Keegan, M.D., FAAFP is a family physician in private practice in Westford, MA. After completing residency at the University of Massachusetts Worcester Family Medicine Residency, she enjoyed an active prenatal practice for three years before backing off to focus on her own family. She maintains clinical interest in the maternal–child dyad and enjoys providing patient-centered care at all stages of life. Clara holds faculty appointments at the medical schools of the University of Massachusetts and Tufts University, and was granted the degree of Fellow of the American Academy of Family Physicians in 2009.

Michael C. Klein, M.D., C.C.F.P., F.C.F.P., F.A.A.P. (Neonatal/Perinatal), F.C.P.S., is Emeritus Professor of Family Practice at the University of British Columbia, Adjunct Professor of Family Medicine McGill University, and Senior Scientist Emeritus at The Child and Family Research Institute in Vancouver. He is best known for his work with Janusz Kaczorowski on the failure of episiotomy as a strategy to prevent perineal trauma, which is credited with contributing to a large drop in routine episiotomy use and a concurrent fall in rectal trauma. His current research includes a four-year study of the beliefs and attitudes of maternity providers and women, a British Columbia study on the role of maternity care in community sustainability in rural settings, and developing a decision-making manual to assist health administrators in low-volume maternity settings. He was head of McGill's Department of Family Medicine for 17 years, where he brought back family practice maternity care from a moribund state, and then was head of the department of family practice at Children's and Women's in Vancouver, where he worked to promote excellence in maternity and newborn practice and to develop maternity care research. He has received the Morris Wood Award for Lifetime Contributions to Primary Care Research from the North American Primary Care Research Group, Family Physician Researcher of the Year from the College of Family Physicians of Canada, the Founders Award from DONA International (the international organization of doulas) and the annual research Award from Lamaze International.

Paul Koch, M.D., M.S., is a faculty family physician with the Medical College of Wisconsin. He graduated from the University of Wisconsin Medical School and completed his family medicine residency program at the University of Massachusetts Medical School in Worcester, MA. He is a fellowship-trained family physician and has earned a M.S. in Epidemiology from Brown University. Paul directs the maternity care training at a family medicine residency program in Milwaukee, Wisconsin in an urban, under-served area. His academic interests include perinatal depression, substance use, postpartum care and operative obstetrics. Paul has been active with the Wisconsin Association for Perinatal Care, a non-profit organization that has raised awareness about perinatal mood disorders and other health issues affecting mothers and infants. He derives great satisfaction from guiding a pregnant woman through her pregnancy and delivery and then working with her and her family to help them with the medical and psychosocial adjustments of raising a child.

Anita Kostecki, M.D., completed an undergraduate degree in biology with a focus on human reproduction at Brown University, and then attended the University of Massachusetts Medical School and did her family medicine residency training at the Family Health Center of Worcester. After a year of obstetrics fellowship at Central Texas Medical Foundation in Austin, TX, she returned to Worcester and began practice at Great Brook Valley Health Center, an urban community health center, where she has provided leadership in prenatal care, colposcopy and family planning programs for a culturally diverse and socioeconomically challenged population. She also works as a part-time staff physician at Planned Parenthood League of Massachusetts. Since 2000, Anita has overseen maternity care for all pregnant inmates at Massachusetts Correctional Institute in Framingham, MA, a state prison for women. Her hospital-based work includes intrapartum care, normal and cesarean deliveries, tubal ligation and dilation and curettage. She serves as the Director of Maternal and Newborn Inpatient Services for Family Medicine at UMass Memorial Health Care.

Lawrence M. Leeman, M.D., M.P.H., completed his family medicine residency at the University of New Mexico and then practiced for six years on the Zuni Reservation in New Mexico. He then completed a fellowship in obstetrics at the University of Rochester (NY) School of Medicine. Larry is now director of the Family Practice Maternal and Child Health clinical service and fellowship at the University of New Mexico. He is co-medical director of the mother–baby unit at the University of New Mexico Hospital in Albuquerque, NM. He is the managing editor of the Advanced Life Support in Obstetrics (ALSO) curriculum of the American Academy of Family Practice and co-editor of the Global ALSO curriculum. Larry's areas of research include rural maternity care, pelvic floor outcomes after childbirth, family planning and vaginal birth after cesarean.

Richard Long, M.D., received his undergraduate degree in Biochemistry from Vassar College and his medical degree from Jefferson Medical College. He completed his family medicine residency at Brown University, and after private practice for two years did a fellowship in Maternal and Child Health at Brown. Rick has been a community health center medical director, the director of the MCH fellowship program, and chairman of a bioethics committee, and has continuously integrated the provision of maternity care into his clinical practice. He has worked extensively in urban community health center networks, and internationally in Nepal, Honduras, Dominican Republic, and Lesotho helping establish the rudiments of primary care. After 15 years in the family medicine residency at Brown, Rick moved to Boston University School of Medicine in 2006 as Clinical Associate Professor of Family Medicine. His research interests include provision of care to under-served populations, spiritual dimensions of healthcare, and collaborative, interdisciplinary care.

Judith S. Mercer, D.N.Sc., C.N.M., F.A.C.N.M., is a Clinical Professor at the University of Rhode Island. She is the former Director of the Nurse-Midwifery Program at Georgetown University and at the University of Rhode Island where she remains on faculty. Judith has a successful research program underway on gentle birth practices and especially the issue of cord clamping time. She is funded by the National Institutes of Health for her research on cord clamping time in preterm infants. She has presented her work nationally and internationally and is widely published. She is a fellow of the American College of Nurse Midwives.

Deana Midmer, R.N., Ed.D, is an Associate Professor and Research Scholar in the Department of Family & Community Medicine, University of Toronto. She is an educational researcher looking at ways to change healthcare provider behavior. Dr. Midmer is the Principal Investigator for the PRIMA (Pregnancy-Related Issues in the Management of Addictions) Project. The PRIMA Project, funded by Health Canada, conducts Train-the-Trainer sessions around problematic substance use in pregnancy in different parts of Canada. Participants attending these sessions return to their home communities to provide knowledge transfer to their colleagues. Significant changes in self-reported clinical competence and confidence have been demonstrated.

Cathleen Morrow, M.D., originally trained as a midwife and then attended medical school at the University of Vermont College of Medicine and family medicine residency at the University of Rochester, NY. She taught full-spectrum family medicine with a focus on women's health, obstetrics, and gynecology for 18 years to family medicine residents in Maine prior to assuming her current position. Cathy has been a residency faculty at Maine Dartmouth Family Medicine Residency since 1994 and currently is the Predoctoral Director at Dartmouth Medical School. She has taught psychosocial family medicine in Vietnam and China and worked providing medical care in Guatemala and Belize.

Elizabeth Naumburg, M.D., graduated from the Mt Sinai School of Medicine in 1979 and completed a residency and chief residency in family medicine at the University of Rochester/Highland Hospital Program. She then practiced full spectrum family medicine at Westside Health Services, a community health center in Rochester, NY until 1986, when she took a faculty position at the Department of Family Medicine in Rochester. She has held several positions in the department including residency director. Her practice includes maternity care, attending deliveries of resident patients as well as her own. In 1998 she became one of four Associate Deans for Advising at the University of Rochester's School of Medicine and Dentistry, a student affairs role with a focus on professional development and student support. Her academic interests include patient interviewing and the affect of class, race, gender and culture on healthcare and medical training. She is the mother of three adults and proud grandmother of two.

Nancy Newman, M.D, L.M.F.T., did her family medicine residency training in Rochester,

NY, where she also trained in marriage and family therapy. She has been on the staff of Hennepin County Medical Center in Minneapolis, Minnesota and on the faculty of the University of Minnesota since 1993. Her clinical work and teaching are predominantly at the HCMC Family Medical Center, which serves mostly low-income patients and families, many of whom speak Spanish. She has a special interest in physician–patient/family interactions in the clinical encounter; her academic interests include cross-cultural care, including the care of people who are gay, lesbian, bisexual or transgender. She lives in St. Paul with her spouse and their two school-age children.

Alice Ordean, M.D., is the Medical Director of the Toronto Centre for Substance Use in Pregnancy (T-CUP) at St. Joseph's Health Centre and Assistant Professor in the Department of Family and Community Medicine at the University of Toronto. She completed medical school in 1998 and family medicine residency in 2000 at the University of Toronto. Subsequently, Alice received a Master of Health Sciences in Family Medicine and Community Health including the Collaborative Program in Alcohol, Tobacco and Other Psychoactive Substances from the University of Toronto in 2005. She is one of the few physicians in Canada with expertise in both addiction medicine and primary care obstetrics. She has given numerous lectures in this area to various hospitals and organizations, and has co-authored several book chapters and articles relating to substance use in pregnancy. Alice is also a principal investigator in numerous research projects including the development of a comprehensive reference guide for healthcare providers and better practice recommendations for the management of problematic substance use in pregnancy.

Stacy Potts, M.D., is a board-certified family physician practicing in a rural Massachusetts community. She graduated from the University of Vermont School of Allied Health Sciences in 1994 and University of Vermont College of Medicine in 1998. She completed the UMass Worcester Family Medicine Residency in 2001 and subsequently a faculty development fellowship in 2002. Stacy has a strong passion for teaching and has been the residency program director since 2008. She has developed expertise in the use of learning portfolios as a strategy in adult education. She is currently a board member of the Family Medicine Education Consortium, a group of committed family medicine educators from the northeast USA. Stacy is also a marathon runner and a mother of four amazing, rapidly growing children.

Debra Rothenberg, M.D., Ph.D., graduated from Cornell University in 1980 and then was a Peace Corps Volunteer in Niger, West Africa, working at a maternal child health center. Upon returning to the United States, she studied both medicine and anthropology at Michigan State University, receiving her M.D. degree in 1990 and completing her Ph.D. in 2001. She completed a residency in family medicine in Rochester, NY and an academic fellowship at the University of Wisconsin Madison. Deb now practices and teaches at Maine Medical Center's Family Medicine Residency Program in Portland where she focuses on maternal–child health. She spends extra efforts reaching out to the growing immigrant community in the Portland area, as well as teaching family medicine residents about cross-cultural issues in healthcare.

Joseph Stenger, M.D., has been on the staff of the Barre Family Health Center in central Massachusetts and on the faculty of the University of Massachusetts Medical School since 1991. His residency in family medicine was in far-northern California, where in 1985 he helped establish Hill Country Community Clinic in a town with a population of 800. Joe participated in creating a Women's Health Curriculum for UMass's Family Medicine Residency Program and has made multiple presentations on men's issues in women's health. He is the father of two young men who give hope for the next generation making headway against patriarchy. Joe and a colleague started the Rural Health Scholars Program at UMass in 2000, and he has been active in rural medical education and rural workforce research. He was a founding member of East Quabbin Alliance (EQUAL), a community health coalition, in 2000. He has educated family medicine residents in end-of-life care and has provided home care for the dying throughout his career.

Rachel Wheeler, M.D., has worked as a family physician in community health centers in Massachusetts for over 30 years. She is also a Clinical Adjunct Assistant Professor in the Department of Family Medicine at the Tufts University School of Medicine where she teaches residents in family medicine. She has been instrumental in helping to develop an academic Department of Family Medicine at the Cambridge Health Alliance, a Harvard Medical School affiliate, and is Associate Chief of the department. Rachel is particularly interested in the development of patient and family-centered services and has presented nationally on this topic. Current work includes active exploration of strategies to increase the power of the patient's voice in service system re-design.

Index